Common Diseases *of* Companion Animals

THIRD EDITION

ALLEICE SUMMERS, MS, DVM

Professor, Veterinary Technology
Cedar Valley College
Lancaster, Texas

COMMON DISEASES OF COMPANION ANIMALS   ISBN: 978-0-323-10126-4

Notice

Knowledge and best practice in this field are constantly changing. As new research and experience broaden our knowledge, changes in practice, treatment and drug therapy may become necessary or appropriate. Readers are advised to check the most current information provided (i) on procedures featured or (ii) by the manufacturer of each product to be administered, to verify the recommended dose or formula, the method and duration of administration, and contraindications. It is the responsibility of the practitioner, relying on their own experience and knowledge of the patient, to make diagnoses and to determine dosages and the best treatment for each individual patient, and to take all appropriate safety precautions. To the fullest extent of the law, neither the Publisher nor the Editor assumes any liability for any injury and/or damage to persons or property arising out of or related to any use of the material contained in this book.

The Publisher

Library of Congress Cataloging-in-Publication Data

Summers, Alleice, author.
 Common diseases of companion animals / Alleice Summers. — Third edition.
   p. ; cm.
 Preceded by: Common diseases of companion animals. 2nd edition. c2007.
 ISBN 978-0-323-10126-4 (pbk. : alk. paper)
 I. Title.
 [DNLM: 1. Dog Diseases—diagnosis. 2. Dog Diseases—therapy. 3. Animal Diseases. 4. Animals, Domestic. 5. Cat Diseases—diagnosis. 6. Cat Diseases—therapy. SF 991]
 SF991
 636.7'0896—dc23

2013021225

Vice President and Publisher: Linda Duncan
Content Strategy Director: Penny Rudolph
Content Manager: Shelly Stringer
Publishing Services Manager: Catherine Jackson
Project Manager: Sara Alsup
Design Direction: Teresa McBryan
Cover Art: "Photo of Bull Terrier" by Rhonda Cassidy

Printed in China

Last digit is the print number: 9 8 7 6 5 4

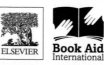

Working together to grow libraries in developing countries

www.elsevier.com • www.bookaid.org

In memory of my parents, Clark and Margaret Toldan, who always believed I could succeed at whatever I attempted. To my husband, Rich, whose support makes my work possible. To my students, past and present, whose questions inspired this book.

Preface

Veterinary technicians serve a wide variety of functions in the clinical setting. Although they are not diagnosticians, they do assist the veterinarian, through assessment and laboratory procedures, in arriving at a diagnosis. Perhaps their most important functions are in treatment planning/implementation and client/patient follow-up and compliance. To perform these duties effectively, they need a strong understanding of diseases.

While teaching a course on small-animal diseases for veterinary technology students, I discovered there was no text written expressly for the veterinary technician that covered this material. I realized that a handy reference was needed that offered a description of the most common diseases encountered in companion animals, including clinical signs, diagnostic tests and laboratory work, treatment, prevention, and client information. Just as important, this book seeks to delineate the role of the technician in all phases of diagnosis, treatment, and client communication.

This third edition of *Common Diseases of Companion Animals* has been expanded. It now covers how basic anatomy and physiology affects the development of disease in many species of companion animals, including horses, goats, reptiles, birds, and small mammals. The equine section has been expanded and all chapters have extra questions and more color pictures. The book is a collection of both clinical and practical information concerning diseases seen frequently in clinical practice. Tech Alerts are included throughout the text to emphasize the role of the technician in the total care of the patient. This book is written as a text for veterinary technology students and as a reference for daily clinical practice. It is not intended to be a comprehensive medical text; rather, the goal of this work is to acquaint veterinary technicians with disease processes and their treatments so that they may better educate their clients.

Organization

The 70 chapters of this book are organized according to organ system. In each chapter, specific diseases that affect each system follow an introductory section. Included in each section are clinical signs, suggested diagnostic tests, treatments, and information for clients. The client information section is designed to help the technician discuss the disease, including treatment and prevention, with the client. The book is written in an informal style, with clinical signs, diagnostic tests, and treatments displayed in a monograph form for easy reference. Because this book is a reference, students are often asked to review anatomy, physiology, surgery, and clinical pathology texts and other works for additional information. It is hoped that the information presented in this book will partner with the education provided to the technician by the veterinarian to provide the technician a fuller appreciation of the disease processes seen in companion animals.

Alleice Summers

Acknowledgments

I would like to thank my colleagues who so generously gave their time to make suggestions for improvements to this book. I would also like to acknowledge my coworkers Bill Lineberry, and Mark Wilson, who supported my work by providing a great working environment that allowed me the freedom to pursue this project. Thanks also to Teri Merchant—she kept calling me about a third edition and to Shelly Stringer who guided the development of this new edition. I thank my clients and their wonderful pets that, over the past 30 years, have provided me with many laughs, tears, and experiences that I will never forget.

Alleice Summers

v

Contents

Section 5   Horses

Section 6   Sheep and Goats

Introduction: The Body Defense Systems—The Body's Response to Disease

Animals, as well as their humans, live their lives in an unfriendly, hostile environment. They are continually assaulted by hordes of microorganisms such as bacteria, viruses, protozoans, fungi, and parasites. Internally, abnormal cells produced by cellular division must be continually removed from the body. If allowed to survive, they become tumors. Some of these tumors may become malignant and spread throughout the body. Tissues within the body are continually being repaired or replaced as they wear out or become damaged. With all this activity going on in the body, it is a wonder that animals and humans survive in this environment.

Immunity

The animal body has developed an efficient system of defense against disease-producing agents: the *immune system*. Components of the immune system patrol the body 24 hours a day looking for foreign and internal enemies. The activities of this system are called immunity; without it, animals could not survive. *Immunity* can be divided into two large categories: nonspecific and specific immunity.

Non-Specific Immunity

Nonspecific immunity is composed of several elements: species resistance, mechanical and chemical barriers, the inflammatory response, interferon, and complement. The term *nonspecific* means that the system responds to all antigenic insults in the same manner, not specifically to any one type of pathogenic organism.

Species Resistance

Species resistance refers to the genetic ability of a particular species to provide defense against certain pathogens. For example, canines do not acquire feline leukemia virus, and felines do not contract canine distemper virus. Neither species can contract plant diseases. Knowledge of species resistance can allow a clinician or veterinary technician to focus on the group of diseases seen in that animal species and not spend time ruling out those conditions that do not appear.

Mechanical and Chemical Barriers

The animal's internal body is protected by a mechanical barrier, the skin and the mucous membranes. If unbroken, this barrier prevents the entry of microorganisms, protecting the underlying tissues from injury. The skin also produces substances such as sebum, mucus, and enzymes that act to inhibit or destroy pathogens. Damage to this barrier allows organisms to reach the internal structures of the body and produce disease. Healthy skin is the animal's best defense against the world of microorganisms. It is called the "first line of defense."

Inflammatory Response

If bacteria or other invaders do gain access to the body, a "second line of defense," known as the *inflammatory response*, exists. When a tissue is invaded by microorganisms or injured in any way, the cells that make up that tissue release enzymes called *mediators;* these mediators attract white blood cells to the area *(chemotaxis)*, dilate blood vessels, and increase the permeability of the vessels in the area. The characteristic signs of inflammation—heat, redness, swelling, and pain—occur as a result of the release of these chemical substances. Specific types of white blood cells (usually neutrophils) attracted to the area will begin to "gobble up" the invading foreign material in a process known as *phagocytosis.* The increased blood flow to the area will increase the temperature of the tissue, inhibiting the growth of new organisms. It also brings in raw materials for the repair of the damaged tissue and clotting factors to assist in hemorrhage control. With time, the body is able to clean up the damage and return the tissue to its normal state.

Interferon and Complement

Chemicals produced by cells invaded by viruses also make up part of nonspecific immunity. Interferon is a substance that interferes with the ability of viruses to cause disease by preventing their replication within the host cell. Complement, another group of enzymes, is activated during infections. Complement binds to the invading cell wall, producing small holes in the membrane. This results in rupture, or *lysis,* of the foreign cell.

Specific Immunity

Specific immunity, the "third line of defense," is conducted by two types of white blood cells called *lymphocytes.* There are two main categories of lymphocytes, B- and T-cell lymphocytes. *B-cell lymphocytes* produce antibodies in response to specific *antigen* stimulation. This is known as the *humoral response. T-cell lymphocytes* interact more directly with the pathogens by combining directly with the foreign agent and destroying it or rendering it incapable of causing disease. Because this response is more direct than that of the B cell, it is known as *cell-mediated immunity.*

Cell-Mediated Immunity

T cells originate in the bone marrow of the animal. After leaving the bone marrow and entering the circulation, they arrive at the *thymus,* a glandular structure found in the mediastinum just cranial to the heart. The thymus is the primary central gland of the lymphoid system and is quite large in young animals, but decreases in size as the animal matures. Here the T cells "go to college," where they are programmed to recognize the markers that are unique on the cells of that specific animal *(self-recognition).* After "graduation," the T cells move out into the spleen and lymph nodes and circulate through the body, constantly on the lookout for invading substances.

Macrophages, a type of white blood cell, also travel through the tissues looking for foreign substances. When they find one, they attach to it and take the invader to the T cell. The T cell then attaches to the receptor site on the invading cell and divides repeatedly. All the new T cells then migrate to the site of the infection and begin to destroy the invading organisms. T-cell response is rapid and deadly to pathogens.

Humoral Immunity

B-cell response (humoral) is a slower type of immune response. Like T cells, B cells originate within the animal's bone marrow or in the bursa of Fabricius in some species. Young, inactive B cells produce *antigen-combining receptor sites over* the surface of their cell membranes. On contact with a specific antigen, the cell divides repeatedly, producing a *clone* of identical B cells. Some of these B cells become *plasma cells* and are stimulated to produce large protein molecules called *antibodies;* others remain as *memory cells,* which have the ability to recognize the antigen if it is ever again presented to them. Each clone of B cells, and hence each antibody, is specific for only one antigen. The antibody produced is a large protein molecule *(immunoglobulin)* whose chemical structure contains an area that is able to lock onto the antigen (Figure I-1). Combining with the antigen may result in rendering the antigen harmless to the body, may cause antigens to clump together *(agglutinate)* and be removed from solution, or may result in the destruction of the antigenic cell. This humoral response is not immediate. It takes time for the B cells to clone and begin to produce antibodies. Within 7 to 10 days after the initial infection, antibodies can be found in the body. However, if the animal has been exposed to the antigen previously and memory cells are present, this period is shorter.

B- and T-cell immunity can be further classified according to the manner in which they develop. *Inherited immunity* occurs as a result of genetic factors that influence the developing animal before birth. Acquired immunity is resistance that develops after the animal is born. *Acquired immunity* may be either natural or

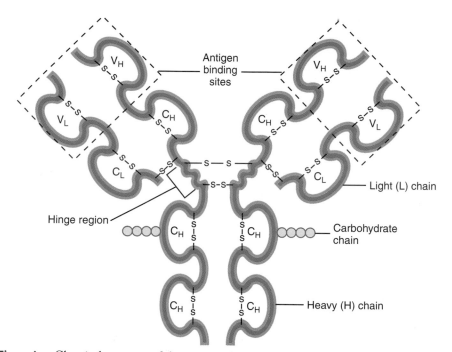

Figure I-1. Chemical structure of the immunoglobulin G class of antibody. Each molecule is composed of four polypeptide chains (two heavy and two light) plus a short carbohydrate chain attached to each heavy chain. The variable chain gives the immunoglobulin its specificity. *C,* Constant region; C_H, constant region of heavy chain; C_L, constant region of light chain; *s-s,* sulfur-sulfur bonds; *V,* variable region; V_H, variable region of heavy chain; V_L, variable region of light chain.

artificial. *Natural immunity* occurs every time the animal is exposed to a pathogen. It is a continual process in the animal world. *Artificial immunity* is usually the result of a deliberate exposure to a pathogen such as with vaccinations. Both natural and artificial immunity can be further divided into either passive or active immunity. In *passive immunity,* antibodies formed in one infected animal are transferred to another animal that is not infected. This transfer provides the uninfected animal with protection against the pathogen. *Active immunity* occurs when the animal's own immune system encounters a pathogen and responds by producing an immune response.

The ultimate result of both specific and nonspecific immunity is that the body eliminates foreign substances, whether they are bacteria, viruses, protozoa, parasites, or the body's own cells that have become harmful. If this system fails or is overwhelmed, disease occurs. Many factors affect the proper functioning of the immune system, such as nutrition, stress, sanitation, and age. Concurrent disease can also weaken the immune system, allowing other organisms to gain access to the body. Veterinary technicians must be familiar with the effects these elements have on the health of the animals in their care and be able to educate pet owners in the areas essential for the healthy life of their pets.

What Happens When the System Does not Function Properly?

This book discusses some of the most commonly seen diseases of domestic animals. The technician should keep the function of the immune system in mind as these diseases are discussed. Disruption of the normal functioning of the immune system results in the clinical illnesses seen in our patients.

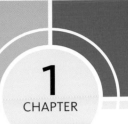

1

CHAPTER

Diseases of the Cardiovascular System

LEARNING OBJECTIVES

When you have completed this chapter, you will be able to:

1. Demonstrate a working knowledge of the anatomy and physiology of the cardiovascular system.
2. Explain to clients how cardiovascular disease affects the patient.
3. Explain diagnostic and treatment plans to clients.
4. Answer clients' questions concerning the medications needed by the patient.

The cardiovascular system plays an important role in maintaining homeostasis throughout the body. It performs this function by regulating the flow of blood through miles of vessels and capillaries. It is in capillaries that vital nutrients are transported into the body cells and removal of waste materials from the cells occurs.

To understand cardiovascular disease, one must first study the anatomy and physiology of the cardiovascular system (refer to an anatomy and physiology text for a detailed description). Simply stated, the cardiovascular system is composed of a pump (the heart) and pipes (vessels). The pump circulates fluid

1

(blood) through vessels, where it delivers its content to the cells and removes waste products. This system is a "closed" system—that is, change in one portion of the system affects other portions of the system.

Anatomy and Physiology

The Pump

At the center of the cardiovascular system is the heart, a four-chambered pump designed to contract, pumping blood to all parts of the body. Two atria (right and left) sit on top of two ventricles (also right and left). The right atrium is separated from the right ventricle by the right atrioventricular valve, also called the *tricuspid valve* because it has three leaflets. The left atrium is separated from the left ventricle by the left atrioventricular valve, or the *mitral valve*. The atrioventricular (AV) septum divides the entire right side of the heart from the left side. Lining tissue of the heart, the endocardium, also covers these valves. Specialized cardiac muscle cells, located in the sino-atrial (SA) node just inside the right atrium, generate an electrical impulse that spreads across both atria and then down the septum to the AV node, where it is slowed down. From there, the impulse travels into the Bundle of His (the AV bundle) and then out to the ventricles along the Purkinje fibers. The arrival of this electrical impulse results in the contraction of the atria and ventricles simultaneously. Blood from the right atrium fills the right ventricle by gravity (80%) and by contraction (20%). Blood from the left atrium fills the left ventricle. The closing of the AV valves produces the first heart sound. Contraction of the ventricles pushes blood *into* the pulmonary artery through the pulmonic valve on the right side of the heart and into the aorta through the aortic valve on the left side and returns blood to the right heart from veins. Closing of the pulmonic and aortic valves creates the second heart sound. This electrical activity can be measured as it moves across the surface of the body by using an *electrocardiograph* (Fig. 1-1). The electrocardiographic instrument measures the electrical activity generated by the heart by the placement of electrodes at specific points on the body surface. Each mechanical contraction of the heart is preceded by an electrical wave front that stimulates heart muscle

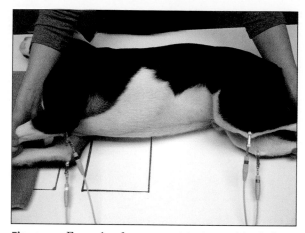

Figure 1-1 Example of correct positioning and lead placement for performing electrocardiography (ECG). Note that the dog is in right lateral recumbency, the limbs are perpendicular to the body, and the white electrode is on the right forelimb, the black electode on the left forelimb, the green electrodes on the right hindlimb, and the red electrode on the left hindlimb. *(From Bassert, J; Thomas, J:* McCurnin's Clinical Textbook for Veterinary Technicians, *ed 8, St Louis, 2014, Saunders.)*

contraction. This electrical wave front begins at the SA node and travels to the muscle cells of the ventricle through the cardiac conduction system. These wave fronts are recorded as the electrocardiogram (ECG). Figure 1-2 shows a normal ECG of a dog. Figure 1-3 represents the normal pathway for electrical conduction through the heart.

The electrical activity of this pump is automatic but can be adjusted by input from the *neuroendocrine system* to meet the demands of the animal's body. Both the sympathetic and the parasympathetic systems augment the rhythmic contraction of the heart.

Many cardiac diseases involve a failure of this pump to function properly. *Congestive heart failure (CHF), cardiomyopathy, valvular disease,* and *congenital malformations* can all affect the pumping efficiency of the heart and, ultimately, the function of the entire body.

The Vessels

Connected to the pump are a series of vessels. Arteries carry oxygenated blood at high pressure

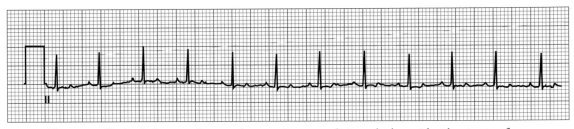

Figure 1-2 Six-lead electrocardiogram documenting normal sinus rhythm with a heart rate of approximately 150 bpm. *(Modified from August, JR: Consultations in Feline Internal Medicine, Volume 6, St. Louis, 2010, W.B. Saunders.)*

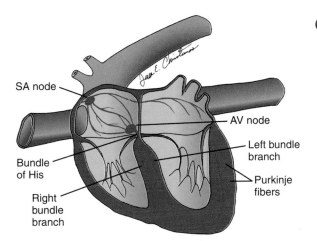

Figure 1-3 Normal pathway for electrical conduction through the heart. *AV,* Atrioventricular; *SA,* sinoatrial. (From McBride DF: *Learning veterinary terminology,* ed 2, St. Louis, MO, 2002, Mosby, by permission.)

(the systolic blood pressure) to arterioles and onto capillaries, where exchange of nutrients and gases occurs. Blood then moves into venules, through veins, and is returned to the right side of the heart via the vena cava. Excessive fluid remaining in the tissue surrounding capillaries is returned to the vascular system via the lymph vessels. Arteries, whose walls contain a large amount of smooth muscle, are capable of dilation and constriction, routing blood to areas where it is needed and away from those areas not in need. Constriction serves to increase blood pressure, and dilation serves to decrease it.

TECH ALERT

The pulmonary artery is the only artery in the body carrying unoxygenated blood, and pulmonary veins are the only veins carrying oxygenated blood!

Vascular diseases affect the flow of blood through the body and, ultimately, its return to the heart. If the volume of blood returning to the heart is abnormal, the heart will compensate by altering the rate of contraction, the strength of contraction, or both to return homeostasis to the circulatory system.

Heart Failure

When the blood returning to the heart cannot be pumped out at a rate matching the body's need, *heart failure* occurs. Many causes for heart failure exist, and the disease is often difficult to explain. The clinical signs of the disease and treatment regimens depend on the diagnosis and evaluation of the *individual* animal. The veterinarian must determine whether the failure is the result of *myocardial dysfunction* (pump failure) or *circulatory failure* (lack of circulating fluid volume).

Myocardial dysfunction is seen in diseases such as the following:
- Cardiomyopathy
- Myocarditis
- Taurine deficiency in cats

Circulatory failure results from the following conditions:
- Hypovolemia (shock, hemorrhage, dehydration)
- Anemia

- Valvular dysfunction
- Congenital shunts or defects

Heart failure is termed *congestive heart failure* when the failing heart allows fluid congestion and edema to accumulate in the body. Most heart failure will become "congestive" as the pump progressively fails.

Today, it is possible for researchers to look into the myocardial cells themselves, even to the level of the deoxyribonucleic acid (DNA) within the nucleus to explain the physiologic changes seen in patients with heart failure. To understand these diseases, the technician needs an understanding of the workings of the myocardial cell in general.

The myocardial cell is striated and involuntary. Each cell contains parallel sarcomeres containing myosin and actin fibers just like skeletal muscle. Movement of these fibers over one another results in a shortening of the cell and contributes to muscle shortening or contraction. Unlike skeletal muscle, myocardial cells have a very small sarcoplasmic reticulum for calcium storage and hence they are dependent on blood calcium for contraction. The myocardial cells are linked to other myocardial cells through strong electrical *intercalated discs*. This network of myocardial cells is able to react as one electrically coupled unit. Cardiac muscle cells have a longer refractory period than skeletal muscle cells to allow for filling of the chambers of the heart during diastole. Researchers have found that disarray of these sarcomeres within the cardiac muscle is often responsible for problems seen in patients with heart failure.

Cardiomyopathies

Canine Dilated Cardiomyopathy

Dilated cardiomyopathy (DCM) is one of the most common acquired cardiovascular diseases of dogs. It is primarily a disease of older, male, large and giant breed dogs such as Scottish Deerhounds, Dobermans, Boxers, Irish Wolfhounds, St. Bernards, Newfoundlands, Afghans, and Old English Sheepdogs. The disease has also been seen in English and American Cocker Spaniels. It is rare in dogs weighing less than 12 kg.

The pathology of the disease involves dilation of all chambers of the heart. This dilation (caused by weak, thin, and flabby cardiac muscle) results in a decrease in cardiac output and an increase in cardiac afterload (blood left in the heart in diastole). The cause of this disease is unknown, although its onset often follows myocardial insult from viral, bacterial, nutritional, or immune-mediated diseases. DCM results in impaired systolic function of the ventricles and, therefore, decreased stroke volume (the volume of blood ejected from the heart with each contraction). The effect on the animal is one of low-output circulatory failure, exhibited by weakness, exercise intolerance, syncope, or shock.

Dogs with DCM frequently experience development of atrial fibrillation (AF), which further contributes to a decrease in cardiac output. Signs of AF include rapid, irregular heart rhythms or sudden death. Patients may remain normal until the atria dilate excessively. The enlarged atria are unable to contract normally, and clinical signs of heart disease become evident. The cause of this dilation appears to be breed related. In Dobermans, the disease appears to be familial, related to an autosomal dominant gene. Great Danes and Irish Wolfhounds also demonstrate a genetic predisposition for this disease. In Cocker Spaniels, a taurine deficiency results in DCM. The disease in Cocker Spaniels appears to be related to diets high in lamb meat and rice and low in taurine. Although DCM is primarily a disease of older dogs, Portugese Water Dogs exhibit a juvenile onset of the disease, which is also genetic. Puppies anywhere from 2 to 32 weeks of age can be affected.

CLINICAL SIGNS

- Giant or large breed male dogs; 4 to 10 years old
- Right-sided heart failure: ascites, hepatomegaly, weight loss, abdominal distension
- Left-sided heart failure: coughing, pulmonary edema, syncope
- Exercise intolerance
- Murmur of mitral regurgitation heard best on left chest
- +/- gallop rhythm
- +/- tachyrhythm

DIAGNOSIS

- Radiographs: may be normal early in the disease. May show enlarged heart later in the disease time line; left ventricular enlargement, enlargement of both atria may be visible
- Echocardiology: test of choice for examination of the heart; will demonstrate left and right atrial wall thinning along with left ventricular dilation
- ECG: may show widened QRS and P waves, rhythm disturbances but is fairly insensitive to changes seen in DCM

LABORATORY TESTS:

- The use of cardiac biomarkers is gaining in popularity for diagnosis of DCM. These tests look for myocardial cell injury seen in DCM.
  - Atrial natriuretic peptide (ANP), brain natriuretic peptide (BNP), and pro-BNP blood tests are commercially available. In DCM, these values will be significantly increased.
  - Troponin 1 (cTn1) will also be increased. (Whole blood is recommended over plasma for this test, but technicians should check with local laboratory before sample collection.)

TREATMENT

- No cure exists for DCM; treatment is aimed at keeping the dog comfortable
- Diuretics: furosemide to decrease fluid load and reduce work of the heart
- Digoxin: to increase cardiac contractility and cardiac output; monitor digoxin blood levels (1 to 2 nanogram per milliliter [ng/mL])
- Enalapril: angiotensin-converting enzyme (ACE) inhibitor prevents the formation of angiotensin II, a potent vasoconstrictor; helps decrease vascular resistance and improve cardiac output
- +/− beta-blockers (β-blockers): metoprolol, propranolol, esmolol are examples
- Pimobendan: a calcium sensitizer with inhibitory properties. It increases the calcium binding capability at cTn1 sites. The result is a more forceful contraction of the myocardial cell. The drug also has an antithrombotic effect and is a positive inotrope. Its use has been shown to slow the progression of the disease and to improve survival times

INFORMATION FOR CLIENTS

- DCM is a progressive disease that is almost always fatal.
- Most dogs will die within 6 months to 2 years.
- Dogs may die suddenly of malignant cardiac arrhythmias.
- The disease does appear to be more prevalent in certain breeds of dogs and has been proven to run in families of many dog breeds. Biomarkers may be of use to diagnose the disease early on.

Canine Hypertrophic Cardiomyopathy

In the rare canine disease hypertrophic cardiomyopathy (HCM), the left ventricular muscle hypertrophies or thickens, decreasing the filling capacity of the ventricle and often blocking the outflow of blood during systole. The cause appears to be heritable.

CLINICAL SIGNS

- Fatigue
- Cough
- Tachypnea
- Syncope
- Presence or absence of cardiac murmurs
- Sudden death
- Some animals may be asymptomatic

DIAGNOSIS

- Echocardiology: indicates concentric thickening and hypertrophy of the left ventricle

TREATMENT

- None routinely used

INFORMATION FOR CLIENTS

- Sudden death and CHF may occur in dogs with HCM.
- The disease may run in families of certain breeds: German Shepherds, Rottweilers, Dalmations, Cocker Spaniels, Boston Terriers, Shih Tzu.

Boxer Right Ventricular Cardiomyopathy

This cardiomyopathy occurs in adult Boxer dogs that present with ventricular arrhythmias, syncope, and sudden death. This is a genetic disease seen within families of Boxers and appears to be an autosomal dominant trait with variable penetration. Some dogs may show no signs of the disease, whereas others may have varying signs.

CLINICAL SIGNS

- Syncope—may be associated with exercise
- Sudden death
- Some dogs will present with left or biventricular heart failure

DIAGNOSIS

Physical Examination

- Many dogs will have a normal physical examination
- Tachyrhythmias, ascites, and murmurs may be present

Laboratory Findings

- Biomarkers may be of value in diagnosing this disease
- Cardiac cTn1 levels will be elevated
- Clinical serum chemistries may be within normal limits

Imaging

- Electrocardiogram: a short recording may be normal. However, these dogs will have ventricular premature contractions on an ECG if the recording is long enough to see them
- Holter monitor: will allow the veterinarian to more accurately diagnose this disease. Increased numbers of ventricular premature complexes (VPCs) should indicate a problem
- Radiographs: usually normal but may show left ventricular enlargement
- Echocardiology: will show left ventricular dilation and systolic dysfunction. Some dogs will have right ventricular enlargement also

TREATMENT

- Mexiletine: to decrease the VPCs
- Pimobendan, ACE inhibitors, if ventricular dilation is present
- Owners should be warned that sudden death of these dogs can occur usually with exercise or excitement

 TECH ALERT

When monitoring anesthesia on Boxer dogs, be alert for the presence of VPCs on the ECG monitor. They should not occur in normal dogs. If they are present, this may indicate the dog needs a further cardiac workup.

Feline Dilated Cardiomyopathy

Before the late 1980s, feline DCM was one of the most frequent cardiac diseases reported in cats. After the association of the disease with taurine deficiency, additional taurine was added to commercial diets, and the incidence of the disease significantly decreased. The pathologic condition is similar to DCM in dogs. Evidence has been found of a genetic predisposition to DCM in cats fed taurine-deficient diets.

CLINICAL SIGNS

- Older, mixed breed cats
- Dyspnea
- Inactivity
- Anorexia
- Acute lameness or paralysis, usually in the rear limbs
- Pain and lack of circulation in the affected limbs
- Hypothermia

DIAGNOSIS

- Clinical signs
- ECG: increased QRS voltages, wide P waves, ventricular arrhythmia
- Echocardiology: dilated heart chambers

TREATMENT

- Oral taurine supplementation: 250 to 500 milligrams per day (mg/day)
- Furosemide: to reduce fluid load on the heart
- Oxygen: to increase oxygen levels to the cells
- Digoxin: to increase cardiac contractility and improve cardiac output
- Enalapril: ACE inhibitor to prevent the formation of angiotensin II and decrease vascular resistance; improves cardiac output
- Pimobendan
- Hydralazine: relaxes vascular smooth muscle and decreases peripheral resistance; improves cardiac output

INFORMATION FOR CLIENTS

- The most dangerous time during treatment of feline DCM is the first 2 weeks.
- Cats that survive the first 2 weeks and respond well to taurine supplementation have a good prognosis.
- Cats that do not respond to taurine supplementation have a poor long-term prognosis.

Feline Hypertrophic Cardiomyopathy

HCM in cats is similar to the disease in dogs, with left ventricular hypertrophy being the predominant pathology. This disease is the most common cardiomyopathy seen in cats. Of the feline cardiac cases, 50% to 70% involve HCM. Neutered male cats between the ages of 1 and 16 years have been found to be most at risk. The cause of the disease may be related to abnormal myocardial myosin or calcium transport within the myocardial cells. The left ventricle becomes thickened and stiff. Mitral regurgitation and aortic embolization occur frequently.

As the atria dilate, the endothelium lining the chambers is damaged, resulting in the release of clotting enzymes, which can result in clot formation. The cats that form thrombi also show evidence of hypercoagulability of their platelets. Thromboembolism occurs in about 16% to 18% of feline HCM. Although the thrombus can lodge in any artery, it appears that the trifurcation of the aorta is a frequent spot resulting in a decrease in circulation to both the rear legs.

CLINICAL SIGNS

- A soft, systolic murmur (grade 2 to 3 or 6)
- Gallop rhythms or other arrhythmia
- Acute onset of heart failure or systemic thromboembolism

DIAGNOSIS

- Radiographs: may show a normal-size heart or mild left atrial enlargement. May see the "valentine" heart shape in the dorsoventral view
- ECG: increased P-wave duration, increased QRS width, sinus tachycardia
- Echocardiology: increased left ventricular wall thickness and a dilated left atrium
- Biomarkers: BNP, pro-BNP, and CTn1 will be increased
- Magnetic resonance imaging (MRI): most accurate method of diagnosis

TREATMENT

- ACE inhibitors
- +/– Propranolol: β-blocker; used to decrease myocardial oxygen demand, decrease sinus heart rate

or

- Diltiazem: calcium channel blocker; inhibits cardiac and vascular smooth muscle contractility; reduces blood pressure and cardiac afterload
- Angiotensin-converting enzyme inhibitors
- Low-dose heparin or low dose aspirin
- Diuretics : furosemide

INFORMATION FOR CLIENTS

- Cats with HCM may experience heart failure, arterial embolism, and sudden death.
- Cats with heart rates less than 200 beats per minute (beats/min) have a better prognosis

compared with cats whose rates are greater than 200 beats/min.
- The median survival time is about 732 days.

Thromboembolism

Thrombus formation is a common and serious complication of myocardial disease in the cat. It is estimated that between 10% and 20% of cats with HCM will experience development of thrombi on the left side of the heart, which may dislodge and become trapped elsewhere in the arterial system. Cats appear to have inherently high platelet reactivity, making clot formation a more likely sequel to endothelial damage and sluggish blood flow occurring with myocardial disease. Approximately 90% of these emboli lodge as "saddle thrombi" in the distal aortic trifucation, resulting in hindlimb pain and paresis. Rarely will a thrombus lodge at other arterial sites such as the renal artery, the coronary arteries, the cerebral arteries, or the mesenteric artery.

The goal of treatment is to dissolve the thrombus and restore perfusion to the area. Several drugs have been tried with varying results. Tissue plasminogen activator (tPA) has shown some success, but it is expensive. Heparin has also been used with some success. Low-dose aspirin therapy can be used prophylactically in cats with myocardial disease.

CLINICAL SIGNS

- Acute onset of rear leg pain and paresis
- Cold, bluish foot pads (decreased circulation)
- Lack of palpable pulses in rear limbs
- History or clinical findings of myocardial disease

DIAGNOSIS

- Clinical signs
- Nonselective angiography, if available

TREATMENT

- TPA (Activase [Genentech]): serves as a fibrolysin resulting in the breakdown of clots already formed in the vasculature
  or
- Heparin: acts on coagulation factors in both the intrinsic and extrinsic coagulation pathways, inhibits the formation of a stable clot
- Prophylaxis: low-dose aspirin

⬤ TECH ALERT

Aspirin use in cats can cause toxicities because of their inability to rapidly metabolize and excrete salicylates. Cats must be dosed carefully and monitored carefully when receiving aspirin therapy.

INFORMATION FOR CLIENTS

- Cats experiencing painful, cold, or paralyzed rear legs should be seen at the hospital immediately.
- The prognosis for cats with thromboembolism is guarded to poor.
- Surgical removal of the thrombus is difficult.

Congenital Heart Disease

Although malformations of the heart and great vessels represent a small cause of clinical heart disease, it is important to identify them in newly acquired pets or those to be used for breeding. Technicians should be encouraged to use their stethoscopes to routinely listen to the heart. With practice, subtle changes will become noticeable, allowing the technician to note abnormalities in the patient's record.

Many malformations have a genetic basis. Breed predilections for congenital heart disease are listed in Table 1-1. The diagnostic approach for congenital heart disease should include a detailed history, with special attention paid to the breed, sex, and age of the patient. Clinical signs of congenital heart failure include failure to grow, dyspnea, weakness, syncope, cyanosis, seizures, and sudden death; however, many animals with congenital malformations may be asymptomatic.

Most cases of congenital abnormalities are identified during the first visit to the veterinarian after the pet has been purchased. On examination, a loud murmur often accompanied by a *precordial thrill* (a vibration of the chest wall) may be heard. With some defects, the clinician may observe pulse abnormalities, cyanosis, jugular pulses, or abdominal distension. Laboratory test results may all be normal. Radiography may suggest cardiac disease in some animals; however, echocardiography can provide an accurate diagnosis of the defect.

Causes of congenital heart disease include genetic, environmental, infectious, nutritional, and drug-related

TABLE 1-1 Canine Breed Predilections for Congenital Heart Disease

Breed	Defect(s)
Basset Hound	P
Beagle	PS
Bichon Frise	PDA
Boxer	SAS, PS, ASD
Boykin Spaniel	PS
Bull Terrier	MVD, AS
Chihuahua	PDA, PS
Chow Chow	PS, CTD
Cocker Spaniel	PDA, PS
Collie	PDA
Doberman Pinscher	ASD
English Bulldog	PS, VSD, TOF
English Springer Spaniel	PDA, VSD
German Shepherd	SAS, PDA, TVD, MVD
German Shorthaired Pointer	SAS
Golden Retriever	SAS, TVD, MVD
Great Dane	TVD, MVD, SAS
Keeshond	TOF, PDA
Labrador Retriever	TVD, PDA, PS
Maltese	PDA
Mastiff	PS, MVD
Newfoundland	SAS, MVD, PS
Pomeranian	PDA
Poodle	PDA
Rottweiler	SAS
Samoyed	PS, SAS, ASD
Schnauzer	PS
Shetland Sheepdog	PDA
Terrier breeds	PS
Weimaraner	TVD, PPDH
Welsh Corgi	PDA
West Highland White Terrier	PS, VSD
Yorkshire Terrier	PDA

AS, Aortic stenosis; *ASD,* atrial septal defect; *CTD,* cor triatriatum dexter; *MVD,* mitral valve dysplasia; *PDA,* patent ductus arteriosus; *PPDH,* peritoneopericardial diaphragmatic hernia; *PS,* pulmonic stenosis; *SAS,* subaortic stenosis; *TOF,* tetralogy of Fallot; *TVD,* tricuspid valve dysplasia; *VSD,* ventricular septal defect.
From Oyama MA, Sisson DD, Thomas WP, Bonagura JD: Congenital heart disease. In Ettinger SJ, Feldman EC, editors: *Textbook of veterinary internal medicine,* ed 6, vol 2, St. Louis, MO, 2005, Saunders.

factors. More is understood of the genetic factors than the other causes. Studies suggest the defects are polygenetic in nature and that they might be difficult to eliminate entirely from a specific breed.

This section discusses the most commonly seen congenital defects. See additional cardiology texts for more detailed descriptions of each defect.

Patent Ductus Arteriosus

Failure of the ductus arteriosus to close after parturition results in blood shunting from the systemic circulation to the pulmonary artery. Normally, the ductus carries blood from the pulmonary artery to the aorta during fetal development. The increase in oxygen tension in the blood at birth results in closure of the path in the first 12 to 14 hours of life. If the ductus remains open, blood will hyperperfuse the lung, and the left side of the heart will become volume overloaded (Fig. 1-4). The resulting cardiac murmur is often referred to as a "machinery murmur"; this type of murmur is heard best over the main pulmonary artery high on the left base.

CLINICAL SIGNS

- Usually, female dogs are most commonly affected, especially Chihuahuas, Collies, Maltese, Poodles, Pomeranians, English Springers, Keeshonds, Bichons Frisces, and Shetland Sheepdogs
- Presence of loud murmur heard best over left thorax
- Some puppies may be asymptomatic

DIAGNOSIS

- ECG: will reveal left ventricular dilation, aortic and pulmonary artery dilation
- Radiographs: overcirculation of the pulmonary tree with left atrial and ventricular enlargement

TREATMENT

- Surgical correction before the age of 2 years

INFORMATION FOR CLIENTS

- The prognosis is excellent with surgical correction.
- It has been estimated that 64% of dogs with patent ductus arteriosus (PDA) will be dead within 1 year of diagnosis without surgical correction.
- The dog *should not* be used for breeding.

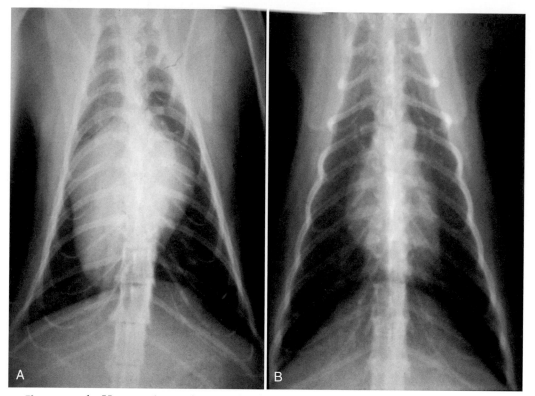

Figure 1-4 A, Hypertrophic cardiomyopathy (HCM) in the feline. **B,** The apex of the heart is shifted to the right with HCM. (From August J: *Consultations in feline internal medicine*, ed 5, St. Louis, MO, 2005, Saunders, by permission.)

Atrial and Ventricular Septal Defects

During fetal development, the atria and the ventricles are joined as a common chamber. The atria are partitioned by two septa and a slitlike opening (the foramen ovale) that allows right-to-left shunting of blood in the fetus. The ventricular septum is formed from several primordial areas. Eventually, the atrial septum and the ventricular septum join in the area of the endocardial cushions. Defects in the structure of these septae result in patencies of the AV septum. This defect is fairly common in the cat. With atrial septal defects (ASDs), blood will typically shunt from left to right, overloading the right side of the heart. In ventricular septal defects (VSDs), the left side of the heart is usually overloaded and enlarged (Fig. 1-5).

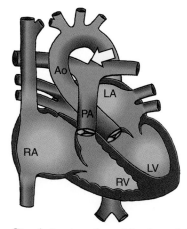

Figure 1-5 Circulation in a dog with a large left-to-right shunting patent ductus arteriosus. The shunt results in pulmonary overcirculation and left ventricular volume overload. *Ao,* Aorta; *LA,* left atrium; *LV,* left ventricle; *PA,* pulmonary artery; *RA,* right atrium; *RV,* right ventricle.

CLINICAL SIGNS

- Typical breed
- ASD: soft, systolic murmur, split-second heart sound
- VSD: harsh, holosystolic murmur, right sternal border
- Signs of CHF before 8 weeks of age

DIAGNOSIS

- Radiology: reveals right-sided heart enlargement with ASD, increased pulmonary vascularity, left atrium normal to slightly enlarged; in VSD, pulmonary overcirculation, left atrium and ventricle enlarged, variable right ventricular enlargement
- Echocardiology: demonstrates the septal defect

TREATMENT

- ASD: medical management of CHF
- VSD: medical management of CHF

INFORMATION FOR CLIENTS

- Repair of these defects requires open-heart surgery or cardiopulmonary bypass. This is uncommon in dogs or cats.
- Most of these animals will *eventually* experience development of CHF and require treatment.

Stenotic Valves (Pulmonic and Aortic Stenosis)

Pulmonic stenosis results when the pulmonic valves are dysplastic or malformed. The lesion results in a narrowing of the outflow tract from the right ventricle. Obstruction to right ventricular outflow causes an increase in ventricular systolic pressure resulting in right ventricular hypertrophy. The right atrium also becomes enlarged. Severe stenosis limits cardiac output during exercise.

CLINICAL SIGNS

- Specific breeds (Chihuahua, Samoyed, English Bulldog, Miniature Schnauzer, Labrador Retriever, Mastiff, Chow Chow, Newfoundland, Basset Hound, Terriers, and Spaniels)
- Age: older than 1 year
- Syncope (fainting)
- Tiring on exercise
- Right-sided congestive heart disease

- Prominent jugular pulse
- Left basilar murmur
- Palpable right ventricular enlargement

DIAGNOSIS

- Radiographs: right ventricular enlargement, poststenotic dilation of the pulmonary artery, pulmonary underperfusion
- ECG: right ventricular hypertrophy and enlargement, increased echogenicity of the pulmonary valves, dilation of the main pulmonary artery

TREATMENT

- Balloon valvuloplasty to relieve the obstruction
- Valvulotomy or partial valvulectomy to open the outflow tract
- Patch graph over the outflow tract to alleviate the obstruction
- Medical management of CHF

INFORMATION FOR CLIENTS

- Affected animals *should not* be used for breeding.
- Dogs with mild-to-moderate pulmonic stenosis can live normal lives.
- Sudden death may occur in dogs with moderate-to-severe pulmonic stenosis.

Subaortic Stenosis

Subaortic stenosis (SAS) occurs predominantly in large-breed dogs. The Newfoundland, Boxer, German Shepherd, Golden Retriever, and Bull Terrier are the most commonly affected. In the Newfoundland, support exists for a genetic basis most compatible with an autosomal dominant mechanism. The lesion develops during the first 4 to 8 weeks of life. The lesion consists of thickening of the endocardial tissue just below the aortic valve. The fibrous thickening results in obstruction to outflow producing left ventricular hypertrophy, left atrial hypertrophy, and dilation of the aorta. Coronary artery circulation may also be affected. Severe SAS may lead to left-sided CHF or sudden death.

CLINICAL SIGNS

- Typical breed
- Soft to moderate ejection murmur in the fourth left intercostal area

- Exertional tiring
- Syncope
- Left CHF
- Sudden death

DIAGNOSIS

- Radiology: normal or left ventricular hypertrophy, widened mediastinum (from aortic dilation)
- ECG: left ventricular hypertrophy, subvalvular fibrous ring, poststenotic dilation of the aorta
- Echocardiography: in advanced stages may indicate left ventricular hypertrophy

TREATMENT

- Restricting exercise
- Balloon catheter dilation of the stenotic ring

Medical

- Propranolol for dogs with syncope and increased pressure gradients

INFORMATION FOR CLIENTS

- These dogs *should not* be used for breeding.
- Most will experience development of left-sided CHF; the onset may be sudden.

- Sudden death is not uncommon in these dogs.
- Endocarditis (inflammation of the lining of the heart) is a risk in all cases of SAS.

Tetralogy of Fallot

Tetralogy of Fallot is a polygenic, genetically transmitted malformation of the heart. Components include right ventricular outflow obstruction (pulmonic stenosis), secondary right ventricular hypertrophy, a subaortic VSD, and overriding aorta (Fig. 1-6). This condition is seen in the Keeshond and the English Bulldog and in cats. It occasionally occurs in other breeds. Symptoms may vary with the severity of the defects.

The presence of these malformations results in increased right-sided resistance and pressure and a right-to-left shunt between the pulmonary and systemic circulations. Because of this pressure gradient, deoxygenated blood from the right ventricle shunts through the VSD to mix with oxygenated blood in the left ventricle. Blood flow to and from the pulmonary vasculature is minimal. This shunting results in hypoxemia, cyanosis, and secondary polycythemia (increased numbers of red blood cells [RBCs]). Right ventricular hypertrophy occurs. The murmur of pulmonic

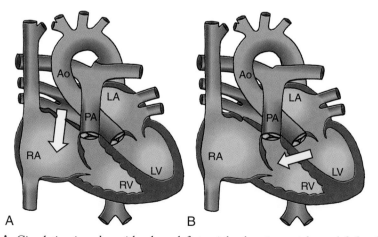

Figure 1-6 A, Circulation in a dog with a large left-to-right shunting atrial septal defect. The shunt results in right ventricular volume overload (*not shown*) and pulmonary overcirculation. There is mild systolic pulmonary hypertension. **B,** Medium-sized ventricular septal defect. The diameter of the defect is less than the diameter of the aorta (*Ao*), so it imposes resistance to blood flow. *LA,* Left atrium; *LV,* left ventricle; *PA,* pulmonary artery; *RA,* right atrium; *RV,* right ventricle.

stenosis usually can be detected on the left hemi-thorax, and less often, the VSD murmur can be heard as well.

CLINICAL SIGNS

- Typical breed
- Failure to grow
- Cyanosis
- Exercise intolerance, shortness of breath
- Weakness
- Syncope, seizures
- Sudden death

DIAGNOSIS

- Radiology: normal-size heart, decreased pulmonary circulation
- ECG: right ventricular hypertrophy, small left chambers, large subaortic VSD, and right outflow obstruction; bubble or Doppler studies indicate right-to-left shunting

TREATMENT

Surgical

- Creation of a systemic to pulmonary systemic shunt has been successful in increasing pulmonary circulation, venous return, left-side heart size, and oxygen saturation in the systemic circulation.

Medical

- Phlebotomy to maintain the packed cell volume between 62% and 68%. Blood volume removed should be replaced with crystalloid fluids to prevent hypoperfusion. Hypoxia can be treated with cage rest and oxygen.

⬤ TECH ALERT

Animals with tetralogy of Fallot may react adversely to sedatives and tranquilizers, acquiring a bradycardia that does not improve with supplemental oxygen therapy.

INFORMATION FOR CLIENTS

- This is a genetically transmitted disorder. These animals *should not* be used for breeding.
- Sudden death is common, but some animals can tolerate the defect for years.

- CHF rarely develops from this disorder.
- Limit stress and exercise for these animals.
- Tranquilizers and sedatives may have an adverse effect on these animals.
- Regular phlebotomy (blood drawing) will be required to maintain a normal RBC level.

Persistent Right Aortic Arch and Other Vascular Ring Anomalies

Persistence of the right fourth aortic arch is a common malformation. The defect results in regurgitation of solid food in weanlings because of obstruction of the esophagus by the retained vascular arch. It is a common defect in German Shepherds, Irish Setters, and Great Danes and is frequently seen in other large breeds.

CLINICAL SIGNS

- Regurgitation of solid food
- Aspiration pneumonia, fever, dyspnea, cough
- Weight loss

DIAGNOSIS

- Barium swallow indicates constriction of the esophagus near the base of the heart on radiographs. Solid food can be mixed with barium to also indicate constriction and retention of the food in the esophagus.

TREATMENT

Surgical

- Surgery should be done early for a better prognosis. Similar to surgery for PDA because the ductus arteriosus is part of the vascular ring anomaly.

Maintenance

- Feed less solid diet or pelleted diet (small amounts frequently)
- Feed from a height to avoid food buildup in the esophagus
- Antibiotics for respiratory infections

INFORMATION FOR CLIENTS

- Without early surgical correction, the prognosis is poor.
- Even with surgical correction, some amount of esophageal dilation will persist. This may

result in vomiting if large boluses of food are consumed.
- These dogs *should not* be used for breeding.

Acquired Valvular Diseases

Chronic Mitral Valve Insufficiency

Chronic mitral valve insufficiency (CMVI), now called myxomatous mitral valve disease (MMVD), is the most commonly encountered cardiovascular disorder in the dog. The prevalence of this disease increases with age with estimates that as many as 75% of all dogs older than 16 years are affected. MMVD is rare in the cat. This disease is a progressive disorder, resulting in an estimated 95% of all cases of CHF in small-breed dogs. The tricuspid as well as the pulmonic and aortic valves may also be affected.

The lesion consists of proliferation of fibroblastic tissue within the structure of the valve leaflets. This results in the nodular thickening of the valvular free edges, which then contract and roll up. The stiff, malformed leaflets fail to close sufficiently during systole, resulting in regurgitation of blood back up into the left atrium. The chordae tendinae are stretched and rupture. There is endothelium loss on the valve surface. The left atrium and infrequently the left ventricle dilate. The dilated atrium may result in pulmonary congestion and compression of the left mainstem bronchus, producing coughing and dyspnea.

Chronic periodontal disease can increase the progression of mitral valvular insufficiency in older animals. Bacteria (mostly gram-negative anaerobes) living in tartar in periodontal pockets are showered into the bloodstream, colonizing the valve leaflets, which become thickened as a result. When the valve leaflets become inflamed and thickened, they fail to close properly, which results in leakage of blood back into the left ventricle. The overload can then result in heart failure over time.

CLINICAL SIGNS

- Small-breed dog or toy breed; male; frequently seen in the Dachshund and King Charles Spaniels
- Age older than 10 years
- Cough: deep, resonant, and usually worse at night or with exercise
- Dyspnea, tachypnea
- Decreased appetite
- Systolic murmur, left apex; "whooping" quality

DIAGNOSIS

- Radiology: if pulmonary edema is present, venous engorgement will be present (vein diameter will be greater than that of the arteries). "Cottonlike" alveolar densities or air bronchograms will be present. Without edema, left atrial and ventricular enlargement, elevation of the thoracic trachea, and loss of the "cardiac waist" can be seen on the lateral view. In the dorsoventral view, the enlarged left auricle can be seen as a bulge in the cardiac silhouette at 2- to 3-o'clock position
- Echocardiology: shows increased diameter of the left atrium and left ventricle. There is marked reduction in left ventricular contractility. The mitral valve leaflets may be thickened or prolapsing

Laboratory Findings
- May have mild increases in liver enzymes
- May demonstrate prerenal azotemia
- Serum cTn1 levels increase with the progression of the disease
- BNP levels will also increase as disease progresses

TREATMENT

- The main goal of treatment is to improve the length and the quality of life for the patient. No therapy will prolong survival or delay the onset of clinical signs. Treatments are adjusted as the disease progresses, thus varying combinations of medications may be used.

Medical
- Diuretics (furosemide): to reduce the circulatory blood volume to the left side of the heart
- Arterial dilators (hydralazine, enalapril): to decrease systemic resistance
- +/- Digoxin: to decrease the heart rate to less than 160 beats/min in small dogs
- ACE inhibitors
- Cough suppressants such as butorphanol, hydrocodone
- Pimobendan

Dietary

- A diet low in sodium will decrease the fluid load in the patient. Overweight patients will experience more problems with respirations; therefore, weight should be maintained within a normal range.

INFORMATION FOR CLIENTS

- MMVD is a progressive disease. The animal will need be reevaluated periodically and medications adjusted to provide it with adequate relief of symptoms.
- No cure exists for this problem.
- A low-salt diet will aid in preventing fluid accumulation in the body. Treats and table foods containing salt should be avoided.
- Eventually, a point will be reached when medications will not relieve the clinical symptoms.

Tricuspid Valve Insufficiency

This disease is exactly similar to mitral valve insufficiency, but the signs are predominantly those of *right*-sided heart failure: pleural effusion, abdominal distension, hepatomegaly, or gastrointestinal signs such as vomiting, diarrhea, or anorexia. Treatment is basically the same as for mitral insufficiency. Repeated abdominocentesis often is required. As the right atrium dilates, animals may develop tachyrhythmias such as AF. Hepatomegaly may be palpated. Cats are more prone than dogs to pleural effusion. Tricuspid insufficiency may be secondary to heartworm disease.

Cardiac Arrhythmias

Arrhythmias may be defined as deviations from the normal heart rate rhythm or rhythms originating from abnormal locations within the heart. Many times there is no observable anatomic pathology in the myocardium that correlates with the rhythm disturbance.

Alterations in normal rhythm result from either *abnormal impulse formation* or *abnormal impulse conduction* within cardiac muscle fibers. (Refer to a physiology text to review nerve conduction and muscle contraction.) Altered impulse formation may occur as a result of ischemia (decreased supply of oxygenated blood), hypocalcemia (low calcium levels), cardiomyopathy, hypercalcemia (high calcium levels), excess catecholamines, or reperfusion injury. Conduction disturbances result when alternate pathways develop for depolarization of cardiac muscle.

Arrhythmias affect the hemodynamics of the body. Cerebral blood flow is reduced as much as 8% to 12% by premature beats, 14% by supraventricular (originating above the ventricles) tachycardias (rapid rates), 23% by AF, and 40% to 75% by ventricular tachycardia (VT).

Many arrhythmias can be easily auscultated and confirmed by ECG. Treatment involves correcting the underlying cause when possible or controlling the arrhythmia when it is not possible to correct the underlying cause.

Supraventricular arrhythmias may be atrial (P-wave positive but abnormal) or junctional (P-wave negative in lead II). This class of arrhythmias includes:

- Supraventricular tachycardia (SVT)
- Atrial premature contractions
- AF

In SVT (or sinus tachycardia), the heart rate typically exceeds 160 to 180 beats/min in the dog, whereas the P-QRS-T complexes remain normal. The heart rate may be slowed by vagal stimulation. Situations such as fear, excitement, exercise, anemia, or hyperthyroidism may cause this arrhythmia. The ECG would display normal complexes with a higher-than-normal heart rate (Fig. 1-7).

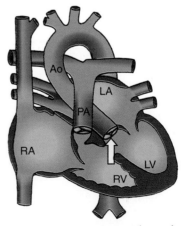

Figure 1-7 Circulation in a patient with tetralogy of Fallot with severe right ventricular outflow obstruction. Systolic pressures in the right ventricle (*RV*), left ventricle (*LV*), and aorta (*Ao*) are identical. *LA,* Left atrium; *PA,* pulmonary artery; *RA,* right atrium.

In atrial premature contractions, abnormal P waves occurring earlier than would normally be expected are seen on the ECG. The P wave is usually followed by a normal QRS complex. These premature contractions may be associated with left atrial enlargement or atrial disease of any type (MMVD). Animals are usually asymptomatic but the technician may palpate a pulse deficit and auscultate a variable heart sound (Fig. 1-8). This arrhythmia may progress to AF.

Atrial Fibrillation (Supraventricular Arrhythmia)

AF occurs when there is no organized atrial contraction. Cardiac output declines because of the loss of atrial "kick" and the rapid ventricular rate. A critical mass of myocardial tissue is required to sustain AF; thus, the larger the heart, the more likely it is to occur. It is therefore more prevalent in large-breed dogs and dogs with cardiac diseases that increase the size of the heart. Cats with AF always have underlying cardiac disease.

Ventricular arrhythmias arise from the fibers of the ventricle, and the QRS complexes are abnormally wide and bizarre. They may or may not be related to the preceding P wave.

CLINICAL SIGNS

- Large-breed dog, with or without concurrent heart disease; may occur in the cat
- Weakness, syncope
- Dyspnea in the cat
- Collapse
- Rapid, irregular heart rate

DIAGNOSIS

- Auscultation of a rapid, irregular heart rate
- ECG: no evidence of P waves, irregular base line; rapid, irregular heart rate

TREATMENT

- Treatment aims to slow heart rate; will not correct the AF
- Digitalis glycosides (digoxin): to slow heart rate

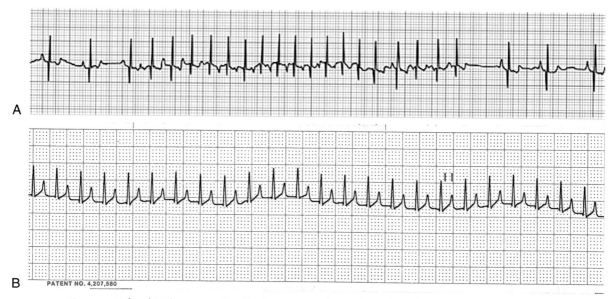

Figure 1-8 A, Atrial tachycardia **B,** Supraventricular tachycardia (dog—lead II; 25 mm/sec; 1 cm/mV). *(A is from Ettinger SJ; Feldman, EC: Textbook of Veterinary Internal Medicine, ed. 7, St Louis, 2010, Saunders. B is from Thomas, JA; Lerche P: Anesthesia and Analgesia for Veterinary Technicians, ed. 4, St Louis, 2011, Mosby.)*

- Calcium channel blockers (diltiazem hydrochloride, verapamil [for dogs only]): to slow atrioventricular node conduction and increase the refractory period

INFORMATION FOR CLIENTS

- Treatment will not cure the AF.
- Concurrent heart disease will progress even with treatment.
- CHF eventually will develop.
- Periodic examinations and reevaluations of the pet will be necessary.
- Report any gastrointestinal upset, anorexia, diarrhea, or worsening of cardiac function (coughing, weakness, collapse) to your veterinarian immediately.
- In an emergency situation, inform the person treating your pet about the drugs your pet has been taking.

Ventricular Tachycardia (Ventricular Arrhythmias)

VT may be associated with many diseases such as cardiomyopathy, CHF, endocarditis or myocarditis, or cardiac neoplasia. Electrolyte and acid-base imbalances will also produce VT. The rapid rate of contraction reduces ventricular filling time and, therefore, decreases cardiac output. If allowed to progress, VT may lead to ventricular fibrillation (VF), a life-threatening condition. VF is equivalent to cardiac arrest, as no blood is moved into the systemic circulation because of inadequate myocardial contractions and poor filling of the ventricles (Fig. 1-9).

CLINICAL SIGNS

- Weakness, collapse, syncope with rapid heart rates
- Sudden death is not uncommon
- CHF with longstanding VTs

DIAGNOSIS

- Auscultation
- ECG: infrequent to frequent widened, bizarre QRS complexes of ventricular origin. In VF, abnormal baseline with no QRS complexes.

TREATMENT

- Treat if the number of ventricular premature contractions is more than 25 per minute, if heart rate is greater than 130 beats/min, if the breed is at risk for sudden death, or if clinical symptoms exist
- Procainamide: decreases myocardial excitability, depresses conduction velocity
- Tocainide: decreases myocardial excitability, automaticity, and conduction velocities (dogs only)
- Lidocaine (2% without epinephrine): decreases automaticity of the heart and decreases myocardial excitability
- Mexiletine to slow heart rate.
- If VF: cardiac defibrillation, IV fluids, sodium bicarbonate; all based on standard cardiopulmonary resuscitation techniques

INFORMATION FOR CLIENTS

- Prognosis is guarded unless the underlying cause of the arrhythmia can be resolved.
- German Shepherds and Boxers are breeds that experience sudden death from VT (Fig. 1-10).

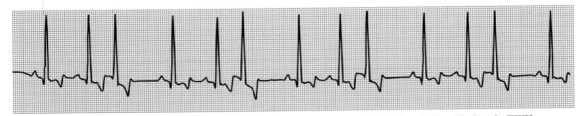

Figure 1-9 Electrocardiogram – atrial premature complexes. *(Modified from Tilley LP; Smith, FWK; Oyama MA; Sleeper MM: Manual of Canine and Feline Cardiology, ed. 4, St Louis, 2008, Saunders).*

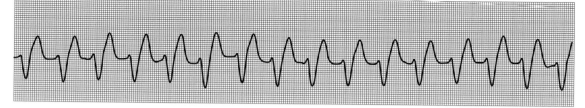

Figure 1-10 Electrocardiogram – ventricular tachycardia. *(Modified from Tilley LP; Smith, FWK; Oyama MA; Sleeper MM:* Manual of Canine and Feline Cardiology, ed. 4, *St Louis, 2008, Saunders).*

Ventricular Fibrillation

In VF, there is a complete lack of well-defined QRS complexes—a lack of heart sounds, blood pressure, and pulse. VF is a life-threatening condition that must be corrected immediately with intubation and respiratory assist, IV fluid therapy, cardiac massage, epinephrine, and possibly electric defibrillation.

Sinus Arrhythmia

Sinus arrhythmia is a common, normal occurrence in dogs. It is related to breathing and alterations in vagal tone that occur during inspiration and expiration. Heart rate increases during inspiration and decreases during expiration. If one listens carefully, this arrhythmia can be heard in almost every dog examined. It is not often seen in cats.

Sinus Bradycardia

Sinus bradycardia is also a commonly seen arrhythmia, especially in large-breed dogs and athletic, highly conditioned animals. The ECG shows normal P and QRS complexes, with a heart rate less than 70 beats/min. Pathologic conditions that may produce this arrhythmia include increased intracranial pressure, hyperkalemia (excess potassium), hypothyroidism, gastrointestinal disturbances, drugs, or any condition that results in increased vagal tone (neck trauma, tumors, etc.).

CLINICAL SIGNS

- Usually none, unless the heart rate declines exceptionally low
- Episodic weakness, syncope, collapse

DIAGNOSIS

- Auscultation
- ECG: slow heart rate with normal P and QRS complexes

TREATMENT

- None, unless clinical signs are present
- Atropine: increases heart rate
- Propantheline bromide: anticholinergic agent similar to atropine in effect
- Placement of an artificial pacemaker

INFORMATION FOR CLIENTS

- This may be a normal finding in athletic dogs.
- Correction of concurrent problems may eliminate the bradycardia.
- Most dogs can live a normal life with this disorder, but if clinical symptoms of weakness or syncope develop, treatment may be necessary.

⊙ TECH ALERT

Brachiocephalic dogs and cats can develop severe bradycardias during intubation. It is important to carefully monitor the patient and avoid traumatic techniques that overstretch the neck or traumatize the vagus nerve.

⊙ TECH ALERT

Postrenal urinary obstruction in cats can elevate potassium levels and cause severe bradycardia that may be life threatening. Avoid using potassium-containing fluids in these cats.

Heartworm Disease

Canine Heartworm Disease

Heartworm disease is of worldwide significance. In the United States, the disease is concentrated in areas within 150 miles of the coastal regions from Texas to New Jersey and along the Mississippi River and its tributaries but can be seen anywhere because of the tremendous mobility of the canine population. The disease is spread by many different species of mosquitoes. Male dogs are more frequently infected compared with female dogs (4:1), and outdoor dogs are more likely to become infected than indoor dogs. The average age at which infections are detected is between 3 and 8 years. Large-breed dogs appear to be more susceptible to infection than small breeds, and cats appear to be somewhat resistant to the disease. (Mosquito bites are less frequent in cats.)

The female mosquito serves as the intermediate host by obtaining a blood meal containing the microfilaria of *Dirofilaria immitis* from an infected dog. These microfilaria develop in the mosquito within 2 to 2.5 weeks and are then injected into the skin of another dog through a bite. The infective larvae migrate within the skin of the new host for about 100 days. Young adults (L5 stage) enter the vasculature and migrate to the pulmonary artery, where they mature into adults. Approximately 6 months after the initial bite, microfilaria can be detected in the blood of the host dog.

Disease severity is partially related to the number of adult heartworms. The presence of adult worms in the pulmonary artery damages the endothelial lining of the vessel and increases the permeability, allowing fluid and proteins to leak into the perivascular tissue. The *physical* presence of the parasites results in right-sided heart enlargement (blockage of the right outflow tract) and pulmonary hypertension.

Heartworm disease is easily detected using immunodiagnostic tests that utilize monoclonal antibodies to heartworm uterine antigen. Microfilaria can be detected using filter techniques, the Knott test or by simply observing a drop of whole blood under the microscope, although these methods may not detect the organisms in as many as 25% of infected dogs.

Treatment previously involved the removal of the adult worms by the use of thiacetarsamide (Caparsolate), which is no longer available. Melarsamine dihydrochloride (Immiticide, Merial) is now the drug of choice for treatment; however, in recent times, this drug has been in short supply. Immiticide is usually followed by a microfilaricide (ivermectin). Animals are then prescribed prophylaxis therapy given monthly.

CLINICAL SIGNS

- Most dogs are asymptomatic and infections are discovered on routine screening during yearly examinations
- Cough, dyspnea
- Exercise intolerance
- Hemoptysis (coughing up blood)
- Signs of right-sided heart failure

DIAGNOSIS

- Positive antigen test
- Positive concentration test
- Radiography: evidence of pulmonary changes consistent with heartworm disease: right ventricular enlargement, increased prominence of pulmonary artery, enlarged lobar arteries, increased perivascular pattern
- Echocardiology: adult worms can be seen in the pulmonary artery and sometimes in the right heart

TREATMENT

- If treatment is elected, the animal should have a pretreatment laboratory workup, which includes a minimum of a complete blood cell count, serum chemistries, and chest radiography.

Adulticide Treatment

- Thiacetarsamide: no longer used; serious side effects seen with its use
- Melarsomine dihydrochloride: given at 24-hour intervals. Injections should be made deep into the lumbar muscles; currently not readily available
- Thiacetarsamide and melarsomine are toxic; signs of toxicity may occur during or after treatment:
  1. Thiacetarsamide: toxicity occurs in approximately 10% to 15% of cases; signs include bilirubinuria, vomiting, anorexia, lethargy, and icterus
  2. Melarsomine hydrochloride: signs of toxicity include respiratory distress, vomiting, panting, excessive salivation, and diarrhea

Treatment of Toxicities

- Thiacetarsamide: stop treatment; IV balanced electrolyte solutions; feed high-carbohydrate, low-fat diet; limit exercise
- Melarsomine dihydrochloride: dimercaprol (British anti-Lewisite [BAL]) in oil

Microfilaricide Treatment

- Given 3 to 6 weeks after the adulticide treatment
- Ivermectin: given as a single dose (dilute 1 mL ivermectin [Ivomec] or Equavalan with 9 mL propylene glycol or water and dose at 1 mL/44 lb)
- Milbemycin oxime: single dose

⦿ TECH ALERT

Use care in treating Collies because they have a genetic susceptibility to ivermectin toxicity.

PREVENTION

- Selamectin (Revolution Spot On)
- Ivermectin (Heartgard)
- Milbemycin oxime (Interceptor)
- Doxycycline
- Microfilaria have a symbiotic parasite, *Wolbachia*, which may be killed by the use of doxycycline. In turn, the death of the parasite adversely affects the adult heartworm. Doxycycline at a dose of 10 mg/kg/day is given for 14 weeks along with weekly ivermectin dosed at four times the label dosage. Studies have not been done on the efficacy of this type of therapy.

⦿ TECH ALERT

Do not use diethylcarbamazine (DEC) in dogs that test positive for heartworms.

Feline Heartworm Disease

In areas where heartworm disease is prevalent, cats are also at risk for infection. Until recently, it has been difficult to diagnose the disease in cats because they are usually negative for microfilaria and the canine heartworm antigen tests are inadequate for detecting the disease in cats.

Cats are somewhat resistant to *D. immitis* infection, having few adult worms, which are eliminated from the host within 2 years. Outdoor male cats are most at risk for infection. The mean age of diagnosis is between 3 and 6 years.

Symptoms in cats differ from those in dogs. Sudden death of an asymptomatic cat is fairly frequently seen. Most symptoms relate to the respiratory system (cough, dyspnea) or the gastrointestinal tract (vomiting, anorexia, lethargy). Acute pulmonary embolism occurs with affected cats demonstrating severe dyspnea, weakness, and anorexia. Ataxia, blindness, and seizures may also be seen.

Prevention is advised and is now available for cats at risk. Treatment regimens are controversial. In most cases, treatment involves supportive care while the cat eliminates the parasite.

CLINICAL SIGNS

- Coughing, dyspnea
- Vomiting
- Anorexia, weight loss
- Lethargy
- Right-sided CHF
- Sudden death or acute development of neurologic signs

DIAGNOSIS

- Feline heartworm antibody immunodiagnostic test (can be done in-house); detection of antibody is missed with this test in many cats
- Feline heartworm antigen immunodiagnostic test: results depend on the sex and number of adult heartworms present
- Radiology: signs are similar to those in the canine but are more difficult to interpret
- Echocardiography: should be done in all cases; will see adult worms in the pulmonary artery

⦿ TECH ALERT

Use caution when performing radiography on dyspneic cats—undue restraint may kill the cat!

TREATMENT

Adulticide treatment is usually *not* recommended in the cat. However, if treatment is prescribed:

- Thiacetarsamide and immiticide both have toxic consequences in the cat and may be fatal.
- Microfilariacide: not needed in cats because of lack of microfilaria
- Cage rest
- Cortisone may be used to decrease the inflammatory component of the disease

⬤ TECH ALERT

Most (half to two thirds) of all cats treated with thiacetarsamide will experience development of signs of toxicity—depression, anorexia, and vomiting. Pulmonary edema is common after treatment. The use of immiticide has not met with great success in naturally infected cats.

PREVENTION

- Milbemycin oxime or ivermectin given monthly

CLINICAL CASES

An adult Boxer was anesthetized for a routine castration. The physical examination and pre-surgery blood work was all within normal limits. During anesthesia induction, the technician noticed occasional ventricular contractions on the monitoring ECG. The surgeon terminated the procedure, and the dog recovered without incident. Repeat ECG studies on the awake dog showed normal sinus rhythm. The dog was adopted and was doing well in his new home. As the owner came home one evening, the dog became excited and experienced cardiac arrest and died. Can you answer the owner's questions?

1. Why did this happen to my healthy dog?
2. If I get another Boxer, is this likely to happen again?
3. What could have been done to prevent this from happening?

REVIEW QUESTIONS

1. A puppy is having a "machinery-like" murmur that is best heard on the left side of the chest. What cardiovascular defect is most likely?
   a. Tetralogy of Fallot
   b. Patent ductus arteriosus
   c. Septal defect
   d. Mitral stenosis
2. While examining a Doberman, you hear a rapid, irregular heart rate with pulse deficits. This arrhythmia is most likely:
   a. Ventricular fibrillation
   b. Ventricular tachycardia
   c. Atrial fibrillation
   d. Sinus tachycardia
3. An owner reports that her Weimaraner puppy is regurgitating undigested food every time the puppy eats. The puppy is losing weight and is coughing. Which of the following abnormalities might this puppy be exhibiting?
   a. Mitral stenosis
   b. Patent ductus arteriosus
   c. Atrial septal defect
   d. Persistent right aortic arch
4. What is the reference range for heart rate in the dog?
   a. 60–180 beats/min
   b. 100–180 beats/min
   c. 100–250 beats/min
   d. 30–75 beats/min
5. What amino acid do cats require in their diet to avoid cardiomyopathy?
   a. Cysteine
   b. Taurine
   c. Guanine
   d. Isoleucine

Answers found on page 551.

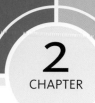

Diseases of the Digestive System

OUTLINE

Anatomy Overview of the Gastrointestinal System
The Tooth and Oral Diseases
Esophageal Diseases
Diseases of the Stomach
Diseases of the Small Intestine
    Diseases of the Large Bowel

Hepatic Disease
Pancreatic Disease
Rectoanal Disease

LEARNING OBJECTIVES

When you have completed this chapter, you will be able to:

1. Explain the basic anatomic arrangement of the mammalian digestive system.
2. Relate changes in the digestive system to the development of disease symptoms.

3. Explain to owners why their pet is ill and how the problem is best treated.

Food is vital for the life of the animal because it provides the source of energy that drives all the chemical reactions in the body. Consumed food is not in a form readily usable by the body. The digestive system breaks down the consumed food to a point where it can be absorbed and used by the animal.

The organs of digestion can be divided into two main groups: (1) the gastrointestinal (GI) tract, a continuous tube beginning at the mouth and ending at the anus, and (2) the *accessory structures*—the teeth, tongue, salivary glands, liver, pancreas, and gallbladder (Fig. 2-1).

A discussion of diseases that affect the GI system can be best approached by dividing the system into regions: oral cavity and esophagus, stomach, small bowel, large bowel, liver, pancreas, and rectum and anus.

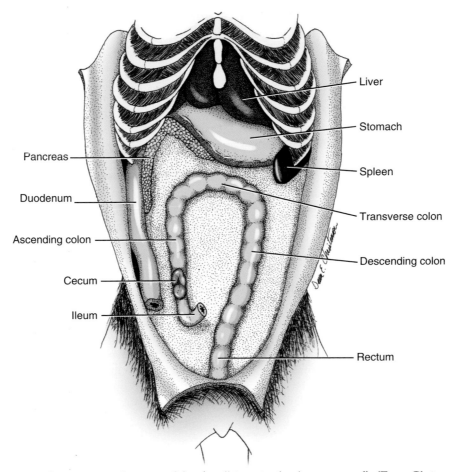

Figure 2-1 Gastrointestinal system of dog (small intestine has been removed). (From Christenson DE: *Veterinary medical terminology*, ed 2, St. Louis, MO, 2009, Saunders, by permission.)

Anatomy Overview of the Gastrointestinal System

The GI system begins with the teeth and the oral cavity. Puppies and kittens are born without teeth, but deciduous teeth begin to erupt from gums at between 3 and 12 weeks of age. As the neonate ages, deciduous teeth are lost and replaced by adult teeth. Adult dogs have 42 permanent teeth, and cats have 30. The last adult teeth to erupt, canine teeth, can be used in aging young animals. These teeth are usually in place by 6 months of age. After this time, it becomes more difficult to estimate an animal's age. Retained deciduous canine teeth are not uncommon in both dogs and cats, and their presence may affect the position of permanent teeth. These "baby" teeth are usually removed at the time of neutering or spaying.

Food in the oral cavity is masticated (chewed) and mixed with saliva to create a bolus, which passes down the esophagus into the stomach through the lower esophageal sphincter, also called the *cardiac sphincter*. The last portion of the esophagus is different in dogs and cats. The cat has smooth muscle in the distal esophagus, whereas the dog has skeletal muscle. This difference predisposes the cat to esophageal injury from oral medications that may "stick" in the distal esophagus and cause inflammation or ulceration. Digestive juices, secreted in the muscular stomach, are composed of hydrochloric acid and enzymes, which further break down the bolus and form a thick emulsion now called *chyme.* Controlled amounts of chyme exit the stomach through the pyloric sphincter and enter the portion of the small intestine called the *duodenum.* In this short area of the small intestine, pancreatic enzymes and bile mix with the chyme, and further breakdown of food occurs. As the chyme passes through the small intestine, amino acids, carbohydrates, and lipids are absorbed through the intestinal lining and enter the bloodstream, where they are carried to the liver for processing. The lining of the small intestine has a large absorptive surface area because of the presence of multiple folds or *villi and microvilli.* Many diseases that affect the GI system involve damage to this absorptive surface. The small intestine also contains an important microbiologic flora which, when disrupted, can result in small bowel disease. From the small intestine, undigested materials are passed into the large intestine for bacterial processing, water re-absorption, and elimination through the rectum. The bacteria in the large bowel also produce valuable vitamins such as vitamin B and vitamin K. Adjunct organs that assist the digestive process include the pancreas, liver, and gall bladder.

The exocrine portion of the pancreas produces digestive enzymes, *pancreatic juices,* that break down proteins, carbohydrates, DNA and RNA (deoxyribonucleic acid and ribonucleic acid), and lipids. Bile, produced in the liver and stored in the gall bladder, makes its way down the common bile duct and joins the pancreatic enzymes in the duodenum. It is not uncommon to see pancreatic, hepatic, and small intestinal signs of disease when any of the three become inflamed. In the small intestine, bile salts form *micelles* with the lipid molecules, making fats soluble in the bloodstream. All these digested and absorbed materials are transported to the liver via the hepatic portal system, where multiple chemical processes further change them to usable *metabolites,* which are "shipped" out to waiting cells and tissues in the body.

The Tooth and Oral Diseases

The tooth begins life as a tooth bud within the gum. Ameloblasts begin to produce enamel, which will eventually cover the crown of the tooth; odontoblasts lay down dentin, which will form the body of the tooth; and the pulp cavity begins to form. As the tooth grows within the gum, the crown is pushed upward, eventually erupting to the surface of the gum. The protective layer of enamel on the crown is hard but very thin and can be damaged when chewing on hard materials. Dogs that chew on rocks, fences, or other hard objects will typically have fractured enamel, which leads to further tooth decay. The roots of the tooth are attached to the alveolar bone of the mandible or the maxilla via the *periodontal ligament.* This ligament not only holds the tooth into the bony socket but also protects the tooth from osteoclastic activity from surrounding bone. The gingiva wraps up onto the surface of the crown, creating a gingival sulcus and protecting the periodontal ligament. Blood vessels, nerves, and lymph channels enter the tooth through the root and pass up into the pulp cavity.

Diseases of the oral cavity most frequently seen in small animals include gingivitis or periodontal disease, lip-fold dermatitis, trauma, salivary mucocele, and oral neoplasms. The clinical signs of these diseases are similar; affected animals are reluctant to eat and have oral pain, halitosis, and excessive salivation.

Gingivitis or Periodontal Disease

Periodontal disease results from infectious inflammation of the gingiva, and it affects all the structures involved in tooth attachment (Fig. 2-2 and Fig. 2-3). This condition is a continuum of disease, beginning with gingivitis and progressing to periodontitis and tooth loss. *Gingivitis,* a reversible process that involves inflammation of the margins of the gums, is caused by accumulation of tartar on teeth and acts as a nidus for bacterial multiplication. Enzymes produced by these bacteria damage the tooth attachments and result in inflammation. Without intervention, gingivitis will progress to *periodontitis,* an irreversible condition that results in loss of gingival epithelial root attachment and alveolar bone resorption. Periodontal disease is estimated to occur in 60% to 80% of dogs and cats.

Periodontal Disease

Periodontal disease is a collective term for plaque-induced inflammation of gums. This inflammation

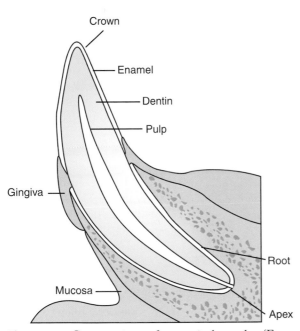

Figure 2-2 Cross-section of a typical tooth. (From Colville T, Bassert JM: *Clinical anatomy and physiology for veterinary technicians*, ed 2, St. Louis, MO, 2008, Mosby, by permission.)

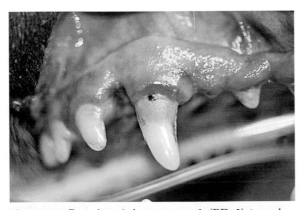

Figure 2-3 Periodontal disease stage 2 (PD 2) in a dog. (From Holmstrom, Steven E. Veterinary Dentistry: A Team Approach, 2nd Edition. W.B. Saunders Company, 2013.)

is progressive and includes gingivitis, gingival hyperplasia, periodontitis with vertical bone destruction, and periodontitis with horizontal bone destruction. The final outcome of periodontal disease is loss of teeth.

Gingivitis

Gingivitis (inflammation of the gingiva) is the earliest sign of periodontal disease. It results from the buildup of dental plaque (tartar) in the gingival sulcus. Bacteria seldom invade gingival tissue directly; however, anaerobic bacteria that comprise much of the subgingival plaque secrete enzymes that result in inflammation of the surrounding gum. The inflammatory response of the host animal results in *gingival hyperplasia*. (Gingival hyperplasia may be breed related or drug induced.) As plaque is mineralized, it becomes dental calculus, which protects the bacterial environment.

Gingivitis is limited to the soft tissue of the gingiva, with sulcal depths remaining within normal limits in both dogs and cats. As the disease progresses to *periodontitis*, pathologic periodontal pockets are formed. The coronal portion of the periodontal ligament is destroyed by inflammation, and alveolar bone resorption begins. If treated early, gingivitis is reversible; however, once periodontal disease progresses, the changes are irreversible. Prevention and treatment of periodontal disease is of utmost importance in the health of companion animals.

CLINICAL SIGNS

- Halitosis
- Reluctance to chew hard food, bones, toys
- Pawing at the mouth
- Head shyness
- Oral pain
- Personality changes
- Sneezing, nasal discharge
- Increased salivation (may be bloody)
- Facial swelling
- Tooth loss

DIAGNOSIS

- Complete oral examination (may require general anesthesia or sedation)
- Increased depth of the gingival sulcus (dogs: >3 mm; cats: >1 mm)
- Presence of tartar on teeth, inflammation

TREATMENT

- Dental scaling, extraction of all loose teeth
- Root planing
- Gingival curettage

- Sublingual lavage
- Antibiotics (clindamycin, enrofloxacin, amoxicillin trihydrate or clavulanate potassium [Clavamox])
- Instruction to owners about developing a good oral hygiene program for their pets

INFORMATION FOR CLIENTS

- Good oral hygiene is a necessity for all pets. It should begin around 2 years of age or when needed.
- Brush the pet's teeth daily to remove tartar and plaque.
- Have routine dental cleanings performed by your veterinarian.
- Have gingivitis treated early, before the development of irreversible signs.
- Some animals may require extraction of all their teeth to remove the source of infection.
- Hard, crunchy foods may promote better dental health by manually removing tartar before it calcifies. Once calcified, tartar must be removed professionally.
- Professional cleaning under anesthesia is required to completely remove tartar and calculus from teeth.

Lip-Fold Dermatitis

Lip-fold dermatitis is commonly seen in breeds with pendulous upper lips and prominent lower lip folds. Breeds such as Spaniels, Setters, Bulldogs, and Bassets are most commonly affected. Constant moisture in these folds from saliva results in increased bacterial growth. Together with the collection of food and hair in the area, the saliva causes increased irritation, erythema, and a fetid odor.

CLINICAL SIGNS

- Halitosis
- Collection of debris in the lower lip folds

DIAGNOSIS

- Clinical signs, especially in breeds predisposed to problems with lip folds
- Complete blood work to rule out other causes of halitosis and lip-fold disease such as periodontal disease, *Demodex* infestation, pemphigus, and renal failure

TREATMENT

- Complete dental cleaning
- Flushing and cleaning of lip folds with 2.5% benzoyl peroxide shampoo
- Surgical resection of lip folds may be required in some cases

INFORMATION FOR CLIENTS

- Keep the lip folds clean and dry.
- Daily cleaning will be required for the life of the animal.
- Drying agents such as cornstarch may help some animals. Dust the agent into the folds several times daily after cleaning.
- Good dental hygiene will benefit these animals.

Oral Trauma

Oral trauma is common in small animals. Falls, fights, burns, blunt trauma, penetration of foreign objects, and automobile accidents account for many injuries to the oral cavity of pets. Head injuries from "high-rise syndrome" (e.g., cats falling from windows of buildings) or from other types of accidents often result in fracture of the mandibular symphysis, maxillary dysfunction, separation of the hard palate of cats, or all of these injuries. The tongue is frequently injured by self-trauma (biting its own tongue), dog fights, penetration of foreign bodies (e.g., splinters, needles, bullets), or strangulation by elastic or stringlike materials. Cats that play with needles and thread may injure the tongue or the frenulum or have a linear foreign body lodged somewhere in the oral cavity. Tongue lacerations have occurred as a result of dogs and cats attempting to eat from discarded tin cans to which the lids are still attached.

Electrical and chemical burns are often seen in young, curious animals that have a tendency to bite electric cords or taste unusual plants or liquids. Electrical burns not only involve the mucosal surface of the oral cavity, but progress deep into the tissue along vessels and wet tissue planes. Contact with caustic chemicals and plants can result in erosion of the oral mucosa, producing pain, inflammation, secondary infection, and necrosis.

Gunshot wounds often result in dental or other oral injuries, as well as shattered bones, teeth, and penetrating wounds of the tongue. Fishhooks of all types attract both dogs and cats. Hooks can become embedded in the lips or the tongue (sometimes both at the same time), resulting in a frantic animal that may require sedation or general anesthesia to properly remove the hook. Round steak bones present a special challenge. These bones typically become lodged behind canine teeth, over the end of the mandible. As the tissue swells, it becomes painful. General anesthesia is required in most cases. The lodged bones must be cut in sections for removal. Cats also have problems with bones; flat chicken bones can become lodged across the upper dental arcade, and sedation of the animal may be required for removal of the bone.

CLINICAL SIGNS

- History or signs of head trauma
- Increased salivation
- Inability to close the mouth
- Reluctance or inability to eat
- Presence of a foreign object

DIAGNOSIS

- Physical examination of the oral cavity (sedation or anesthesia may be required)
- Radiography to rule out the presence of an embedded linear foreign body

TREATMENT

- Treatment depends on the extent of the damage
- Control of bleeding
- Supportive treatment: fluids, pain relief
- Maintenance of adequate airway
- Lavage with copious amount of water in the case of chemical burns
- Repair or extraction of damaged teeth
- Surgical repair of fractures

INFORMATION FOR CLIENTS

- Young animals should never be left alone. Protect animals from accidental electrical burns and ingestion of caustic chemicals by confining them when they cannot be watched.
- Keep pets fenced or on a leash to prevent roaming and the possibility of gunshot wounds.
- Limit cats' access to thread and needles.

- Avoid feeding bones to dogs and cats.
- Seek veterinary assistance in case of any head injury.
- Advances in dental repair make it possible to cap and repair damaged teeth.
- Animals can function well even with loss of large amounts of tongue tissue.

Salivary Mucocele

The salivary mucocele is the most common clinically recognized disease of the salivary glands in dogs, although it may also occur secondary to trauma in cats. A mucocele is an accumulation of excessive amounts of saliva in the subcutaneous tissue and the consequent tissue reaction that occurs. This disease occurs most often in dogs between the ages of 2 and 4 years; German Shepherds and Miniature Poodles are most commonly affected. The initial cause of the accumulation usually is unknown. Owners report a history of a slowly enlarging, fluid-filled, painless swelling on the neck. The animal may have respiratory distress or difficulty swallowing secondary to the partial obstruction of the pharynx. In cats, a ranula (a large fluid-filled swelling under the tongue) may be seen.

CLINICAL SIGNS

- Slowly enlarging, painless, fluid-filled swelling on the neck or under the tongue
- Reluctance to eat
- Difficulty swallowing
- Blood-tinged saliva
- Respiratory distress

DIAGNOSIS

- Clinical signs
- Paracentesis shows a stringy, blood-tinged fluid with a low cell count
- Sialography by retrograde infusion of a water-soluble angiographic contrast material (Renografin: 0.055–0.110 mL/kg body weight [BW]) into the duct of the salivary gland

TREATMENT

- Aspiration of fluid
- Surgical drainage
- Removal of the gland, followed by placement of a Penrose drain for 5 to 7 days

INFORMATION FOR CLIENTS

- The cause of the development of mucoceles in animals is unknown, although trauma may be involved in some cases.
- Without removal of the gland, excessive amounts of fluid will continue to accumulate.
- Some cases may resolve spontaneously.

Oral Neoplasms

Oral neoplasms are relatively common in dogs and cats, with malignant melanomas and squamous cell carcinomas being the most common. In general, older animals are more commonly affected, and male animals are at an increased risk for malignant melanoma and fibrosarcoma. Dogs with heavily pigmented oral mucosa are also at greater risk for malignant melanoma compared with dogs having pink oral mucosa.

Benign neoplasms such as papillomas and epulides are seen in dogs (Fig. 2-4). Papillomas, which are pale-colored, cauliflower-like growths, have a viral cause and may be removed surgically or may regress spontaneously. Epulides occur in the gingiva near incisors. They are generally slow growing, but some may be locally invasive and involve bone destruction.

Malignant melanomas are rapidly growing tumors characterized by early bone involvement. They metastasize early to the lungs and regional lymph nodes. These lesions are dome shaped or sessile and may be

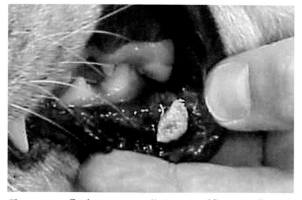

Figure 2-4 Oral canine papillomatosis. (Courtesy Patrick Hensel and Tracey Gieger, University of Georgia, Athens, GA. IN Greene C: *Infectious diseases of the dog and cat,* ed 3, St Louis, 2006, Elsevier.)

black, brown, mottled, or unpigmented. Squamous cell carcinomas are ulcerative, erosive neoplasms. They invade the mucosa and often bone and metastasize to regional lymph nodes.

Treatment for oral neoplasia includes surgical removal, chemotherapy, radiation therapy, or all. The prognosis for malignant oral neoplasms is guarded to poor.

CLINICAL SIGNS

- Signs depend on location and size of growth
- Abnormal food prehension
- Increased salivation
- Halitosis
- Tooth loss
- Oral pain

DIAGNOSIS

- Diagnosis is by histology of the mass
- Complete blood cell count (CBC) or serum chemistries
- Radiography to rule out visceral metastases and to evaluate bone involvement
- Lymph node biopsy

TREATMENT

- Surgical excision with a 2-cm tumor-free margin
- If bone is involved or metastasis is suspected, a hemimaxillectomy or a hemimandibulectomy should be performed. Extensive removal of bone and soft tissue can be performed without harm to the animal
- Radiation therapy
- Chemotherapy
  - Cisplatin for dogs with squamous cell carcinomas
  - Doxorubicin or cyclophosphamide for cats with squamous cell carcinomas and fibrosarcomas

INFORMATION FOR CLIENTS

- The prognosis for animals with malignant neoplasia is guarded to poor even with aggressive treatment.
- Benign lesions have a good prognosis after surgical resection, radiation therapy, or both.
- Animals (especially cats) with maxillectomies or mandibulectomies may need nutritional support such as a feeding tube.

Esophageal Diseases

Diseases of the esophagus include megaesophagus (see Chapter 8), esophagitis or gastroesophageal reflux (GER), vascular ring anomalies (see Chapter 1), and foreign body obstruction.

Esophagitis or Gastroesophageal Reflux

Esophagitis is an inflammation of the esophageal wall and is most often associated with contact of irritants with the mucosa of the esophagus. Acids, alkalis, drugs, and hot materials can produce lesions of varying severity in the esophagus. The extent of the lesion will depend on several factors: (1) the type of material, (2) the length of contact with the mucosal surface, and (3) the integrity of the esophageal mucosal barrier. Physical trauma by foreign bodies or chemical damage from chronic vomiting may predispose the esophagus to further damage.

The esophagus has a great ability to withstand injury. The mucosa–gel barrier, tight cell junctions, and a bicarbonate-rich layer all serve to protect the mucosal lining from damage. One of the most common causes of esophagitis is GER. In healthy animals, the lower esophageal sphincter prevents reflux of gastric contents back into the esophagus. Gastric acid, pepsin, and trypsin found in gastric fluid will damage the mucosal lining if allowed to remain in contact with it for prolonged periods. Once inflammatory damage to the esophagus has occurred, lower esophageal sphincter function becomes abnormal, perpetuating the problem.

CLINICAL SIGNS

- Anorexia
- Dysphagia
- Excessive salivation
- Regurgitation
- Concurrent signs of respiratory disease (calicivirus in cats)

DIAGNOSIS

- Endoscopy will demonstrate mucosal inflammation and the presence or absence of ulceration. The lower esophageal sphincter may be open abnormally in animals with GER. Fluoroscopy may be required to document actual reflux.

TREATMENT

- The goal of treatment is to decrease inflammation and to protect the lining from further damage.

Ingestion of Irritant Substances

- *Do not* induce vomiting. It may cause further damage to the esophagus.
- Administer neutralizing compounds (e.g., activated charcoal, egg white, sodium bicarbonate, olive oil), or check the container for information on accidental ingestions.
- Bathe or flush the skin with water to prevent further ingestion.
- Use intestinal absorbants such as activated charcoal to decrease further toxic effects.
- Rest the esophagus by withholding food and water for several days.
- You may need a gastrostomy tube in severe cases.
- Sucralfate: Dissolve a 1-g tablet in 10 mL of warm water; then give 5 to 10 mL of the solution orally three times daily.
- Administer broad-spectrum antibiotics.
- Corticosteroids: Use at antiinflammatory doses.

Gastroesophageal Reflux

- Dietary changes: recommend weight loss and use of a high-protein, low-fat diet to normalize gastric emptying
- Sucralfate (see previous section for dose)
- Histamine 2 (H_2) receptor blockers or proton pump blockers:
  - Cimetidine (Tagamet): three times daily
  - Ranitidine (Zantac): three times daily
  - Omeprazole (Prilosec): daily
- Metoclopramide (Reglan): three to four times daily to increase lower esophageal pressure and esophageal motility

INFORMATION FOR CLIENTS

- Prevent access to irritant materials such as cleaning liquids, chemicals, paint thinners, and medications. Avoid feeding foods heated in the microwave because they may contain hot spots that can result in burns to the esophagus; always stir well to mix and cool the food.
- Proper weight management will prevent pets from becoming obese. A good exercise program will

help most pets keep the weight in the proper range.

- Healing of the esophagus is a slow process, and treatment may be required for a long period.

⬤ TECH ALERT

When administering oral medications to cats, ensure that the medication is washed down with water to prevent the tablet or capsule from sticking in the lower portion of the esophagus and causing irritation.

Esophageal Obstruction

Ingestion of nondigestible foreign objects is more common in dogs than in cats, with young animals being more likely to be affected. Bones and small toys commonly lodge at the thoracic inlet, cardiac base, or distal esophagus. The degree of damage to the esophagus depends on the size of the object, the shape, and the time spent in contact with the esophageal mucosal lining.

Prompt removal is important to prevent serious damage. Endoscopy will allow the clinician direct visualization of the object, and most foreign bodies can be removed by endoscopic retrieval. Those that cannot be removed orally can often be pushed into the stomach and removed surgically. Surgical removal of foreign objects directly from the esophagus has a less favorable prognosis because of the poor healing qualities of the esophagus and the potential for stricture formation.

CLINICAL SIGNS

- Exaggerated swallowing movements
- Increased salivation
- Restlessness
- Retching
- Anorexia
- History of chewing on foreign objects

DIAGNOSIS

Endoscopy

- Use a flexible or rigid endoscope. A basket or retrieval forceps may be used to grasp the object for removal. Once the object is removed, the mucosal lining of the esophagus can then be examined for damage.

Radiology

- If the object is radiopaque, it may be seen on a radiograph. Contrast material can be used to outline radiolucent objects. Iodated contrast agents should be selected if a perforation is suspected.

TREATMENT

- Prompt removal of the foreign object is imperative.
- Fast the animal for 24 to 48 hours after removal to allow the esophagus to rest and begin healing.
- After 48 hours, resume feeding with soft foods for several days.
- Treat the esophagitis that may be present (see previous section).
- If damage to the esophagus is extensive, placement of a percutaneous endoscopic gastrostomy tube may be required.

INFORMATION FOR CLIENTS

- Limit access to bones and small toys that can be swallowed.
- String and needles present a special hazard for cats.
- The prognosis usually is good for affected animals if serious damage to the esophagus can be prevented.

Diseases of the Stomach

The stomach is located in the left cranial abdomen and stores ingesta, mixing it with gastric juices and then propelling it into the duodenum at a controlled rate. Anatomically, the stomach wall is composed of three layers of tissue: (1) the mucosal (epithelial) lining, (2) the muscular (smooth muscle) layer, and (3) the serosa. The mucosal lining contains glands that secrete mucus, parietal glands that secrete hydrochloric acid, chief cells that secrete pepsinogen, and argentaffin cells that secrete gastrin. Gastric mucosal cells also secrete bicarbonate.

Gastric motility depends on two motor control centers in the stomach and also on external control from the autonomic nervous system. Emptying of solids depends on caloric density and pyloric resistance. The presence of fats and proteins will delay gastric emptying.

The normal bacterial flora of the stomach consists of spirilla (*Helicobacter* spp. and *Gastrospirillum hominus*). In addition, cats may have a nonpathogenic *Chlamydia* living in the mucosal lining of their stomachs.

Disruption of the gastric mucosal barrier (the mucosal lining, mucous coating, and bicarbonate layer) or motility disorders can result in damage to the stomach. The most commonly seen disorders include gastritis, both acute and chronic; ulceration; foreign body obstruction; gastric dilatation or volvulus; hypermotility; and neoplasia.

Acute Gastritis

One common cause of vomiting in dogs and cats is acute gastritis. Causes of acute gastritis include diet (spoiled food, change in diet, food allergy, or food intolerance), infection (bacterial, viral, or parasitic), and toxins (chemicals, plants, drugs, or organ failure). Ingestion of foreign objects may also result in gastritis. Whatever the cause, once the mucosa is damaged, inflammation occurs, and clinical symptoms develop.

CLINICAL SIGNS

- Anorexia
- Acute onset of vomiting
- Presence or absence of dehydration
- Presence or absence of painful abdomen
- History of dietary change, toxin ingestion, or infection
- History of internal parasites

DIAGNOSIS

- Based on history and the physical examination
- CBC may indicate a stress leukogram and dehydration
- Serum chemistries to rule out metabolic imbalances or organ failure
- Radiography may reveal changes in the stomach wall

TREATMENT

- Nothing by mouth for 24 to 36 hours
- Fluid therapy may be given subcutaneously (SQ) or intravenously (IV), depending on the severity of the dehydration (66 mL/kg/day plus additional fluids to offset loss from vomiting)
- After 36 hours, start feeding with a low-fat diet such as Hill's i/d canned food, low-fat cottage cheese (1 part) and boiled rice (2 parts), or well-drained boiled meat (1 part) and boiled rice (3 parts)
- Antiemetics:
  - Chlorpromazine: dog, intramuscularly (IM) every 8 hours; cat, IM every 8 hours
  - Metoclopramide: every 6 hours orally (PO), IM, SQ
- Antibiotics are seldom necessary but are frequently prescribed because vomiting can upset the normal flora of the GI tract

INFORMATION FOR CLIENTS

- Avoid abrupt changes in diet for your pet. Mix the new diet with the old, and slowly increase the amount of the new food in the diet for the first week. After the first week, you may feed only the new food.
- If your pet vomits two to three times, do not provide food and water for 24 hours. If the vomiting continues, call your veterinarian.
- Dogs and cats do not need a varied diet. They can be satisfied with the same food every day. Avoid feeding table scraps and human food because these can cause gastritis.
- Avoid giving pets objects that can be swallowed or chewed into small, abrasive pieces.

Immune-Mediated Inflammatory Bowel Disease (Chronic Gastritis, Enteritis, Colitis)

Immune-mediated inflammatory bowel disease (IBD) is the result of the accumulation of inflammatory cells within the lining of the small intestine, stomach, or the large bowel and is seen most commonly in cats, although it occurs in dogs as well. The etiology of the disease is unknown, but it is thought that a disruption of the immunologic tolerance to the normal bacterial flora of the small intestine or to dietary substances develops resulting in an inflammatory response with cellular infiltration. The range of symptoms reported with this disease is related to the location and type of infiltrate. Diagnosis is made from intestinal and gastric biopsies. Treatment begins with daily administration of dietary modification and antibacterial and immunosuppressive therapies. If the patient has a good response, as measured by decreased clinical symptoms, then the amount administered may be slowly decreased over 1 to 2 weeks. More severe cases may require azathioprine or cyclophosphamide. Hypoallergenic diets should be prescribed for these animals.

CLINICAL SIGNS

- Chronic vomiting
- Weight loss
- Diarrhea
- Straining to defecate, mucus in stool

DIAGNOSIS

- CBC: may show neutrophilia or eosinophilia
- Serum chemistries are usually normal
- Urinalysis
- Fecal sample for culture if bacterial problem suspected; fecal float
- Feline leukemia virus (FeLV) or feline immunodeficiency virus testing
- Cobalamin and serum folate levels
- All of the above, to rule out other causes of chronic vomiting and diarrhea
- Endoscopic evaluation of the stomach, small intestine, and colon lining together with biopsies of each area provide a definitive diagnosis and confirm the type of infiltrate present

TREATMENT

- Prednisone: every 12 hours for several months, then in tapering doses for maintenance
- Azathioprine: PO daily for 1 week, then every 48 hours
- Cyclophosphamide (reserved for severe cases)
- Sulfasalazine: dog, PO every 8 to 12 hours; cats, every 8 to 12 hours; best for disease involving the colon
- Hypoallergenic diet: a diet free of preservatives or additives, with a highly digestible protein source not commonly used for the species (rabbit, lamb, tofu, chicken, etc.); home-made diets that are rice based work well; commercial diets are now available

INFORMATION FOR CLIENTS

- The diagnosis of IBD requires a complete laboratory workup to rule out other causes of the clinical symptoms.
- A definitive diagnosis requires an intestinal biopsy.
- Therapy will be required for the life of the animal.
- The pet will require a special diet for life. The owner must eliminate all other food sources from the animal's diet. This may mean eliminating flavored vitamins, treats, and table food.
- The immunosuppressive drugs used to treat this disease have side effects in animals. Polyuria, polydipsia, polyphagia, weight gain, and skin and urinary infections may occur. The animal must be closely monitored by the veterinarian, and the lowest possible dose of antiinflammatory drug must be used.
- Nursing care for these animals includes keeping the perianal area clean and soothed (if diarrhea is present).

Gastric Ulceration

Gastric ulceration and erosion is commonly the result of drug therapy in dogs and cats. Nonsteroidal antiinflammatory drugs (NSAIDs) are the most commonly implicated drugs, which produce ulceration in humans as well as in dogs. These drugs, which include aspirin, ibuprofen, flunixin meglumine, and phenylbutazone, disrupt the normal gastric mucosal barrier, resulting in ulceration. Stress, as seen in severely traumatized animals or animals in strenuous training, can also result in gastric erosion. Renal failure, hepatic failure, and hypoadrenocorticism may also result in gastric erosion or ulceration.

CLINICAL SIGNS

- Can vary from absence of symptoms to vomiting of blood
- Anemia
- Edema
- Melena
- Anorexia
- Abdominal pain
- Septicemia, if perforation has occurred

DIAGNOSIS

Radiology

- Contrast studies using multiple positions and barium sulfate (unless a perforation is suspected) may show ulcerations in the mucosa of the stomach

Endoscopy

- Allows direct observation of ulcerated areas; more expedient for assessing the extent of the problem (Fig. 2-5)

TREATMENT

- Fluid therapy, if animal is dehydrated
- Restriction of oral intake of food and fluids
- Oral antacids containing aluminum hydroxide or magnesium hydroxide given four to six times daily may help
- H$_2$ antagonists: cimetidine, PO two to three times daily; ranitidine, twice daily
- Omeprazole: PO once daily
- Sucralfate (Carafate): PO two to four times daily; sucralfate binds to the ulcer site, protecting it from damage; it can also bind other drugs and should not be given at the same time as other medications
- Misoprostol: PO two to three times daily; this drug protects against gastric mucosal damage and decreases acid secretion

INFORMATION FOR CLIENTS

- Do not use NSAIDs in animals without veterinary supervision.
- *Never* administer ibuprofen, naproxen, or aspirin to a dog or cat without a prescription.

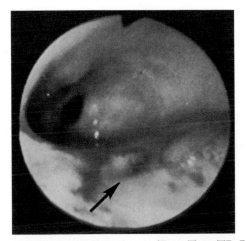

Figure 2-5 Gastric ulcers in the cat. (From Tams TR, Rawlings, CA: *Small animal endoscopy*, ed 3, St. Louis, MO, 2011, Mosby.)

- If your veterinarian prescribes these medications for your pet, ask if you may give the medication with a meal or antacids to prevent gastric irritation.

Gastric Dilation with Volvulus

Gastric dilation with volvulus (GDV) is primarily a disease of 2- to 10-year-old large and giant breed, deep-chested dogs, but it can occasionally occur in small breeds. The exact mechanism for the disease remains unclear, but diet and exercise have been implicated in its development. Delayed gastric emptying, pyloric obstruction, aerophagia, and engorgement may predispose dogs to dilation and volvulus. Recent studies indicate that affected dogs may have gastric dysrhythmias that predispose them to GDV.

The stomach is similar to a bag with openings at each end. As the stomach fills with air, food, fluid, or both, the outflow tracts can become occluded. Further distension results in simple dilation (an air-filled stomach), or the air-filled stomach may twist along its longitudinal axis (volvulus). The pylorus usually passes under the stomach and comes to rest above the cardia on the left side of the abdomen. The enlarged tympanic stomach pushes against the diaphragm, making breathing difficult and blocking venous return of blood through the hepatic portal vein and the posterior vena cava. The increased luminal pressure within the gastric wall results in ischemia and subsequent necrosis of the wall.

The spleen may also be involved and can become congested. Endotoxins that accumulate in the GI tract activate the inflammatory mediators. The end result is the development of hypovolemic, endotoxic shock in patients with GDV.

CLINICAL SIGNS

- Weakness, collapse
- Depression
- Nausea
- Nonproductive retching
- Hypersalivation
- Abdominal pain and distension (distension may not be evident in very large dogs)
- Increased heart rate and respiratory rates

DIAGNOSIS

- History and physical examination demonstrate a depressed, weak animal with prolonged capillary refill time (CRT) and abnormal mucous membranes.
- Radiographs of right lateral view best define torsion. The stomach will appear air filled (Fig. 2-6). The pylorus will be gas filled and seen dorsal and cranial to the gastric fundus. A compartmentalization is frequently observed between the pylorus and the fundus.
- Electrocardiographic monitoring may indicate a ventricular arrhythmia or sinus tachycardia.
- CBC and serum chemistries are necessary for correction of electrolyte and pH imbalances and for proper fluid therapy.

TREATMENT

- The goal of treatment is to decompress the stomach, stabilize the patient, and prepare the patient for surgical intervention.

Aggressive Treatment of Shock

- 14- to 16-gauge jugular catheter or two cephalic catheters should be placed
- Crystalloid IV fluids at 45.5 ml/kg over a 15-minute period
- Corticosteroids: IV (Solu-Delta, Cortef) or flunixin meglumine (0.5–1 mg/kg IV)
- Bicarbonate: total carbon dioxide (CO_2) is less than 12 milliequivalents (mEq). The dose may be calculated if using the formula: body weight (kg) $\times$ (12 − patient's HCO^{-3}) $\times$ 0.3. Give this amount IV over 30 to 60 minutes.

Alleviate Distention

- In an emergency situation, an 18-gauge needle may be used as a trocar to relieve the pressure in the stomach. Clip and scrub a small area caudal to the costal arch. Insert the needle through the skin and into the stomach to allow gas to escape.

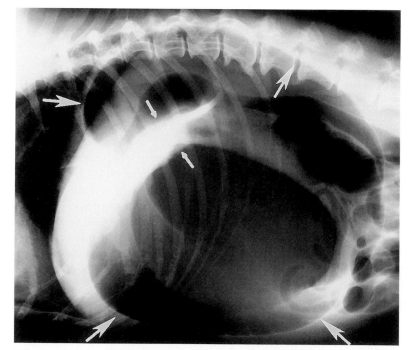

Figure 2-6 Lateral radiograph of a dog with gastric dilation with volvulus. The stomach is dilated (*large arrows*), and there is a "shelf" of tissue (*small arrows*), demonstrating that the stomach is malpositioned. Radiographs obtained from the right lateral position appear superior to those of other views in demonstrating this shelf. If the stomach were similarly distended but not malpositioned, the diagnosis would be gastric dilation. (From Nelson RW, Couto CG: *Small animal internal medicine*, ed 4, St. Louis, MO, 2009, Mosby, by permission.)

- Pass a stomach tube and decompress the stomach. Care must be taken not to perforate the already compromised stomach or the distal esophagus. Place the animal in sternal or lateral recumbency, and use a large-bore tube.
- If surgery must be delayed, placement of a temporary gastrostomy tube can be performed.
- Perform gastric lavage to remove all the remaining food and fluid.

Antibiotics
- Antibiotics targeted against gram-negative and anaerobic microorganisms are given IV (cefoxitin 20 mg/kg IV every 6 hours; or ampicillin 20 mg/kg IV every 6 hours).

Continuous Monitoring of the Electrocardiogram
- Treat ventricular arrhythmias with lidocaine (2 mg/kg IV), if necessary. If the arrhythmia is lidocaine responsive, a constant rate infusion of 30 to 80 microgram per kilogram per minute (mcg/kg/min) can be established. If the arrhythmia is not lidocaine responsive, procainamide can be given IV at a dose of 6 to 10 mg/kg in 2-mg/kg boluses every 5 minutes. If effective, continue constant-rate infusion at 25 to 40 mcg/kg/min.

Potassium
- Potassium supplementation may be required if potassium levels are less than 3 mEq/L.

Surgical Correction
- Surgery should be considered as soon as the patient is stable.

Postoperative Nursing Care
- Continuous ECG monitoring for at least 24 hours.
- Serial observation of hemodynamic parameters; mean arterial pressure >70 mm Hg, systolic pressure >110 mm Hg
- Pain management: oxymorphone 0.05 to 2 mg/kg every 4 hours or to effect
- Monitoring of urine output and fluid input using a closed catheter system
- Monitoring of serum electrolytes and acid-base status every 8 hours

- Continuation of antibiotics
- Gastric atony and ileus may produce vomiting: metoclopramide 2 to 5 mg/kg every 8 hours SQ to control
- Maintaining good body temperature and turning patient frequently to prevent skin and muscle damage
- Providing parenteral nutritional support if vomiting occurs; oral fluids started in small volumes at 12 hours after surgery if no vomiting occurs; low-fat canned food the day after surgery unless resection of the stomach or bowel has been performed

INFORMATION FOR CLIENTS
- Predisposition to GDV may be genetic or familial.
- Avoid feeding large dogs one huge meal per day. Several small meals will prevent gastric overload.
- Limit exercise immediately after eating.
- Feed a high-quality-protein, low-fat diet. Avoid easily fermentable diets.
- The average hospital stay for dogs with GDV is about 3 to 7 days.
- The mortality rate for this disease is between 15% and 18%.
- Surgical correction and tack-down procedures (gastropexy) are not a guarantee against future episodes of GDV.

Gastric Neoplasia

Gastric neoplasia is fairly uncommon in dogs and cats. Malignant tumors are more common than benign lesions, and malignant neoplasias are more frequent in males than in females.

The most common malignant canine gastric tumor is the adenocarcinoma. This type of tumor is most commonly found in older animals, and because the clinical signs are relatively nonspecific (vomiting and weight loss), the tumor may be well advanced before it is diagnosed.

Gastric lymphoma is the most commonly diagnosed feline gastric tumor. Polyps and gastric leiomyomas, both benign tumors, may also be seen in dogs and cats.

CLINICAL SIGNS
- Weight loss
- Vomiting, with or without blood

- Obstruction
- Usually seen in older animals

DIAGNOSIS

- Endoscopy is performed to locate the lesion. A biopsy is required for diagnosis. In some cases, a full-thickness biopsy from a surgical approach may be required for a definitive diagnosis.

TREATMENT

- Surgical removal is the treatment of choice; however, many tumors are too advanced at the time of diagnosis and are inoperable. Cats with a single lesion (e.g., lymphosarcoma) usually respond well to removal of the single mass
- Chemotherapy: long-term response is not good
- Radiation: not successful for treatment of these tumors

INFORMATION FOR CLIENTS

- The prognosis for malignant gastric tumors is guarded to poor. Gastric neoplasia is a fatal disease.
- Supportive care, control of vomiting, and maintenance of a good nutritional status is important for keeping these animals comfortable.

Diseases of the Small Intestine

Disease of the small intestine involves impairment of the absorptive villous surface of the small intestine, which causes diarrhea, malabsorption, and weight loss. Types of intestinal damage may include villous atrophy, disruption of the microvilli, and disruption or defects in villous proteins and disruption of the microflora. Diarrhea, defined as an increase in frequency, fluidity, and volume of defecation, may result any time the flux of fluid or nutrients across the absorptive membrane is altered. It may be classified in several ways: *acute* or *chronic*; *osmotic* (resulting from decreased digestion or absorption that increases the osmotic solute load in the bowel), *secretory* (caused by hypersecretion of ions), *exudative* (resulting from an increased permeability with loss of plasma proteins), or *dysmotile* (resulting from abnormal motility).

Diarrhea may also be classified with respect to the causative agent: parasitic, viral, bacterial, or dietary intolerance or sensitivity.

Acute Diarrhea

Acute diarrhea is one of the most commonly seen types of diarrhea in the small-animal clinic. Frequently, the cause is a change of diet, drug therapy, or any stressful situation that may result in disruption of the normal bacterial flora within the bowel. Acute diarrhea is easily managed with supportive and symptomatic treatment.

CLINICAL SIGNS

- Abrupt onset of diarrhea
- Presence or absence of vomiting
- Other than preceding signs, a normal-appearing animal

DIAGNOSIS

- Rule out other causes of diarrhea
- Fecal sample for direct and flotation examination
- Hematocrit (HCT) to monitor hydration

TREATMENT

Supportive

- Replace fluid and electrolytes (SQ, PO, or IV)
- Nothing by mouth for 24 to 48 hours; water is allowed if the animal is not vomiting
- Intestinal absorbants: Pepto-Bismol 1 mL/5 kg every 8 hours
- Loperamide: every 6 hours
- +/− Antibiotics: choose a broad-spectrum drug

Dietary

- Start on a bland, low-fat diet after 24 to 48 hours.
- Feed Hill's i/d canned food.
- Chicken and rice or beef and rice: Boil the meat and drain well. Mix 1 part meat with 4 parts boiled rice. Feed small amounts for 2 to 3 days until stool returns to normal, then return to regular diet.

Parasitic Diarrhea

Intestinal parasites may be the primary cause of diarrhea in the small animal. The technician should review the life cycles and pathophysiology of the common intestinal parasites. Common parasite eggs and protozoans are shown in Figure 2-7.

CLINICAL SIGNS

- Diarrhea
- Presence or absence of blood

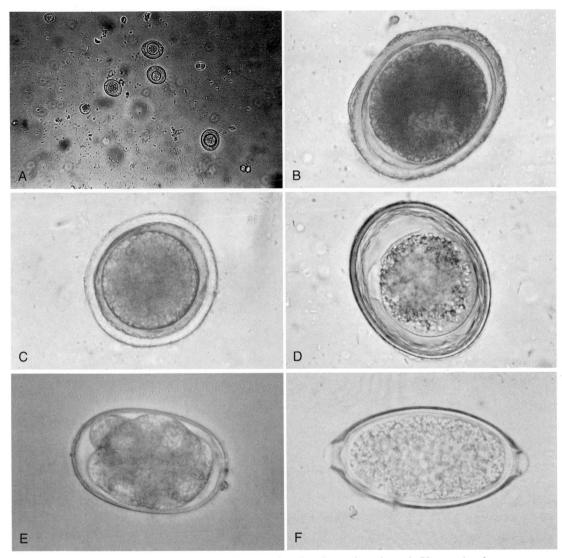

Figure 2-7 Common parasite eggs and oocysts found in dog and cat feces. **A,** Unsporulated oocysts of *Isospora* species. *Isospora canis* (large oocysts) and *Isospora bigemina* (small oocysts) are present. **B,** Egg of *Toxocara canis*. **C,** Characteristic egg of *Toxocara cati* is similar in structure to that of *T. canis* but smaller in diameter. **D,** Eggs of *Toxascaris leonina*. These eggs have a smooth outer shell and hyaline, or "ground glass," central portion. **E,** These eggs of hookworm species may represent one of several genera that parasitize dogs and cats: *Ancylostoma caninum*, *Ancylostoma tubaeforme*, *Ancylostoma braziliense*, and *Uncinaria stenocephala*. **F,** Characteristic egg of *Trichuris vulpis*.

Continued

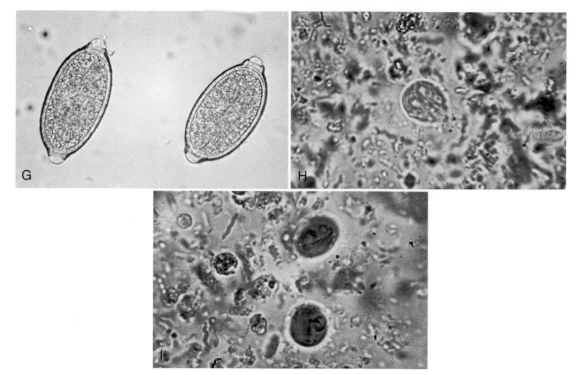

Figure 2-7, cont'd G, Egg of *Eucoleus aerophilus* (*Capillaria aerophila*). **H,** Cysts of *Giardia* species. **I,** Motile trophozoite of *Giardia* species. (From Hendrix CM, Robinson E: *Diagnostic parasitology for veterinary technicians,* ed 4, St. Louis, MO, 2012, Mosby, by permission.)

- Presence or absence of vomiting
- Weight loss
- Poor hair coat
- Listlessness
- Anorexia

DIAGNOSIS

- Fecal sample for direct and flotation examination
- ELISA (enzyme-linked immunosorbant assay) test for *Giardia*

TREATMENT

Anthelmintics for a Specific Parasite
- Fenbendazole: orally for 3 consecutive days
- Pyrantel pamoate: orally, repeat in 10 to 14 days

Antiprotozoal Medication
- *Giardia:* metronidazole, twice daily for 5 to 10 days PO; albendazole, twice daily for 2 days

- *Coccidia:* sulfadimethoxine (Albon), oral loading dose followed by maintenance dose for 9 days

Viral Diarrhea

Viral diarrheas are seen in young animals and in animals not vaccinated against the common offenders such as parvovirus, distemper, coronavirus, or feline panleukopenia virus.

CLINICAL SIGNS

- Diarrhea with or without blood
- Presence or absence of vomiting
- Patient may or may not be febrile
- Anorexia
- Depression

DIAGNOSIS

- Parvovirus: ELISA (CITE or IDEXX)
- Canine distemper titer

- Panleukopenia with a white blood cell (WBC) count <500 WBC/µL

TREATMENT

Supportive
- Intravenous fluids
- Antidiarrheal therapy
- Antibiotics having gram-negative spectrum

Prevention
- Vaccination

Nursing Care

● TECH ALERT

These animals are immunosuppressed.
- Avoid giving fluids subcutaneously because infections and skin necrosis can develop.
- Keep the animal clean and dry. Avoid letting fecal matter collect on the coat or the perianal skin.
- Keep the animal warm. If using a heating pad, take care to turn the animal frequently to prevent thermal injury to the skin. Never leave an animal on a heating pad without supervision.
- Wear protective clothing and shoe covers when handling these animals. These animals and all materials that they come in contact with may be infectious to other patients in the clinic.
- Have an isolation area in the clinic specifically for these patients. Keep all necessary materials for treatment and maintenance of these patients in the isolation area. Never bring the patient into the main clinic area. All disposable materials from the contaminated area should be disposed of directly into the outdoor trash receptacle.

INFORMATION FOR CLIENTS
- The sick animal may infect other dogs or cats in the household.
- Coronavirus diarrhea is usually not fatal.
- The prognosis with parvovirus depends on the severity of the disease (estimated by the decrease in the WBC count).
- The mortality for canine distemper is about 50%, and the prognosis for feline panleukopenia (feline distemper) is guarded to poor.
- These viruses can be spread by contact with feces. Avoid areas where high concentrations of

unvaccinated animals may congregate (parks, boarding kennels, beaches, dog shows). Make sure that your pet is properly vaccinated, and make sure that your kennel, animal hospital, dog show, and other relevant places require current vaccination records on all animals.

Bacterial Diarrhea

Pathogenic bacteria produce intestinal disease by invading and damaging the intestinal epithelium by releasing enterotoxins that stimulate secretions, attaching to the mucosal surface, producing cytotoxins, or both. Bacteria such as *Salmonella*, *Shigella*, *Campylobacter*, and some strains of *Escherichia coli* invade the mucosa, whereas *Clostridium* produces cytotoxins. *Staphylococcus* induces hypersecretion and also invades the mucosal lining.

CLINICAL SIGNS
- Diarrhea with or without blood
- Patient may or may not have fever
- Anorexia

DIAGNOSIS
- Rule out parasites with a fecal examination.
- The presence of gram-negative, slender, curved rods in stained fecal smears or S-shaped motile organisms with darting or spiral movement in fresh saline smears can indicate *Campylobacter*.
- Perform fecal cytotoxin assay for *Clostridium* with a titer >1:20.
- *E. coli*: No reliable way to serotype this organism in animals is available.

TREATMENT
- Oral antibiotics (if disease is severe)
- Enrofloxacin: twice a day
- Trimethoprim or sulfa: twice a day
- Erythromycin: three times a day
- Metronidazole: twice a day
- Fluid and electrolyte replacement (IV or SQ)

Dietary Intolerance or Sensitivity Diarrhea

Dietary-induced intestinal disease is common in small animals. The cause may be immune mediated (dietary sensitivity) or nonimmunologic (dietary intolerance). Identification of a specific cause is often difficult. Dietary sensitivity can be diagnosed after a complete clinical and dietary history, and a thorough laboratory examination is performed to rule out other causes of vomiting, diarrhea, abdominal discomfort, and weight loss. Endoscopic biopsies should be used to assess the damage to the intestinal mucosa.

Dietary intolerance is seen in animals that are unable to handle certain substances in their diet such as carbohydrates, fats, or milk products. This condition is most often seen in animals that are fed large amounts of table food or who raid the garbage for scraps. Some animals are intolerant of processed animal foods that contain milk products or large amounts of fats.

Symptoms of dietary indiscretion are also seen in pets that ingest foreign materials such as paper, tin foil, rubber bands, and other household substances.

CLINICAL SIGNS

- Diarrhea
- Vomiting
- Abdominal pain or discomfort
- Weight loss

DIAGNOSIS

- History of sensitivity to specific foods
- History of a recent diet change
- Physical examination and laboratory work to rule out all other causes of symptoms
- CBC and serum chemistries
- Fecal examination
- Radiography to rule out partial bowel obstructions
- Fecal culture and sensitivity
- Trypsin-like immunoreactivity test

TREATMENT

- Dietary trial: feeding of an exclusion diet for a minimum of 6 weeks; this diet should contain a protein source not usually eaten by the animal (e.g., chicken, rabbit); the diet should contain no milk products and no preservatives (Table 2-1)
- Oral prednisone twice a day for 2 to 4 weeks, followed by a dose reduction at 2-week intervals

INFORMATION FOR CLIENTS

- Prevent pets from gaining access to garbage and any foreign objects that can result in irritation to the bowel.
- Commercial diets that contain novel protein sources are readily available. These must be fed for adequate periods to see clinical response (2 to 3 months).
- Treats and some medications contain additives to which the pet may be sensitive. Avoid using these items while your pet is on a restricted protein source diet.
- Longhaired pets should have the hair shaved around the rectum to prevent loose stool from accumulating on the hair.
- It may take significant trial and error attempts to determine the cause of this problem. Be patient with your veterinarian.

Chronic Enteropathies

Chronic IBD in the dog and cat is commonly seen in small-animal practice. Lymphocytic-plasmocytic enteritis, seen in both dogs and cats, represents the most common form of this disease. Chronic antigenic stimulation within the intestinal lumen (from a variety of causes) results in excessive infiltration of the lamina propria with lymphocytes and plasma cells. Infiltration results in damage to the mucosa and abnormal intestinal absorption. Management and treatment are aimed at eliminating the antigen and decreasing the immune response.

CLINICAL SIGNS

- Usually nonspecific
- Chronic, intermittent vomiting with or without diarrhea
- Listlessness
- Weight loss
- Older animals
- Polyuria (Pu) or polydipsia (Pd)
- Borborygmus
- Halitosis

TABLE 2-1   Home-Prepared Diets for Intestinal Disease (Approximately 10-kg Dog)

Highly Digestible, Low-Fat Exclusion Diets (Single-Source Protein)
Supplies 675–700 kcal (20%–34% of calories from protein, 46%–48% from CHO, and 19%–22% from fat)

Lamb	Venison	Rabbit
6 oz lean lamb	6 oz venison	6 oz rabbit
No corn oil	2 teaspoons corn oil	1 teaspoon corn oil
10 oz boiled white rice	10 oz boiled white rice	10 oz boiled white rice
1 teaspoon dicalcium phosphate	1 teaspoon dicalcium phosphate	1 teaspoon dicalcium phosphate
1 teaspoon lite salt	1 teaspoon lite salt	1 teaspoon lite salt
½ capsule Centrum Adult multivitamins	½ capsule Centrum Adult multivitamins	½ capsule Centrum Adult multivitamins

Highly Digestible Moderate- and High-Fat Diets
Supplies 680 kcal (chicken: 33% of calories from protein, 37% of calories from carbohydrates (CHO), and 30% from fat; beef: 33% of calories from protein, 24% from CHO, and 43% from fat)

Chicken (Moderate-Fat)	Beef (High-Fat)
6 oz chicken	6 oz hamburger (lean)
8 oz boiled white rice	6 oz boiled white rice
2 teaspoons corn oil	No corn oil
1 teaspoon dicalcium phosphate	1 teaspoon dicalcium phosphate
1 teaspoon lite salt	1 teaspoon lite salt
½ capsule Centrum adult multivitamins	½ capsule Centrum adult multivitamins

Ingredients for each diet should be well mixed and cooked in a microwave oven or casserole before being served.

- Flatus
- Symptoms are progressive, becoming more frequent over time

TECH ALERT

Vomiting hairballs is an important clinical sign of disease in cats.

DIAGNOSIS

Physical Examination
- Physical examination is usually unremarkable.
- Edema or ascites may be seen if serum protein levels are low.

Laboratory Tests
- CBC and serum profile: panhypoproteinemia, neutrophilia, hypocalcemia (cats may have normal serum protein)
- Fecal examination to rule out intestinal parasites
- Biopsy to identify lymphocytic-plasmacytic infiltrates within the lamina propria (customarily reported as mild, moderate, or severe)

TREATMENT

Medical
- Oral prednisolone: every 12 hours for a month followed by 50% reduction every 2 weeks
- Azathioprine: daily in dogs and a lower dose daily in cats for 3 to 9 months; monitor WBC counts every 2 to 4 weeks while the animal is taking medication
- Metronidazole: twice a day for 2 to 4 weeks, then once daily
- Intestinal protectants: sucralfate three times a day; cimetidine three times a day to decrease erosive disease and protect against excessive protein loss in dogs
- Vitamin therapy to replace fat-soluble vitamins A, D, K, and B

Dietary

- Limit carbohydrates, and avoid lactose. (Rice is a good source of carbohydrates, especially for dogs.)
- Restrict dietary fats.
- Feed a good-quality protein (animal derived).
- Dietary therapy alone is seldom successful in the cat, although commercial hypoallergenic diets may be tried.

INFORMATION FOR CLIENTS

- Treatment for this disease may be prolonged and expensive.
- A cure is not usually obtained.
- Pets receiving antiinflammatory therapy will need to be monitored on a routine basis (WBC counts) to prevent the occurrence of bone marrow suppression.

Intestinal Lymphangiectasia

Intestinal lymphangiectasia is a chronic protein-losing intestinal disease of dogs that is characterized by impaired intestinal lymphatic drainage resulting from obstruction of normal lymphatic flow. The backup of lymph releases fluid into the intestinal lumen, causing a loss of lipids, plasma protein, and lymphocytes.

CLINICAL SIGNS

- Edema and effusion
- Ascites or hydrothorax
- Presence or absence of light-colored diarrhea
- Weight loss, progressive emaciation
- Progressive symptoms

DIAGNOSIS

- CBC and serum chemistry profile showing lymphopenia, hypocholesterolemia, hypoglobulinemia, decreased serum albumin and globulin levels, and hypocalcemia
- Biopsy showing chyle-filled lacteals and intestinal lymphatics with ballooning distortion of villi and mucosal edema

TREATMENT

- The aim of treatment is to decrease the loss of intestinal protein.

Medical

- Prednisolone: twice a day; adjust after remission is achieved
- Metronidazole: twice a day

Dietary

- Choose a food with minimal fat and good-quality protein source.
- Divide food into two or three feedings.
- Supplement diet with fat-soluble vitamins.

Surgical

- Surgery may be necessary to relieve any obvious obstructions to lymph flow.

INFORMATION FOR CLIENTS

- This disease is usually progressive, and although remissions can be achieved, most dogs will experience a relapse and finally succumb to protein depletion, diarrhea, or severe effusions.
- Treatment may be prolonged and will require dietary management to achieve remission.
- No cure currently exists for most animals.

Intestinal Neoplasia

Intestinal adenocarcinomas account for about 25% of all intestinal neoplasms in dogs and 52% in cats. Lymphosarcomas, the next most common neoplasm, account for 10% of the GI neoplasms in dogs and 21% in cats. Mast cell tumors occur in the cat as well. Clinical signs are usually progressive and are related to the location and growth rate of the tumor. Widespread metastasis may occur. Adenocarcinomas typically occur in the older animal, whereas lymphosarcomas may be found in animals of any age, although middle-aged to older animals are most commonly affected.

CLINICAL SIGNS

- Weight loss
- Signs of partial GI obstruction
- Presence or absence of melena
- Signs of malabsorption, maldigestion with or without vomiting and diarrhea
- Abdominal discomfort
- Anorexia

DIAGNOSIS

Physical Examination

- Abdominal mass may be palpable in the intestines, or the intestinal wall may feel thickened. Mesenteric lymph nodes may be enlarged.

Radiography

- Contrast studies may show mucosal irregularity, thickened wall, or abnormal luminal diameter ("apple core" sign).

Biopsy

- Endoscopic biopsy is possible for lesions in the upper GI region, but surgical biopsy is usually required for most animals.

Laboratory Tests: Complete Blood Cell Count and Serum Profile

- Anemia
- Hypoproteinemia
- Leukocytosis with a left shift
- Serum tests may show the involvement of other organ systems

TREATMENT

- Surgical removal of the tumor, if possible
- Dogs respond poorly to chemotherapy; cats may do well receiving the COP (cytoxan, oncovin, prednisolone) protocol
- Supportive care should include effective nutritional management and transfusions, if needed
- Antibiotics to control bacterial overgrowth during chemotherapy
- For mast cell tumors: prednisone, cimetidine, antibiotics

INFORMATION FOR CLIENTS

- The prognosis for adenocarcinoma is poor, with mean survival times (with treatment) of 7 months to 2 years.
- Cats with lymphosarcoma respond well to chemotherapy with remissions lasting up to 2 years.
- For animals with cancer, supportive care is important. Nutritional support is critical. High-quality, easily digestible diets are required to maintain cellular repair.

Diseases of the Large Bowel

The large bowel may be divided into the cecum, the colon, and the rectum. The cecum is a small, sigmoid-shaped diverticulum located near the ileocolic junction. The colon can be divided into the short, ascending portion (the right side of the abdomen); the transverse portion (cranial abdomen); and the long, descending portion (the left side of the abdomen). Histologically, the wall is similar to that of the small intestine but with no villi. Crypts of Lieberkühn contain epithelial, mucous, and endocrine cells. Large numbers of goblet cells in the colon produce mucus when stimulated.

The main function of the colon in the dog and the cat is water and electrolyte resorption. The colon also serves to store feces while microorganisms ferment undigested material and produce vitamins K and B.

The most common signs of large-bowel disease are diarrhea, straining to defecate, and blood in the stool. Diagnosis is by colonoscopy and histopathologic evaluation of mucosal samples.

Inflammatory Bowel Disease

A diagnosis of IBD is often made when an excessive number of inflammatory cells are found in mucosal samples from the GI systems of dogs and cats. The cause is unknown but is probably multifactorial. Colonic inflammation disrupts mucosal integrity and results in decreased absorption of sodium and water. Inflammation also increases motility, resulting in more frequent defecation.

CLINICAL SIGNS

- Diarrhea, with little weight loss
- Increased frequency of defecation and decreased fecal volume
- Tenesmus
- Hematochezia
- Increased mucus
- Mild fever

DIAGNOSIS

Laboratory Tests

- CBC or serum chemistry profile, to rule out other causes of diarrhea; usually no consistent pattern of abnormalities are seen with IBD

- Complete fecal examination to rule out parasites

Radiographs
- May show gas-filled loops of intestine

Histopathology
- Increased numbers of lymphocytes and plasma cells in the lamina propria of the large bowel

TREATMENT

Medical
- Sulfasalazine:
  - Dogs: 20 to 50 mg/kg to maximum of 1 g every 8 hours; decrease dose after fourth week of no diarrhea; decrease the dose 50% after 4 additional weeks free of diarrhea; side effects include vomiting, so the drug must be given with food; keratoconjunctivitis sicca (KCS) may develop over a period of 6 to 8 months of treatment
  - Cats: must be used with caution because of sensitivity to salicylates: 10 to 20 mg/kg every 12 hours
- Prednisone: every 24 hours (dogs); lower dose every 24 hours (cats)
- Mesalamine: every 8 hours (dogs); similar dose in cats (may also cause KCS)
- Metronidazole: every 8 hours
- In cases refractory to treatment: azathioprine every 24 hours (dogs); much lower dose every 48 hours (cats)
- Tylosin: every 12 hours

Dietary
- Hypoallergenic diets low in fat are recommended.
- Hill's Science Diet–Maximum Stress
- Prescription diet (dermatology diet [d/d], canine diet [c/d], reducing diet [r/d])
- Home diets low in fat and high in fiber

INFORMATION FOR CLIENTS
- Treatment for this condition may be prolonged.
- The goal of treatment is control of symptoms.
- Animals with IBD may have to be taken outside many times daily to defecate.

Intussusception

The cause of intussusception is usually idiopathic but can be the result of parasitic infestation, foreign bodies, infections, and neoplasia. Intussusception occurs when the smaller, proximal segment of the intestine at the ileocolic junction invaginates into the larger, more distal segment of the large bowel. This "telescoping" produces a partial to complete blockage and compromises the blood supply to the segments, causing bowel necrosis.

CLINICAL SIGNS
- Vomiting
- Anorexia
- Depression
- Diarrhea with or without blood in dogs

DIAGNOSIS
- Palpation of a sausage-like mass in the cranial abdomen
- Ultrasonography shows multilayered concentric rings representing bowel wall layers

TREATMENT
- Surgical reduction or resection of necrotic bowel
- Restore fluid and electrolyte balance, if necessary
- Broad-spectrum antibiotics after surgery
- Restrict solid food for 24 hours after surgery, then resume a bland diet for 10 to 24 days to allow healing of the intestinal wall

INFORMATION FOR CLIENTS
- Recurrence of intussusception is infrequent.
- The prognosis depends on the amount of bowel involved and the extent of damage to that bowel.
- Puppies should be treated for parasites on a proper schedule to prevent bowel irritation and intussusception. Ask your veterinarian for preventive treatment recommendations.

Megacolon

Although the literature reports megacolon to be an uncommon condition, it is seen frequently in cats. Of the many reasons suggested for feline obstipation, approximately 62% are attributed to idiopathic megacolon. The typical affected cat is middle-aged to older and obese; the presenting symptom is straining to defecate. Some cats are able to pass a liquid stool that contains blood, mucus, or both. These cats are usually dehydrated and may be vomiting. Palpation demonstrates a markedly distended colon packed with firm feces. Radiography confirms the diagnosis. Medical and dietary management are usually unrewarding in the long term, and surgery should be considered in cases with repeat episodes. The cause of this disorder has been thought to involve a defect in the neurostimulation mechanism that promotes colon evacuation. Other causes such as hypokalemia, hypothyroidism, pelvic deformities, or prolonged, severe colonic distension for any reason can disrupt normal motility and result in megacolon (Fig. 2-8).

CLINICAL SIGNS

- Straining to defecate (must be distinguished from straining to urinate in the male cat)
- Vomiting
- Weakness
- Dehydration
- Anorexia
- Small, hard feces or liquid feces with or without blood and mucus

DIAGNOSIS

- Physical examination: distended colon is filled with firm, packed feces
- Radiography: shows colon width greater than the length of the lumbar vertebra
- CBC or serum chemistries: show dehydration, increased HCT; may also show dysfunction of other organ systems.

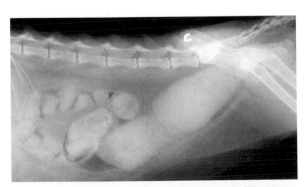

Figure 2-8 Megacolon in the cat. (From Little SE: *The cat: Clinical medicine and management*, ed 2, St. Louis, MO, 2012, Mosby, by permission.)

TREATMENT

Medical

- Stool softeners may be effective only if constipation is mild.
  - Dulcolax: one to two pediatric suppositories or 5 mg every 24 hours PO
  - Docusate (Colace): one to two pediatric suppositories or 50 mg every 24 hours PO
- Lactulose (Cephulac): every 8 to 12 hours
- Enemas: 5 to 10 mL/kg warm water mixed with 5 to 10 mL dioctyl sodium succinate (DSS) and gentle digital removal of feces, if necessary
- Cisapride (Propulsid): every 8 to 12 hours PO

⬤ TECH ALERT

Propulsid has been removed from the market because of serious medical complications in humans. Cats respond well to the medication and experience few negative side effects. It can be obtained from compounding pharmacies.
- Correct dehydration and electrolyte imbalances.
- Provide antibiotics to protect against sepsis through the damaged colonic wall.
- Treat any underlying disease.

Dietary

- Increase fiber in the diet.
- Add raw, canned pumpkin to diet.
- Use high-fiber diet (prescription r/d or w/d).
- Provide soft food (canned).
- Increase water intake by salting food.

Surgical

- Subtotal colectomy, if disease is refractory to medical management

Hospital Care

- Anesthesia is required for severely constipated cats. These cats should be rehydrated and have electrolyte imbalances corrected before administering anesthesia to avoid problems.
- Manual removal of the feces from the colon must be performed with care. Use a well-lubricated, gloved finger, and take care not to scrape or use excessive pressure against the already compromised colon wall.

- Radiography should be performed after feces removal to ensure the colon is empty.
- Postevacuation: Use a soothing ointment or cream around the rectum, and make sure the patient is wiped clean and dried. Keep the patient warm.
- Animals will pass excess enema fluid after the procedure. Make sure the perineal area is kept clean while the animals are in the hospital.

INFORMATION FOR CLIENTS

- Without surgery, this problem will recur in most cats.
- Medical treatment of the cat will be lifelong.
- After surgical correction, cats respond well and often pass fairly normal feces within several months.

Constipation (Canine)

Many times owners will call the veterinarian asking what they can give their constipated animals. Because true constipation is uncommon in dogs and cats, the technician (and the veterinarian) should be wary of prescribing laxatives without examining the animal.

The presence of foreign objects, tumors, pelvic injury, anal sac abscesses, urinary obstruction, dehydration, and a number of other factors can result in the failure to pass feces. Giving laxatives in the presence of mechanical obstruction or metabolic dysfunction may only complicate the situation. The owner should be advised to have the animal examined before medicating.

CLINICAL SIGNS

- Straining to defecate
- Anorexia
- Passing small amounts of hard, dry stool
- Presence or absence of vomiting

DIAGNOSIS

- Palpation of a distended colon with an otherwise normal physical examination
- Radiography confirms that the colon is full of feces with no physical obstruction
- Serum chemistries and CBC should be done to rule out other organ disease and to monitor hydration
- Rectal palpation confirms adequate pelvic canal opening

TREATMENT

- Enema with warm water and DSS
- Oral laxatives: Dulcolax, Colace
- Restore fluid and electrolyte balance, as necessary
- Manual removal of feces under anesthesia, if required

INFORMATION FOR CLIENTS

- Prevent access to small foreign objects that may obstruct the bowel if swallowed (bones, small toys, rocks, etc.).
- Make sure pets always have access to water.
- Do not treat "constipated" animals without a complete physical examination by a veterinarian.
- High-fiber diets may help pets prone to constipation.

Liver Disease

The liver plays a major role in a number of biologic processes within the animal body. It has been estimated that the liver performs at least 1500 functions essential for survival. Because the liver has a large functional reserve and significant regenerative capabilities, liver injury must be severe before laboratory tests show the presence of disease.

Signs of liver disease are usually vague in the early stages. These signs include anorexia, vomiting, diarrhea or constipation, weight loss, polyuria, polydipsia, and pyrexia. Cats often display hypersalivation. Some animals may experience development of bleeding tendencies because of vitamin K malabsorption. (Vitamin K requires bile acids for absorption.) Jaundice may develop as the disease progresses.

Liver diseases can be categorized as follows: drug- or toxin-induced liver disease, infectious liver disease, feline hepatic lipidosis, neoplastic liver disease, and congenital portosystemic shunts.

Drug- or Toxin-Induced Liver Disease (Acute)

Acute liver failure occurs when at least 70% to 80% of functional liver mass is injured. The liver is most susceptible to damage from ingested toxins because it receives 100% of the portal venous blood from the stomach and the intestine. Toxins may be specific for hepatocytes or may simply be toxic to all cells, but they reach the hepatocytes first. Some are made more toxic after they are metabolized inside the hepatocytes.

The species and sex of the animal, dose of toxin, route of administration, and duration of exposure are all factors that affect the extent of liver damage. Although toxicosis is not a frequent occurrence in dogs and cats, drugs that are most commonly implicated are acetaminophen, phenobarbital, thiacetarsamide sodium (Caparsolate), antifungals, diethylcarbamazine, anabolic steroids, and halothane or methoxyflurane (Metofane). Acute onset of hepatic disease usually results from an overdose of these medications, whereas chronic damage may occur with long-term use at clinical doses.

CLINICAL SIGNS

- Acute onset of symptoms
- Anorexia
- Vomiting
- Diarrhea or constipation
- Pu or Pd
- Presence or absence of jaundice
- Melena, hematuria, or both
- Signs of central nervous system involvement: depression, ataxia, dementia, blindness, seizures, and coma

DIAGNOSIS

- History of recent drug administration
- Palpation of painful liver, which may be increased in size
- Serum chemistries:
  - Markedly increased alanine aminotransferase (ALT)
  - Increased alkaline phosphatase (ALP)
  - Increased total bilirubin
  - Increased fasting and postprandial serum bile acids
  - Hypoglycemia
  - Hyperammonemia
  - Coagulopathy
- Radiography
- Ultrasonography shows decreased echogenicity of the liver that is usually diffuse
- Liver biopsy: unless coagulopathy is suspected

TREATMENT

Antidotes

- Available only for acetaminophen
- Induce vomiting
- Activated charcoal should be given
- *N*-acetylcysteine 20% IV

Supportive Therapy

- Aggressive replacement of fluids and electrolytes (IV) with B-complex vitamins added (1 mL/L)
- Glucose may be added if needed (2.5% to 5%)
- Vitamin K therapy
- Cimetidine SQ, IV; or ranitidine SQ, IV
- Antibiotics: amikacin every 8 hours and ampicillin every 8 hours or enrofloxacin intramuscularly (IM) every 12 hours and ampicillin

Nutritional Support

- Dogs: Hill's Prescription Canine k/d or u/d
- Cats: Hill's Prescription Feline k/d

Drug- or Toxin-Induced Liver Disease (Chronic)

Long-term use of drugs such as anticonvulsants (phenytoin, phenobarbital, primidone), glucocorticoids, diethylcarbamazine, methimazole, antifungals, and NSAID-like drugs such as carprofen and phenylbutazone can result in chronic liver damage.

CLINICAL SIGNS

- Weight loss
- Anorexia
- Weakness
- Ascites
- Jaundice
- Pu or Pd

DIAGNOSIS

- History of long-term use of a hepatotoxic drug
- Serum chemistries:
  - Increased ALP (2–12 times normal)
  - Increased ALT (2–5 times normal)
  - ALT increase greater than ALP increase
  - Increased serum bile acids
  - Hypoalbuminemia
  - Hypocholesterolemia

- Liver biopsy: hepatocellular hypertrophy, cirrhosis (anticonvulsants), and vacuolated hepatocytes (steroids) may suggest hepatotoxic disease

TREATMENT

- *Stop* the medication!
- Begin a low-protein diet.
- Force-feeding or gastric feeding tube may be required if the animal is not eating.
- Maintain adequate hydration.
- If neurologic signs are present, administer lactulose: dogs, 2.5 to 15 mL PO every 8 hours; cats, 2.5 to 5 mL PO every 8 hours.
- Administer antibiotics as in acute hepatotoxicity.

Nursing Care

If using an indwelling feeding tube, make sure to flush with clear water after each feeding. If the tube becomes clogged, a small amount of carbonated beverage can be placed into the tube for flushing out the obstruction. Keep the tube and point of entry through the skin clean. Dogs and cats require 50 to 100 mL of water daily. Animals must receive adequate calories known as the *resting energy requirement (RER)*. This may be calculated using the following formula:

$$RER = (30 \times BW_{kg}) + 70$$

where *BW* is the animal's body weight in kilograms.

Animals that are ill or under stress will require more energy than do healthy animals. Therefore, you must multiply the calculated RER by a factor of 1.2 to 1.5 (the value depends on the amount of stress to the animal) to compensate for this increased energy requirement. The equation then becomes:

$$1.5 \times RER$$

or

$$1.5 \times ([30 \times BW_{kg}] + 70)$$

Hill's Prescription Diet a/d or Eukanuba Veterinary Diet Recovery Formula (canned) can be used to prepare a gruel or for liquid feeding.

Infectious Canine Hepatitis

Infectious canine hepatitis (ICH) is caused by canine adenovirus 1 and has long been recognized as a cause of hepatic necrosis in dogs. Owing to effective vaccination programs, the disease is uncommon today. However, unvaccinated dogs and feral animals are still susceptible to the virus. Infection occurs via the oronasal route. Viral replication occurs in the tonsils and regional lymph nodes. Viruses released into the body localize in the liver.

CLINICAL SIGNS

- Petechial hemorrhages
- Lethargy
- Fever >103°F
- Depression
- Pale mucous membranes
- Abdominal pain
- Anorexia
- Corneal opacities ("blue eye")
- Bloody diarrhea
- Hepatomegaly

DIAGNOSIS

- CBC: neutropenia, lymphopenia with WBC count <2500 in severe cases; thrombocytopenia
- Serum chemistry: increased ALT
- Serum titers for ICH: elevated and increasing

Treatment

- Intravenous fluids
- Force feeding, if necessary
- Blood transfusion, if necessary

INFORMATION FOR CLIENTS

- Vaccination is the best prevention for ICH. Make sure your pet is vaccinated properly.
- ICH is a viral infection, and it will not respond to antibiotic therapy. Supportive therapy is the only means of treatment that will help the animal.

Leptospirosis

Leptospirosis is caused by infection with antigenically distinct serovars of *Leptospira interrogans*. Domestic and wild animals serve as reservoirs of infection for humans and other animals. Recently, the number of cases of leptospirosis has increased. Serotypes previously not associated with clinical disease are now being isolated from infected dogs. Serovars *canicola* and *icterohemorrhagica* have classically been the cause of canine renal and liver disease. Currently, serovars *pomona*, *grippotyphosa*, and *bratislavia* are also being isolated from dogs with symptoms of leptospirosis. Typically, dogs are incidental hosts for these serovars, with skunks, raccoons, opossums, and pigs being the natural hosts.

Clinical symptoms of leptospirosis include acute renal failure with or without hepatic involvement (Fig. 2-9). Leptospirosis should be considered in any dog that exhibits these symptoms.

Animals with leptospirosis may pose a health hazard for humans and other animals. Infected animals should be isolated, and anyone handling them should wear protective clothing and practice strict hygiene. Laboratory technicians should take care when handling body fluids.

CLINICAL SIGNS

- Acute renal failure
- Dehydration
- Vomiting
- Fever
- Increased thirst
- Reluctance to move
- Jaundice
- Peracute shock and death

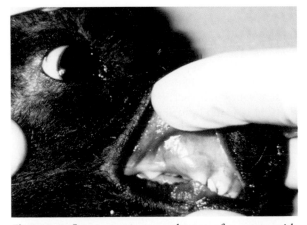

Figure 2-9 Icteric mucous membranes of a puppy with leptospirosis. (Courtesy University of Georgia, Athens, GA. IN. Greene C: *Infectious diseases of the dog and cat,* ed 3, St Louis, 2006, Elsevier)

DIAGNOSIS
Serology

- Microscopic agglutination test: A fourfold increase in titer over 4 weeks is a positive diagnosis.
- Fluorescent antibody test will not identify serovar.
- Polymerase chain reaction (PCR) allows identification of serovar but is not readily available.

Complete Blood Cell Count

- Leukocytosis, thrombocytopenia

Serum Chemistry

- Increased blood urea nitrogen (BUN), creatinine
- Increased ALT
- Bilirubinuria

TREATMENT
Supportive Treatment

- Intravenous fluids
- Furosemide, if oliguric

Antibiotics

- Penicillin: every 24 hours IV or IM for 14 days followed by doxycycline
- Doxycycline: PO twice a day for 14 days to eliminate the carrier state

INFORMATION FOR CLIENTS

- Animals with leptospirosis are contagious to humans and other animals.
- Supportive care is important.
- Treatment and diagnosis are expensive.
- Vaccinations do not protect your dog from other serovars which it may come in contact with.

Cholangiohepatitis

Cholangiohepatitis is a common hepatobiliary disorder of cats, but it is less common in dogs. This condition is a complex of disorders that involve cholangitis, cholangiohepatitis, and biliary cirrhosis.

Bile duct inflammation leads to hepatocyte involvement, which progresses to cirrhosis. The exact cause is unknown, although ascending biliary infections from the GI tract and immune-mediated mechanisms have been suggested. Persian cats appear to have a predisposition for this disorder.

A chronic pancreatitis is commonly seen in cats with cholangiohepatitis.

CLINICAL SIGNS

- Anorexia
- Depression
- Weight loss
- Vomiting
- Dehydration
- Fever
- Jaundice
- Ascites as the disease progresses
- Hepatomegaly

DIAGNOSIS

Complete Blood Cell Count
- Neutrophilia with a left shift
- Mild, regenerative anemia

Serum Chemistry
- Mild-to-moderate increase in ALT
- Normal to increased ALP (increased ALP is strongly related to cholestasis in cats)
- Mild-to-moderate increase in gamma-glutamyl transferase (GGT) (also related to cholestasis)
- Normal to increased fasting serum bile acids
- Hypoalbuminemia in later stages
- Decreased BUN in later stages

Radiology
- Hepatomegaly, choleliths may be observed.

Liver biopsy
- Cellular infiltrates in and around bile ducts with or without portal fibrosis is the definitive diagnosis.

TREATMENT

- Antibiotics based on culture or sensitivity (bile should always be cultured)
- Ampicillin: PO, IV, SQ every 8 hours for as long as 3 months
- Amoxicillin: PO, SQ twice a day
- Metronidazole: PO every 12 hours
- Ursodeoxycholic acid: PO every 24 hours
- Prednisolone: PO every 24 hours for 1 to 2 weeks, then taper to every 48 hours
- Fluid and electrolyte corrections

- Nutritional support as for other liver disorders
- Vitamin therapy

INFORMATION FOR CLIENTS

- The prognosis for this disease is variable.
- Treatment may be prolonged and expensive.
- Permanent damage to the liver may occur.

Feline Hepatic Lipidosis (Idiopathic)

Idiopathic hepatic lipidosis (IHL) is the most common hepatopathy seen in cats. IHL affects adult, obese cats of any age, sex, or breed. The exact cause of the disease is unknown, but stress seems to trigger the syndrome. Any diet change, boarding, illness, or environmental change resulting in anorexia can precipitate the event. If the anorexia is prolonged for longer than 2 weeks, an imbalance between the breakdown of peripheral lipids and lipid clearance within the liver can occur, resulting in excess accumulation of fat within hepatocytes. Other proposed mechanisms for this disease include hormonal abnormalities (leptin, insulin), impaired formation and release of very-low-density lipoprotein from the liver, and decreased oxidation of fatty acids in the liver. The resulting clinical signs are those of hepatic failure. Early diagnosis and aggressive treatment is important for recovery. Complete recovery has been achieved in about 60% to 65% of reported cases.

CLINICAL SIGNS

- Anorexia
- Obesity
- Weight loss (often >25% of body weight)
- Depression
- Sporadic vomiting
- Icterus
- Mild hepatomegaly
- Presence or absence of bleeding tendencies (i.e., tendency to hemorrhage spontaneously from gums, petechial hemorrhages on ears, abdomen)

DIAGNOSIS

Complete Blood Cell Count
- Nonregenerative anemia
- Stress neutrophilia
- Lymphopenia
- Poikilocytes are frequently present

Serum Chemistry
- Markedly increased ALP
- Increased ALT, aspartate aminotransferase
- Hyperbilirubinemia
- Hypoalbuminemia
- Increased serum bile acids

Radiography
- Liver mildly enlarged

Ultrasonography
- Liver hyperechoic when compared with falciform fat

Liver Biopsy
- Severely vacuolized hepatocytes; fat is confirmed using Oil Red O stain on formalin-fixed liver tissue (Fig. 2-10)

TREATMENT

Nutritive Support
- Provide high-protein, calorie-dense diet. Avoid feeding until vitamin and electrolyte balance has been normalized.
- Animals usually require a feeding tube (Fig. 2-11):
  - Nasogastric tube for short-term, liquid diets

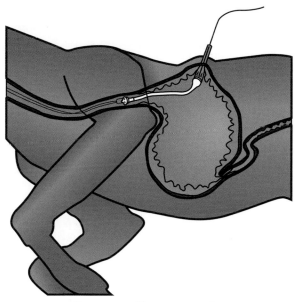

Figure 2-11   Gastrostomy tube.

- Gastrostomy tubes are best if the cat can handle anesthesia
  - Gastroesophageal tube is not well tolerated by all cats
- Tubes may need to remain in place for up to 3 to 6 weeks (no less than 10 days).
- Diets for nutritional support include Hill's Prescription a/d, c/d, p/d, Purina CNM Feline CV Formula, and Iams Nutritional Recovery Formula.
- Mix 1 oz water with 1 oz food.
- Daily caloric needs may be calculated using the following formula:

$$RER = 1.5\,([30 \times BW_{kg}] + 70)$$

Example: A 5-kg cat would require 330 Kcal/day or about four fifths of a 15.5-oz can of c/d.
- Divide the total amount into six feedings for the first several days to allow the stomach to adjust to the presence of food. Then slowly decrease the number of feedings to three per day.
- Flush tube with water before and after feeding (10–15 mL).
- If vomiting occurs, feed a smaller volume, warm the food, or provide medication.

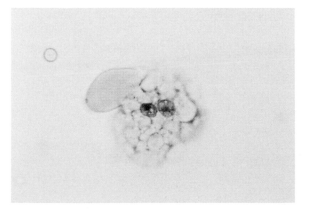

Figure 2-10   Feline fatty liver. Swollen hepatocytes contain small clear vacuoles representing lipid accumulation and fine intracytoplasmic granular clumps of bile pigment. (From Willard MD, Tvedten H: *Small animal clinical diagnosis by laboratory methods*, ed 5, St. Louis, MO, 2012, Saunders.)

Medications

- Intravenous fluids to maintain hydration: avoid Lactated Ringer solution
- Potassium supplement (if necessary)
- Metoclopramide: SQ about 15 minutes before feeding at a dose of 0.4 mg/kg
- Diazepam as an appetite stimulant: seldom successful in the long term and may increase hemolysis
- Vitamin B1, thiamine oral therapy
- Vitamin B12 therapy, carnitine and taurine orally

Monitoring

- Recheck weekly to assess progress.
- CBC, serum chemistries every 2 weeks. Expect to see decreases in ALP and ALT in 1 to 2 weeks.
- Owners may have to skip a tube feeding as laboratory values become normal. Many cats enjoy the tube feedings and will not eat on their own unless challenged. Try special treats or favorite foods. When the cat is eating well, the tube may be removed.
- Withhold food for 8 hours before tube removal and 12 hours after removal.

Nursing Care

- Feeding tubes must be flushed before and after feeding.
- Keep tube capped.
- Keep site clean, and apply antiseptic ointment around the tube to protect the skin.
- After removing the tube, instruct the client on how to clean and care for the wound until healing is complete.

INFORMATION FOR CLIENTS

- Avoid stress in obese cats.
- Early intervention is essential.
- A cat that usually eats well then stops eating is at risk; therefore, owners should monitor the food intake under stressful conditions and have the cat seen immediately by a veterinarian if problems arise.
- Cats do not respond well to frequent diet changes.
- Prevent obesity by feeding your cat properly.
- Although the prognosis is guarded, with early intervention and aggressive treatment, the cure rate for IHL is about 60% to 65%.

TECH ALERT

- Avoid using propofol in these cats. Both valium and propofol will increase hemolysis. Also avoid jugular venipuncture because of increased bleeding tendency.
- When calculating fluid and drug doses, base them on the lean body weight of the cat, not the actual weight.

Neoplasia

Primary and metastatic tumors are a significant cause of liver disease in dogs and cats. Metastatic tumors arising from the pancreas, lymph nodes, spleen, mammary glands, bone, lungs, thyroid gland, or the GI tract are more common than primary liver tumors. Primary tumors are usually epithelial in nature and are derived from hepatocytes or biliary epithelium. Hepatocellular adenomas and adenocarcinomas are most common in dogs, whereas bile duct neoplasms are most common in cats.

Carcinomas may occur in three forms: (1) massive—a single large mass in one liver lobe; (2) nodular—discrete nodules in several liver lobes; and (3) diffuse—infiltration throughout a large mass of liver tissue. Metastases are frequent.

Primary hepatic neoplasm is most common in animals older than 10 years. Clinical signs are usually nonspecific and vague and may not be noticed until the tumor is advanced. Surgical removal of a single mass is the preferred treatment. Nodular and diffuse neoplasms respond poorly to chemotherapy and carry a poor prognosis.

CLINICAL SIGNS

- Anorexia (especially in cats)
- Lethargy (especially in cats)
- Weight loss
- Pu or Pd
- Vomiting (especially in dogs)
- Abdominal distension (dogs)
- Jaundice
- Presence or absence of diarrhea
- Presence or absence of bleeding

- Pale mucous membranes
- Hepatomegaly

DIAGNOSIS

Complete Blood Cell Count
- Anemia, usually nonregenerative

Serum Chemistry
- Increased ALT, ALP (mild to marked; cats may have a normal ALP)
- Hyperbilirubinemia
- Hypoalbuminemia
- Hypoglycemia
- Increased serum bile acids
- Hyperglobulinemia
- Azotemia (especially in cats)

Radiology
- Symmetric or asymmetric hepatomegaly
- Presence or absence of ascites
- Rule out metastasis to thorax with chest radiography

Ultrasonography
- Focal, multifocal, or diffuse changes in echogenicity of the liver

Biopsy
- Best done through laparotomy or fine-needle aspiration for diffuse lesions

Abdominal Tap
- May show tumor cells

TREATMENT

Surgical
- Remove affected lobe if a single lesion is present.

Chemotherapy
- Primary liver tumors respond poorly to chemotherapy. Better response may be obtained with metastatic tumors.

Supportive
- Correct fluid and electrolyte imbalances.
- Maintain a good nutritional level.
- Treat symptoms of nausea and diarrhea.

INFORMATION FOR CLIENTS
- These tumors carry a guarded to poor prognosis.
- Survival times of 195 to 1025 days have been reported for single masses removed by partial hepatectomy.
- Chemotherapy is unsuccessful in the treatment of these cancers.
- Early detection affords the best chance for survival. Routine physical examinations of pets are important.

Portosystemic Shunts (Congenital)

Vascular communications between the portal and systemic venous systems that allow blood to bypass the liver are known as portosystemic shunts (PSSs). Because blood carrying toxins from the GI tract of animals with this defect bypasses hepatic detoxification, systemic toxin levels increase, causing hepatic encephalopathy. The livers of affected animals appear small and atrophied. The PSSs may be intrahepatic or extrahepatic and singular or multiple. The single intrahepatic PSS is most common in large-breed dogs, whereas the single extrahepatic PSS is most common in cats and small-breed dogs. Intrahepatic PSS is usually caused by failure of the ductus venosus to close at birth. Congenital PSS occurs more commonly in purebred dogs, especially Miniature Schnauzers and Yorkshire Terriers, and in mixed breed cats. Clinical signs usually develop by 6 months of age. Diagnosis is by demonstration of a shunting of portal blood directly into the systemic circulation. Complete or partial ligation of the shunt is the preferred treatment.

CLINICAL SIGNS

Signs of Central Nervous System Involvement
- Anorexia
- Depression
- Lethargy
- Episodic weakness
- Ataxia
- Head-pressing
- Circling, pacing, blindness
- Seizures
- Coma
- Hypersalivation (cats)
- Bizarre aggressive behavior (cats)

Gastrointestinal Signs
- Vomiting
- Diarrhea
- Stunted growth and failure to thrive
- Pu or Pd (dogs)

Urinary Signs
- Urate urolithiasis in breeds other than Dalmatians
- Hematuria
- Ammonium biurate crystals in sediment
- Isosthenuria or hyposthenuria if Pu or Pd is present

DIAGNOSIS

Complete Blood Cell Count
- Microcytosis
- Target cells
- Poikilocytosis (especially in cats)
- Mild, nonregenerative anemia

Serum Chemistry
- Hypoproteinemia
- Hypoalbuminemia
- Hypoglycemia
- Decreased BUN
- Increased ALT, ALP (mild, two to three times normal)
- Increased serum bile acids
- Hyperammonemia

Radiographs
- Microhepatia: can use contrast portography to detect the shunt. Rectal portal scintigraphy is also being used.

TREATMENT

Medical
- Seldom successful
- Low-protein diet
- Lactulose
- Neomycin or metronidazole
- Fluid therapy

Surgical
Surgical ligation is the preferred treatment. However, total ligation of most shunts may result in serous portal hypertension. In many cases, partial ligation (60% to 80%) can be performed. Closure of the shunt forces blood back through the atrophic liver, resulting in hypertension, abdominal pain, ascites, ileus, endotoxic shock, and cardiovascular collapse. Therefore, partial occlusion is often followed with a second surgery to totally close the shunt, allowing the liver time to adjust to the increased blood flow.

Animals should be closely monitored for 24 hours after. If signs of portal hypertension develop, a second surgery should be performed to remove the ligation, and emergency treatment with shock doses of fluids and glucocorticoids together with antibiotics should be given.

Postsurgical
- Systemic antibiotics
- Fluid therapy
- Oral lactulose: PO every 6 hours (dogs); 0.25 to 1 mL PO (cats)
- Protein-restricted diet

INFORMATION FOR CLIENTS
- The prognosis for resolution of symptoms after surgical ligation of the shunt is excellent.
- Surgery yields the most successful prognosis if performed before the dog is older than 1 year.
- The shunt may recanalize after surgery, resulting in relapses (more common in cats).
- Animals with partial ligations of the shunt may require a low-protein diet to avoid clinical signs of hepatic encephalopathy.
- This surgical procedure may be expensive and requires a referral center with specialized techniques.

Pancreatic Dysfunction (Exocrine)

The major function of the exocrine pancreas is the secretion of digestive enzymes into the small intestine. It also secretes bicarbonate to neutralize stomach acid, assists in inhibiting bacterial overgrowth in the lumen of the small intestine, and aids in the absorption of vitamin B_{12} and other nutrients.

The pancreas is closely associated with the stomach, liver, and duodenum. The right lobe lies along the descending duodenum; the left lobe accompanies the pyloric portion of the stomach. The left and right lobes join the body at the cranial end of the duodenum near the liver. Pancreatic ducts open into the duodenum at the major duodenal papilla together with the bile duct and at the minor duodenal papilla.

Digestive enzymes, produced and stored within the acinar cells of the pancreas, are released into the small intestine on a routine basis. When stimulated by the presence of food, the volume of secretion increases. The enzymes are secreted in an inactive form to protect the pancreas from autodigestion. (The inactive forms of the enzymes usually have a prefix of *pro-* or an *-ogen* suffix.) Once in the lumen of the small intestine, the enzymes are activated chemically by enteropeptidase, which removes the protective segment of their polypeptide chain.

The digestive enzymes produced in the pancreas include trypsinogen, chymotrypsinogen, proelastase, procarboxypeptidase, prophospholipase, α-amylase, lipase, procolipase, and pancreatic secretory trypsin inhibitor. Amylase and lipase leak from the gland into the blood of healthy animals and are cleared by the kidneys. Clinically, these enzymes are used as a measure of pancreatic health although amylase is not definitive for pancreatic dysfunction.

Pancreatitis

Inflammation of the pancreas is known as *pancreatitis*. Pancreatitis may be acute or chronic, and it is believed to develop when digestive enzymes are activated *within* the gland, resulting in pancreatic autodigestion. Once autodigestion develops, the gland becomes inflamed, resulting in tissue damage, multisystemic involvement, and often death.

Pancreatitis is more prevalent in obese animals. Diets high in fat may predispose animals to the disease. In cats, pancreatitis has been associated with hepatic lipidosis. Drugs such as furosemide, azathioprine, sulfonamides, and tetracycline have been suspected of causing pancreatitis. In addition, edema of the duodenal wall, parasites, tumors, and trauma may also result in pancreatitis. Disruption of the bacterial flora in the small intestine may also be involved in the inflammation or infection of the pancreas.

The disease is unpredictable, with varying levels of severity. Some animals recover fully, whereas others experience development of fulminating disease and die.

CLINICAL SIGNS

- An older, obese dog or cat with a history of a recent fatty meal
- Depression
- Anorexia
- Vomiting
- Presence or absence of diarrhea
- Dehydration
- Fever
- Presence or absence of abdominal pain
- Shock and collapse may develop

DIAGNOSIS
Complete Blood Cell Count

- Leukocytosis
- Increased packed cell volume (PCV)
- Serum chemistries
- Azotemia
- Increased ALT
- Mild hypocalcemia
- Hyperlipemia
- Normal to increased amylase, increased lipase
- Increased serum trypsin-like immunoreactivity, a pancreas-specific test
- Serum *canine pancreatic lipase immunoreactivity (cPLI)*, a recently introduced serum test (developed at Texas A&M), may be the most accurate blood test for identifying pancreatitis

TREATMENT

- Maintain adequate fluid and electrolyte balance.
- Replace potassium, if necessary.
- Suspend all oral intake for 3 to 4 days.
- Antibiotic therapy:
  - Trimethoprim-sulfadiazine: SQ once a day (dogs) and SQ every 12 to 24 hours (cats)
  - Enrofloxacin: IM every 12 hours
- Butorphanol tartrate for analgesia: SQ every 6 hours
- Plasma or albumin: 50 to 250 mL
- 1 to 2 days after vomiting stops, start back on a high-carbohydrate diet; as the animal improves, add a low-fat dietary food

◉ TECH ALERT

Pancreatitis is commonly a postholiday disease. Feeding table scraps from turkey, ham, or roast drastically increases an animal's dietary fat, resulting in acute signs of the disease. Warn your clients to avoid providing these treats!

INFORMATION FOR CLIENTS

- To prevent obesity, avoid overfeeding your pets.
- Feed only low-fat treats.
- Most animals will recover with prompt treatment; however, some dogs may die even after prompt and proper treatment.

Exocrine Pancreatic Insufficiency

Exocrine pancreatic insufficiency (EPI) develops with a progressive loss of acinar cells followed by inadequate production of digestive enzymes. Because the pancreas has considerable reserves, clinical signs may not develop until 85% to 90% of the secretory ability has been lost. Pancreatic acinar atrophy (PAA) is the most common cause of the disease in dogs. PAA may occur spontaneously in the dog, especially in young German Shepherds, a breed with a genetic predisposition to PAA. In cats, EPI is primarily the result of chronic pancreatitis.

Lack of normal pancreatic secretions affects the mucosal lining of the small intestine and decreases its absorptive power. Bacterial overgrowth that occurs also interferes with absorption. Disruption of the normal acinar architecture of the pancreas may affect insulin production, leading to glucose intolerance.

Clinical signs of EPI include weight loss in spite of a good appetite; diarrhea with a gray, fatty, foul-smelling stool; flatulence; and poor hair coat. Treatment is aimed at replacing digestive enzymes.

CLINICAL SIGNS

- Mild to marked weight loss
- Polyphagia
- Coprophagia, pica, or both
- Diarrhea, fatty stool (light in color)
- Flatulence

DIAGNOSIS

Complete Blood Cell Count
- Normal CBC

Serum Chemistries
- Increased ALT (mild to moderate)
- Decreased total lipid
- Serum trypsin-like immunoreactivity; detects both trypsin and trypsinogen; levels are decreased to <2 microgram per liter (mcg/L) in EPI

Fecal Tests
- Fecal tests are unreliable for diagnosis.

Fecal Proteolytic Activity
- Decreased in EPI

TREATMENT

- Supplement pancreatic enzymes with each meal: commercial product such as Pancrezyme or Viokase-V (2 tsp/20 kg body weight added to food) or chopped raw ox or pig pancreas (3–4 oz/20 kg body weight)
- Low-fiber diet with high digestibility
- Medium chain triglyceride (MCT) oil: 0.5 to 4 tsp/day with food
- Vitamins
  - Tocopherol: 400 to 500 international units (IU) given once daily with food for 30 days
  - Cobalamin: 250 mcg IM or SQ every 7 days for several weeks
- Antibiotic therapy to decrease bacterial overgrowth in the small intestine
  - Oxytetracycline: every 12 hours for 7 to 28 days
  - Metronidazole: every 12 to 24 hours for 7 days or
  - Tylosin: with each meal
- Prednisolone may be used if response to the above treatments is poor

INFORMATION FOR CLIENTS

- EPI is irreversible and will require lifelong treatment.
- Pancreatic enzyme replacements are expensive.
- With enzyme replacement, most dogs will regain their weight, and the diarrhea will resolve.
- Enzyme replacements must be given with every meal.

Rectoanal Disease

Three conditions involving the rectoanal area are commonly seen in small-animal medicine: (1) perineal hernia, (2) perianal fistula, and (3) perianal gland adenoma. Anal sac problems are covered in Chapter 6.

Perineal Hernias

Perineal hernias, seen most commonly in intact male dogs older than 8 years, are associated with neurogenic atrophy of the levator ani muscle and herniation of the rectum and other pelvic organs into the ischiorectal fossa.

CLINICAL SIGNS

- Reducible perineal swelling
- Tenesmus
- Dyschezia (painful or difficult defecation)
- Constipation or obstipation
- Some dogs have signs of urethral obstruction if the bladder is involved

⬤ TECH ALERT

Brachiocephalic breeds show a predisposition to this problem.

DIAGNOSIS

- Rectal palpation will reveal the hernia sac.

TREATMENT

Medical
- Stool softeners such as Colace (DSS) (seldom effective for long-term maintenance)
- Enemas (seldom effective for long-term maintenance)

Surgical
- Herniorrhaphy to correct the weakness in the pelvic diaphragm
- Castration usually recommended

INFORMATION FOR CLIENTS

- Ensuring that the stool is well formed but soft may help decrease straining.

- Castration is usually recommended because the role of the hormone testosterone in this disease is unknown.

Perianal Fistulas (Anal Furunculosis)

Perianal fistulas are characterized by single or multiple ulcerated sinuses that may involve up to all of the perianal tissue. Their presence can result in pain, bleeding, self mutilation, dyschezia, and anal stenosis.

CLINICAL SIGNS

- Tenesmus
- Dyschezia, pain on examination
- Fecal incontinence
- Licking of perianal area
- Bleeding
- Foul odor to anal area
- Typically a large-breed dog

DIAGNOSIS

- Examination to rule out anal sac disease and perirectal tumors

TREATMENT

- Medical: Medical management is usually not successful.
- Topical tacrolimus: has shown promise in these cases but is expensive and has the potential for severe immunosuppression.
- Surgical: No one technique has been consistently successful. Recently carbon dioxide laser surgery has been reported to be very effective, with a 95% remission rate but a 25% recurrence rate. En bloc removal of the affected tissue has a higher remission rate.

INFORMATION FOR CLIENTS

- These animals will have pain around the anal area; be careful to avoid getting bitten when treating them.
- Keep the involved area clean and dry. Spray antibiotics can be used to decrease the level of infection.
- Long-term oral antibiotics may be required for maintenance.

Perianal Gland Adenomas

Because growth and development of perianal gland adenomas are related to plasma androgen levels, 85% are seen in older, intact male dogs. Most lesions are firm, single, or multiple masses that may ulcerate. The lesions may result in intense pruritus and can interfere with defecation. They are not invasive or metastatic.

CLINICAL SIGNS

- Pruritus in anal area
- Bleeding
- Firm nodule in perianal integument, tail root, or the prepuce

DIAGNOSIS

- Palpation and location of lesion
- Biopsy

TREATMENT

- Surgical removal
- Radiation
- Cryosurgery
- Castration results in regression of tumors and decreases the risk for new tumor development

INFORMATION FOR CLIENTS

- Pets with perianal fistulas or ulcerated adenomas need to be kept clean. Gently cleanse the area daily using a baby wipe or damp cloth.
- Castration of male dogs at an early age can help prevent this disease.

CLINICAL CASE HISTORY

Fred, a 2-year-old gray tabby Domestic Short Hair cat was presented to the local veterinarian for castration. The technician who was taking a history noticed that the cat's ears were yellow and immediately called for the doctor to examine the cat. Blood was drawn for a complete blood count (CBC), hand differential, serum chemistries and a feline leukemia virus (FeLV) test. Can you list three possible causes of icterus in the cat and the tests that would be the most valuable in making a diagnosis? See page 559 for the laboratory results and diagnosis.

REVIEW QUESTIONS

1. Gingivitis is a reversible disease.
   a. True
   b. False
2. A normal gingival sulcus in a cat should measure:
   a. Greater than 4 mm
   b. Less than 1 mm
   c. Between 1 and 3 mm
3. A cauliflower-like growth near the oral cavity of young dog might be:
   a. Epulide
   b. Carcinoma
   c. Papilloma
   d. Sarcoma
4. Signs of acute gastritis would most likely include (list all that apply):
   a. Vomiting
   b. Seizures
   c. Dehydration
   d. Anorexia
   e. Fever
   f. Diarrhea
5. What is the most frequent side effect of NSAID administration in dogs and cats?
   a. Nausea
   b. Diarrhea
   c. Gastric ulceration
   d. Drowsiness
6. After surgical correction for a gastric dilatation or volvulus, what is the most frequently seen cardiac arrhythmia?
   a. Ventricular arrhythmia
   b. Supraventricular arrhythmia
   c. Atrial fibrillation
   d. Premature atrial contractions
7. Cardiac arrhythmias arising after surgery with GDV may be treated using:
   a. Digitalis
   b. Propofol
   c. Lidocaine
   d. Epinephrine

8. A laboratory examination of a patient with diarrhea should always include:
   a. A stool culture and sensitivity
   b. A serum chemistry profile
   c. A thyroid function test
   d. A fecal examination
9. The majority of feline intestinal neoplasias in the cat are:
   a. Adenocarcinomas
   b. Lymphosarcomas
   c. Melanomas
   d. Papillomas
10. Unformed feces that contain excess mucus may be seen with:
    a. Small-bowel disease
    b. Large-bowel disease
    c. Gastric disease
11. What percentage of cases of megacolon in the cat are thought to be idiopathic?
    a. 25%
    b. 62%
    c. 90%
    d. 56%

12. IHL in adult, obese cats may be triggered by:
    a. Stress
    b. Diet change
    c. Illness
    d. All of the above
13. What may develop as a sequel to pancreatitis?
    a. Diabetes insipidus
    b. Diabetes mellitus
    c. Cushing's disease
    d. Addison's disease
14. An increased trypsin-like immunoreactivity test result indicates dysfunction of the:
    a. Adrenal gland
    b. Small intestine
    c. Liver
    d. Pancreas
15. Exacerbation of neurologic signs after a high-protein meal may indicate:
    a. Patent ductus arteriosus
    b. Epilepsy
    c. Portosystemic shunt
    d. Polycystic renal disease

Answers found on page 551.

Diseases of the Endocrine System

LEARNING OBJECTIVES

When you have completed this chapter, you will be able to:
1. Explain the interrelationship between the nervous system and the endocrine system.
2. Understand the clinical pathologic changes that occur with each endocrine disease.
3. Describe how the absence of a specific hormone can have clinical effects on the animal.
4. Explain to owners the treatment regime necessary for their pets.

Anatomy of the Endocrine System

The endocrine system can be divided into three main levels: (1) the central control, (2) the glands, and (3) the target organs. The pituitary gland and the hypothalamus make up the central control level of the system. The hypothalamus is responsible for two hormones, *antidiuretic hormone* (vasopressin) and *oxytocin*. These hormones are stored in the posterior pituitary. A variety of releasing hormones formed in the hypothalamus stimulate hormone production in the anterior pituitary. The anterior pituitary then manufactures and releases a variety of hormones classified as *stimulating hormones*. These stimulating hormones travel through the bloodstream to target glands, which are stimulated to produce their hormones. This is the second level of endocrine control. Glandular hormones are then carried to target tissues, where they finally produce their end effects.

The cells of the body must maintain *homeostasis* (equilibrium) with their internal environment because the chemical processes conducted at the cellular level can occur only under specific conditions. The endocrine system works together with the nervous system to achieve a stable internal environment; each system may work independently, or the systems may act together to accomplish this task. The hypothalamus and the pituitary gland regulate the release of chemical messengers called *hormones* (chemicals secreted directly into the bloodstream) to signal target cells to perform certain functions in response to changes in homeostasis. As hormone concentrations in blood increase, the system is signaled to reduce hormone production; this *negative feedback system* works much the same way as a thermostat controls the heating system in a house.

Ideally, the glands that regulate the release and balance of hormones work continuously to maintain homeostasis. When one or more of these glands work ineffectively, incorrectly, or not at all, the potential for problems develops. The endocrine glands most commonly involved in diseases of small animals are the thyroid gland, adrenal gland, pancreas, parathyroid gland, and gonads (testes and ovaries) (Fig. 3-1).

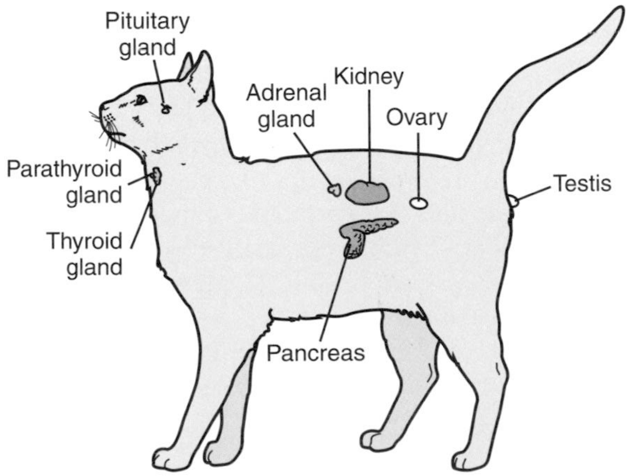

Diseases that affect the pituitary gland or the hypothalamus cause multiple irregularities in the body; they are discussed in this chapter only in the context of their relationship to other syndromes.

Thyroid Gland

The thyroid gland is located in the ventral cervical region along the lateral margins of the trachea. The gland is not usually palpable in a healthy animal. The gland is composed of follicles that produce the thyroid hormones *triiodothyronine* (T_3) and *tetraiodothyronine* (T_4). These hormones are produced by the follicular cells and stored in the gland until they are needed by the body. A third hormone, *calcitonin*, is produced by the parafollicular cells in the thyroid gland. Calcitonin acts to increase calcium deposition within bone to decrease blood calcium concentration, whereas T3 and T4 function to control all of the body's metabolic processes.

Two common diseases of small animals involve the thyroid gland (Fig. 3-2): (1) hypothyroidism (insufficient thyroid hormone) and (2) hyperthyroidism

Figure 3-1 Locations of major endocrine glands in the cat. (From Colville T, Bassert JM: *Clinical anatomy and physiology for veterinary technicians*, ed 2, St. Louis, MO, 2008, Mosby.)

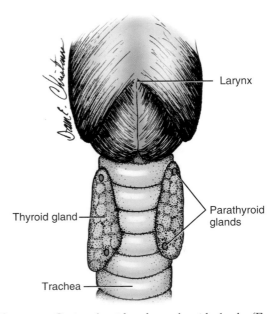

Figure 3-2 Canine thyroid and parathyroid glands. (From Christenson DE: *Veterinary medical terminology*, Philadelphia, PA, 2009, Saunders, by permission.)

(excessive thyroid hormone). *Hypothyroidism* is most commonly seen in the canine (1 in 156 to 500 animals). *Hyperthyroidism* is seen primarily in cats.

Hypothyroid Disease

Primary acquired hypothyroidism is the most common type of hypothyroid disease seen in dogs and usually follows thyroid atrophy or lymphocytic thyroiditis. Central acquired hypothyroidism is rare and develops when the pituitary or hypothalamus is diseased.

CLINICAL SIGNS

- Breeds predisposed to this disease: Golden Retrievers, Dobermans, Irish Setters, Schnauzers, Cocker Spaniels, and Dachshunds
- Common in middle-aged dogs (4–10 years of age); female-to-male ratio is 2.5:1
- Weight gain with no change in diet
- Bilaterally symmetric alopecia; "rat tail" (loss of hair on the tail)
- Cold intolerant
- Recurrent skin infections
- Reproduction problems

● TECH ALERT

Hypothyroid disease and Cushing disease are the only known diseases that produce this alopecia pattern:
- Dry hair or excessive shedding
- Lethargy
- Anestrus (infertility, testicular atrophy)
- Hyperpigmentation of the skin
- Cold intolerance
- Anemia
- Hypercholesterolemia

DIAGNOSIS

- 66% to 75% of animals will have increased cholesterol level.
- 25% to 40% of animals have a mild, nonregenerative anemia.
- Thyroid hormones usually measured include total T_4 (TT_4), total T_3 (TT_3), free T_4 (fT_4).

● TECH ALERT

Thyroid hormones are stable up to 5 days if stored in plastic containers and not in glass containers. Serum should be transported to the laboratory in plastic vials.

- Thyroid-stimulating hormone (TSH) tests are expensive and often unavailable. Recommended doses of TSH for this test are 0.396 units/kg body weight intravenously (IV), 0.099 units/kg intramuscularly (IM), or 1 unit IV to 10 units IV, IM, or subcutaneously (SQ). Take blood sample at 6 hours. The normal response shows an increase of T4 concentration greater than 2 micrograms per deciliter (mcg/dL) above baseline concentration
- Measurement of thyroid hormone antibody concentration
- Thyroid ultrasonography
- Thyroid biopsy

TREATMENT

- Life long supplementation with thyroid replacement hormone
- *Dogs:* Initially use trade name products at a dose of 22 mcg/kg twice daily; reevaluate in 4 to 8 weeks for clinical response and adjust the dose, as needed; some dogs may need only one dose daily
- *Cats:* 17-22 mcg/kg daily; reevaluate in 4 to 6 weeks and adjust the dose

Products

- Levothyroxine sodium tablets: 0.1-, 0.2-, 0.3-, 0.4-, 0.5-, 0.6-, 0.7-, 0.8-mg sizes
- Levothyroxine sodium products approved for use in animals: Soloxine (Daniels), Thyro-Tabs (Vet-A-Mix), Thyro-Form (Vet-A-Mix) chewable tablets
- Levothyroxine sodium products approved for use in humans: Synthroid (Knoll Pharmaceuticals), 0.025 to 0.3 mg; Levo-T (Lederle), Levothroid (Forest Laboratories)
- Thyroxyl: oral solution of levothyroxine sodium; allows for easy dosing at any level

INFORMATION FOR CLIENTS

- Oral supplementation will be required for the life of the animal.

- Daily dosing is required to maintain normal concentration of thyroid hormone.
- Excess medication can produce signs of hyperthyroidism: increased thirst and urination, nervousness, weight loss, excessive panting, weakness, and increased appetite. If any of these signs are noticed, stop the medication, and call your veterinarian.
- Follow-up blood tests may be required to ensure adequate hormone concentration.
- Certain drugs may decrease thyroid hormone concentration. Inform your veterinarian if your animal is currently taking any of these medications: cortisone, aspirin, flunixin (Banamine), ketoprofen, meloxicam, furosemide (Lasix), or phenobarbital.

Hyperthyroid Disease

Hyperthyroidism is the most commonly seen endocrine disorder in cats; however, it is rarely seen in dogs except as a result of neoplasia. The disease was first documented in the late 1970s to the early 1980s, with incidence increasing steadily. The excess of both T3 and T4 results in a multisystemic disease seen primarily in older cats. Bilateral thyroid gland enlargement occurs in approximately 70% of cases and is the result of a functional thyroid adenoma. Thyroid carcinoma is rarely seen in cats, comprising only 1% to 2% of all cases of hyperthyroidism.

CLINICAL SIGNS

- Middle-aged to older cat
- Weight loss
- Polyphagia
- Vomiting
- Increased appetite
- Tachycardia with or without murmurs
- Aggressive behavior, hyperactivity
- Palpable enlarged thyroid
- Increased systolic blood pressure
- Blindness with retinal detachment

DIAGNOSIS

- Check for palpable enlarged thyroid.
- Test for increased serum T4 concentration.
- Perform serum chemistries to rule out other organ system failures that may be present. Increased alanine aminotransferase (ALT), alkaline phosphatase

TECH ALERT

Make sure to palpate the ventral neck area of every older cat to detect early enlargement of the thyroid gland.

(ALP), and lactate dehydrogenase (LDH) levels are usually seen; increased blood urea nitrogen (BUN) and creatinine level may be seen.
- Packed cell volume is often in the high to normal range on the stress leukogram.
- Check for abnormal thyroid radionuclide uptake imaging using either iodine-131 (131I) or technetium (99mTc).

TREATMENT

- Control of excessive excretion of thyroid hormones can be accomplished by three methods. Choice of treatment depends on the severity of the disease, the age and physical status of the cat, and facilities available.

Surgery

- Removal of the thyroid gland provides a cure for the disease, but it is important to preserve the parathyroid glands when removing thyroid tissue.

Radioactive Iodine-131

- Radioactive ^{131}I is the treatment of choice. Diseased tissue in the thyroid gland will take up larger amounts of radioactive ^{131}I compared with normal tissue. This uptake results in the destruction of the tissue, reducing thyroid hormone concentration. Cats should remain hospitalized until their wastes (especially urine) are below hazardous radiation levels (1 to 3 weeks).

Antithyroid Drug Therapy

- Antithyroid drugs: inhibit the synthesis of thyroid hormone by disrupting the incorporation of iodine
- Methimazole (Tapazole) or carbimazole: initially administer daily, adjusting the dose every 2 to 3 weeks (monitor T4 concentration). Gradually increase the dose until the desired effect is achieved
- Propranolol: to control tachycardias
- Calcium ipodate: administer daily orally (PO)

Hyperthyroidism in Dogs

Hyperthyroidism is uncommon in dogs and is usually related to a functional tumor in the thyroid gland. The disease occurs in middle-aged to older dogs with Beagles, Golden Retrievers, and Boxers overrepresented. Diagnosis is by palpation and measurement of total T_4 concentration. Surgical removal of the thyroid may not correct the problem, since these tumors are highly invasive to structures in the neck area. Radiotherapy may be successful in some cases.

INFORMATION FOR CLIENTS

- Surgery or radioactive iodine is the only cure for hyperthyroidism.
- The cause of this disease is unknown.
- Medical management produces side effects in many cats. Report negative effects to your veterinarian.
- Treatment to decrease thyroid hormone concentration may unmask concurrent diseases such as renal failure. This renal disease may be life threatening if not recognized.
- Concurrent diseases may need to be corrected before surgery.
- Bilateral removal of the thyroid glands may result in hypothyroidism, which will require daily treatment.
- All animals with hyperthyroidism should have their blood pressure checked routinely. If the use of methimazole (Tapazole) does not result in reduction of blood pressure, then other antihypertensive agents should be added.

Pancreas

The pancreas is located adjacent to the greater curvature of the stomach, extending onto the duodenal small intestine. The gland has both endocrine and exocrine functions. The exocrine function is discussed in Chapter 3. The endocrine portion consists of pancreatic islet cells (formerly called the *islets of Langerhans*). These islets are dispersed throughout the gland and produce several important hormones: beta-cells (β-cells) that produce *insulin* , the most well-known hormone; alpha-cells (α-cells) that secrete *glucagon*; and delta cells that produce *somatostatin*. F-cells secrete *pancreatic polypeptides*. Disruption of any of these hormone-producing cells can affect hormone levels (Fig. 3-3).

Diabetes Mellitus

Cells need glucose as a fuel. Through the processes of glycolysis, the citric acid cycle, electron transport, and oxidative phosphorylation, glucose is chemically converted into energy in the form of adenosine triphosphate, carbon dioxide, and water. It is, therefore, important for the body to regulate the concentration of glucose in circulation. Levels must be kept within certain limits to ensure that adequate fuel is always available for energy production. The endocrine pancreas aids in this regulation; β-cells in the pancreatic islets (islets of Langerhans) produce the hormone insulin, which facilitates the entry of glucose into the cell for the process of glycolysis. Diabetes mellitus results when these β-cells stop producing insulin in adequate amounts or when the cells in specific body tissues become resistant to the action of insulin. The incidence of diabetes mellitus in dogs and cats is reported to be between 1 in 100 and 1 in 500. The cause of the disease is unknown, although chronic pancreatitis, immune-mediated disease, and hereditary predisposition have been suggested as possible causes.

Almost 100% of dogs and about 50% of cats will have *insulin-dependent diabetes (type I)* at examination. As many as 50% of presenting cats will have *non–insulin-dependent diabetes (type II)*, which does not require insulin therapy.

Therapy for diabetes mellitus in most animals includes dietary regulation (usually a high-fiber diet) and daily insulin replacement. In cats with non–insulin-dependent diabetes, drug therapy and diet restriction are somewhat successful in managing the disease.

The type of insulin chosen for therapy depends on the severity of the disease and animal needs. Treatment should be tailored to the species of the animal involved. (Feline insulin most resembles beef insulin, and canine insulin resembles pork and human insulins.) Although it would be ideal to match the structure of each species' insulin, it is not easy to do

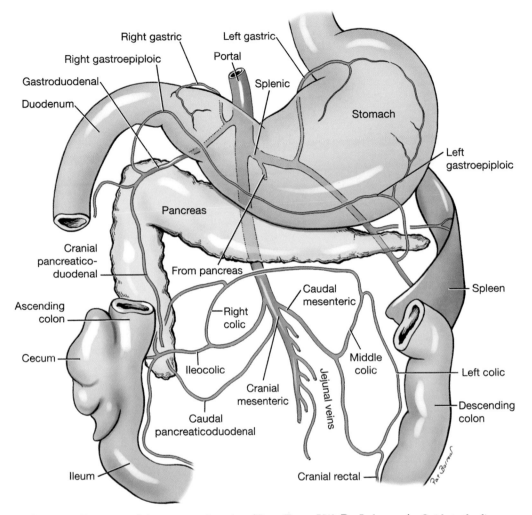

Figure 3-3 Location of the pancreas in a dog. (From Evans HE, De Lahunta A: *Guide to the dissection of the dog*, ed 7, St. Louis, MO, 2010, Saunders.)

this. Beef and pork insulins and their combinations have virtually disappeared from the market since the late 1990s; Vetsulin has taken their place, but it has been discontinued because of problems related to stability and possibly sterility.

Animals with diabetes whose sugar concentration remains uncontrolled may become *ketotic*. Cells begin to use fat as fuel for energy production, yielding *ketone bodies* that accumulate in blood. Acidosis, dehydration, and electrolyte imbalances can occur as a result of ketosis.

CLINICAL SIGNS

Nonketotic Diabetes

- *Dogs:* 4 to 14 years of age, female dogs are twice as likely to be affected
- *Cats:* all ages, with neutered male cats most affected
- Breeds predisposed to the disease: Poodles, Schnauzers, Keeshonds, Cairn Terriers, Dachshunds, Cocker Spaniels, and Beagles
- Polyuria (Pu) or polydipsia (Pd)
- Weight loss (especially in cats)
- Polyphagia

- Sudden cataract formation
- Dehydration
- Plantigrade posture in cats (walking on hocks)

Ketotic Diabetes

Clinical signs include all of the preceding symptoms plus the following:
- Depression
- Weakness
- Tachypnea
- Vomiting
- Odor of acetone on the breath

DIAGNOSIS

- Evaluate clinical signs present in animal.
- Observe for documented fasting blood glucose concentration greater than 200 mg/dL.
- Test urine for glycosuria.
- Perform complete serum chemistry to rule out other concurrent disease.
- Obtain serum blood glucose curve.

TREATMENT

Dietary Management

- Restrict animal to a diet high in fiber and complex carbohydrates, such as Prescription Diet r/d or w/d (Hill's), Fit and Trim (Purina), or Science Diet Light (Hill's). This type of diet helps avoid postprandial increases of glucose concentration and allows for better regulation of blood glucose concentration.

Insulin Therapy

- Two types of insulin are available: (1) human (Humulin, Eli Lilly and Company) and (2) beef-and-pork combination (Iletin I, Eli Lilly and Company). Most treatment regimens involve the use of neutral protamine Hagedorn (NPH, intermediate-acting) or Ultralente (long-acting) insulins.

● TECH ALERT

These forms of insulin recently have been removed from the market by Eli Lilly and Company. Animals that must be switched to another form of insulin should be monitored carefully. It is recommended that doses be reduced when switching until the animal's glucose levels stabilize.

- Oral therapy: Glipizide can be used in cats that do not require insulin to control their blood glucose concentration (type II). The exact mechanism of action is unknown; however, it is believed that the sulfonylureas may stimulate the existing β-cells to secrete more insulin. Animals may become resistant to this therapy and need insulin.
- Recommended therapy doses:
  - *Dogs:* initially NPH insulin daily; can be increased to twice daily if necessary
  - *Cats:* ultralente insulin (Humulin, Eli Lilly and Company) daily or beef-and-pork lente insulin (Iletin, Eli Lilly and Company) twice daily
- Insulin therapy should be monitored using improvement in clinical signs as a guide. Blood glucose concentration can be checked weekly to assist in adjusting the insulin dose. Animals whose glucose levels do not regulate will require a glucose curve to adjust their insulin therapy.
- Serum fructose concentration can be monitored and will provide an evaluation of the average blood sugar concentration over time. Samples should be frozen and shipped in cold packs. This value can be used to separate "stress hyperglycemia" from chronic hyperglycemia and is perhaps more valuable in regulating the condition in animals compared with spot checks on blood glucose.

Exercise Regulation

Exercise regulation will help to regulate insulin requirements. By normalizing the exercise routine for the animal, closer control of glucose levels can be achieved. If excessive exercise is expected, as with hunting dogs and show dogs or for other reasons, the insulin dose may need to be decreased to maintain adequate glucose levels.

INFORMATION FOR CLIENTS

- This disease will require lifelong insulin replacement therapy.
- Insulin is administered by injection.
- Because it is a protein molecule, insulin can be damaged by heat, rough handling, or chemicals. Refrigerate, mix gently, and avoid syringes that have been cleaned with soap or other cleaning agents.

- The formation of cataracts is the most common complication seen in animals with diabetes. The process is irreversible once it occurs. However, 80% to 90% of dogs can re-gain their sight following cataract surgery.
- Consistent feeding and exercise routines will make regulation easier.
- Animals will require periodic monitoring of blood glucose concentration for life.
- If untreated, the disease will progress and may lead to death.

Insulin Shock (Insulin Overdose)

Animals with diabetes that receive insulin therapy will need to live a closely regulated lifestyle. Consistent feeding (both type and amount of food), exercise, and monitoring will make insulin regulation easier for the owner and safer for the pet. Animals that experience fluctuations in diet (do not eat consistent amounts or change foods frequently with loss of appetite) or who are allowed to exercise to excess can experience insulin shock. Exercise increases the need for glucose by body cells. This increased need uses up the exogenous insulin quickly, forcing glucose into the cells rapidly and reducing the blood concentration of glucose significantly. This rapid decline in glucose concentration in the blood results in lack of glucose for the brain. Symptoms of weakness, restlessness, incoordination, seizures, and coma may develop. (These same symptoms may be seen in animals mistakenly given an excessive dose of insulin.) The following schedule is recommended for feeding animals receiving insulin therapy:

- Monitor urine or blood glucose concentration at the same time each day.
- Base insulin dose on the current blood glucose measurements.
- Feed the animal one third of its total daily diet with insulin administration.
- Feed the remainder of the diet about 8 hours later (or at the time of measured peak insulin activity).
- Try to maintain a consistent daily exercise program, but avoid excessive exercise. If the animal is expected to be more active than normal, administer less insulin that day.

Owners should have a handy supply of sugar in the event of insulin shock (Karo syrup, oral glucose solution or paste, treats). Owner should give these to the pet if any signs of insulin shock are present.

● TECH ALERT

Hyperglycemia is never acutely fatal, whereas hypoglycemia can be life threatening!

Insulinoma

Functional tumors of the β-cells of the pancreas secrete insulin or proinsulin independent of the negative feedback effect. Hyperinsulinemia results in the development of hypoglycemia. Prolonged or severe hypoglycemia can result in irreversible brain damage, weakness, ataxia, seizures, or complete collapse. Insulin-secreting tumors typically occur in middle-aged or older dogs; however, the disease has been reported in dogs as young as 3 years. There appears to be a greater incidence of occurrence in certain breeds (Standard Poodle, German Shepherd, Irish Setter, Boxer, and Fox Terrier). Although rare in cats, the disease has been described in a Siamese cat.

CLINICAL SIGNS

Many of the clinical signs may occur intermittently or for short periods because of the body's compensatory mechanisms for increasing blood glucose concentrations. Most signs will be exacerbated by exercise, fasting, or excitement.

- Seizures
- Weakness or collapse
- Ataxia
- Bizarre behavior
- Depression or lethargy

DIAGNOSIS

- Complete blood cell count (CBC), urinalysis, and the majority of blood chemistries will all be normal; blood glucose levels may be in the range of 15 to 78 mg/dL
- Ultrasonography: detection of a mass lesion in the pancreas may help to confirm suspicions of a β-cell tumor

- Demonstration of Whipple's triad:
  1. Symptoms occurring after fasting or exercise
  2. At the time of symptoms, blood glucose concentrations less than 50 mg/dL
  3. Symptoms corrected by administration of glucose
- Plasma insulin concentration: greater than 20 microunits/mL in a dog with blood glucose levels less than 60 mg/dL and clinical symptoms strongly supports insulinoma
- Amended insulin/glucose ratios:
  - Plasma insulin (microunits/ml) $\times$ 100
  - Plasma glucose (mg/dL): 30
  - Amended insulin-to-glucose ratios greater than 30 are considered diagnostic for insulin-secreting tumors

TREATMENT

Surgical

- Removal of a single mass or resection of multiple sites can result in a "cure" or improvement of this disease. Surgery may not be recommended for aged animals or animals with many metastatic lesions.

Medical

- Acute hypoglycemic crisis: if the animal is at home, the owner should apply Karo syrup to the oral mucous membranes, which will increase the blood glucose concentration quickly. If the animal responds to oral glucose, it should be fed a small, high-protein meal and kept quiet until veterinary attention can be obtained. If the animal is in the hospital when the crisis occurs, slow intravenous administration of 50% dextrose will alleviate the symptoms. The animal should then be maintained with diet and drug therapy.
- Chronic hypoglycemia: to reduce the frequency and severity of clinical signs and to avoid acute hypoglycemic crisis:
  - Provide frequent feedings (3-6/day) of a high-protein, low-fat food.
  - Limit exercise to leash walking.
  - Glucocorticoid therapy: glucocorticoids antagonize the effects of insulin at the cellular level. Prednisone is most often used in daily divided doses. If signs of hypercortisolism occur, alternative therapy should be added.

- Diazoxide: inhibits the secretion of insulin and tissue use of glucose to promote hyperglycemia. Dosage is adjusted to maintain normal blood glucose concentrations. Side effects may include anorexia and vomiting.
- Octreotide (Sandostatin) injections: an analog of somatostatin that inhibits the synthesis and secretion of insulin by both normal and neoplastic β-cells.
- Streptozocin: a nitrosourea antibiotic that selectively destroys β-cells in the pancreas. The adverse effects of this drug, including acute renal failure and vomiting, may outweigh its benefits in the treatment of insulinomas.

INFORMATION FOR CLIENTS

- By the time most dogs are diagnosed with insulinoma, metastasis has occurred. The prognosis is poor.
- With proper medical treatment, survival time may range from 12 to 24 months.
- Always limit exercise and excitement in animals with insulinoma.
- Feed multiple, small meals throughout the day. Keep sugar or food in your pockets when walking or exercising the dog.
- Keep Karo syrup on hand for emergencies. Rub the syrup on the oral mucous membranes for a quick glucose boost.
- Even with surgery, most dogs survive for less than 1 year.
- Avoid placing a hand or object into an animal's mouth during a seizure because you are likely to be bitten.

Adrenal Glands

The adrenal glands are located dorsally and cranially to the kidneys, embedded in the perirenal fat (Fig. 3-4). They are composed of two distinct regions: (1) the *medullary* or *central area* and (2) the *cortical* or *outer area*, each of which produces distinct hormones.

The cortex produces three families of hormones: (1) the *glucocorticoids*, (2) the *mineralocorticoids*, and (3) the *androgenic hormones (sex hormones)*. Glucocorticoids promote gluconeogenesis, suppress inflammation, suppress the immune system, and inhibit cartilage growth and development. They are not essential for life but

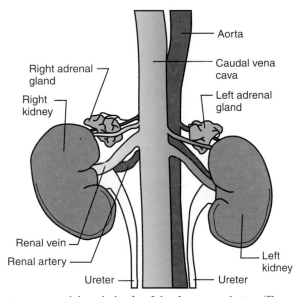

Figure 3-4 Adrenal glands of the dog: ventral view. (From Colville T, Bassert JM: *Clinical anatomy and physiology for veterinary technicians*, St. Louis, MO, 2008, Mosby, by permission.)

are important for maintaining normal homeostasis. *Hyperadrenocorticism*, also known as *Cushing syndrome*, occurs when excess glucocorticoids are produced by the adrenal gland.

Aldosterone is the principal mineralocorticoid. This hormone regulates electrolytes and has a potent effect on water metabolism within the body. Lack of this hormone is life threatening. *Hypoadrenocorticism*, or *Addison disease*, is seen primarily in dogs and rarely in cats.

The androgenic hormones produced by the adrenal glands are identical to those produced by the testicle. The small amount produced limits their effect on the animal.

The medullary area produces two hormones: (1) *epinephrine* and (2) *norepinephrine*. Both hormones affect the sympathetic nervous system and are involved in the "fight-or-flight" response.

The two most common diseases involving the adrenal glands are Addison disease and Cushing syndrome.

Hypoadrenocorticism (Addison Disease)

Primary hypoadrenocorticism, most often classified as idiopathic, involves atrophy of the adrenal cortex,

causing decreased production of both glucocorticoids and mineralocorticoids (loss of aldosterone is responsible for most of the clinical signs). An immune mechanism has been suggested for this disease. The disease is not common in dogs and is even rarer in cats. Other causes of hypoadrenocorticism include trauma, fungal infection, neoplasm, and hereditary tendencies (Standard Poodles and Labrador Retrievers). Excess amounts of the drug o,p-DDD (mitotane) can also produce this disease. Secondary hypoadrenocorticism, resulting from lack of adrenocorticotropic hormone (ACTH), is a much less frequent cause of clinical disease. Aldosterone production in the adrenal cortex depends on the renin–angiotensin axis (Fig. 3-5), the plasma potassium concentration, and the plasma ACTH and sodium concentration. The entire system is stimulated by a decrease in blood pressure or vascular volume, resulting in an increase in angiotensin II and an increase in production of aldosterone by the adrenal gland. Mineralocorticoids are responsible for sodium–potassium (Na-K) exchange in the renal tubules and are important for the conservation of sodium within the body. Abnormal levels of aldosterone produce signs

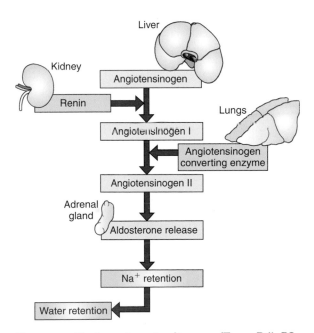

Figure 3-5 Renin-angiotensin diagram. (From Bill RL: *Clinical Pharmacology and therapeutics for the veterinary technician*, ed 3, St. Louis, MO, 2006, Mosby.)

of disease that include hyponatremia and hyperkalemia. An abnormal Na:K ratio of less than 24 has been used as a bench mark for diagnosis of this disease; however, animals may present with normal Na:K ratios and still have *atypical hypoadrenocorticism.*

CLINICAL SIGNS

- Middle-aged, female dogs (usually <7 years)
- Vague signs of depression, lethargy, weakness, anorexia, and weight loss
- Vomiting and diarrhea
- Pu or Pd
- Symptoms frequently wax and wane over time
- Bradycardia in about one third of all animals
- Dehydration

DIAGNOSIS

Serum Chemistry Panel

- Test for a Na:K ratio of less than 27:1 (normal is between 27:2 and 40:1).
- Nonregenerative anemia, lymphocytosis
- Verify increased BUN, creatinine, and calcium levels.
- Check for decreased blood glucose and albumin concentrations.
- Evaluate for acidosis.

Adrenocorticotropic Hormone Stimulation Test

- The ACTH stimulation test provides a definitive diagnosis of hypoadrenocorticism. ACTH gel (CortaGel 40, Savage Labs) or synthetic ACTH (Cortrosyn, Organon) is given to the animal in the following doses:
  - *Gel:* 2.2 units/kg IM with plasma cortisol samples at 0 and 120 minutes in dogs and 0, 60, and 120 minutes in cats
  - *Synthetic:* 0.25 mg IM for dogs or 0.15 mg IM for cats with samples at 0 and 60 minutes in dogs and 0, 30, and 60 minutes in cats; animals with hypoadrenocorticism typically have low resting cortisol concentration, which remains essentially unchanged after ACTH stimulation
- *Endogenous ACTH concentration* testing must be done carefully because ACTH is not stable over long periods. Concentrations will be increased in dogs with primary (nonpituitary) hypoadrenocorticism.

TECH ALERT

When determining the diagnosis in a vomiting dog with a high BUN and no kidney disease, think Addison disease.

TREATMENT

Acute Crisis Management

- Normal saline is the preferred fluid for intravenous administration; give 44 to 88 mL/kg initially.
- Administer dexamethasone sodium phosphate IV or prednisolone sodium succinate (Solu-Delta-Cortef) IV.
- Desoxycorticosterone pivalate (Percorten-V) IM or SQ or fludrocortisone acetate (Florinef) daily PO can also be used.

Chronic Management

- Give oral glucocorticoids for 3 to 4 weeks, tapering dose gradually. Prednisolone or prednisone should be given in daily doses, divided every 12 hours.
- Mineralocorticoid replacement requires Florinef in divided daily doses every 12 hours.
- Monitor electrolytes, BUN or creatine concentration, and clinical signs.

INFORMATION FOR CLIENTS

- Lack of mineralocorticoids is life threatening.
- Prognosis is excellent with medical treatment.
- Your pet will require periodic serum chemistry reevaluation.
- Most animals will need glucocorticoid supplementation in times of stress.
- In case of trauma, surgery, or other stressful situations, make sure that the treating veterinarian knows your pet has hypoadrenocorticism so that appropriate treatment can be provided.

Hyperadrenocorticism (Canine Cushing Syndrome)

Hyperadrenocorticism is rarely seen in cats, but it is common in dogs (Fig. 3-6). The term *canine Cushing syndrome* is applied to any disease state that results in hypersecretion of cortisol. Excessive secretion of cortisol may result from a pituitary lesion (excess ACTH)

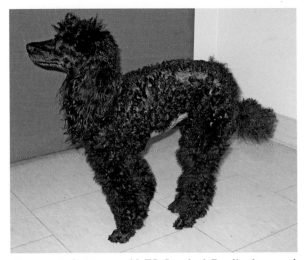

Figure 3-6 A 14-year-old FS Standard Poodle diagnosed with Cushing disease and demonstrating Cushing myopathy. Note the rigid extension in both thoracic and pelvic limbs. (From Lorenz MD, Coates JR, Kent M: *Handbook of veterinary neurology*, ed 5, St. Louis, MO, 2011, Saunders.)

or an adrenal tumor (excess cortisol). Hyperadrenocorticism frequently can be the result of overmedication with corticosteroids.

Pituitary-dependent hyperadrenocorticism (PDH) is seen most commonly in dogs weighing less than 20 kg. Breeds such as Poodles, Dachshunds, Terriers, Beagles, and German Shepherds are affected. Boston Terriers and Boxers have been reported to be at increased risk for development of this disease. Abnormal cells within the pituitary gland secrete excessive amounts of ACTH; this results in hyperplasia of the adrenal glands, which is subsequently followed by oversecretion of cortisol. Although increased cortisol concentration usually serves to cause the pituitary to discontinue ACTH secretion, in these dogs, the pituitary tissue does not respond normally.

Functioning adrenal tumors secrete excessive amounts of cortisol independent of pituitary control. Dogs with this form of the disease are typically Toy Poodles, German Shepherds, Dachshunds, Labrador Retrievers, and some Terrier breeds, with 45% to 50% weighing more than 20 kg.

Clinical signs of either type of Cushing disease are the result of excess cortisol. They are usually slow to develop and often go unnoticed by the owner.

CLINICAL SIGNS

- Dog >6 years of age (60%–65% are female)
- Pu or Pd
- Polyphagia
- Excessive panting
- Abdominal enlargement (related to abdominal muscle weakness); obesity
- Muscle weakness, lethargy, lameness
- Bilateral, symmetric alopecia; pruritus; pyoderma
- Calcinosis cutis (firm plaques of calcium under the skin), but infrequent
- Abnormal gonadal function: lack of estrus; soft, small testicles

DIAGNOSIS

Serum Chemistry Panel Abnormalities
- Increased ALP
- Increased ALT
- Increased cholesterol level
- Increased blood glucose concentration
- Decreased BUN concentration
- Lipemia

Urine Cortisol:Creatinine Ratios
- Increased urine cortisol:creatinine ratios
- Good for screening only

ACTH Stimulation Test
- Procedure is described in earlier section on hypoadrenocorticism (Addison disease).
  - PDH: 80% to 85% will be abnormal
  - Adrenal tumor: 20% to 40% may be normal

> **TECH ALERT**
>
> Hyperadrenocorticism may not be distinguishable from PDH and adrenal tumor.

Dexamethasone Suppression Test
- In the healthy animal, dexamethasone will suppress the pituitary secretion of ACTH, which, in turn, will decrease cortisol concentration within 2 to 3 hours and keep them suppressed for 8 to 24 hours.

- *Low Dose*
  - PDH: no change in cortisol concentration at 8 hours after injection
  - Adrenal tumor: no change in cortisol concentration

⬤ **TECH ALERT**

Procedure: Administer 0.01 mg/kg dexamethasone IV with samples at baseline (preinjection), 4 hours, and 8 hours after injection.
- High Dose
  - 0.1 mg/kg IV with samples at baseline and 8 hours after injection
  - PDH: suppression seen at high doses; 75% to 80% of dogs with PDH will have 50% suppression of cortisol concentration
  - Adrenal tumor: no suppression seen

TREATMENT

Surgical Removal
- One or both adrenal glands are removed.

Medical Management
- The most frequent treatment choice is o,p-DDD therapy (Lysodren, mitotane). The drug results in the necrosis of the zona fasciculata and zona reticularis; excessive doses will also affect the zona glomerulosa and reduce aldosterone concentration, producing Addison disease.
- The initial therapy requires mitotane, 50 mg/kg/day in divided doses, given after meals for 8 days. Monitor clinical signs for decrease in polyphagia and Pu or Pd. Repeat ACTH stimulation test every 7 to 10 days until cortisol concentrations are normal.
- Prednisone may be given during the loading dose regimen.
- Maintenance therapy requires the administration of o,p-DDD at a dose of every 7 days.
- Trilostane acts to inhibit adrenal synthesis of progesterone, a precursor of cortisol; has fewer side effects than mitotane; and must be given daily for the life of the patient.
- Other drugs used for treatment include the following:
  - Ketoconazole: twice daily for 7 days; if no side effects appear, increase to twice daily for 14 days

  - ʟ-Deprenyl (Selegiline): orally each day for pituitary dependent hyperadrenocorticism

INFORMATION FOR CLIENTS
- This is a serious disease.
- Animals will require lifelong treatment.
- Periodic monitoring is required.
- Overdoses with o,p-DDD are common.
- Clinical signs are identical to those in Addison disease. Report any lethargy, weakness, vomiting, or diarrhea.
- Prognosis: Average life expectancy is about 20 to 30 months, with frequent recurrence of clinical symptoms.

Parathyroid Disease

Parathyroid glands (two glands associated with each thyroid lobe) secrete parathyroid hormone (PTH), which controls serum calcium concentrations. PTH stimulates bone resorption (increases osteoclastic activity) and renal calcium resorption, and mediates intestinal calcium absorption. The action of PTH controls serum calcium levels within narrow limits.

Primary Hyperparathyroidism

Primary hyperparathyroidism is typically diagnosed in older dogs (7 to 11 years of age) and is infrequently diagnosed in cats. Keeshonden appear to be overrepresented in studies of the disease. (German Shepherds, Poodles, Retrievers, and Dobermans have also been reported.) No sex predilection appears to exist. Hypercalcemia results from the excessive secretion of PTH, which is usually caused by the presence of parathyroid adenoma or carcinoma. The disease may also be evident if the parathyroid gland is hyperplastic.

CLINICAL SIGNS

Many animals will show no clinical signs of primary hyperparathyroidism, and hypercalcemia will be diagnosed on routine serum chemistry examination. Signs usually appear as organ dysfunction occurs.
- Anorexia
- Vomiting
- Constipation
- Pu or Pd
- Listlessness, obtundation, coma, or all
- Urinary calculi, cystitis, or both

- Incontinence
- Weakness, exercise intolerance

DIAGNOSIS

Serum Chemistries

- Low to low-normal phosphorus concentrations
- BUN–creatinine concentration may be normal, unless renal involvement
- Serum alkaline phosphatase (SAP) level may be mildly increased
- Hypercalcemia is the hallmark of parathyroid disease (serum total calcium levels >12 mg/dL). However, other causes for hypercalcemia may need to be ruled out before making a diagnosis. Other causes for hypercalcemia include the following:
  - Sample error
  - Acidosis
  - Neoplasia (especially lymphosarcoma)
  - Addison disease
  - Rodenticide toxicosis
  - Acute renal failure
  - Septic bone disease
  - PTH "two-site" assay:
  - All dogs and cats with primary hyperparathyroidism have excessive concentrations of serum PTH. Results of this assay should be evaluated in conjunction with serum calcium levels

TECH ALERT

If calcium levels are increased, PTH levels should be decreased. Be suspicious if PTH levels are normal in the presence of increased calcium levels.

- Cervical ultrasonography: Results will depend on operator skill and experience. Most masses will be large enough to be visualized with ultrasonography (4–6 mm).

TREATMENT

- Surgical removal of affected parathyroid gland(s)
- Ultrasound-guided heat or chemical ablation of the parathyroid mass

Postoperative Management

- Postsurgical decreases in PTH levels may predispose animals to hypocalcemia. Animals should be hospitalized for 5 to 7 days to monitor total serum calcium concentrations daily. Postsurgical hypocalcemia is more likely in dogs whose presurgical calcium levels were greater than 14 mg/dL. These animals should receive vitamin D with or without calcium therapy immediately after recovery from surgery.
- Clinical signs of hypocalcemia include the following:
  - Panting
  - Muscle tremors, leg cramping, pain
  - Ataxia, stiff gait
  - Facial rubbing, biting of the feet
  - Focal or generalized seizures
- Calcium therapy
  - Calcium carbonate tablets
  - Calcium gluconate tablets, syrup
  - Calcium glubionate syrup
- Vitamin D therapy
  - Vitamin D2 capsules
  - Calcitriol (vitamin D3) capsules

INFORMATION FOR CLIENTS

- Most animals diagnosed with primary hyperparathyroidism show no clinical signs.
- Because hyperparathyroidism is often diagnosed on routine serum chemistry evaluation, it is important to obtain laboratory profiles yearly for all older animals.
- The prognosis for primary hyperparathyroidism is dependent on the severity of any secondary changes induced by increased calcium levels.
- Treatment with vitamin D and calcium will be lifelong. It must not be discontinued.

Hypocalcemia or Hypoparathyroidism

Numerous causes of hypocalcemia in dogs and cats have been reported. Parathyroid-related disease, chronic renal failure, acute pancreatitis, and puerperal tetany (eclampsia) are among the most common causes. Therapy for hypocalcemia resulting from parathyroid-related disease, chronic or acute renal failure, or acute pancreatitis includes correction of the underlying cause and vitamin D and calcium supplementation.

Parathyroid-Related Disease

The most common cause of hypocalcemia related to the parathyroid gland involves inadvertent surgical removal of the glands during a thyroidectomy or other neck surgery. Primary hypoparathyroidism is an uncommon disorder in both dogs and cats.

Chronic or Acute Renal Failure

Chronic renal failure is an extremely common disorder in dogs and cats and represents a common explanation for mild-to-moderate hypocalcemia. Hypocalcemia is usually related to the metabolic acidosis that develops with renal failure.

Acute Pancreatitis

Precipitation of calcium soaps within the pancreatic tissue may be related to the development of mild hypocalcemia.

Puerperal Tetany (Eclampsia)

Puerperal tetany secondary to hypocalcemia occurs most commonly in the postpartum period but may be seen in late gestation. It can be life threatening. Predisposing factors include improper perinatal nutrition, heavy lactation, and inappropriate calcium supplementation. The disease is seen most commonly in dogs and is uncommon in cats. Recognition of the clinical signs of eclampsia is important because therapy should begin immediately. The goal of treatment is to increase blood calcium levels with administration of intravenous infusions containing calcium.

The prognosis for eclampsia is good if treatment is prompt. An effort should be made to correct nutritional deficiencies and to diminish lactational demands of the dam. Hand-feeding or early weaning of the puppies, or both, is encouraged. Recurrence of eclampsia with subsequent pregnancies has been reported.

CLINICAL SIGNS

- Irritability
- Restlessness
- Salivation
- Facial pruritus
- Stiffness, ataxia
- Hyperthermia
- Tachycardia
- Muscle tremors and tonic-clonic contractions
- Seizures

DIAGNOSIS

- Treatment should not wait for laboratory confirmation of hypocalcemia
- Total serum calcium levels less than 6.5 mg/dL

TREATMENT

- Slow, intravenous infusion of 10% calcium gluconate solution (monitor heart rate and rhythm while administering calcium solutions)
- Diazepam IV to control seizures
- Oral supplementation of calcium should be started once the immediate symptoms are controlled
- Calcium carbonate tablets or capsules
- Calcium glubionate (Neo-Calglucon) syrup
- Improve the nutritional plane of the dam by feeding a balanced diet

INFORMATION FOR CLIENTS

- Avoid excessive calcium supplementation during pregnancy.
- Feed a well-balanced dog food; increase amounts fed as pregnancy progresses.
- Development of signs in a pregnant animal is an emergency situation. Call your veterinarian immediately.
- This disease may reoccur with subsequent pregnancies. Owners should reconsider using animals predisposed to eclampsia for breeding.
- Hand-feeding of puppies with supplemental feeds may be required until the dam's calcium levels stabilize. Early weaning may also be desired.

REVIEW QUESTIONS

1. Regulation of hormone levels within the body is through a _____ feedback system.
   a. Negative
   b. Positive
   c. Neutral
2. _____ is the most frequently seen disorder of the thyroid in dogs, whereas _____ is more common in cats.
   a. Hyperthyroidism; hypothyroidism
   b. Hypothyroidism; hyperthyroidism
   c. Hyperthyroidism; euthyroidism
   d. Euthyroidism; hypothyroidism

3. The treatment of choice for thyroid disease in cats is _____.
   a. Radioactive iodine therapy
   b. Surgical removal of the entire thyroid
   c. Tapazole given orally
4. Which laboratory test provides an accurate evaluation of the average blood glucose concentration over a specific period and may be used to monitor animals with diabetes?
   a. Urine dip sticks
   b. Daily serum glucose concentration
   c. Serum fructose concentration
5. An insulinoma is a functional tumor of the _____ cells of the pancreas.
   a. α
   b. β
   c. γ
6. Na:K ratios of <27:1 are indicative of:
   a. Cushing disease
   b. Addison disease
   c. Thyroid disease
   d. Diabetes mellitus
7. Only two endocrine diseases produce bilaterally symmetric alopecia. What are the two diseases?

8. The drug mitotane is primarily used to treat which type of hyperadrenocorticism?
   a. Pituitary-dependent hyperadrenocorticism
   b. Non–pituitary-dependent hyperadrenocorticism
   c. Both types
9. What is generally the long-term prognosis for dogs with an insulinoma?
   a. Excellent
   b. Good
   c. Poor
   d. Grave
10. In what period of gestation does eclampsia occur most commonly?
    a. Early
    b. Middle
    c. Late
    d. Postpartum
11. Serum calcium levels >12 mg/dL indicate disease of the:
    a. Thyroid gland
    b. Parathyroid gland
    c. Adrenal gland

Answers found on page 551.

4

CHAPTER

Diseases of the Eye

LEARNING OBJECTIVES

When you have completed this chapter, you will be able to:

1. Explain the structures of the eye and the purpose of each.
2. Describe how changes from normal result in clinical disease.
3. Discuss and demonstrate the proper treatments for common eye problems in small animals.

Special structures that exist in all animals help them survive in their environments. The special senses—sight, hearing, smell, and taste—are extensions of the central nervous system and are different from each other in their forms and functions. Problems involving sight and hearing are frequently seen in dogs and cats. This chapter focuses on ocular problems commonly seen in small-animal practice. The topic of deafness is discussed in Chapter 8.

The eye, made up of the globe and its accessory structures (Fig. 4-1), is perhaps the most highly developed of all the special senses. Its structure converts light into electrical impulses that travel to the brain and are interpreted as visual pictures.

The function of the eye depends on all components of the visual system functioning properly. Disruption of any of these components can result in abnormal vision for the animal. Although most pets can live

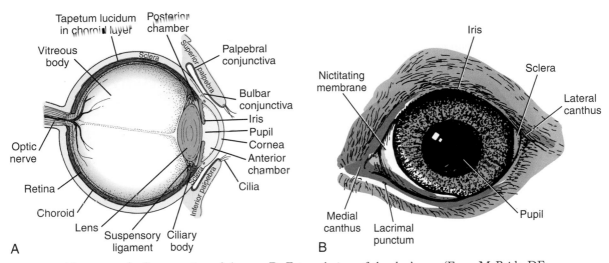

Figure 4-1 A, Cross-section of the eye. **B,** External view of the dog's eye. (From McBride DF: *Learning veterinary terminology,* ed 2, St. Louis, MO, 2002, Mosby, by permission.)

quality lives with a loss of vision, proper diagnosis and quick treatment of eye problems is essential if sight is to be preserved.

Diseases of the eye may be divided into three main categories:

1. Diseases that involve the accessory structures
2. Diseases that involve the structures within the globe
3. Disease that involves the retina and the neural pathways

Anatomy of the Eye

The structure of the animal eye is essentially the same as the human eye with some small differences. The globe of the eye is a three layered sphere. The outer layer of the globe is the *fibrous layer*, which is composed of the sclera (the white, caudal portion of the globe) and the cornea (the clear window that makes up the front of the sphere). The sclera is composed of tough fibrous tissue, which helps maintain the shape of the eye. The cornea is also part of the fibrous layer but is entirely different in appearance from the sclera. The cornea is transparent, lacking blood vessels but well supplied with nerve endings.

The outer surface of the cornea is composed of corneal epithelium. The inner surface of the cornea,

the basement membrane, is known as *Descemet membrane*. In between is the corneal stroma. Like epithelium elsewhere in the body, the cornea heals quickly when damaged. The space between the underside of the cornea and the iris (the colored portion of the eye) is called the *anterior chamber*. This space is filled with a waterlike substance that is continually being produced by the choroid. This fluid is drained from the anterior chamber through the *canal of Schlemm*, which is located at the junction of the cornea and the iris. This fluid is responsible for the *intraocular pressure*, and production of too much fluid or too little drainage results in *glaucoma*.

The second layer of the globe is the vascular layer. This layer is composed of the choroid, the ciliary bodies, and the iris. The choroid contains blood and lymph vessels plus pigment. Like the inside of a camera, the choroid's black color decreases stray light reflection in the interior of the eye. At the anterior portion of the choroid is a thickening of the tissue to form the ciliary bodies. Within this tissue lies the small ciliary muscle composed of both radial and circular smooth muscle fibers that close and open the pupil. Folds in the ciliary bodies form the ciliary processes, to which are attached the suspensory ligaments that blend with the capsule of the lens. By shortening, these ligaments cause the lens to change shape, allowing the eye to focus near and far with little effort (known as *accommodation)*. The fluid found in the anterior chamber is produced by these ciliary bodies. The iris is the last component of the vascular layer. The posterior surface of the iris is brown-black, like the choroid, but the anterior surface is what makes the eye beautiful. Whether the animal has emerald green, sky blue, or deeply brown eyes, it is often the first thing we notice when looking at our pets. In the middle of the iris is the pupil. Oblong, rectangular, or round, pupil shape varies by species and acts as the passageway for light from the anterior portion of the eye to the retina. Just behind the pupil sits the lens. By thickening or thinning, the lens lets the eye adjust for varying distances. Compression of lens fibers with age results in the gray cloudiness seen in older animals' eyes. This aging change, known as *lenticular* or *nuclear sclerosis*, is different from the thickened lens that results from disease states such as diabetes mellitus. A *cataract* is the result of changes that occur in the energy metabolism of the lens stroma. The change in the metabolism produces a structural change in proteins within the lens that result in it becoming less transparent.

The last layer of the globe is the nerve layer, the retina. Light entering the eye must pass completely through the retina to reach the photopigments responsible for generating electrical (nerve) impulses. These impulses must then pass back through the entire retina to reach the optic nerve. From there, impulses move toward the brain, decussating at the optic chiasm before entering the brain. Although it is unknown exactly what an animal sees, it is possible to say that its vision is somewhat different from ours. Canine and feline retinas have few cones that are responsible for color vision but have many rods, giving them good vision even in dim light. Dogs have *two* types of cones that allow them to see only in the blue and yellow-green range of the spectrum. Cats, however, have *three* sets of cones, similar to those found in humans, but probably see less color compared with their human counterparts. Experiments have shown that both dogs and cats see objects better if they are moving than if stationary.

The back of the animal eye has a structure not found in the human eye. The *tapedum* is a highly reflective area of the retina that reflects light within the eye allowing the animal to have much improved vision even in dim light conditions.

Diseases of the Accessory Structures

Diseases that involve the eyelids, conjunctiva, tear ducts, third eyelid, and the lacrimal glands may be included in the group of diseases of the accessory structures. Trauma to or infection of these tissues is a common reason for small animals to be presented to the veterinary hospital. Typical presenting signs include red eyes, blepharospasm (squinting), and ocular discharge. Many eye problems present with similar signs; a thorough clinical examination is needed before a treatment plan can be formulated.

Conjunctivitis

Canine conjunctivitis, or inflammation of the conjunctiva, is rarely a primary disease process; therefore, it is important for the veterinarian to discover the underlying cause to treat this condition effectively.

The conjunctiva is a highly vascular tissue. When injured, it responds by developing hyperemia (redness), chemosis (swelling), and ocular discharge. Dogs typically develop noninfectious conjunctivitis. Causes of noninfectious conjunctivitis in dogs include immune-mediated follicular conjunctivitis, allergic conjunctivitis (atopy), and anatomic conjunctivitis (ectropion or entropion). Bacterial conjunctivitis can develop in the dog as a result of the disruption of normal tear production, injury, or foreign bodies.

Feline conjunctivitis is primarily infectious. Feline herpes virus (FHV) is the most common cause of bilateral conjunctivitis in young kittens and is typically seen in conjunction with upper respiratory tract symptoms. FHV-1 virus replicates best in epithelial tissue that is slightly cooler than body temperature and therefore tends to infect the superficial epithelial tissues of the nasal, oral, and conjunctival regions.

Calicivirus may also cause a mild conjunctivitis in cats. *Chlamydia psittaci* infection may present as a unilateral problem with marked chemosis in some cats. Mycoplasmas have also been isolated from cases of feline conjunctivitis.

CLINICAL SIGNS

- Chemosis
- Hyperemia
- Ocular discharge (serous or purulent)
- Presence or absence of other signs of upper respiratory tract disease

DIAGNOSIS

- A complete physical examination is necessary to diagnose the primary disease.
- A thorough visual examination of the conjunctiva must be conducted to rule out foreign bodies or the presence of follicles.
- The Schirmer tear test is useful in recurrent cases.
- Conjunctival scraping may need to be performed, including cytology, culture, and sensitivity.

TREATMENT

- Treat to resolve the underlying systemic disease.
- Topical antibiotic ointments can be used:
  - Neomycin, bacitracin, or polymyxin B ointment: two to four times daily (general cases)
  - Gentamicin ophthalmic ointment: two to four times daily for bacterial infections
  - Antibiotic ointment with cortisone for cases that involve follicular or atopic conjunctivitis
- Nonsteroidal ointments and solutions may be necessary:
  - Ketorolac tromethamine 0.5%: four times daily for allergic conjunctivitis
  - Lodoxamide tromethamine 0.1%: four times daily for allergic conjunctivitis
- Keep eyes clear of dried exudate by cleaning with warm water and a cloth or a cotton ball.
- For viral conjunctivitis in cats, the following can be used:
  - Idoxuridine (IDU, Stoxil) 0.5%, every 4 to 5 hours
  - Viroptic Ophthalmic Solution 1% (Trifluridine) (B-W) 3%, 1 drop every 2 hours

INFORMATION FOR CLIENTS

- Prevent irritation of the conjunctiva in dogs by not allowing them to ride in cars with their heads out of the windows.
- Keep dried ocular discharge from accumulating in the medial canthus of the eye. Keep the area clean and dry. Remove excess hair that may trap exudate.
- Vaccinate kittens against respiratory viral disease per your veterinarian's schedule.
- When using ophthalmic medications, make sure not to touch the tip of the applicator to the eye; this will contaminate the container.
- Ointments provide longer tissue contact compared with solutions.
- Ophthalmic preparations must be applied frequently to be effective.
- Ask your technician to demonstrate the proper method for administering eye medication (Fig. 4-2).
- Discard any unused eye medications as soon as treatment is no longer needed. Do not save them for future use!

Epiphora

Epiphora, an overflow of tears, may be the result of overproduction of tears or faulty drainage by the lacrimal system. Overproduction of tears is always the result of ocular pain or irritation. Faulty functioning of the lacrimal drainage system may occur for several reasons, including blockage of the lacrimal duct by

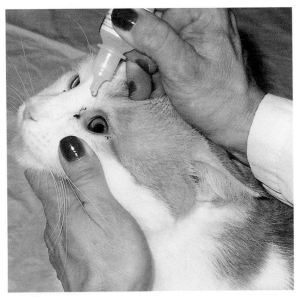

Figure 4-2 Placing eye medication on the lower palpebral border in a cat. (From McCurnin DM, Bassert JM: *Clinical textbook for veterinary technicians*, ed 7, St. Louis, MO, 2010, Saunders, by permission.)

swelling or inflammatory cells, imperforate puncta, or trauma.

Brachycephalic dogs and cats have large globes in shallow orbits, leaving little room for the accumulation of tears. Subsequently, tears spill out onto the face. Accumulations of hair or face folds may wick the tears onto the face in some animals. An entropion or ectropion may also result in faulty drainage of tears.

Surgical correction of lid position is the treatment of choice in animals with entropion or ectropion. Keeping the facial hair cut shorter may also be beneficial. Obstruction of the lacrimal puncta may occur in animals as a result of inflammation, the presence of foreign bodies, or accumulation of debris. Cocker Spaniels and Poodles typically have imperforate puncta (no opening to provide drainage). Many times, the obstruction can be removed by flushing the nasolacrimal ducts or surgically removing the tissue covering the puncta.

Facial hair or cilia originating from the meibomian glands of the lid may rub against the cornea, creating irritation and often corneal ulceration. Epiphora then results as a reflex against the pain created by the irritation. Treatment includes removal of the cilia or shortening of the facial hair and topical therapy.

CLINICAL SIGNS

- "Watering" of the eye—may be acute or chronic
- Wet facial hair in the medial canthus
- Secondary bacterial infection of the skin underlying the hair at the medial canthus
- Discoloration of the facial hair at the medial canthus

DIAGNOSIS

- Perform a complete eye examination to find the source of pain.
- Apply fluorescein dye to the eye. Dye that exits the nares indicates a patent nasolacrimal system in most patients.
- Dacryocystorhinography can be performed in recurring cases.

TREATMENT

- Treat the primary cause of ocular pain and irritation.
- Flush the lacrimal ducts to remove any obstructions (Fig. 4-3).
- Surgically open imperforate puncta.
- Apply a topical antibiotic ointment for 7 to 10 days.
- Keep facial hair trimmed to prevent contact with the cornea.

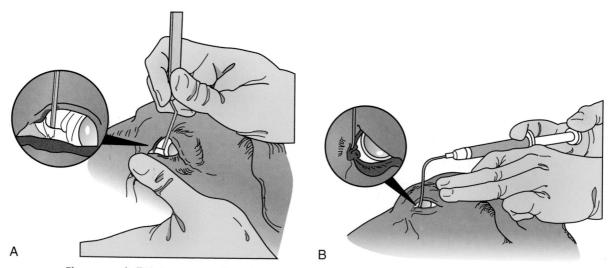

A   B

Figure 4-3 A, Dilating puncta of nasolacrimal duct with blunt metal probe. **B,** Flushing nasolacrimal duct.

- Keep facial hair trimmed in the eye area to prevent wicking of tears and accumulation of debris in the corner of the eye.
- The red stain seen on the hair of white or light-colored dogs is not blood but a pigment contained in the tears. It will not hurt the dog.
- In some breeds, epiphora may be a lifelong problem requiring continual maintenance.

Eyelid Diseases

The eyelids are important for ocular health. They protect the globe, help remove debris from the eye, shade the eye during sleep, and spread lubricating secretions over the eye. Eyelashes project from the border of each lid. At the base of each lash is a sebaceous gland, which produces a lubricating fluid for the hair follicles (glands of Zeis, or meibomian glands).

An abscess of the sebaceous gland is called a *hordeolum*, and it is usually the result of a staphylococcal infection. When the inflammation involves the meibomian glands and granuloma formation occurs, it is called a *chalazion*. Therapy for both these swellings includes warm compresses, manual expression, topical antibiotic ointment, and possibly surgical curettage.

When the eyelids themselves become inflamed, *blepharitis* results. Causative factors include bacterial infections (*Staphylococcus*), parasitic infections (*Demodex, Notoedres*), and mycotic infections (dermatophytes). Atopy may frequently present with inflamed and pruritic eyelids.

Eyelid neoplasms are frequently seen in older animals. Most tumors of the eyelids are benign and can be treated by surgical resection. Eyelid neoplasms in the cat are usually malignant. Squamous cell carcinomas are the most common type of tumor.

Blepharitis

Blepharitis is defined as a swelling of the eyelids. Causes include exposure to allergens, nutritional deficiencies, viral infections, or dermatitis from any cause. Symptoms include edema of the lids with redness, discharge, and spasms of the lids.

- Swelling at the lid margin or generalized swelling of the lid

- Periocular pruritus
- Periocular alopecia
- Rubbing of the eyes

- Careful examination of the eyes and the lids must be made; this may require magnification.
- Skin scraping of periorbital area is often necessary.
- Fungal cultures should be obtained.
- Bacterial cultures should be obtained.

- Warm compresses should be applied to reduce swelling.
- Express hordeolum, or remove chalazion.
- Topical antibiotic ointments or systemic antibiotics can be applied:
  - Chloramphenicol (ophthalmic)
  - Gentamicin (ophthalmic ointment or drops)
  - Tetracycline (ophthalmic)
  - Bacitracin, neomycin, or polymixin B (Schering-Plough)
  - Mycitracin
  - Optiprime
  - Trioptics
  - Neo-Predef
- Corticosteroid: prednisolone twice daily for 10 to 14 days, then gradually reduce dose
- Mycotic: topical antifungal solutions such as Conofite or Tresaderm (before you apply these around the eye, place protective ointment into the eye)

- Warm packs applied to the swollen, painful eyelids may provide relief for the animal. Use a cotton ball soaked in warm water, soak a cloth in warm water and ring well to remove excess water, or use a hot pack *warmed* in the microwave (take care not to make it too hot).
- Remove exudate from the corners of the eye several times daily using a soft, wet cloth or cotton ball.

Entropion and Ectropion

Entropion and ectropion defects involve eyelids that either roll in against the cornea (entropion) or roll outward, exposing the cornea (ectropion). In either case, the lids are incapable of performing their protective functions for the eye, and disease may result.

Entropion is common in dogs but less common in cats. Entropion exists in three main forms: (1) congenital (inherited), (2) acquired nonspastic, and (3) acquired spastic. The congenital form includes those breeds predisposed to entropion because of large orbits with deep-set eyes, which provide inadequate lid support. The lid droops over the lower orbital rim and inverts. Collies, Great Danes, Irish Setters, Doberman Pinschers, Golden Retrievers, Rottweilers, and Weimaraners are breeds that exhibit congenital entropion.

Several breeds are predisposed to poor muscular development that involves the ocular muscles. Chesapeake Bay Retrievers, Labrador Retrievers, Chow Chows, and Samoyeds may exhibit this condition, although it is not well documented. A large number of breeds are predisposed to entropion from primary lid deformities.

The cause of acquired nonspastic entropion is usually surgical or traumatic, resulting in scarring of the lid with contraction. This causes the lid to turn inward toward the globe. The third form of entropion, acquired spastic, is the most commonly observed form in cats. This form of entropion usually occurs secondary to painful corneal lesions, conjunctival inflammation, or both.

Ectropion is the reverse of entropion. In this condition, the lid is excessive and droops outward. Ectropion is a natural breed characteristic in Basset Hounds, Bloodhounds, Cocker Spaniels, Clumber Spaniels, English Bulldogs, and Saint Bernards. In these animals, the condition is usually asymptomatic. In any breed, however (even the ones listed above), ectropion can develop clinical symptoms. Acquired ectropion can form secondary to muscular disease in senile dogs that lose muscle tone and in dogs that have had overcorrection of an entropion.

CLINICAL SIGNS

Entropion
- Rolling inward of the lid margin(s)
- Epiphora
- Chemosis
- Conjunctival erythema, conjunctivitis
- Blepharospasm

- Pain
- Presence or absence of corneal ulceration
- Photophobia

Ectropion
- Lid eversion
- Conjunctivitis
- Epiphora
- Keratitis, usually from exposure
- Purulent exudate

DIAGNOSIS

- Observe the lids and their interaction with the globe.
- Complete an evaluation of other structures of the eye, especially the cornea, conjunctiva, and lid margins.
- The evaluation of lid inversion or eversion should be done while the patient is awake to prevent overcorrection or undercorrection of the defect.

TREATMENT

Entropion
- Surgical correction is suggested:
  - Temporary vertical mattress suture placement to evert the eye (young animals)
  - Lateral canthoplasty to shorten the lid
  - Hotz–Celsus procedure: an elliptical piece of tissue is removed from under the eye to evert the lid into a normal position

Ectropion
- Surgical correction is recommended if clinical signs are present:
  - V plasty procedure to shorten the lid
  - Lateral blepharoplasty
  - V-Y plasty if scar tissue has contracted the lid in an everted position

INFORMATION FOR CLIENTS

- You may want to avoid purchasing breeds predisposed to entropion or ectropion.
- Carefully examine puppies for these defects before purchasing them. Dogs usually do not "outgrow" these conditions.
- Correction of these defects will provide normal lid function and save the globe from damage by

preventing overexposure to the environment and by reducing contact with the lid margins.

Hypertrophy of Nictitans Gland (Cherry Eye)

The nictitating membrane (third eyelid) is important as a protective structure. It assists in spreading the precorneal tear film and covers the eye to protect it from injury. It also produces about 50% of the lacrimal fluid.

The membrane is composed of a T-shaped cartilaginous skeleton embedded in the superficial gland of the third eyelid. The tissue undergoes what has been described as passive forward displacement when the eye is withdrawn into the orbit. This action results in prolapse of the third eyelid.

Hypertrophy of the gland (cherry eye) occurs only in dogs. The cause is unknown; however, there is a breed predisposition (Basset Hound, Beagle, Boston Terrier, Cocker Spaniel). When this condition is present, the medial canthus is filled with the red, swollen, nictitating membrane, which resembles a small cherry. This is usually seen in young dogs (< 2 years old). When the condition occurs in older animals and in cats, the cause is usually related to neoplasia of the tissue comprising the third eyelid.

CLINICAL SIGNS

- Reddened enlargement of tissue in the medial canthus of the eye
- Mild irritation, usually no pain
- Epiphora
- Presence or absence of conjunctival irritation

DIAGNOSIS

- Clinical signs
- Predisposed breed
- Tumor has been ruled out in older dogs and cats

TREATMENT

- Surgical replacement of the gland using tack-down procedures
- *Avoid* excision of the gland, as it will predispose the animal to keratoconjunctivitis sicca (KCS) later in life. Excision should be used only in cases of neoplasia of the gland.

INFORMATION FOR CLIENTS

- Surgery is the only method of correction.
- Without surgery, the animal may suffer corneal damage, which may affect eyesight.

Diseases of the Eye

Glaucoma

The eyeball represents a relatively closed system housed in a bony orbit. An increase in the contents of the globe results in increased intraocular pressure (IOP) because expansion is limited. In the healthy eye, the production of aqueous fluid is equal to the amount leaving the eye, and the IOP remains fairly constant. If more aqueous fluid is produced than leaves the eye, glaucoma results.

Normal canine and feline IOP ranges from 12 to 22 mm Hg. Values greater than 30 mm Hg are diagnostic of glaucoma. Most canine glaucoma cases result from decreased outflow of aqueous fluid as opposed to increased production. IOP may be measured by using a Schiotz tonometer or a Tono-Pen (Tono-Pen Vet, Medtronic).

Glaucoma may be primary or secondary. Primary glaucoma is an inherited defect that affects both eyes. Cocker Spaniels, Basset Hounds, and Chow Chows are predisposed to primary glaucoma. Secondary glaucoma results from obstruction of the drainage angles secondary to another disease process such as a neoplasm, uveitis, lens luxation, or hemorrhage.

Glaucoma may also be acute or chronic. Acute development of severely elevated IOP (>60 mm Hg) can produce blindness within hours because of disruption of retinal ganglion cells and retinal circulation. The goal of treatment is to decrease IOP rapidly to prevent permanent injury.

Sustained IOP in chronic glaucoma produces a painful, blind eye, which is unresponsive to medical therapy. Salvage procedures to make the pet more comfortable are the only recommended treatments.

CLINICAL SIGNS

Acute
- Ocular pain
- Conjunctival and episcleral injection (vascular congestion)

- Diffuse corneal edema
- Dilated pupil, unresponsive or sluggish to light
- Animal may or may not be blind on presentation

Chronic

- Buphthalmus (enlarged globe)
- Corneal striae
- Optic disk cupping
- Pain
- Blindness

DIAGNOSIS

- Measured IOP 30 mm Hg
- Clinical signs
- Rule out lens luxation as cause

TREATMENT

Acute

 TECH ALERT

This is a true emergency.

- Latanoprost (Xalatan 0.005%): 1 drop every 24 hours to facilitate aqueous outflow
- Intravenous (IV) mannitol: slowly over 20 to 30 minutes
- Oral dichlorphenamide (Daranide; Merck, Whitehouse Station, N.J.): every 8 hours orally (PO); decreases aqueous humor production
- Topical pilocarpine (pilocarpine 2%): instill into the eye every 8 hours; used to increase aqueous outflow
- Timolol 0.5% (Timoptic, Merck): can be used in combination with carbonic anhydrase inhibitors such as Daranide
- Treatment may include one or more of the preceding drugs depending on the clinical presentation and personal experience

Surgical

- Procedures that decrease aqueous production by destroying part of the ciliary body:
  - Transscleral cryosurgery
  - Laser cyclophotocoagulation

TECH ALERT

Transscleral cryosurgery and laser cyclophotocoagulation may cause postoperative increases in IOP that may result in permanent blindness. The laser method seems to produce better results with fewer side effects.

- Procedures that increase outflow of aqueous fluid: These are usually expensive and require referral to a specialty practice.

Chronic

- For a blind, painful eye, surgery is the treatment of choice to relieve the pain.
  - Enucleation
  - Intraocular evisceration with an implant
  - Ciliary ablation using gentamicin intravitreal injection

INFORMATION FOR CLIENTS

- Have your pet examined immediately when signs of a red, swollen, painful eye occur. This may be a true emergency, and vision can be quickly lost if treatment is postponed.
- This condition will require lifelong treatment.
- The disease is progressive.
- Even with proper treatment, vision may be lost in the affected eye as the disease progresses.
- Blind animals can live happy, comfortable lives. Their extra senses allow them to adjust well to the loss of sight.
- Avoid moving or changing a blind pet's environment too rapidly. They need time to adjust.
- Breeds that are predisposed to glaucoma include Cocker Spaniels, Basset Hounds, Miniature Poodles, Boston Terriers, Dalmatians, Arctic breeds, and Beagles.
- Enucleation (removal of the affected eye) will relieve the severe pain that results from glaucoma and will greatly improve the animal's quality of life.
- Glaucoma is a bilateral disease even if one eye shows no symptoms. The asymptomatic eye must be monitored.

Ulcerative Keratitis (Corneal Ulcers)

The cornea is the "window" of the eye and is composed of four layers: (1) the epithelium, (2) the stroma, (3) Descemet membrane, and (4) the endothelium. The epithelial covering provides a barrier to microorganisms entering the eye. A corneal ulcer is a full-thickness loss of corneal epithelium that exposes the underlying stroma. Causes of ulceration include trauma, chemicals, foreign objects, diseases such as KCS, and conformational abnormalities. In cats, herpes virus can directly invade the corneal epithelium and produce ulceration.

Patients usually present with pain, epiphora, blepharospasm, and conjunctival hyperemia. Diagnosis involves using fluorescein dye, which is absorbed well by the corneal stroma but not by intact corneal epithelium. The ulcerated area will fluoresce green when exposed to light with a cobalt blue filter.

Corneal epithelium will heal rapidly as cells divide and migrate. Treatment of uncomplicated ulcers includes application of topical atropine ointment to decrease pain and a topical antibiotic ointment. In most cases, ulcers will heal within several days. If the ulcers do not heal, alternative methods of treatment should be considered.

Distichiasis (hairs from the meibomian glands on the inner lid surface), ectopic cilia, and trichiasis (normal hairs that rub on the cornea) are frequent causes of ulcers in some breeds. A thorough examination of the eyelids is required (under magnification) to find these culprits.

Infected ulcers may also heal slowly. A culture and sensitivity should be obtained if infection is suspected. Indolent ulcers (Boxer ulcers) fail to heal even after weeks of therapy. The epithelium is usually undermined at the edge of the ulcer, preventing migration of healing tissue across the lesion. Treatment may involve a grid keratectomy or a superficial keratectomy.

CLINICAL SIGNS

- Epiphora
- Blepharospasm
- Hyperemia of conjunctiva

DIAGNOSIS

- Fluorescein dye applied to the cornea will have a green fluorescence under cobalt blue light if epithelium is not intact.

- Complete a thorough eye examination—look for aberrant cilia or hairs and foreign material. Be sure to look under the third eyelid.
- Perform a culture and sensitivity if you suspect an infectious agent.

TREATMENT

- Topical atropine 1% ointment can be used to decrease pain and blepharospasm.
- Topical broad-spectrum antibiotic ophthalmic ointment can be used four to six times daily.
- Surgery is another option:
  - Grid keratotomy (does not appear to improve healing time in cats)
  - Superficial keratotomy
  - Eyelid flaps
  - Conjunctival flaps
  - Contact lenses
- Serum: Prepare patient serum from a blood sample. Apply 1 drop into the eye every 2 to 4 hours daily. Recheck in 24 to 48 hours for healing.

INFORMATION FOR CLIENTS

- Most ulcers will heal quickly with treatment.
- Avoid using old medications you may have in the refrigerator to treat a red, watering eye.
- Medications that contain cortisone will retard healing and make the ulcer worse.
- Discard any ophthalmic medications after the prescribed period of use.
- Ulcers that involve dissolution of the corneal epithelium, indolent ulcers, or ulcers that involve Descemet's membrane are serious and will require aggressive treatment.
- When using ophthalmic medications, take care not to touch the eye or the tissue around the eye with the end of the medicine container. This will result in contamination of the medication.
- Frequent rechecks by your veterinarian are necessary to follow the healing of your pet's ulcer.

Chronic Superficial Keratitis (Pannus)

The term *pannus* is used to describe superficial corneal vascularization and infiltration of granulation tissue. The disease is progressive, bilateral, and degenerative, and potentially can result in blindness. Lesions typically begin at the limbus and progressively enlarge to involve the entire cornea. The cause is thought to be immune mediated, and middle-aged animals living at elevations greater than 5000 feet are most susceptible. Increased levels of ultraviolet light also increase incidence. Breeds commonly associated with the development of pannus include the German Shepherd, Belgian Tervuren, Border Collie, Greyhound, and Siberian Husky. Lesions typically involve infiltration of the cornea with lymphocytes and plasma cells. Treatment is lifelong and is aimed at lesion regression and control.

CLINICAL SIGNS

- Breed predisposed to disease with opaque lesion beginning at the limbus and extending into the cornea (may be pink or tan)

DIAGNOSIS

- Perform a corneal scraping. Positive cytology will show lymphocytic–plasmocytic infiltrate.
- Complete a thorough eye examination to rule out KCS, corneal ulcers, or other pathologies.

TREATMENT

- Antiinflammatory agents for the life of the patient include the following:
  - Topical cyclosporine A (Optimmune) four times daily
  - 1% prednisolone acetate (AK-Tate)
  - 1% prednisolone sodium phosphate (AK-Pred)
  - 0.1% dexamethasone ophthalmic (AK-Dex)
- Subconjunctival injection may be necessary: triamcinolone acetonide (Vetalog) 0.1 mL for 2 weeks or methylprednisolone acetate (Depo-Medrol): g/mL; 0.2 mL for 3 weeks
- Cryosurgery with liquid nitrogen is also an option.
- Superficial keratectomy will be required if all other treatments fail and loss of vision occurs.

INFORMATION FOR CLIENTS

- No cure exists for pannus. Treatment to maintain regression of the lesion will be lifelong.
- If treatment is inconsistent or discontinued, the lesion will return and continue to expand.
- Dogs living at higher altitudes and exposed to ultraviolet radiation (sunlight) are at greater risk of acquiring this disease.

Keratoconjunctivitis Sicca

Continuous production and distribution of tears are necessary for maintaining a healthy cornea. Tears clean, lubricate, nourish, reduce bacteria, and aid in healing. The tear film is composed of three layers. The lipid layer is secreted by the meibomian glands and aids in tear distribution. The aqueous layer, which is produced by the lacrimal glands and makes up the bulk of tear volume, contains immunoglobulins, enzymes, glucose, proteins, ions, and salts. The mucous, or innermost, layer is secreted by the conjunctival goblet cells and aids in the adhesion of the tear layer to the corneal surface.

Dogs and cats have two lacrimal glands, one located in the lateral superior orbit and one at the base of the third eyelid. Approximately 70% of the total tear volume is produced by the orbital gland. The nictitans is responsible for the remaining 30% of production. Loss of both glands (atrophy) produces KCS.

Causes of KCS include viral infections, drug-related toxicities, immune-mediated disease, inflammation, breed predisposition, and congenital anomalies. Most cases are idiopathic, but the disease tends to occur in older animals (usually >7 years). The disease is more common in neutered animals because loss of sex hormones decreases tear production. Diagnosis requires a complete medical history and a comprehensive physical examination. Treatment is aimed at restoring tear production and controlling secondary infections.

CLINICAL SIGNS

- Recurrent conjunctivitis, corneal ulcers, keratitis
- Cornea and conjunctiva appear dull, dry, and irregular
- Tenacious mucoid ocular discharge on lid margins and in the medial canthus
- Blepharospasm
- Crusty nares
- Diagnosis
- Schirmer tear test: values >15 mm/min on repeat testing (reference values: dogs: 15–25 mm/min; cats: 11–23 mm/min)
- Corneal fluorescein staining to show ulcers

TREATMENT

- Tear stimulation: cyclosporine (Optimmune), apply to eye every 8 hours; oral pilocarpine 2%,

1 to 2 drops/9 kg body weight in food twice daily (side effects include salivation, vomiting, diarrhea, and bradycardia)
- Topical artificial tear ointments:
  - Duolube (Bausch & Lomb, Rochester, NY)
  - Hypo Tears (IOLab, Claremont, CA)
  - Lacri-Lube (Allergan, Buckinghamshire, United Kingdom)

◉ TECH ALERT

Ointments remain in contact with the cornea longer than solutions and require less frequent applications.

- Topical antibiotic ointments (broad spectrum): neomycin-bacitracin-polymyxin
- *Avoid* atropine, contact lenses, topical anesthetics, and corticosteroids if ulceration is present
- Surgery: if all other medical treatments are unsuccessful—parotid duct transposition

INFORMATION FOR CLIENTS

- The prognosis for resolution is guarded.
- Treatment will need to continue for the life of the animal.
- About 15% to 20% of patients may exhibit remission with return of tear production.
- Failure to treat these animals will result in blindness.

Cataracts

The most common disease involving the lens is cataract formation. A *cataract* may be defined as an opacity of the lens sufficient to cause a reduction in visual function. Cataracts are a frequent cause of blindness in dogs but also are seen occasionally in cats. Most cataracts in dogs are inherited, but cataracts may also occur secondary to diabetes mellitus, hypocalcemia, trauma, nutritional deficiencies, electric shock, uveitis, or lens luxation.

Cataracts must be differentiated from senile nuclear (lenticular) sclerosis, a normal change in aging animals. Aging cells within the lens become dehydrated and overlap each other, producing a central change in the reflection of light. The lens may appear gray and opaque; however, with lenticular sclerosis, vision is maintained, and the ocular fundus is visible by ophthalmoscopy.

Surgical removal of a primary cataract is the only means of treatment and should be considered if the animal has bilateral cataracts with significantly impaired vision or if the animal is unable to maintain a normal lifestyle. Before surgery, it is important to establish the integrity of the retina and visual pathways. Removal of a cataract is unnecessary if vision has been lost to concurrent retinal or optic nerve disease. The electroretinogram (ERG) provides the most reliable criteria for retinal evaluation; however, it is limited to use in referral centers. If visual pathways are intact, cataract surgery can successfully restore the animal's sight.

Cataracts that result secondary to other disease states will require medical management of those diseases before surgical removal.

CLINICAL SIGNS

- Progressive loss of vision
- Opaque pupillary opening (usually noticed by owner)
- Signs related to systemic diseases such as diabetes mellitus or hypocalcemia

DIAGNOSIS

- Perform a complete ophthalmologic examination.
- Assess vision based on completion of an obstacle course, lack of menace response, and failure to track visual responses (use cotton balls).
- Pupillary light response is usually normal.
- Test serum chemistries to rule out concurrent systemic disease.
- ERG should be used to rule out retinal degeneration or optic nerve disease.

TREATMENT

- Surgical removal of the cataract is necessary.
- Treatment of any other disease that may result in the formation of the cataract must be completed first.

INFORMATION FOR CLIENTS

- Most cataracts are inherited, so affected animals should not be used for breeding.
- Certain breeds are prone to cataract, retinal degeneration, or both.

- Many animals can have quality lives even with bilateral cataracts.
- To decrease the chance of postoperative complications, most surgeons will remove only one cataract.
- Surgery requires referral to a veterinary ophthalmologist with special training; this is expensive.
- Function of the visual pathway must be ensured before surgery.

Anterior Uveitis

The uvea is the pigmented vascular tunic located between the fibrous and nervous tunics. It includes the iris, the ciliary body, and the choroid. Inflammation of this tissue is known as *uveitis*.

Anterior uveitis may have several causative factors: trauma, extension of local infections, foreign bodies, neoplasm, or thermal trauma. Bacterial, viral, and mycotic diseases may undergo hematogenous spread to the uvea. Parasites and protozoa also may affect the tissue. Some cases may be immune mediated. Whatever the cause, the symptoms will be similar; prompt treatment will be needed to prevent permanent damage to the eye.

CLINICAL SIGNS

- Epiphora
- Blepharospasm
- Photophobia
- Presence or absence of vision defects
- Corneal edema (cornea will be gray or white)
- Chemosis of the conjunctiva
- Scleral injection
- Prolapsed third eyelid
- Pain
- Change in color of the iris, if chronic

DIAGNOSIS

- Clinical signs
- History
- Complete blood cell count, serum chemistries to rule out systemic disease
- Immunology screening panel to rule out brucellosis, toxoplasmosis, blastomycosis, cryptococcosis, leptospirosis, infectious canine hepatitis (ICH), feline infectious peritonitis, and feline leukemia virus (FeLV) infection
- Radiography or ultrasound examination of the eye

- Tonometry: IOP may be low (4–8 mm Hg) or increased (>27 mm Hg)

TREATMENT

- Identify and eliminate the immediate cause of the uveitis, if possible.
- Control inflammation.
  - Topical steroids: dexamethasone ophthalmic ointment every 4 to 6 hours
  - Flunixin meglumine (Banamine): IV in dogs only, once daily

⬤ TECH ALERT

Do not use Banamine in dogs taking aspirin.

- Aspirin: three times daily in dogs; q48h in cats (only under a veterinarian's supervision)
- Atropine 1% ophthalmic ointment helps restore the integrity of vascular permeability and prevent adhesions of the lens to the iris by dilating the pupil. Use every 4 hours until dilated, then decrease to maintain mydriasis (dilation).

INFORMATION FOR CLIENTS

- The prognosis is excellent for uncomplicated cases.
- Most of the diseases that can result in secondary anterior uveitis are extremely serious and may not be curable.
- Diagnosis and treatment of the initial disease may be costly and prolonged.
- Without treatment, vision will eventually be lost.

Progressive Retinal Atrophy

The inner posterior portion of the eye is composed of the retina, the neural tunic of the eyeball where the visual pathway begins. Located within the optic disc, the optic nerve exits each eye and extends toward the brain. Arteries and veins fan out from the nerve to nourish the anterior surface of the retina. Within the retina are the photoreceptor cells (rods and cones) that are responsible for light sensing. Rods are functional for black-and-white vision and low-light situations, whereas the cones are bright-light receptors and are responsible for color vision. The retina must be functioning normally for vision to occur.

Progressive retinal atrophy is the term used to describe a group of hereditary retinal disorders seen in many breeds of dogs. The disease is common in Toy Poodles, Miniature Poodles, Golden Retrievers, Irish Setters, Cocker Spaniels, Miniature Schnauzers, Collies, Samoyed, Gordon Setters, and Norwegian Elkhounds. Inheritance has been shown to be by an autosomal recessive gene in several of these breeds. There is no sex predilection. Signs of the disease can be detected in some breeds of dogs as young as 6 months old (Irish Setters, Collies) and in others by middle age (Poodles). Clinical signs are usually slow to develop; a loss of night or low-light vision occurs first. As the disease progresses, day vision may be affected. Cataracts often develop in the affected eye. Diagnosis is through a complete ophthalmoscopic examination and an ERG. The end-stage lesions are those of retinal thinning with retinal nerve atrophy and vascular attenuation. No cure or treatment exists.

Retinal atrophy does occur in cats but not as frequently as in dogs. Central retinal degeneration in cats is related to a taurine-deficient diet.

CLINICAL SIGNS

- Defective night vision
- Slowly progressive loss of day vision
- Cataract formation

DIAGNOSIS

- Perform complete blood count and serum chemistries to rule out other causes of cataracts or loss of vision, or both.
- Ophthalmologic examination of the retina early on will show a gray, granular appearance of the peripheral tapetal retina. Under bright light, the area may appear hyperreflective. As the disease progresses, the retina will become thinner, resulting in increased reflectivity. End-stage lesions will include severe vascular attenuation and optic nerve atrophy.
- ERG is abnormal.

TREATMENT

- No treatment currently exists.

INFORMATION FOR CLIENTS

- Progressive retinal atrophy is an inherited disease. Avoid buying breeds affected by this defect unless the animal has had a complete eye examination by a board-certified veterinary ophthalmologist and the animal is certified free of the disease.
- Blind animals seem to adapt well to their familiar environment and will have trouble only when placed in strange surroundings.
- Cats must be fed a taurine-rich diet to avoid retinal degeneration.

REVIEW QUESTIONS

1. Progressive retinal atrophy should be screened for in puppies of (list all that apply):
   a. Collies
   b. Golden Retrievers
   c. Basset Hounds
   d. Beagles
2. With entropion, the eyelids would tend to:
   a. Roll outward away from the cornea
   b. Roll inward toward the cornea
   c. Contain excess cilia
   d. Lack meibomian glands
3. An abscess of the meibomian gland is called a:
   a. Hordeolum
   b. Chalazion
   c. Keratoma
4. "Cherry eye" (benign hyperplasia) occurs only in the dog.
   a. True
   b. False
5. Normal intraocular pressure (IOP) in the dog and cat is:
   a. Between 5 and 10 mm Hg
   b. Between 12 and 22 mm Hg
   c. Between 22 and 30 mm Hg
   d. Between 30 and 45 mm Hg
6. Acute glaucoma with pressures greater than 60 mm Hg can result in blindness within:
   a. Less than 15 minutes
   b. 1 hour
   c. After 24 hours
   d. Several hours
7. Which types of cells within the cornea accumulate in chronic superficial keratitis (pannus)?
   a. Neutrophils and lymphocytes
   b. Mast cells and monocytes
   c. Plasma cells and lymphocytes
   d. Eosinophils and monocytes

8. Lenticular sclerosis must be differentiated from what other lens dysfunction?
   a. Luxation
   b. Cataract
9. What medication is used to increase tear production in the disease known as keratoconjunctivitis sicca (KCS)?
   a. Triple antibiotic ophthalmic
   b. Cyclosporine ophthalmic
   c. Gentamicin ophthalmic
   d. Daranide ophthalmic

10. What is the most common cause of bilateral conjunctivitis in young kittens?
    a. Feline leukemia virus
    b. Calicivirus
    c. Feline viral rhinotracheitis
    d. Feline immunodeficiency virus

Answers found on page 551.

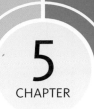

Hematologic and Immunologic Diseases

Anemia
Antibody
Antigen

Dyscrasia
Endemic
Methemoglobinemia

Spherocytes
Thrombocytopenia

OUTLINE

Blood
Red Cells (Erythrocytes)
Erythrocyte Disorders
 Anemia Caused by Hemorrhage
 Iron-Deficiency Anemia
 Hemolysis
 Blood-Borne Parasites
 Toxin-Induced or Heinz Body Anemias
 Immune-Mediated Hemolytic Anemia
Thrombocytes (Platelets)
 Immune-Mediated Thrombocytopenia

Leukocytes
 Ehrlichiosis
 von Willebrand Disease
Lymphoma
 Feline Lymphoma
 Mediastinal Lymphoma
 Alimentary Lymphoma
 Multicentric Lymphoma
 Canine Lymphoma
 Feline Immunovirus (Feline Acquired
  Immunodeficiency Syndrome)

LEARNING OBJECTIVES

When you have completed this chapter, you will be able to:

1. Describe the cellular components of blood.
2. Relate changes in blood components to common blood diseases seen in dogs and cats.

3. Discuss with owners treatment options for specific blood dyscrasias seen in dogs and cats.

Immune-mediated and hematologic disorders are commonly seen in veterinary practice. Although these diseases may be interrelated in some cases, this chapter discusses the most important diseases as individual entities. Knowledge of hematology and the functions of the immune system will assist the student in understanding these diseases.

Blood

Blood is the only liquid connective tissue in the body. It is a multifunctional tissue, and without it, the animal cannot survive. The functions of blood include temperature regulation, pH balance, nutritional transport and waste disposal, hormone transport, and immune response. Blood is composed of the cellular components: *erythrocytes* (red blood cells [RBCs]), *leukocytes* (white blood cells [WBCs]) and *thrombocytes* (platelets), and the liquid component, *plasma*. In the majority of our companion animals the cellular components make up about 45% of the blood, whereas the plasma fraction is close to 55% of the total blood volume. The approximate total blood volume of any animal can be calculated using the following formula:

$$\text{Body weight (lb)} \times 0.08 \times 500 \text{ mL/lb} = \text{approximate blood volume}$$

or

$$\text{Body weight (kg)} \times 0.08 \times 1000 \text{ mL/kg} = \text{approximate blood volume}$$

Red Blood Cells (Erythrocytes)

RBCs are produced in the red bone marrow found in the epiphyses of long bones and in flat bones such as the ribs, the sternum, or the pelvis. Each RBC is packed with an oxygen-carrying pigment called *hemoglobin* but no organelles. After leaving bone marrow as reticulocytes, they mature into adult RBCs, unable to reproduce and destined for removal within 100 days or so. Because the life of each RBC includes millions of trips through small capillaries, the cell membrane of the RBC is very flexible; however, as the cell ages, it tends to lose its flexibility and eventually is removed from circulation by the spleen or the liver to be replaced by new, fresh, flexible cells. Stem cells within bone marrow constantly replace lost or damaged RBCs. The main job of the RBC is to carry oxygen from the lungs to cells and to remove carbon dioxide and waste products from tissues.

The number of RBCs remains fairly constant throughout the life of the animal and can be estimated as the *packed cell volume (PVC)* or calculated as the *hematocrit (HCT)*.

Erythrocyte Disorders

Erythrocyte disorders are frequently diagnosed in dogs and cats and may be associated with decreased production, increased destruction, or inappropriate loss of RBCs (hemorrhage). Included in this category of disorders are anemias, hemorrhage, and neoplasia.

Anemia is one of the most common laboratory findings encountered in veterinary medicine and is usually secondary to a primary disorder elsewhere in the body. The major causes of anemia are varied and include hemorrhage, hemolysis, blood parasites, iron deficiencies, immune-mediated disease, and toxins.

A systematic diagnostic approach to anemia is necessary and should include a thorough history, physical examination, and a complete blood count (CBC), including blood films. Treatment should be aimed at correcting the primary disorder and supporting the patient. Therefore, it is important to establish whether the anemia is *regenerative* or *nonregenerative*. This can be done by evaluating the reticulocyte count. Regenerative anemias are usually the result of hemorrhage or hemolysis, whereas nonregenerative cases may involve bone marrow.

Anemia Caused by Hemorrhage

The most common cause of hemorrhage is trauma, although platelet abnormalities and abnormal clotting chemistries must be considered when determining the diagnosis. Acute hemorrhage that occurs as a result of trauma or laceration is usually an easily diagnosable problem. With acute blood loss internally, the hematocrit does not reflect the severity of the problem, and as fluid shifts occur to compensate for blood loss, shock may result. Treatment should consist of controlling the hemorrhage and volume replacement.

Thrombocytopenia accounts for many cases of generalized bleeding in pet animals. In these cases, it may be more difficult for the veterinarian to diagnose blood loss. Signs of platelet deficiency include petechial hemorrhages on earflaps, mucous membranes, and nonhaired areas such as the abdomen. Treatment involves steroid therapy, platelet-rich or whole-blood transfusions, and avoidance of trauma.

Iron Deficiency Anemia

Dogs experiencing chronic external blood loss can experience development of iron deficiency anemia. Severe flea infestation, gastrointestinal (GI) parasites, gastric ulceration, and bleeding neoplasms can cause significant blood loss over time. The iron and hemoglobin lost with this external bleeding result in the formation of altered RBCs with decreased life spans. Treatment consists of correcting the cause of the blood loss and oral iron supplementation for 30 to 60 days.

Hemolysis

When immune components attach directly or indirectly to the RBC membrane, they alter its structure. The body, in an attempt to regain homeostasis, begins to remove these altered cells. Macrophages interact with the altered cells, resulting in extravascular hemolysis. This disease, when seen in dogs, appears to be related to the presence of an underlying inflammatory process. Affected animals acutely develop exercise intolerance, pale mucous membranes, tachycardia, and icterus if the condition is severe. In cats, the most common cause of hemolytic anemia is hemobartonellosis. Chronic infections with feline leukemia virus (FeLV) may also stimulate immunohemolytic disease in the cat.

Treatment is aimed at suppressing the immune system (steroid therapy) and supportive therapy. Transfusion should be considered if the HCT of the cat declines to life-threatening levels. Tetracycline or doxycycline should be used to treat cats with hemobartonellosis.

A special form of immune-mediated hemolytic disease is seen in neonates. This occurs in horses and, rarely, in cats and dogs. The dam passes antibodies against fetal RBCs in her colostrum. The neonate's RBCs are attacked and lysed because they are coated with these antibodies. This problem can be avoided by blood-typing breeding animals and by fostering the young born to incompatible dams.

Blood-Borne Parasites

Several commonly seen blood parasitic diseases produce anemia through hemolysis. *Mycoplasma hemofelis* is a common cause of anemia in cats. The parasite attaches to the erythrocyte membrane, causing increased destruction of the cells. Animals that have nonspecific signs of weight loss, anorexia, fever, hepatomegaly, and splenomegaly should have blood films examined for the presence of this microorganism. Some of these animals may be icteric on examination.

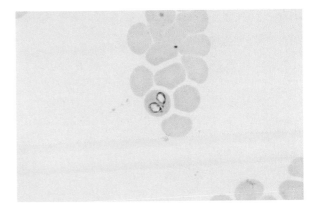

Figure 5-1 Trophozoites of *Babesia canis* within canine red blood cells. (Cowell RL, Taylor RD, Meinkoth JH, DeNicola DB: *Diagnostic cytology and hematology of the dog and cat*, ed 3, St. Louis, MO, 2007, Mosby.)

Babesia canis and *Babesia gibsoni* both produce hemolytic disease in dogs (Fig. 5-1). The brown dog tick *Rhipicephalus sanguineus* transmits these parasites. The presence of this intracellular parasite results in hemolysis of the infected RBCs. Diagnosis is accomplished by finding the intracellular organism on blood films or by serology testing. Symptoms exhibited in dogs include hemoglobinuria, dehydration, fever, anorexia, and depression. Treatment involves tetracycline administration (for *M. hemofelis*) and supportive care.

Cytauxzoon felis, a protozoal organism from the southern United States (Florida to Texas and Oklahoma), is responsible for a fatal disease in cats. The intracellular form of the disease produces anemia, whereas the extracellular form proliferates within the macrophages lining the vascular system, resulting in blood stasis and vascular occlusion (Fig. 5-2). Cats die within days of the development of clinical signs.

Toxin-Induced Anemias or Heinz Body Anemias

Drugs can be the source of anemias in small animals. Exposure of the erythrocyte to oxidants in plasma can result in the formation of reversible and nonreversible hemichromes. When the nonreversible form is present, hemoglobin denaturation continues, forming aggregates of the irreversible hemichromes called *Heinz bodies*. These aggregates may be seen as large

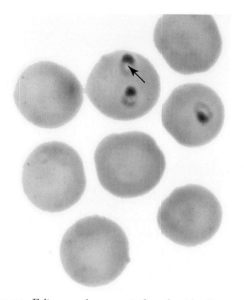

Figure 5-2 Feline erythrocytes infected with *Cytauxzoon* piroplasms. (From Greene CE: *Infectious diseases of the dog and cat*, ed 4, St. Louis, MO, 2012, Saunders.)

eccentric pale structures within the feline RBC or as multiple small structures within the canine RBC. Cats are considered more susceptible to Heinz body formation because of the structure of their hemoglobin. One of the most common causes of Heinz body anemia in dogs is onion toxicity, primarily arising from owners treating dogs to table scraps. Clinical signs may appear several days after ingestion and are usually those of a mild anemia. Acetaminophen toxicity also results in methemoglobinemia and anemia in dogs and cats. Toxic doses are usually the result of the owner medicating the animal. As little as half a tablet can result in clinical signs. Methylene blue, which is a urinary antiseptic used in cats, has long been known to produce Heinz body anemia when given to healthy cats. Specific diseases of clinical significance include immune-mediated hemolytic anemia (IMHA), immune-mediated thrombocytopenia (IMTP), ehrlichiosis, and von Willebrand disease (vWD).

Immune-Mediated Hemolytic Anemia

Although the specific cause of IMHA is unknown, the accelerated RBC destruction occurs because of the presence of antibodies that attach to the RBC membrane. These cells are then removed by the immune system, resulting in anemia. The antibodies may bind directly to the cell membrane or may attach to a microorganism or drug that has previously been bound to the membrane receptor sites. Adherence of these antibodies activates the complement system, causing agglutination and destruction of the RBC.

IMHA is found most commonly in dogs 2 to 8 years of age. A breed predisposition exists in Poodles, Old English Sheepdogs, Irish Setters, and Cocker Spaniels. The disease is four times more prevalent in female dogs than in male dogs.

Clinical syndromes seen with IMHA include immune-mediated extravascular hemolysis, intravascular hemolysis, and cryopathic IMHA.

CLINICAL SIGNS

- Anorexia
- Listlessness, weakness
- Depression
- Tachycardia, tachypnea
- Presence or absence of icterus (if intravascular)
- Presence or absence of hepatomegaly, splenomegaly (if extravascular)
- Necrosis of distal extremities (cryopathic form)
- Pale mucous membranes

DIAGNOSIS

- CBC: leukocytosis; absolute neutrophilia with a left shift; regenerative anemia

> ### ● TECH ALERT
>
> Spherocytes are commonly found on complete blood count.

- Serum chemistries are usually unremarkable.
- Agglutination test: Mix 1 drop of anticoagulated blood and 1 drop of saline on a clean glass slide. If antibody molecules are present, agglutination will be observed.
- Direct Coombs test: Must be species specific. False-positive and false-negative results are common. Take clinical signs into account when interpreting a positive result.

- Direct immunofluorescence assay: Detects antibodies against immunoglobulin G (IgG), IgA, IgM, and complement C3.

TREATMENT

- Treatment should be aimed at improving tissue oxygenation and managing immune response
- Glucocorticoids: dexamethasone intravenously (IV) every 12 hours; prednisone or prednisolone orally (PO) every 12 hours
- Cimetidine or misoprostol to prevent gastric ulceration from cortisone:
  - Cimetidine: PO every 6 to 12 hours
  - Misoprostol: PO every 6 to 8 hours
- Sucralfate to protect gastric ulcerations: 1 gram (g) PO every 8 hours
- Danazol: A synthetic testosterone that works synergistically with cortisone: PO every 12 hours
- Heparin to prevent thromboembolism or disseminated intravascular coagulation (DIC): SQ three times daily

INFORMATION FOR CLIENTS

- The prognosis for animals with this disease is guarded.
- Approximately 30% to 40% of all dogs will die despite aggressive treatment.
- Relapses are common.
- Your veterinarian may suggest an ovariohysterectomy for your intact female dog.

Thrombocytes (Platelets)

Thrombocytes or platelets are not actually cells. They are fragments of a larger cell found within bone marrow. Thrombocytes are formed from stem cells that develop into megakaryocytes. These large cells fragment as they pass out of bone marrow into smaller units called *platelets*. Platelets are necessary for blood clotting. They may be small, but they are packed with chemicals that are involved in both hemostasis and blood clotting. Shortly after vascular injury, platelets become activated and begin to stick together, forming a platelet plug that blocks the vessel and prevents hemorrhage. Chemicals contained within the thrombocyte are also necessary for the activation and maintenance of the blood clotting

cascades. When platelet levels decrease below normal, bleeding becomes a problem for the animal.

Immune-Mediated Thrombocytopenia

As in IMHA, IMTP occurs when platelets become coated with antibodies or complement–antibody complexes. Destruction may occur in the spleen, bone marrow, or liver. The inciting cause is usually unknown, but some drugs such as sulfonamide, chlorothiazide, arsenicals, digitoxin, and quinidine have been associated with the development of IMTP. The disease typically appears in dogs 5 to 6 years of age; female dogs are twice as likely to be affected as male dogs.

As platelet numbers decline to less than 30,000 thrombocytes/mm3 blood, bleeding problems develop. Animals are usually presented for bleeding, most commonly epistaxis. Petechial hemorrhages may appear on mucous membranes, earflaps, and other mucocutaneous surfaces. Bloody stool or blood in vomitus is seen occasionally.

CLINICAL SIGNS

- Petechial and ecchymotic hemorrhages on skin and mucosal surfaces
- Weakness, lethargy

DIAGNOSIS

- Rule out other causes of thrombocytopenia such as DIC, lymphoma, and myeloproliferative disease.
- Bone marrow examination indicates actively budding megakaryocytes and increased plasma cells.
- Clinical signs and response to treatment confirm diagnosis.

TREATMENT

- Prednisone: divided twice daily
- Vincristine: IV repeated one to two times at weekly intervals
- Platelet-rich transfusion
- Danazol and cimetidine as for IMHA

INFORMATION FOR CLIENTS

- The prognosis for animals with IMTP is guarded to good. About 20% of affected animals will die.
- Relapses may occur.
- Splenectomy may be required in refractory cases.

- Owners of intact female animals should consider having the pet spayed to decrease hormonal stress.

Leukocytes

There are five types of leukocytes or WBCs: the granulocytes—neutrophils, basophils, and eosinophils—and the agranulocytes—lymphocytes and monocytes. Leukocytes are formed in the red bone marrow and in the thymus and lymph system. Each cell type has a special job within the blood and tissues. The neutrophils and monocytes are predominately phagocytic cells, active in inflammatory responses to disease. Basophils contain histamine and heparin, which are chemicals involved in immune response and blood clotting, respectively, and eosinophils are seen increased in allergic responses and in parasitic infections. Lymphocytes can be divided into two types, T-lymphocytes and B-lymphocytes, each with a different job. After formation in the bone marrow, the cells destined to become T-lymphocytes migrate through the thymus and are trained to recognize "self." The T-lymphocytes are active in *cell-mediated* immune responses. They respond directly to destroy invaders recognized as "non-self." There are several different types of T-cells: helper T-cells, cytotoxic T-cells, and natural killer T-cells. Natural killer T-cells are active against tumor cells, as are the cytotoxic T-cells. Helper cells assist B-lymphocytes in the inflammatory response to microbes. B-lymphocytes make up the *humoral* response system. After activation, they produce antibodies specifically designed to destroy the invader. They are also responsible for activation of adjunct mechanisms such as *complement activation* and *opsonization* of microorganisms.

The leukocyte count makes up part of the CBC and should be a part of every clinical diagnostic plan.

Ehrlichiosis

Ehrlichia canis was first recognized in the United States in 1963. The disease gained prominence because of the large losses among military working dogs stationed in Vietnam. The disease is seen primarily in tropical and subtropical environments throughout the world.

This rickettsial disease is spread by the tick vector *Rhipicephalus sanguineus*, the brown dog tick, and is most commonly diagnosed in dogs living in the southeastern and southwestern United States, which are areas with large tick populations. Infection occurs when the organism is transmitted via the tick saliva during a blood meal. It may also be transmitted by blood transfusion from an infected animal to a noninfected animal. After infection, the organism multiplies within mononuclear cells, both circulating and fixed (liver, spleen, and lymph nodes). The infected circulating cells can infect other organs. Infection results in vascular endothelial damage, platelet consumption, and erythrocyte destruction. Suppression of bone marrow also occurs, resulting in aplastic anemia.

Dogs unable to mount an adequate immune response become chronically infected.

CLINICAL SIGNS

Acute Phase

- Depression, anorexia
- Fever
- Weight loss
- Ocular and nasal discharge
- Dyspnea
- Edema of the limbs or scrotum
- Lymphadenopathy

Chronic Phase

- Bleeding tendencies
- Severe weight loss
- Debilitation
- Abdominal tenderness
- Anterior uveitis, retinal hemorrhages

DIAGNOSIS

Hematology

- Pancytopenia
- Aplastic anemia
- Thrombocytopenia (most common sign)
- Anemia
- Positive Coombs test
- Increased serum proteins
- Finding the organisms within peripheral blood smears (Fig. 5-3)

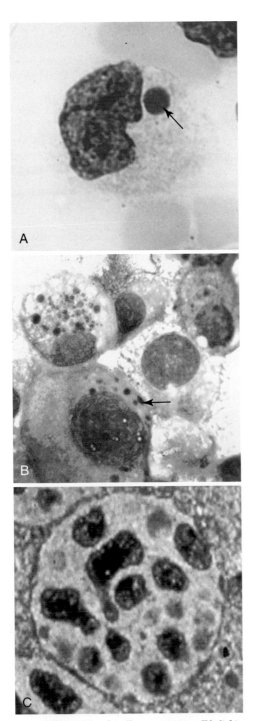

Figure 5-3 White blood cells containing *Ehrlichia canis*. (Courtesy Dr. Itamer Aroch, Koret School of Veterinary Medicine, The Hebrew University of Jerusalem, Israel. IN Greene CE: *Infectious Diseases of the Dog and Cat*, ed. 4, St. Louis, 2012, Saunders)

Serology
- Immunofluorescent antibody (IFA) test

TREATMENT
- Tetracycline: three times a day for 14 days is the treatment of choice
- Doxycycline: for 14 days has been used in refractory cases
- Tetracycline: daily use as prophylaxis in endemic areas

INFORMATION FOR CLIENTS
- The prognosis for this disease is generally good.
- Because dogs do not mount a protective immune response, reinfection may occur.
- Long-term tetracycline prophylaxis may be required in endemic areas.
- Tick control is important to prevent disease.

von Willebrand Disease

Canine vWD is the most common inherited disorder of hemostasis. In healthy dogs, the von Willebrand factor (vWF) promotes platelet clumping, whereas decreased amounts or lack of the factor results in a bleeding disorder. vWD has been identified in 54 breeds in the United States with Doberman Pinschers, German Shepherds, and Labrador Retrievers being overrepresented. In most dogs, the inheritance is autosomal dominant with incomplete penetrance. Dogs that carry the gene will demonstrate variable signs and severity with respect to bleeding tendencies.

Dogs with this disorder should not be used for breeding. Special care must be taken at surgery to ensure adequate hemostasis; thus, it is recommended that breeds that can carry the affected gene have a buccal mucosal bleeding time evaluation performed before surgery.

CLINICAL SIGNS
- Easy bruising in breeds predisposed to the disease
- Prolonged bleeding during estrus
- Prolonged bleeding from venipuncture

DIAGNOSIS
- Buccal mucosal bleeding time prolonged >4 minutes
- Low levels of vWF in plasma

- Deoxyribonucleic acid (DNA) confirmation of the gene defect
- Positive enzyme-linked immunosorbent assay (ELISA)

TREATMENT

- Bleeding episodes can be managed with plasma or cryoprecipitate infusion.
- Desmopressin acetate can be used to control bleeding during surgery (administer 20 to 30 minutes before surgery). Effect lasts about 2 hours. Dose is 1 mcg/kg SQ.

INFORMATION FOR CLIENTS

- This disease is inherited. You should not use this animal for breeding.
- Any trauma or stress may precipitate a bleeding episode.
- Surgery will require special precautions to control hemorrhage.
- When purchasing one of the affected breeds, always purchase dogs whose parents have been found to be free of the disease.

Lymphoma

Feline Lymphoma

Lymphoma accounts for approximately 90% of all feline hematopoietic tumors. Most feline lymphomas are induced by FeLV, with 70% of lymphoma cases being FeLV-positive cats. The average age for development of the disease in FeLV-positive cats is 3 years, whereas in FeLV-negative cats, the disease develops later in life (7 years of age). Cats with the multicentric form of the disease have the greatest incidence of FeLV-positive status (80%).

Lymphomas may be classified in one of two ways: (1) by anatomic location or (2) according to the extent of the disease. Both schemes complement each other. This chapter concentrates on the classification system using anatomic location.

Mediastinal Lymphoma

The mediastinal, or thymic, form of lymphoma is seen in young cats (2 to 3 years of age). Most of these cats are FeLV positive (80%). Clinical signs associated with this form of the disease are those of a space-occupying mass within the mediastinum and include dyspnea, tachypnea, regurgitation, cough, anorexia, depression, weight loss, and pleural effusion.

Alimentary Lymphoma

The alimentary form of lymphoma occurs in older cats, and the majority of these cats are FeLV negative (70%). Clinical signs are related to an intestinal mass and include vomiting, diarrhea, weight loss, and intestinal obstruction.

Multicentric Lymphoma

Multicentric disease is the most commonly observed form of lymphoma. Most cats with multicentric lymphoma are FeLV positive, with the average age of presentation being 4 years. Clinical signs are variable and depend on the location and the size of the tumors. Many cats may be asymptomatic, whereas others may have anorexia, weight loss, and lethargy. Peripheral lymph nodes may become visibly enlarged but are nonpainful on palpation. Because a majority of these cats are also FeLV positive, anemia is also prevalent.

CLINICAL SIGNS

Clinical signs depend on the location and size of the tumors but can include the following:
- Dyspnea
- Anemia
- Vomiting
- Diarrhea
- Lethargy
- Weight loss
- Visibly enlarged peripheral lymph nodes

DIAGNOSIS

- Cytology is the best method for diagnosis. Fine-needle aspiration or surgical biopsy will provide a diagnosis. Cytology will demonstrate a monomorphic population of immature lymphocytes.

TREATMENT

- Chemotherapy is the preferred method of treatment. Drug protocols are divided into four phases: (1) induction of remission, (2) intensification, (3) maintenance, and (4) rescue.

Induction of Remission

- COP (Cytoxan, Oncovin, prednisone) protocol:
  - Cyclophosphamide (Cytoxan): given PO on days 1 and 22 of the month
  - Vincristine (Oncovin): given IV on days 1, 8, 15, and 22 of the month
  - Prednisone: once daily

TECH ALERT

Remission rates of up to 80% have been reported with this protocol; the duration of remission ranges from 42 days to 42 months.

- COAP (Cytoxan, Oncovin, cytosine arabinoside, prednisone) protocol:
  - Cyclophosphamide (Cytoxan): PO 4 days/ week given every other day
  - Vincristine (Oncovin): IV once each week
  - Cytosine arabinoside (Cytosar-U): given by intravenous drip or SQ for only 2 days
  - Prednisone: PO daily for 7 days, then every other day
- Use protocol for 6 weeks, then switch to maintenance therapy

Intensification

- Add L-asparaginase (Elspar) SQ for one dose.

Maintenance

- LMP (Leukeran, methotrexate, prednisone) protocol:
  - Chlorambucil (Leukeran): PO every other day or PO every other week
  - Methotrexate: PO two to three times weekly
  - Prednisone: PO every other day

Rescue

- Protocols are available that add drugs such as adriamycin and dacarbazine (consult oncology texts for further information)
- *Additional drugs* used in the treatment of lymphomas in the cat include the following:
  - Idarubicin: for 2 consecutive days every 21 days
  - Doxorubicin: IV every 3 weeks

RADIATION THERAPY

- Radiation therapy is useful in cases of localized lymphomas.

TECH ALERT

Note that radiation doses are in milligrams per square meter (mg/sq.m). Body surface area is a more accurate method of dosing toxic materials.

- All the chemotherapeutic agents induce side effects in animals undergoing treatment. Negative side effects include the following:
  - Anorexia: use cyproheptadine two to three times daily to stimulate appetite
  - Vomiting
  - Leukopenia: check blood cell count 1 week after each dose of Cytoxan; reduce the dose by 25% if segmented neutrophil count is <1000 cells per microliter (cells/µL).
  - Renal toxicity: monitor renal function
  - Hemorrhagic cystitis: this is uncommon but can occur with Cytoxan therapy

INFORMATION FOR CLIENTS

- There is no cure for this disease. The goal of therapy is to induce remission, make the cat more comfortable, and prolong life.
- Cats that achieve complete remission live a median of 5 months (with a range of 2 to 42 months); all animals will have a relapse of the disease eventually.
- Maintenance therapy and follow-up is important to the success of the treatment protocol.
- Nutritional support is important with the alimentary form of the disease; a feeding tube may be needed.
- All therapy protocols will produce some toxicity that may need to be treated.
- Wear gloves when handling chemotherapeutic drugs to prevent absorption through skin.

TECH ALERT

Clinicians and technicians should consult with oncology specialists for optional protocols in the treatment of this disease.

Canine Lymphoma

Malignant lymphoma (lymphosarcoma) is the most common hematopoietic tumor of the dog. More than 85% of cases treated by veterinarians involve regional or generalized lymphadenopathy. Survival times for untreated dogs are short, and most die within 4 to 6 weeks after diagnosis. With treatment, remission rates can approach 90%; the duration of remission normally lasts longer than 6 months.

Therapy involves two phases of treatment: (1) the induction and maintenance phase and (2) the rescue phase. Combined drug protocols provide the best response rates and duration of remission. Dogs treated initially with only prednisolone have shorter remission periods and decreased survival times. (See the literature for the various protocols that are available.) Eventually, most dogs will require rescue therapy. The duration of the new remissions is generally poor because of the emergence of drug-resistant tumor cells.

Alternative therapies such as monoclonal antibody therapy or bone marrow transplantation show some promise for future treatment of malignant lymphoma in the dog.

CLINICAL SIGNS

- Enlarged peripheral lymph nodes
- Lethargy
- Weight loss
- Vomiting, diarrhea, or both

DIAGNOSIS

- Cytology or biopsy (as for cats)

TREATMENT

- Several combined drug therapy protocols are available. The following protocol is from the University of Wisconsin at Madison:
  - Vincristine: IV at weeks 1, 3, 6, and 8
  - L-Asparaginase: IM at week 1
  - Prednisone: PO daily at weeks 1, 2, 3, and 4 in decreasing doses
  - Cyclophosphamide (Cytoxan): IV at weeks 2 and 7
  - Doxorubicin: IV at weeks 4 and 9
- *Other treatments* that may result in less successful remissions include the following:
  - Prednisone: PO; this treatment has been shown to help for a short period (30 days), but use of

it may make it more difficult to reestablish remission a second time
  - Cytoxan: PO for 4 consecutive days weekly; administer with prednisone
  - Doxorubicin: IV every 3 weeks for a total of five treatments

Maintenance Therapy

- Vincristine: IV
- Chlorambucil: PO
- Methotrexate IV or doxorubicin IV (alternate these two drugs until a total doxorubicin dose of 180 mg/m^2 is attained, then use methotrexate alone):
  - Begin on week 11 and alternate these three treatments every 2 weeks
  - After week 25, alternate every 3 weeks
  - After week 49, alternate every 4 weeks
  - Discontinue after 2 years if the dog is in complete remission

Rescue Therapy

- Actinomycin D: IV every 2 to 3 weeks
- Mitoxantrone: every 3 weeks
- Doxorubicin (IV at day 1) and dacarbazine (IV at days 1–5); cycle every 21 days

INFORMATION FOR CLIENTS

- Most dogs eventually will experience relapse.
- Durability of new remissions is usually poor; life expectancy ranges from 2 to 5 months.
- Medications used in chemotherapy will cause suppression of the immune system and blood cell counts need to be monitored frequently.
- Boxers, Bullmastiffs, Basset Hounds, Saint Bernards, and Scottish Terriers have a predisposition for this disease.
- Without treatment, most dogs die within 4 to 6 weeks after diagnosis.
- With proper treatment, survival time may approach 1 year.

Feline Immunodeficiency Virus (Feline Acquired Immunodeficiency Syndrome)

In 1987, Pederson and colleagues first isolated feline immunodeficiency virus (FIV). The virus, a lentivirus, interacts with lymphocytes (predominantly CD4 cells and macrophages), changing their ability to function normally in the immune response process. The resulting lymphopenia, loss of memory cell function, and decrease in antibody production from T-cell–stimulated lymphocytes leaves the cat open for opportunistic infections.

FIV is endemic in most of the United States. Outdoor, free-roaming cats are at greatest risk, with male cats being 1.5 to 3 times more likely to become infected compared with female cats. This is probably related to their fighting behavior and territorial aggressiveness. The average age at the time of diagnosis is between 6 and 8 years. Incidental transmission through food bowls, mutual grooming, or other fomites is unlikely in multiple-cat households. Kittens can become infected with the virus while nursing queens that are experiencing the acute phase of the disease (FIV passed in milk). With the availability of the FIV vaccine, it has become more difficult to diagnose a clinical infection versus a vaccine antibody titer. Antibodies can be detected as early as 2 weeks after vaccine administration, and ELISA is not able to distinguish between the two.

FIV can be divided into three stages: (1) acute infection (3–6 months), (2) subclinical infection (months to years), and (3) chronic clinical infection (months to years).

- *Acute stage:* usually mild symptoms of recurrent fever, lethargy, anorexia, and generalized lymphadenopathy
- *Subclinical stage:* usually no clinical signs shown in infected cats; however, the disease is progressing
- *Chronic clinical stage:* A variety of signs involve the establishment of opportunistic infections throughout the body and symptoms related to viral infection:
  - Chronic stomatitis and weight loss
  - Recurrent upper respiratory tract infections
  - Chronic enteritis
  - Persistent dermatomycosis
  - Ocular disease: anterior uveitis, retinal degeneration or hemorrhage, transient conjunctivitis
  - Tumors
  - Chronic wasting syndrome: cats lose up to 30% of body weight in several weeks
  - Neurologic signs: altered behavior, paresis, weakness

Therapies focus on preventing exposure to pathogens and supportive care. The average time from diagnosis to death is approximately 5 years.

CLINICAL SIGNS

- Febrile episodes
- Lymphadenopathy
- Persistent infections unresponsive to treatment
- Weight loss
- Gingivitis
- Ocular lesions
- Slow-healing traumatic wounds
- Behavior abnormalities
- Chronic upper respiratory infections
- Anemia

DIAGNOSIS

- In-house serology: Membrane-bound ELISA test (CITE test, Idexx) is sensitive and specific for the presence of antibodies.

TREATMENT

- Reverse transcriptase inhibitors are expensive, but easily available:
  - Azothiouridine (AZT Retrovir, Burroughs Wellcome): three times daily
  - Interferon-α: PO every 24 hours for 5 days on alternate weeks

Supportive Care

- Limit contact with other cats to decrease exposure to secondary pathogens.
- Avoid routine vaccinations.
- Limit vaccines to rabies as required by law.

PREVENTIVE

- Keep cats inside; avoid contact with feral cats.
- Vaccination: may result in a cat that tests positive on future FIV tests.

INFORMATION FOR CLIENTS

- This is a progressive disease.
- The average life span from diagnosis to death is about 5 years.
- To prevent this disease, keep cats indoors and limit contact with feral or free-roaming cats.
- Test all new additions to the cat's household.
- Incidental infection among cats in a household is unlikely.
- FIV has not been found to grow in human cells.

REVIEW QUESTIONS

1. When determining whether an anemia is regenerative or nonregenerative, one must look at the:
   a. Complete blood count
   b. Absolute reticulocyte count
   c. Red blood cell count
   d. Red blood cell morphology
2. What is the tick vector responsible for the spread of canine ehrlichiosis?
   a. *Dermacentor variabilis*
   b. *Amblyomma americanum*
   c. *Rhipicephalus sanguineus*
   d. *Boophilus annulatus*
3. A buccal mucosal bleeding time longer than 4 minutes in a healthy, young Doberman might indicate the presence of:
   a. Heinz body anemia
   b. von Willebrand disease
   c. Immune-mediated hemolytic anemia
   d. Iron deficiency
4. Few cats with feline lymphoma will test positive for FeLV.
   a. True
   b. False
5. List three drugs that are useful in the treatment of canine lymphosarcoma.

6. According to the new protocols for vaccination, all cats should be vaccinated for FIV.
   a. True
   b. False
7. What is the main disadvantage to vaccinating young cats for FIV?
8. When dosing toxic drugs, _____, instead of weight, should be used to determine the dose.
   a. Body surface area
   b. Blood volume
   c. Body height
   d. Liver function test value
9. *Haemobartonella felis* is now called _____.
   a. *Haemobartonella cati*
   b. *Mycoplasma hemofelis*
   c. *Haemobartonella macrofilia*
   d. *Mycobacterium cati*
10. Animals demonstrating intravascular hemolytic disease will have _____ plasma.
    a. Yellow
    b. Milky
    c. Red
    d. Brown

Answers found on page 551.

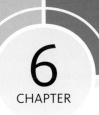

Diseases of the Integumentary System

Alopecia
Amelanotic
Benign
Carcinoma
Ectoparasites

Erythema
Flaccid paralysis
Mitacide
Myiasis
Pruritus

Pyodermia
Sarcoma
Stratum
Squamous epithelium
Systemic

Anatomy of the Skin
Ectoparasites
    Ear Mites
    Fleas (*Ctenocephalides* spp.)
    Ticks (*Ixodes* spp. and *Argasid* spp.)
    Mange Mites
    Demodectic Mange
    Sarcoptic Mange (Scabies)
    Cuterebra "Warbles"
    Myiasis (Maggots)
    Lice
Superficial Dermatomycoses (Fungal Infections)
    Microsporum canis Infections
Pyodermas
    Superficial Pyodermas
    Acute Moist Dermatitis ("Hot spots")
    Impetigo

    Acne
    Skinfold Pyoderma
    Deep Pyodermas
Anal Glands
Tumors of the Skin
    Benign Skin Tumors
        Lipoma
        Papillomas (Warts)
        Sebaceous cysts
    Malignant Skin Tumors
        Fibrosarcomas (not vaccine-induced)
        Feline fibrosarcomas (vaccine-induced)
        Mast cell tumors
        Melanoma (benign or malignant)
        Perianal tumors (adenomas and adenocarcinomas)
        Squamous cell carcinoma

When you have completed this chapter, you will be able to:
1. Describe the arrangement and importance of the skin as an organ.
2. List common ectoparasites that produce skin disease in companion animals.
3. Demonstrate the ability to explain parasite control for the most common ectoparasites.
4. Relate diagnosis and treatment of skin lumps and bumps, for example, tumors, abscesses, and cysts.

The skin makes up the largest organ system in the body. It comprises approximately 24% of the total body weight of a newborn puppy and about 12% of the body weight of an adult animal. It consists of three distinct layers: (1) the *epidermis*, (2) the *dermis*, and (3) the *hypodermis*, or the subcuticular layer (Fig. 6-1). The skin serves as a barrier between the animal's body and the environment. It not only protects the animal from physical, chemical, and microbiologic injury, but the sensory organs found in the skin allow the animal to feel pain, heat, cold, touch, and pressure. The skin is also a storage depot for electrolytes, water, proteins, fats, and carbohydrates, and it assists in the activation of vitamin D by solar energy.

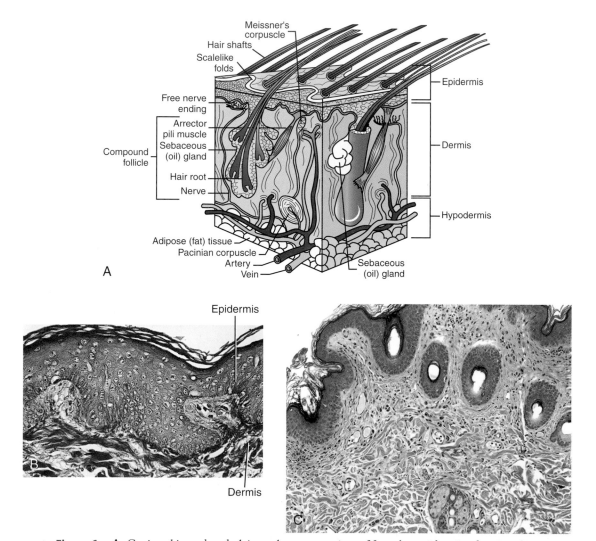

Figure 6-1 A, Canine skin and underlying subcutaneous tissue. Note that epidermis of canine skin includes folds from which compound hairs arise. **B,** Normal canine skin. **C,** Normal feline skin. Note the thin epidermis and compound hair follicle arrangement of both species. (**A,** From Colville T, Bassert JM: *Clinical anatomy and physiology for veterinary technicians*, St. Louis, MO, 2008, Mosby, by permission; **B,** From Scott DW, Miller WH, Jr., Griffin CE: *Muller and Kirk's small animal dermatology*, ed 6, Philadelphia, PA, 2001, Saunders. **C,** From Norris AJ, Griffey SM, Lucroy MD, Madewell BR: Cyclin D3 expression in normal fetal, normal adult and neoplastic feline tissue. *Journal of Comparative Pathology*, *132:4*, 329-339, 2005.)

The hypodermis stores fat for insulation and energy reserves. The animal's skin has many functions:

- *Enclosing barrier:* protects the internal environment of the body from water and electrolyte loss
- *Environmental protection:* protects the internal environment from the external environment
- *Temperature regulation:* maintains the animal's coat and regulates the blood supply to the cutaneous tissues, which regulate heat dissipation and retention
- *Sensory perception:* contains sense organs for touch, temperature, and pain
- *Motion and shape:* allows for motion and provides a definition to the body
- *Antimicrobial:* contains antimicrobial and antifungal properties
- *Blood pressure control:* the peripheral vascular beds within the skin help control blood pressure
- *Secretion:* contains both apocrine and sebaceous glands
- *Adnexa:* produces hair, nails, hooves, and horny layers of the epidermis
- *Storage:* stores electrolytes, water, vitamins, fat, proteins, carbohydrates, and other substances
- *Pigmentation:* processes within the skin (e.g., melanin formation) help to determine coat and skin color and provide solar protection
- *Excretion:* the animal's skin has a limited excretory function
- *Vitamin D production:* the skin is essential for solar energy activation of vitamin D, which is necessary for normal calcium absorption

⬤ TECH ALERT

The skin is an important indicator of internal disease.

Any physical condition that disrupts the normal functions of this barrier can result in disease. Increased moisture, chemical exposure, increased temperature, hormonal change, and physical damage can produce a breach in the barrier, allowing the invasion of disease-producing microorganisms.

Problems relating to the skin are the most frequent complaints presented in small-animal medicine. Technicians deal with these complaints daily as clients ask questions and seek help for the treatment and prevention of skin diseases afflicting their pets. This chapter focuses on the most commonly seen skin problems of companion animals.

Anatomy of the Skin

Undisturbed, the skin is a perfect barrier protecting the underlying tissues and organs from microbiologic and environmental intrusions. In most humans and animals, it is difficult to maintain the integrity of the skin and, hence, to remain immune to invasion. The top layer of the skin, the epidermis, is formed from multiple layers of squamous epithelium. As with all epithelial tissues, it consists of a deep basement membrane and a superficial edge open to the environment. Between the two are multiple layers of epithelial cells slowly moving from the deeper layers toward the surface and to death. Just above the basement membrane is the *stratum basale,* a single layer of cuboidal cells that rapidly undergo mitosis and form all the cells found in the more superficial layers of the epidermis. Above the stratum basale are 8 to 10 layers of the *stratum spinosum,* and 2 to 5 layers of the *stratum granulosum,* dying cells filling with keratohyalin granules. Above these two layers are the *stratum lucidium,* clear cells that contain a precursor of keratin, eleidin, and the *stratum corneum* or the horny layer. The stratum corneum comprises of mostly dead cells filled with keratin fibers imbedded with glycophospholipids, forming a tough, waterproof covering of the body. Cells continuously migrate from the deeper layers of the epidermis toward the surface where they slough off. In humans, the regeneration time for this process is around 35 days.

The *dermis* is located under the epidermis. The two are linked together through the basement membrane and a polysaccharide gel-type glue. Located within the dermis are hair follicles, sweat glands, blood and lymph vessels, nerves, and other sensory receptors. The *hypodermis,* or *subcuticular layer,* lies under the dermis. It is composed mostly of loose connective tissues and adipose cells. In humans, the subcuticular space is very small but in animal species, it is quite large making subcutaneous (SQ) injections of medications and fluids safer and more efficient.

Paw pads, claws and hoofs, fur, and tactile hairs are structures found within the skin of companion animals but not in humans. Thickened areas of the epidermis occur on areas of the body exposed to continued use, for example, the pads of the paw. The thickened skin in these areas provides protection from constant abrasion. Claws develop from keratinized epithelial cells that grow from the stratum spinosum and the stratum granulosum in the nail bed. The claw has good vascular and nerve supply and may be pigmented or non-pigmented, depending on the species. The claw is a constantly growing living tissue and is either worn down by the animal walking on it or must be trimmed by the owner or the veterinary staff.

Hair begins its growth in the hair follicle found in the dermis. Epidermal cells migrate down into the hair follicles during gestation. Their continual mitotic activity and keratinization forms the hair root pushing the cells upward to form the hair shaft. Like claws, hairs are continually lost and replaced during the life of the animal. Pigments are incorporated into the hair shaft during formation giving the hair coat the characteristic coat color of the species.

Ectoparasites

External parasites are responsible for many skin problems seen in small-animal medicine (see a parasitology text for detailed information on the life cycles of the individual parasites discussed in this chapter). The most commonly diagnosed ectoparasites are as follows:
- Ear mites (*Otodectes cynotis*)
- Fleas (*Ctenocephalides* spp.)
- Ticks (*Ixodes* spp. and others)
- Mange (*Demodex canis, Sarcoptes scabiei, Notoedres cati*)
- Warbles (*Cutebrae* spp.)
- Myiasis (fly maggots)
- Lice (*Linognathus setosus*)

Some of these parasites live on the skin; some live within or under the skin; and some pierce the skin, sucking blood meals that produce severe cutaneous reactions. These reactions include inflammation, edema, and itching. In many cases, the animal itself is responsible for increased damage to the skin through licking, chewing, and scratching.

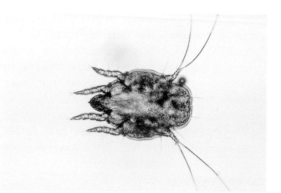

Figure 6-2 Adult male ear mite, *Otodectes cynotis*. (From Hendrix CM, Robinson E: *Diagnostic parasitology for veterinary technicians*, ed 3, St. Louis, MO, 2012, Mosby.)

Ear Mites (*Otodectes cynotis*)

Ear mites live on the surface of the skin in the external ear canal, feeding on epidermal debris (Fig. 6-2).

CLINICAL SIGNS
- Ear canals may be filled with a brown-black, crusty exudate.
- Mites are extremely irritating, so animals will scratch their ears.
- Scrapes (wounds) may be visible on the side of the face or head.

DIAGNOSIS
- Under an otoscope, the large, white, adult mites can be seen crawling on the surface of the crusty exudate.
- Adult mites and eggs can be seen on microscopic examination of smears of the exudate.

TREATMENT
Many otic products contain ingredients that will kill mites. The technician should first carefully clean the exudate from the ear canal and then apply a miticide into the canal. Recommended miticides include the following:
- Ivermectin (off-label uses): 300 mcg/kg subcutaneously (SQ) or orally (PO) (*repeat in 14 days*)

TECH ALERT

Owners must be informed that ivermectin is not licensed for subcutaneous use in companion-animal species.

INFORMATION FOR CLIENTS

- The life cycle of the parasite is 3 weeks. Eggs hatch every 10 days, so treatment must be continued for no less than 30 days.
- This parasite is highly contagious. All animals that have had contact with the infested animal should be treated.
- Humans do not become infested by this parasite in most cases.
- The mites may spend time elsewhere on the animal's body, especially on a cat's tail. If infestations recur, treat the entire animal with dip or shampoo.

Fleas (*Ctenocephalides* spp.)

Fleas are blood-sucking ectoparasites that feed sporadically on mammals and birds (Fig. 6-3). Fleas produce severe skin irritation as a result of their frequent bites. Flea saliva is highly antigenic in some animals and will produce an allergic dermatitis. Fleas can act as vectors for diseases and as intermediary hosts for the dog tapeworm (*Dipylidium caninum*). Pets, as well as their environments, can become infested with massive numbers of fleas.

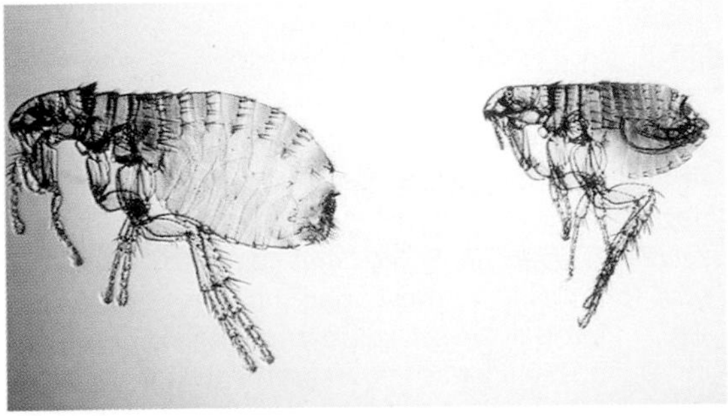

Figure 6-3 Adult male and female *Ctenocephalides felis*, cat fleas, the most common flea found on dogs and cats. (From Hendrix CM, Robinson E: *Diagnostic parasitology for veterinary technicians*, ed 3, St. Louis, MO, 2012, Mosby, by permission.)

CLINICAL SIGNS

- Animals infested with fleas will continually scratch or bite their skin.
- Areas commonly affected include the tail-head area and the inner thigh region of the animal. These areas may be red, inflamed, and scabbed. In cats, small scabs may cover the entire dorsum (miliary dermatitis).
- Small, pepperlike granules may be found on the skin and hair coat. When placed on white paper wet with alcohol or water, the granules give off a red color. These granules are dried flea excrement and contain blood products.

DIAGNOSIS

- Finding fleas on the animal
- Finding flea dirt on the animal
- Finding lesions consistent with flea infestation

TREATMENT

- Several flea products currently are available on the market. They can be categorized into those that are applied topically (sprays, dips, powders, and shampoos) and those that are applied systemically (spot-ons, oral, or injectable). All these products act at some point in the flea's life cycle to interrupt development of the adult flea or to repel the adult flea from the animal.

Sprays and Powders

- Many products that contain a combination of ingredients are on the market. Most act to repel or kill the adult flea. Each product has specific species and age specifications; therefore, you must read the label carefully before use. Become familiar with the products sold in your clinic.

Shampoos

- Shampoos provide no residual effect. The product will kill fleas that come into contact with the shampoo, but it will not remain on the skin after rinsing. Read the label carefully for species specifications.

Dips

- Dips provide residual effect on the animal. These products are more toxic than other topical preparations. Read the label carefully for species specifications and proper dilution techniques. Animals should not be rinsed off or towel dried after being dipped.

Systemics

Systemics are one of the newest treatments for fleas. These products are absorbed and distributed within the skin to kill the flea when it feeds, or to render reproduction impossible (Box 6-1).

● TECH ALERT

The product Promeris for Dogs has been removed from the market because of adverse reactions in some dogs. The product has been implicated in the development of a pemphigus folliaceus. Avoid use of this product.

INFORMATION FOR CLIENTS

- Control of ectoparasites such as fleas can be a frustrating task. Environmental factors, geographic location, and species sensitivity affect the development of disease.
- Treatment of the environment is essential in preventing flea infestation. Fleas spend most of their life cycle off the host.
- If one animal in the house has fleas, all other animals have fleas, too!

- Flea infestation results in damage to the skin, allowing other skin problems to develop.
- Fleas will bite and feed on humans if animals are not available.
- Some fleas can remain dormant in the environment for months if conditions are suitable. You must clean the environment by vacuuming and treating with sprays or foggers.

Ticks (*Ixodes* spp. and *Argasid* spp.)

Ticks are seen commonly on outdoor dogs and cats, especially during the summer months. These blood-sucking, arthropod parasites are not host specific and will infest all warm-blooded animals in the area (including humans). Heavy infestation may produce anemia in the host. Ticks also can transmit many bacterial, viral, rickettsial, and protozoan diseases. Lyme disease is one high-profile example of tick-borne disease. Ticks are divided into two main families: (1) *Ixodidae* (hard ticks) and (2) *Argasidae* (soft ticks). Most of the commonly found ticks belong to the *Ixodidae* family. Some of the best known members of this family include *Rhipicephalus sanguineus* (the brown dog tick (Fig. 6-4), *Dermacentor variabilis* (the American dog tick), and *Amblyomma* spp. All but *Rhipicephalus* spp. gain access to the host outdoors. *Rhipicephalus* spp. typically inhabit buildings and kennels. One soft tick, the spinose ear tick (*Otobius megnini*), can be found in the ear canals of dogs and cats in the southwestern United States.

BOX 6-1   Common Brands of Systemics

Advantage: A once monthly spot-on helps to kill adult fleas and prevent reproduction; it is dosed according to weight and species.

Program: Lufenuron, the active ingredient, is absorbed by the fatty tissue and slowly distributed to the bloodstream. This ingredient interferes with the synthesis of chitin, a necessary element in flea development. It is given by tablet once monthly or every 6 months by injection to cats. It takes 30 to 60 days to reach full effectiveness. Adult fleas may continue to be seen on the animal.

Frontline: Apply monthly to skin.

Sentinel: Contains lufenuron; also contains milbemycin for heartworm prevention. It is dosed by weight in dogs.

Revolution (selamectin; Pfizer, Cambridge, MA): Kills fleas for 1 month by preventing the eggs from hatching. It is also used to treat heartworms, ear mites, intestinal parasites, and sarcoptic mange in dogs and cats older than 6 weeks. It is dosed by body weight.

Advantix (imidicloprid, permethrin, Bayer): Kills adult fleas and ticks.

Comfortis (spinosad, Lilly): Kills adult fleas.

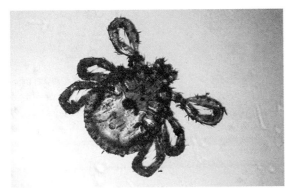

Figure 6-4 *Rhipicephalus sanguineus* (brown dog tick) invades both kennel and household environments. (From Bassert JM, McCurnin DM: *McCurnin's clinical textbook for veterinary technicians*, ed 7, St. Louis, MO, 2010, Saunders.)

Ticks injure animals by several means: irritation of the actual bite, as vectors of disease, and through a neurotoxin found in the saliva of 12 different *Ixodes* species. This neurotoxin causes *tick paralysis*, an ascending, flaccid paralysis of dogs.

CLINICAL SIGNS

- Owners report a tick or "a lump" attached to the animal
- Weakness or pale mucous membranes when infested with large numbers of ticks
- Ascending, flaccid paralysis
- Arthritis-like symptoms of lameness, joint and muscle pain, fever (Lyme disease)

DIAGNOSIS

- Finding a tick on the animal is the definitive diagnosis.
- A history of exposure to wooded, grassy areas known to have tick infestations suggests the diagnosis.

TREATMENT

- Manual removal of all ticks. Soak the tick in alcohol; firmly grasp the head parts using a curved mosquito hemostat, and pull to remove the tick. Destroy the tick by crushing or soaking in alcohol. One should never use bare hands to remove a tick or crush a tick because the blood contained within the tick may contain infectious microorganisms.

Never use a lighted cigarette, gasoline, or kerosene to remove a tick because the use of such substances will result in serious damage to the animal's skin.

- Topical treatments (dips, sprays, and powders): The following list is only a sample of some of the more commonly used products:
  - Paramite Dip (Vet-Kem)
  - Pyrethrin Dip (VetMate)
  - Durakyl Pet Dip (DVM Pharmaceuticals, Miami, FL)
  - Adams Flea and Tick Dust
  - VIP Flea and Tick Powder (Veterinary Products Laboratories, Phoenix, AZ)
  - Adams Flea and Tick 14-day Mist
- Collars: Preventic collar (Virbac, Inc., Fort Worth, TX) is the only collar that is effective against ticks (even though others claim to be effective). These collars are effective for about 3 months if they do not get wet.
- Topical systemic treatments: Frontline is a spot-on product that is effective against fleas.
  - Advantix
  - Revolution
  - Frontline Topspot
  - Frontline Plus
  - Vectra
- Environmental treatments include the following:
  - Adams Home and Kennel Spray
  - Vet-Fog Fogger
  - Siphotrol Plus Fogger
  - Permectrin Pet, Yard, and Kennel Spray (Bio-Ceutic, St Joseph, MO)
  - Some yard sprays and garden sprays will also kill ticks
- The tick population in the environment can be decreased by removing brush, limiting rodent populations, and keeping grassy areas cut.

INFORMATION FOR CLIENTS

- Routinely check all animals for ticks, especially after they spend time outside during the spring and summer. Check around the ears and between the toes, as these are areas where ticks are commonly found.
- Do *not* use gasoline, kerosene, or lighted cigarettes to remove ticks from the animal.

- Do *not* use your bare hands to remove or crush ticks.
- You will need to treat the environment to prevent reinfestation of your pets.
- If infestation is severe, you may need to call a professional exterminator.
- Ticks are not species specific; they will feed on humans whenever they get the chance. They can carry disease.
- Destroy outdoor habitat by cutting brush, trimming trees, and eliminating rodents. Repellant collars and sprays may help keep ticks off pets while outdoors.

Mange Mites

Three primary diseases called "mange" are seen in the dog and cat: (1) demodectic mange, (2) sarcoptic mange, and (3) notoedric mange. These diseases are the result of tiny mites living on or in the skin, where they produce irritation and inflammation. The symptoms for each of the diseases are distinct, and diagnosis must include identification of the mite through skin scrapings or biopsy.

Demodectic Mange

Demodex canis, a cigar-shaped mite, lives within the hair follicles of most dogs and some cats (Fig. 6-5). These mites spend their entire life cycle on the host. In most dogs, the immune system holds the number of mites in check; however, in dogs with compromised immune systems (such as puppies with poor nutrition or other parasites, or dogs with chronic disease), the number of mites becomes excessive, causing disease. A hereditary predisposition to demodectic mange seems to exist, and certain breeds seem to be at greater risk.

Demodectic mange occurs in two forms: (1) *localized*, the more commonly seen form, and (2) *generalized*, the more severe but less common form.

CLINICAL SIGNS (LOCALIZED *DEMODEX*)

- Animal is almost always a young dog (3 months to 1 year). When found in the localized form in adults, the animals have a history of the disease earlier in life.
- Alopecia (hair loss) appears especially on the face, around the eyes, mouth, and ears. The next most frequently involved areas are the forelegs and, occasionally, the trunk.
- Erythema (redness) is common; the patches are red and sometimes crusty. This type of mange has been called *red mange*.

⬤ TECH ALERT

The animals are *nonpruritic* (not itching). This is an important distinguishing characteristic to help differentiate demodectic mange from other types of mange.

CLINICAL SIGNS (GENERALIZED *DEMODEX*)

- Animals usually will be febrile.
- The entire body surface will be involved.
- Secondary bacterial skin infections with pustules will be seen.

DIAGNOSIS

- Diagnosis is by mite identification, usually through skin scrapings. Place a drop of mineral oil on the lesion, and firmly scrape while squeezing the skin. Transfer the material to a clean glass slide, and examine under a microscope. This mite is found easily (Fig. 6-6).
- Culture and sensitivity of the skin lesions may be necessary if a secondary bacterial infection is present.

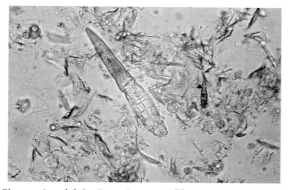

Figure 6-5 Adult *Demodex canis*. These mites resemble eight-legged alligators. (From Hendrix CM, Robinson E: *Diagnostic parasitology for veterinary technicians*, ed 3, St. Louis, MO, 2012, Mosby, by permission.)

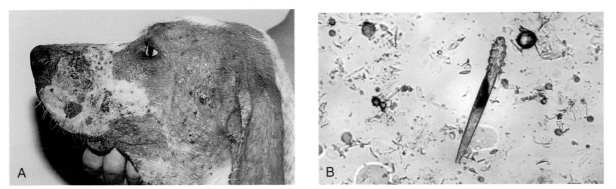

Figure 6-6 A, Generalized demodicosis in a dog. **B,** Microscopic image of *Demodex injai*. (From Hnilica KA: *Small animal dermatology: A color atlas and therapeutic guide*, ed 3, St. Louis, MO, 2011, Saunders.)

TREATMENT

- Treatment of *Demodex* depends on the age of the patient, the extent of the lesions, and veterinarian preference.

Localized

- Rotenone (Goodwinol ointment): Apply to lesions daily.
- Rotenone (Canex): Apply to lesions daily.

Generalized or Severe Localized

- Mitaban dips (Amitraz): Clip the dog closely to remove hair. Bathe the entire animal in a mild soap and towel dry. Treat the entire animal with the dip at the proper dilution (1 bottle/2 gallons water). Do not rinse or towel dry the animal. Three to six treatments may be required, each treatment given 14 days apart and continued until skin scrapings are negative.
- Ivermectin: *Use of this drug in the dog is "off-label"; therefore, client release forms should be signed.* Give 0.3 mg/kg SQ or PO. Repeat in 14 days.
- Interceptor: Administer monthly for a minimum of 90 days.
- Oral antibiotics: Choice is based on culture and sensitivity.

INFORMATION FOR CLIENTS

- Many animals will outgrow mange as they age.
- *Demodex* is not contagious to humans and other animals.

- Treatment will never completely remove the mites from the skin. The goal of treatment is to reduce the number of mites on the animal and to improve the general health of the pet.
- Breeders should not use previously infected animals in their breeding programs.
- Treatment may be prolonged in some animals.
- The generalized form may be fatal in some animals.

Sarcoptic Mange (Scabies)

Scabies is an intensely pruritic, contagious disease of animals. The mite, *Sarcoptes scabiei* var. *canis*, has a rounded body with four pairs of legs (Fig. 6-7). The female mite burrows into the epidermis and lays eggs. This burrowing produces intense itching and inflammation within the skin. Scabies can occur in dogs of any age, sex, or breed. Humans may experience development of visible lesions after exposure to infected animals; however, the mites do not survive off the animal host for longer than a few days. If the owner experiences development of small, red papules on his or her skin, a medical doctor should be consulted.

CLINICAL SIGNS

- Typical red, crusty lesions appear on the ears, elbows, and elsewhere on the trunk of the animal.
- Scabies is *intensely pruritic!* This distinguishes it from *Demodex*.
- Secondary bacterial skin infections may be present owing to self-trauma.
- The disease will progressively become more severe.

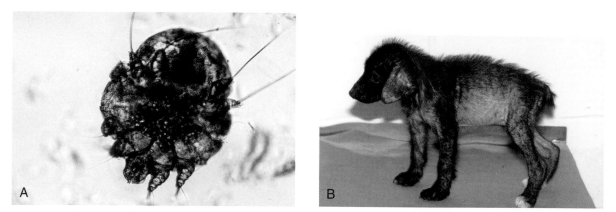

Figure 6-7 Canine scabies. **A,** Mite. **B,** Disease in the canine. (From Hnilica KA: *Small animal dermatology: A color atlas and therapeutic guide*, ed 3, St. Louis, MO, 2011, Saunders.)

DIAGNOSIS

- Identification of the mite through skin scrapings. These mites are difficult to find in many cases because they are located deep in the epidermis. Scraping should be deep to maximize the chance of finding the mite. Multiple scrapings of the same animal may be necessary to locate the mite. Mites can also be seen on skin biopsies.

TREATMENT

- *Remove the mites!* Dips are frequently used for this purpose.
- Paramite Dip (Vet-Kem): Dip every 14 days until the clinical signs resolve.
- Ivermectin: SQ or PO; repeat in 14 days. This constitutes "off-label" use of this drug.
- Paramite Dust (Vet-Kem): Administer per package instructions. Rub through entire coat. Do not treat puppies younger than 12 weeks.
- Revolution topical: Apply topically at 2-3 week intervals until the skin scrapings are negative.

INFORMATION FOR CLIENTS

- Scabies is a highly contagious disease among dogs.
- Humans frequently experience development of visible lesions appearing as small, red papules. Owners should contact their physicians if this occurs.
- Mites do not remain on humans for longer than a few hours.

- A similar disease is seen in cats, but the mite is not the same. *N. cati* produces lesions in cats similar to those seen with sarcoptic mange in dogs. The dog mite will rarely infect the cat.
- Species variants of the sarcoptic mite infest almost all species of haired animals.

Cuterebra "Warbles"

The *Cuterebra* fly lays eggs in the soil. These eggs mature into a larval stage similar to a grub that directly penetrates the host's skin (Fig. 6-8 and Fig. 6-9). Here, in a subcutaneous pocket, the larva continues to mature, finally leaving the wound to become an adult fly. A fistula or opening in the swelling allows the larva to breathe while maturing; the larva can be seen moving up and down in the opening to the fistula.

DIAGNOSIS

- This disease is usually seen in young puppies, kittens, and rabbits.
- Owners may notice a large swelling behind the ears, on the neck, or around the face. In rabbits, the lesion may be in the nasal cavity.
- The swelling has an opening (a fistula) through which the larva can be seen (Fig. 6-10).

TREATMENT

- The fistula opening should be incised to allow removal of the larva. Using a curved mosquito

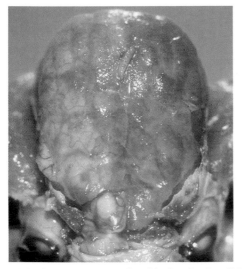

Figure 6-8 *Cuterebra* species, "warbles" or "wolves," found in the skin of dogs or cats. (From Hendrix CM, Robinson E: *Diagnostic parasitology for veterinary technicians*, ed 3, St. Louis, MO, 2012, Mosby, by permission.)

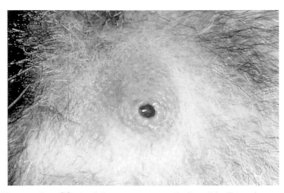

Figure 6-9 Typical lesion seen with "warbles" in the cat. (From Hendrix CM, Robinson E: *Diagnostic parasitology for veterinary technicians*, ed 3, St. Louis, MO, 2012, Mosby.)

hemostat, carefully remove the intact larva. Avoid crushing or tearing the larva because release of larval protein can cause allergic reactions in the host.
- The wound should be flushed; use diluted povidone-iodine (Betadine; Purdue Frederick, Norwalk, CT) or chlorhexidine diacetate (Nolvasan; Fort Dodge, Madison, NJ) solution.

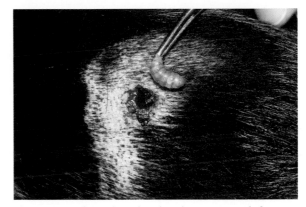

Figure 6-10 Cuterebra that has been removed from its tract. (From Hnilica KA: *Small animal dermatology: A color atlas and therapeutic guide*, ed 3, St. Louis, MO, 2011, Saunders.)

- Oral or topical antibiotics should be given to combat skin infection.

INFORMATION FOR CLIENTS
- Keep young animals in clean, fly-free areas to avoid infection.
- Fly repellant gels may help prevent the disease. Apply to ears and around the neck area (read the label for restrictions).
- Even after removal of the larva, the wound may heal slowly.

Myiasis (Maggots)

Many adult forms of dipterous flies often deposit eggs on the wet, warm, or damaged skin of animals. These eggs hatch into larvae known as *maggots*, which are highly destructive, producing punched-out areas in the skin. These lesions often coalesce to form even larger ulcerated areas. Large numbers of maggots may be found in wounds that have gone unnoticed by owners. Heavy coats and neglect predispose animals to this problem.

DIAGNOSIS
- Owners often report matted hair, a bad odor, or a painful reaction when the animal is petted in a specific area.
- Maggots may be found on physical examination.

TREATMENT

- Clip hair from all lesions.
- Flush the areas with copious amounts of water to remove larvae.
- Manually remove larvae not washed off.
- Daily wound cleaning and treatment must be done.
- Administer oral antibiotics to combat the infection; use one with a good spectrum for skin (Keflex, cephalexin, triple sulfas).
- Keep the pet indoors to prevent reinfestation.

INFORMATION FOR CLIENTS

- Myiasis is a disease of neglect. Owners need to check their outdoor pets frequently, especially during the summer months.
- Heavy-coated animals should be clipped during the hot, humid summer months to avoid damage to the skin.
- Avoid using toxic dips or sprays on wounds to remove larvae.
- Keep pets indoors during peak fly hours to prevent infestation (usually early morning and late afternoon).
- Keep pet's outdoor environment clean to avoid attracting flies.

Lice

Lice are host specific and spend all their lives on that host (Fig. 6-11). They are found on debilitated, dirty, ill-kept animals and are also commonly seen on poultry and pigeons. Lice infestation is a disease of neglect.

DIAGNOSIS

- Pet may become ill-tempered and agitated because of the presence of lice.
- Lice cause intense itching.
- Anemia can develop from blood-sucking lice.
- Presence of lice or nits on the hair coat is diagnostic (Fig. 6-12).

TREATMENT

- Treat all the animals in the house using an insecticide dip, shampoo, or dust. Clip all the hair on the animal. Bathe with a good shampoo. Treat with an insecticide dip, dust, or spray.
- All bedding and grooming tools must be washed thoroughly.
- Ivermectin can be used orally. *However, this use is "off-label"; therefore, a signed release should be obtained from the owner.*

INFORMATION FOR CLIENTS

- Humans cannot get lice from pets.
- The pet cannot get lice from humans.
- Clean the environment to prevent reinfestation.
- Improve the coat care of the pet by including routine bathing and grooming.

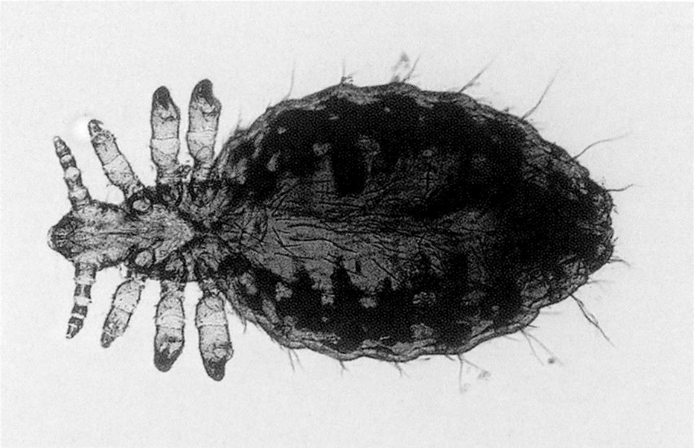

Figure 6-11 Sucking louse *Linognathus setosus* of dogs. (From Hendrix CM, Robinson E: *Diagnostic parasitology for veterinary technicians*, ed 3, St. Louis, MO, 2012, Mosby.)

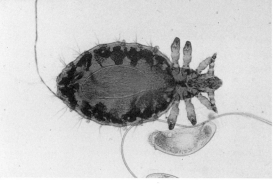

Figure 6-12 *Linognathus setosus*: gravid female sucking louse and associated nit on hair shaft collected from a dog. Nits are oval, white, and usually found cemented to hair shaft. (From Hendrix CM, Robinson E: *Diagnostic parasitology for veterinary technicians*, ed 3, St. Louis, MO, 2012, Mosby.)

Superficial Dermatomycoses (Fungal Infections)

Infections by fungal elements usually occur when the dermatophyte penetrates the skin and begins to proliferate on the surface of the hair shaft. Three species of fungi typically cause disease in the dog and cat: (1) *Microsporum gypseum*, (2) *Trichophyton mentagrophytes*, and (3) *Microsporum canis*. The latter organism is the most commonly isolated dermatophyte of dogs and cats. This fungus may also produce lesions in humans. Infections are usually the result of contact with the organism, and young or debilitated animals appear to be most susceptible. The fungus produces enzymes that result in hypertrophy of the surrounding epidermis. Lesions become scaly with excessive keratin.

Microsporum canis Infections

CLINICAL SIGNS

- The appearance of a rapidly growing circular patch of alopecia indicates *M. canis* infestation; some areas will be red, raised, and crusty (Fig. 6-13, Fig. 6-14, and Fig. 6-15).
- Lesions are most frequently seen on the face and head.

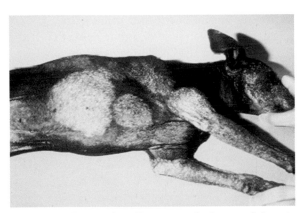

Figure 6-13 Dog with well-circumscribed areas of alopecia and grayish crusts caused by *Microsporum canis*. (From Scott DW, Miller WH, Jr., Griffin CE: *Muller and Kirk's small animal dermatology*, ed 7, Philadelphia, PA, 2013, Saunders.)

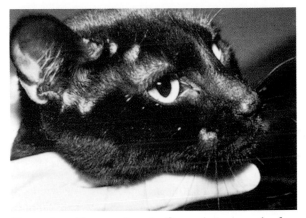

Figure 6-14 Dermatophytosis: Crusty lesions on the face and head of a cat. (From Scott D: *Muller and Kirk's small animal dermatology*, ed 6, St. Louis, MO, 2013, Saunders.)

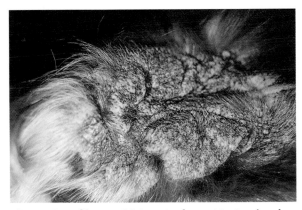

Figure 6-15 Chronic *Malassezia* dermatitis in the dog. (From Gaudiano F: *Veterinary dermatology*, Oxford, U.K., 2005, Elsevier.)

- Hairs in the lesion may appear broken.
- Pet owners may describe similar lesions on themselves.

DIAGNOSIS

- A Wood's light examination may show infected hair shafts that fluoresce. Approximately 50% of *M. canis* organisms will be fluorescent on examination. (Hair shaft will glow yellow-green under ultraviolet light. Ointments and creams applied topically may also fluoresce, producing a false-positive result.)

- Potassium hydroxide (KOH) slide preparation: Place hairs and skin scraping on a clean microscope slide and add a few drops of 10% KOH. Apply a coverslip and heat gently for a few seconds. Observe for fungal elements.
- Culture: Fungal cultures are the most accurate method of diagnosis. Fungal growth is slow, and it may be 10 to 14 days before results are seen.
- Products such as Fungassay and Sab-Duets (Bacti-Labs, Mountain V, CA) may be used in the clinic. A color change from yellow to red occurs with the growth of pathologic organisms. Dermatophyte colonies will be white to cream colored. Cultures should be checked daily for results:
  - Place plucked hairs on the surface of the medium.
  - Label with client or patient identification and the inoculation date.
  - Leave the cap loose to allow oxygen for dermatophyte growth.
  - Place in a warm, out-of-the-way area.

TREATMENT

Localized Lesions

- Clip the affected areas to remove contaminated hair shafts. (Clippers will be contaminated.)
- Treat local areas twice daily with a topical antifungal medication. Continue treatment for 2 weeks after lesions clear. Recommended medications include the following:
  - Miconazole nitrate (Conofite; Pitman-Moore; Mallinckrodt Veterinary Inc., Mundelein, IL)
  - Tresaderm (MSD Agvet; Merck, Whitehouse Station, NJ)
  - Miconazole (Micatin Cream Advanced Care)
  - Miconazole (Monistat; Ortho-McNeil Pharmaceuticals, Raritan, NJ)
  - Lotrimin (Schering-Plough, Kenilworth, NJ)
  - Clotrimazole (Mycelex; Miles Pharmaceuticals, West Haven, CT)
  - Dilute Clorox solution (Clorox Company, Oakland, CA)

Generalized Lesions

- Clip the entire coat. Bathe animal in a medicated shampoo such as Nolvasan. Treat entire body with antifungal preparations 1 to 2 times weekly until cultures are negative. This may take 4 to 16 weeks or longer. Antifungal preparations include the following:
  - Lyme Dyp (DVM Pharmaceuticals)
  - Nolvasan
  - Betadine
  - Clorox
- Oral therapy:
  - Griseofulvin (microsize): PO every 24 hours (Fulvicin U/F; Schering-Plough)
  - Griseofulvin suspension (pediatric) (Ortho-McNeil Pharmaceuticals): two times a day for 4 to 6 weeks; griseofulvin may cause vomiting and diarrhea and is contraindicated in pregnant animals
  - Ketoconazole (Nizoral; Jansen; Janssen Pharmaceuticals, Titusville, NJ): PO every 12 to 24 hours with food; side effects may include depression, anorexia, vomiting and diarrhea, increased alanine aminotransferase, and jaundice

INFORMATION FOR CLIENTS

- *M. canis* infection disease is contagious through contact with the organism.
- Fungal hairs remain infective on shed hairs of the animal for as long as 18 months. Environmental cleaning is a necessity to prevent reinfection. Carpets and furniture should be vacuumed weekly with the bag being discarded each time. Hard surfaces should be cleaned using a 1:10 Clorox solution or Nolvasan solution. Repaint surfaces that cannot be easily cleaned. Throw away toys and equipment not easily cleaned.
- Handle infected animals as little as possible.
- Some cats may be carriers of fungal infection while not exhibiting any clinical signs.
- See your doctor if lesions develop on family members.

Pyodermas

Pyoderma is the term applied to bacterial infections that involve the skin. Pyodermas may be primary or secondary, superficial or deep. The disease is recognized as part of several distinct clinical syndromes.

Superficial Pyodermas

Clinically seen diseases in the superficial pyoderma category include acute moist dermatitis ("hot spots"), impetigo, acne, and skinfold pyodermas. The lesions typically involve only the superficial epidermis, with healing occurring without scarring. The disease is usually of short duration. The animal is rarely systemically ill. The skin around the lesion remains normal, whereas the affected portions may be ulcerated or traumatized by the animal.

Acute Moist Dermatitis ("Hot Spots")

Acute moist dermatitis occurs secondary to skin trauma (usually self-inflicted). Lesions appear rapidly as well-demarcated, red, moist, hot, and painful areas. The condition is common in heavy-coated, water-loving breeds such as Golden Retrievers, Labrador Retrievers, Newfoundlands, German Shepherds, and Saint Bernards. The incidence of the disease appears to be seasonal, being worse in the hot, moist summer months.

CLINICAL SIGNS

- Rapid appearance of red, hot, moist, painful patches
- Hair loss over the area
- Pruritus

DIAGNOSIS

- Visual inspection of the affected area shows typical lesions (Fig. 6-16).

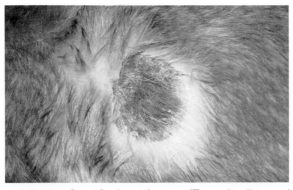

Figure 6-16 Superficial pyodermas. (From *Small animal dermatology: A color atlas and therapeutic guide*, ed 3, St. Louis, MO, 2011, Saunders [Fig 3-21].)

TREATMENT

- Carefully clip the hair from the lesions. Clip area large enough to expose the edges of the lesion. If lesions are large, consider using sedation.
- Gently cleanse the skin using a medicated shampoo:
  - Etiderm (Allerderm, Phoenix, AZ)
  - ChlorhexaDerm (DVM Pharmaceuticals)
- Apply topical medications to lesions twice daily. Avoid medications that dry or attract attention to the site because this will increase self-trauma from licking or rubbing. Although topical medications are not frequently recommended, gentamicin (Gentocin) spray has been of some use.
- Treat the original disease that induced the self-trauma to the skin (e.g., fleas, allergy).
- Cortisone and systemic antibiotics may speed healing:
  - Prednisone: daily for 1 week
  - Cephalexin: twice a day
  - Enrofloxacin: once daily or divided in two doses/day
  - Amoxicillin or clavulanic acid: twice a day

INFORMATION FOR CLIENTS

- Gentle cleansing of the area on a daily basis will speed recovery.
- Owners should wash their hands after treating an infected animal to prevent contamination with *Staphylococcus*. Although human infections are rare, the microorganism could present a danger to owners who are immunosuppressed.
- Lesions may be slow to heal.
- Owners should use an Elizabethan collar to prevent the animal from traumatizing the area.

Impetigo

Impetigo is seen most commonly in young dogs as a secondary infection related to malnourishment, debilitation, and poor hygiene. *Streptococcus* is the usual organism involved, although staphylococci are occasionally cultured from lesions. This disease is not contagious.

CLINICAL SIGNS

- Lesions are seen in young dogs.
- Lesions are commonly seen on the abdomen.

- Lesions include pustules that rupture to form honey-colored crusts.
- Lesions are nonpruritic and nonpainful.

DIAGNOSIS

- Physical appearance in a young animal
- Culture and sensitivity

TREATMENT

- Improve the animal's general health.
- Systemic antibiotics based on culture or sensitivity or an antibiotic with good gram-positive spectrum:
  - Cephalexin: twice a day
  - Enrofloxacin: once daily or divided in two doses/day (avoid use in young animals)
  - Amoxicillin or clavulanic acid: twice a day
- Gently cleanse the lesions using an antibacterial shampoo such as ChlorhexaDerm (DVM Pharmaceuticals) or Etiderm (Allerderm): Use at 2- to 3-day intervals after initial cleaning.
- Topical antibiotic creams may be applied to lesions.

INFORMATION FOR CLIENTS

- Impetigo is not contagious.
- Programs for the elimination of parasites, improvement of the diet, and better sanitation should be implemented to improve the general health of the animal.
- Continue treatment for at least 2 weeks after the lesions disappear.

Acne

Although canine acne is fairly common in young (3 to 12 months of age), short-coated breeds, the disease presents few problems clinically. As dogs mature, lesions spontaneously heal. However, feline acne is clinically significant and often becomes a chronic problem. Acne can occur in cats of all ages.

CLINICAL SIGNS

- The chin may be swollen and painful to the touch.
- Owners may report seeing "dark spots" on the chin and be concerned about neoplasia.
- Large comedones (blackheads) may be present on the chin.
- Cats severely affected may be febrile.

DIAGNOSIS

- Characteristic appearance is diagnostic.
- Rule out other skin infections such as bite abscess.

TREATMENT

- Gently clip the hair on the chin.
- Cleanse with an antibacterial soap.
- Large comedones may require extraction under sedation.
- Clean daily with a human acne product such as Stridex pads (benzoyl peroxide).
- Provide systemic antibiotics for 14 to 21 days (see previous section on impetigo for antibiotic choices and doses). The product should have a good gram-positive spectrum.

INFORMATION FOR CLIENTS

- This problem may become chronic.
- Daily cleaning of the chin may prevent further damage.

Skinfold Pyoderma

Skinfold pyoderma can occur wherever skin is plentiful: lips, facial folds, vulvar folds, and tail folds. The redundant tissue in these folds traps moisture and heat, whereas constant rubbing results in trauma and secondary infection. Facial folds may also present a danger to the cornea of the eye as the hairs on the fold rub across the surface of the cornea.

Skinfold pyodermas are usually a chronic problem that requires long-term medical treatment. Surgical removal of the excess skin is the only effective cure.

DIAGNOSIS

- Presented with a commonly affected breed: Spaniels and Setters (lip fold), Pekingese and Pugs (facial fold), Boston Terriers and Pugs (tail fold), and obese dogs of any breed (tail and vulvar folds).
- Report of a foul odor or discharge from the affected area can be diagnostic.
- Affected area will be moist, red, and ulcerated.

TREATMENT

- Relief of symptoms is the goal of treatment:
  - Clip and clean the area.
  - Dry the lesions. Topical drying agents may be used (e.g., cornstarch).
  - Topical antibiotic ointments may be of some use.

- Surgical removal of the excess skin is the only real cure for the problem.
- Encourage weight reduction for obese animals through diet and exercise programs.

INFORMATION FOR CLIENTS

- Skinfold pyodermas will require long-term medical treatment.
- The affected areas need to be kept dry and clean.
- Weight reduction is mandatory for those animals with tailfold and vulvarfold pyodermas.
- On dogs with facial folds, keep hair away from the eyes, and monitor the appearance of the cornea for signs of injury.

Deep Pyodermas

Deep pyodermas present a greater challenge clinically compared with superficial infections. Deep pyodermas tend to become chronic infections, often resistant to treatment. It has been speculated that these pyodermas may occur in animals with some degree of immunosuppression or allergy. A great many of these cases involve the microorganism *Staphylococcus intermedius*, previously known as *S. aureus*, which produces toxins and enzymes that cause severe tissue damage. Diseases seen clinically include juvenile pyoderma (puppy strangles), interdigital pyoderma (interdigital cysts), and generalized pyoderma (German Shepherd pyoderma). The clinical signs and treatments of all deep pyodermas are similar.

CLINICAL SIGNS

- Appearance of papules and pustules with crusting in characteristic locations is diagnostic.
- Dogs are often febrile.
- Draining fistula tracts with severe infection may exist.

DIAGNOSIS

- Clinical signs
- Culture and sensitivity
- Biopsy

TREATMENT

- Thorough and gentle daily cleaning of the infected areas

- Topical, water-based antibiotic creams, sprays, or solutions applied two to four times daily
- Systemic antibiotics chosen from the culture or sensitivity results or a good gram-positive spectrum drug. Therapy may be needed for 3 months or longer in many cases (see Superficial Pyoderma section for dosing guidelines):
  - Clavamox
  - Enrofloxacin
  - Cephalexin
- Staphylococcal bacterin is given weekly:
  - Staphage Lysate (Delmont Laboratories, Swarthmore, PA)

INFORMATION FOR CLIENTS

- The organism that is responsible for deep pyodermas is often drug resistant.
- Treatment may be prolonged and expensive in large-breed dogs.
- Underlying conditions that predispose the animal to these infections should be investigated. Diabetes mellitus and Cushing disease are two conditions that may present as recurrent skin infections.
- Some animals will never recover.

Anal Glands

The anal sacs create a special set of problems in companion animals. Three commonly seen anal sac problems are impaction, chronic infection, and rupture or abscessation. The anal sacs are located between muscle layers of the anus at the 4 and 8 o'clock positions. Each sac connects to the surface through a narrow duct. The sacs are lined with abundant sebaceous glands that produce an oily brown fluid that has a characteristic odor (foul smelling). When feces pass over the sacs, the sacs are compressed, expelling some of the fluid onto the surface of the fecal material. The odor of this fluid may have the function of social marking among dogs and cats. If the fluid produced becomes too thick or blockage of the duct occurs, the sacs will overfill. As water is reabsorbed from the fluid, the material dries out, causing impaction of the sac. Infections and impactions may result in anal sac rupture or abscessation. This condition is usually seen in small-breed dogs.

CLINICAL SIGNS

- History of scooting the rear end across the floor or licking excessively at the perianal area (Fig. 6-17)
- Foul odor

DIAGNOSIS

- Digital palpation of distended anal sacs (may be performed rectally or externally)

TREATMENT

- Express contents of the distended sac (the dog may need sedation).
- Lavage the infected sac with lactated Ringer solution.
- Instill antibiotic ointment into the sac.
- Treat abscessed sacs aggressively with lavage and cleaning.
- Oral antibiotics may speed healing time.
- Chronically infected sacs should be surgically removed.
- *Remember:* Empty the opposite sac also when you are treating a unilateral infection.

INFORMATION FOR CLIENTS

- Owners should be shown how to check their pet's anal sacs. If they request, demonstrate how to empty them.
- Scooting on the floor does not usually mean that the pet has worms.

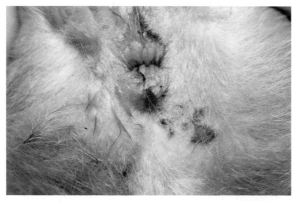

Figure 6-17 Anal sac disease. (From *Small animal dermatology: A color atlas and therapeutic guide*, ed 3, St. Louis, MO, 2011, Saunders [Fig 13-78].)

- Blood under the tail may indicate a ruptured anal sac.
- These impactions and infections tend to recur.
- Cats can develop impactions, which may abscess.

Tumors of the Skin

The word *tumor* may be defined as a new growth of tissue characterized by progressive, uncontrolled proliferation of cells. Tumors can be *benign* (do no harm) or *malignant* (may result in death) and localized or invasive. Malignant tumors usually consist of poorly differentiated cells that metastasize to other parts of the body and are usually invasive to surrounding tissues. Malignant tumors of the skin are usually *carcinomas* (those of epithelial origin) or *sarcomas* (those of connective tissue origin). An estimated 37% of canine tumors and 24% of feline tumors involve the skin.

Although no clear-cut cause of tumors has been found, certain trends are worth mentioning:
- Most skin tumors occur in older dogs (>6 years) and cats (>4 years).
- Younger dogs are more likely to acquire viral-induced tumors.
- Certain breeds such as Boxers and Cocker Spaniels appear to be more susceptible to tumor development.

Although the role genetics plays in the development of neoplastic disease (neoplasia) is still under investigation, neoplasia may be a result of a combination of events that allow a mass of unregulated cells to proliferate within the tissues of the body.

Benign Skin Tumors

Histiocytomas

CLINICAL SIGNS

- Found almost exclusively in young dogs
- Small, buttonlike nodules, usually pink
- Usually hairless and may be ulcerated
- Found on the face, legs, lips, and abdomen
- Rapidly growing lesion

DIAGNOSIS

- General appearance
- Biopsy

TREATMENT

- Local surgical excision
- Many tumors regress spontaneously

INFORMATION FOR CLIENTS

- Histiocytomas are not malignant and do not metastasize.
- This tumor is not seen in cats.
- Lesions may regress spontaneously; however, surgical excision is the treatment of choice.

Lipoma

CLINICAL SIGNS

- Obese, older dogs commonly affected
- Female dogs more commonly affected than male dogs
- Round or oval subcuticular masses
- Encapsulated and slow-growing masses
- Lesions are soft
- Many lesions are freely movable

DIAGNOSIS

- Biopsy
- Fine-needle aspiration will provide a presumptive diagnosis. (A gray, greasy, mucoidlike substance is removed from the slide by the fixing step of staining.)

TREATMENT

- Surgical excision is the treatment of choice.
- Care should be taken to close the tissue space that results from removal of the mass.

INFORMATION FOR CLIENTS

- These masses rarely become malignant.
- They may recur after removal.
- A change in diet will probably not affect existing lipomas.
- These are benign tumors, even though they may grow large.

Papillomas (Warts)

CLINICAL SIGNS

- Young dogs are commonly affected.
- Lesion begins as a smooth, white, elevated lesion in the oral mucosa that develops into a cauliflower-like growth (may be few or multiple).
- Regression of the lesion may occur spontaneously.

DIAGNOSIS

- General appearance
- Biopsy

TREATMENT

- Surgical excision of large masses may stimulate regression of others.
- Autogenous vaccines can be made by grinding tumor tissue (1:4 weight-to-volume) in 0.5% phenol. Inject 1 to 5 mL intradermally weekly for 3 weeks.
- Lesions usually will regress without treatment.

INFORMATION FOR CLIENTS

- Papillomas are caused by a deoxyribonucleic acid (DNA) virus.
- Disease may last as long as 21 weeks or more.
- Cats are not affected.
- Older dogs are resistant.
- This disease usually regresses spontaneously, and adult animals become immune for life.

Sebaceous Cysts

CLINICAL SIGNS

- Sebaceous cysts may occur in dogs of any age or sex. The cysts are more common in Cocker Spaniels.
- Cysts are encapsulated, round, and fluctuate on palpation. When compressed, they may exude a gray, cheeselike material.
- Cysts slowly enlarge and may spontaneously rupture.
- Cysts may be found on the back, legs, chest, and neck of the animal.

DIAGNOSIS

- Characteristic contents of the cyst
- Histology of cyst wall

TREATMENT

- Surgical removal of entire encapsulated cyst

INFORMATION FOR CLIENTS

- These growths are formed by degenerative changes in the glandular area surrounding the hair follicle.

- Sebaceous cysts are benign growths.
- Surgical removal will cure the problem.
- These lesions are usually slow growing.
- Dogs may have multiple lesions at varying times, especially in breeds that are predisposed to this problem.

Malignant Skin Tumors

Basal Cell Carcinoma

CLINICAL SIGNS

- Basal cell carcinoma is a common tumor of adult animals.
- A single, discrete lesion that is round, firm, and often ulcerated is found.
- This lesion is most commonly found on the head (around the eyes), ears, lips, neck, and legs.
- These lesions are slow growing.

DIAGNOSIS

- Biopsy

TREATMENT

- Wide surgical excision

INFORMATION FOR CLIENTS

- These tumors rarely metastasize.
- Local recurrence after surgery is possible.
- A less favorable prognosis exists if there are multiple lesions.

Fibrosarcomas (not Vaccine-induced)

CLINICAL SIGNS

- Older dogs are affected.
- Face, legs, and mammary glands are the most common sites.
- Tumors range in size, feel firm but rubbery on palpation, are unencapsulated, and feel adhered to underlying tissues.

DIAGNOSIS

- Biopsy

TREATMENT

- Wide surgical excision is necessary, and recurrence is common.

INFORMATION FOR CLIENTS

- Generally the prognosis for fibrosarcomas is poor because the tumors are invasive and metastasize readily.
- Recurrence is common.
- Other therapies such as radiation and chemotherapy are not usually effective.
- Wide surgical excision may require amputation of the limb.

Feline Fibrosarcomas (Vaccine-induced)

Until the late 1980s, feline fibrosarcomas were unrecognized. During that time, a killed rabies vaccine and the feline leukemia vaccine became available to practitioners. The incidence of vaccination-related tumors began to increase to between 1:1000 and 1:10,000 vaccinated cats. With an estimated 20 million vaccines administered to pet cats throughout the world, this tumor development has become a significant problem for feline practitioners and owners. These tumors are rapidly developing, highly invasive, and malignant. They occur at the site of vaccination, usually within 4 to 6 weeks after the vaccine has been given. After routine surgical removal, they often recur. By the time many owners act, it is too late to provide successful treatment for the cats. In an effort to prevent or reduce the incidence of this disease, the Vaccine-Associated Sarcoma Task Force has issued the following guidelines for feline vaccination:

1. Use single-dose vaccines, whenever possible. Intranasal vaccines should be chosen when available. Never vaccinate between the shoulder blades.
2. Rabies vaccine should be given as low on the *right* rear leg as possible, leukemia vaccine low on the *left* rear leg, and the distemper combinations on the *right* shoulder.
3. Any swelling not resolved within 6 weeks should be removed by radical surgical excision.

CLINICAL SIGNS

- Swelling over the site of a recent vaccination in a cat
- Rapidly growing, firm, often elongated mass

DIAGNOSIS

- Biopsy or needle aspiration may confirm suspicion.

TREATMENT

- Radical surgical excision, which may involve limb amputation, is the treatment of choice.

INFORMATION FOR CLIENTS

- Feline fibrosarcoma has a poor prognosis if not detected early and treated aggressively.
- Some individual cats or breeds of cats may be genetically at risk for this disease.
- Inflammatory lumps do develop over vaccine sites in many cats; however, they usually disappear within 1 to 2 weeks. If the lump does not resolve in 4 to 6 weeks, see your veterinarian.

⬤ TECH ALERT

The vaccine most often suspected of causing these tumors has been the adjuvant rabies vaccine containing aluminum. Newer nonadjuvant rabies vaccines are on the market and should be used, when possible.

Mast Cell Tumors

CLINICAL SIGNS

- Isolated, firm nodules form in the skin. About 50% are found on the rear legs, perineum, or external genitalia.
- Tumors may be ulcerated and edematous.
- These tumors are usually seen in dogs older than 6 years and cats older than 10 years.
- Siamese and male cats are usually predisposed.
- Lesions may appear crusty in cats.
- When crusts are removed, ulcerated surfaces are exposed.

DIAGNOSIS

- Biopsy
- Impression smears may demonstrate mast cell granules for presumptive diagnosis

TREATMENT

- Surgical excision with a lymph node examination to rule out metastasis
- Chemotherapy (using the following drugs):

⬤ TECH ALERT

Animals requiring chemotherapy may best be handled by a referral to an oncology specialist.

- • Vinblastine: once weekly
  - • Cytoxan: once every 4 days
  - • Prednisolone: daily for 1 week
- Prednisolone: PO every 24 hours for 14 days, then half that dose for 14 days, then half dose every 48 hours for 5 months
- Radiation and cryosurgery
- Cimetidine: 4 mg/kg every 6 hours in cases of lymph node involvement or gastric ulceration or irritation
- Premedication with diphenhydramine (Benadryl IM) has been recommended to block the histamine release caused by manipulation of the tumor at surgery

INFORMATION FOR CLIENTS

- Mast cell tumors do not usually metastasize; however, up to 30% may metastasize.
- The prognosis depends on the amount of cell differentiation within the tumor. In dogs, the survival times range from 18 to 51 weeks; in cats, the lesions are usually benign.
- Recurrence at the surgical site is possible.
- A virus may cause these tumors.

Melanoma (Benign or Malignant)

CLINICAL SIGNS

- Benign lesions are usually small, slow-growing, hairless growths with dark pigmentation.
- Malignant growths are usually large, dome-shaped, sessile growths of varying pigmentation.
- Tumors most commonly occur in the highly pigmented tissues of the canine (oral, skin, and digits) although amelanotic tumors do occur.

DIAGNOSIS

- Biopsy

TREATMENT

- Surgical resection

INFORMATION FOR CLIENTS

- Tumors of the oral cavity and digits tend to be malignant.
- These tumors metastasize readily.
- Because of early metastasis, the prognosis is often poor.
- Recurrence after surgery is common.
- In dogs with small lesions, median survival time is 12 months (54% are dead within 2 years). With large lesions, survival time is 4 months (100% are dead within 2 years).

Perianal Tumors (Adenomas and Adenocarcinomas)

CLINICAL SIGNS

- Adenomas are most commonly seen in male dogs older than 8 years.
- Carcinomas occur with equal frequency in male and female animals.
- Lesions are small, slow-growing, single or multiple lumps close to the anus.
- Lesions are frequently ulcerated, and owners may report seeing blood under the tail.
- Cocker Spaniels, Beagles, Samoyeds, and German Shepherds appear to be predisposed to perianal tumors.

DIAGNOSIS

- Clinical appearance and location
- Biopsy

TREATMENT

- Complete surgical excision is recommended.
- Castration aids in preventing recurrence of adenomas.
- Radiation and cryosurgery are both effective in treating these tumors.

INFORMATION FOR CLIENTS

- Castration of the intact male dog is highly recommended to prevent recurrence of adenomas.
- Adenomas rarely become malignant.
- Adenocarcinomas are usually highly invasive to surrounding tissue.
- Without a biopsy, it may be difficult to distinguish an adenoma from an adenocarcinoma.

Squamous Cell Carcinoma

CLINICAL SIGNS

- Older dogs and cats (>9 years of age)
- Lesions seen on the head, ears, oral cavity, nose, and neck of cats; trunk, toes, and scrotum of dogs (nonpigmented areas)
- Tumor appears as a raised, ulcerated, cauliflower-like mass with a necrotic odor
- Affected animals have a history of being "sunbathers"

DIAGNOSIS

- Biopsy

TREATMENT

- Surgical excision
- Cryosurgery
- Radiotherapy (photodynamic therapy)

INFORMATION FOR CLIENTS

- These tumors occur most frequently in sun-damaged skin.
- Most tumors are locally invasive but slow to metastasize.
- Recurrence after surgery is common.
- Preventing chronic exposure to the sun will prevent the development of the tumors.
- The degree of malignancy determines the prognosis, especially in cats whose poorly differentiated tumors have a poor prognosis.

REVIEW QUESTIONS

1. Because of the development of vaccine-induced feline sarcomas in some cats, it is recommended to administer the feline leukemia virus vaccine:
   a. Between the shoulders
   b. Low on the right shoulder
   c. Low on the left rear leg
   d. Low on the right rear leg
2. What benign tumor is found exclusively in young dogs and is usually a rapidly growing, hairless mass found on the face or legs?
   a. Mast cell tumor
   b. Histiocytoma
   c. Squamous cell carcinoma
   d. Fibrosarcoma

3. It is possible to fully eliminate the *Demodex* mite from the animal with treatment.
   a. True
   b. False
4. What tick typically inhabits buildings and kennels?
   a. *Dermacentor variabilis*
   b. *Amblyomma* spp.
   c. *Rhipicephalus sanguineus*
5. Patients having mast cell tumors surgically removed are often premedicated with _____ to block histamine released by tumor manipulation.
   a. tripelennamine
   b. diphenhydramine
   c. chlorpheniramine
   d. trimeprazine
6. The recurrence of perineal adenomas may be prevented by castration.
   a. True
   b. False
7. What growths are formed by degenerative changes in the glandular area surrounding the hair follicle?
   a. Basal cell carcinomas
   b. Squamous cell carcinomas
   c. Sebaceous cysts
   d. Papillomas

8. Approximately _____ of *M. canis* organisms will be fluorescent when examined with Wood's light.
   a. 20%
   b. 40%
   c. 100%
   d. 50%
9. Most dermatophyte media change color with the growth of pathogenic organisms. The color change is from _____ to _____.
   a. Red; yellow
   b. Yellow; red
   c. Brown; green
   d. Blue; green
10. Technicians should avoid tearing the *Cuterebra* larva when removing it from the swelling on the animal because this can result in an anaphylactic reaction.
    a. True
    b. False

Answers found on page 552.

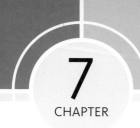

7
CHAPTER

Diseases of the Musculoskeletal System

LEARNING OBJECTIVES

When you have completed this chapter, you will be able to:

1. Describe how muscles and bones act together to result in purposeful movement.
2. List various musculoskeletal problems with respect to bone, muscle, joint, or combinations of each as the cause.
3. Discuss various musculoskeletal problems, treatments, therapy with clients.
4. Know what diagnostic tests are needed for the diagnosis of musculoskeletal diseases.

The musculoskeletal system is responsible for movement and shape in all animals. Animals must be able to move, find food, seek shelter, and escape predators to survive. Without a rigid frame (the skeleton), flexible articulations (joints), and a system of pulleys (muscles, tendons, and ligaments), animals would be little more than lumps of tissue. The integration of these systems provides *movement*, one of the basic characteristics of life.

Disruption of the musculoskeletal system can occur as a result of the following:

- Trauma—fractures, ligament ruptures
- Degenerative disease—osteochondritis dissecans (OCD), degenerative joint disease (DJD), non-united anconeal process
- Inflammation—myositis, panosteitis
- Poor conformation—luxating patella
- Neoplasia

Anatomy of the Musculoskeletal System

A complete review of the anatomy of the musculoskeletal system is beyond the scope of this text; however, a brief overview of bone and muscle metabolism and joint function is necessary to appreciate how disease of this system affects the health of the animal. Often, the muscular and skeletal systems are combined because without one the other cannot function.

Bone

Long bone begins its formation in the fetus as a cartilage model. As the fetus develops, that cartilage is converted to bone through a process called *endochondral ossification.* The cartilage is replaced with osteoblasts, osteoclasts, and osteocytes, all of which are active in producing and shaping new bone. Long bones such as the humerus and the femur have shafts (diaphysis) comprising compact bone, whereas the ends (epiphysis) are filled with spongy bone. Spongy bone is also called *cancellous bone.* Flat bones such as those found in the skull also begin as cartilage but are converted to bone in a manner different from long bones. These bones are formed through intramembranous ossification (Fig. 7-1). Bone formation takes place here in a connective tissue membrane, which is then converted at multiple sites into both cancellous

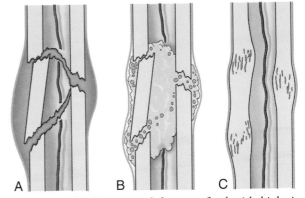

Figure 7-1 A, Comminuted fractures fixed with biologic techniques of indirect reduction, major segment alignment, and optimal stabilization appear to heal with a combination of direct differentiation of mesenchymal cells to osteoblasts and endochondral ossification. **B,** The fracture site fills with endosteal and bridging callus. **C,** Resorption of woven bone and formation of lamellar bone at the fracture sites result in remodeling of bony callus to cortical bone (From Fossum, TW: Small Animal Surgery, ed. 4, St Louis, 2013, Mosby, by permission).

(internal) and compact bone (superficial). Students are familiar with bone from the anatomy models, but they seldom think of bone as a living tissue! In the body, bone is constantly being broken down, remodeled, and produced, and as the animal uses bone, it strengthens along the lines of stress, becoming stronger with use. Bone is also a large storehouse for calcium, phosphorus, and certain minerals. Epiphyseal bone is active in red blood cell (RBC) production. Bones are important for movement, protection of underlying tissues, and support. The hormones calcitonin and parathyroid hormone balance the level of calcium in both blood and bone, constantly adjusting levels to meet the needs of the animal.

Muscles

Skeletal muscle tissue combines with bones to form the musculoskeletal system. This muscle tissue is striated and voluntary. The striations are formed from the overlap of the actin and myosin fibers found in the sarcomere, the contractile unit of the muscle. Contraction of these muscle fibers occurs in the presence of neuronal stimulation at the neuromuscular junction (cholinergic) and with increased calcium released within the muscle fiber in response to this stimulation (Fig. 7-2). Contraction of multiple muscle fibers simultaneously moves the bones attached to those muscles.

Injuries that involve the musculoskeletal system are painful, and analgesics should be used to increase the comfort of the patient. A pain-free patient will not only be more comfortable while healing, but will be able to function normally again more rapidly. Any disease or malfunction of this system compromises the animal's ability to maintain homeostasis with its environment.

Joints

Muscles and bones form lever systems such as joints. Bone makes up the *lever*, and joints serve as the *fulcrum* for the system. When contracting, the muscle moves the lever (bone) around the joint's fulcrum. The manner in which different muscles are placed with respect to bone determines the motion of that joint. Along with muscles, bones are connected to tendons and ligaments, which also support the movement of the joint. This lever system provides a mechanical means of movement for the limbs.

Long Bone Fractures

At least three fourths of long bone fractures occur as a result of motor vehicle accidents. Other causes include indirect violence, bone disease, or repeated stress. These fractures may be classified as *open* (bone exposed through the skin) or *closed* (bone not exposed through the skin), *simple* or *comminuted* (splintered or fragmented), and *stable* or *unstable* (Fig. 7-3). The type of fracture and its location determine the best method of repair.

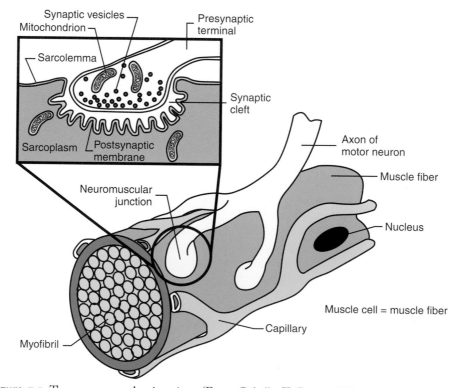

Figure 7-2 The neuromuscular junction. (From Colville T, Bassert JM: *Clinical anatomy and physiology for veterinary technicians,* ed 2, St. Louis, MO, 2008, Mosby.)

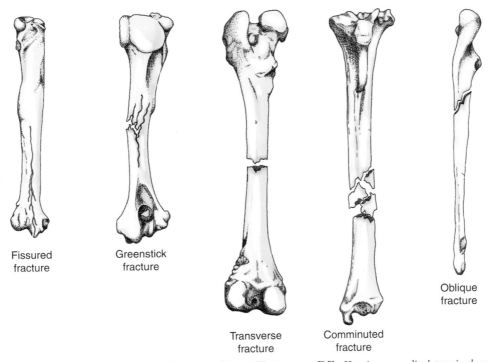

Fissured fracture

Greenstick fracture

Transverse fracture

Comminuted fracture

Oblique fracture

Figure 7-3 Common traumatic fractures. (From Christenson DE: *Veterinary medical terminology*, Philadelphia, PA, 2009, Saunders, by permission.)

The job of the veterinary technician is to quickly assess the patient, especially in the case of motor vehicle accidents. After treatment for shock, hemorrhage, and soft tissue trauma, the possibility of fractures should be addressed. Technicians should always be aware that fractures might exist. They should take care when moving the animal, protect any areas of suspected fractures with support bandages (such as a Robert Jones), if possible, and be careful not to make the injury worse by restraint methods or handling when obtaining radiographs.

CLINICAL SIGNS

- History of trauma
- Pain or localized tenderness
- Lameness
- Deformity of the bone
- Loss of function
- Crepitus
- Localized swelling or bruising

DIAGNOSIS

- Radiographs, at least two views, are required to diagnose and characterize the fracture.
- Radiographs of the opposite limb may be of use for comparison.

TREATMENT

- Reduction and fixation of the fracture should be accomplished as soon as the patient is stable.

Methods of Fixation

- Splints:
  - A mold of material that surrounds the affected area is placed to hold the fracture segments in the reduced position while healing occurs.
  - Use is usually limited to limbs.
  - Make sure to use adequate padding to prevent the split from causing soft tissue injury.
  - Keep the splint dry, and restrict activity.

- Evidence of problems with the splint includes a foul odor, swelling, pain, fever, chewing at the splint, and generalized depression.
- Casts:
  - Casts are made of plaster of Paris or other rigid, moldable material.
  - Their function is similar to splints.

TECH ALERT

Casts and splints may not prevent rotation or overriding of fracture pieces and may result in delayed healing or nonunion in some fractures.

- Intramedullary pins:
  - Provide good rigidity to fracture site (Fig. 7-4)
  - May be used in combination with other methods to prevent rotation
  - Usually require removal after the fracture has healed
  - Must be inserted under sterile conditions
  - Promote healing (adult dogs) in 7 to 12 weeks
- Bone plates:
  - Work well on most long bone fractures, particularly in large dogs or a semidomesticated species
  - Should always be removed after healing is complete; however, most are left in place unless

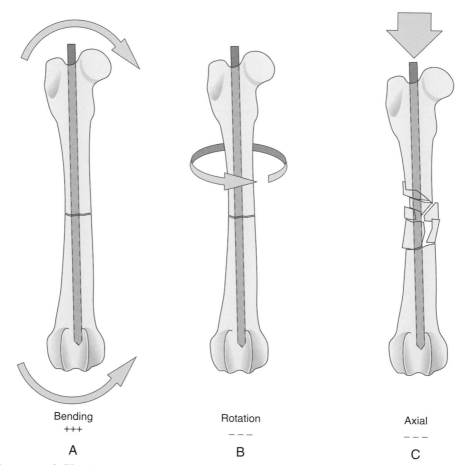

Bending
+++

A

Rotation
– – –

B

Axial
– – –

C

Figure 7-4 A, The biomechanical advantage of intramedullary pins is that they are equally resistant to bending loads applied from any direction because they are round. **B** and **C,** Biomechanical disadvantages of intramedullary pins include poor resistance to rotational or axial (compressive) loads and lack of fixation (interlocking) with bone. (From Fossum TW: *Small animal surgery,* ed 3, St. Louis, MO, 2007, Mosby, by permission.)

they break, interfere with normal bone growth in young animals, or become irritating or infected
- Can usually be removed after bone union in adult dogs (5–12 months)
- Require specialized instrumentation and surgical technique for correct application (Fig. 7-5)
- Provide an early return to function

INFORMATION FOR CLIENTS

- Activity must be restricted while bone is healing. Leash walking and cage rest may be required for 5 to 8 weeks.
- Report any evidence of drainage, swelling, or heat in the affected limb.
- Bone plates and intramedullary pins are stronger than surrounding bone, and refracture of bone may occur in some cases. Report any change in use of the limb.
- Follow-up radiographs are required to assess healing. Surgery may be required to remove the pin or plate after healing has been completed.

- Some animals suffer cold sensitivity to plates and pins. If this occurs, the plates and pins may have to be removed.
- Physical therapy will prevent muscle atrophy and keep the joints supple.

Cruciate Ligament Injury

The *anterior* and *posterior cruciate ligaments* are intraarticular structures that help stabilize the stifle joint. Rupture of the cranial cruciate ligament is possibly the most common injury to the stifle of the dog and is a major cause of DJD in the stifle joint (Fig. 7-6). The ligament may rupture completely, resulting in gross instability of the joint, or it may tear, producing minor instability. Both injuries result in degenerative changes within the joint within a few weeks.

Cruciate ligament injuries are usually seen in middle-aged, obese, inactive animals that suddenly hyperextend their stifle joint while exercising. Rupture may also occur in animals engaged in athletic endeavors (such as racing or jumping), resulting in

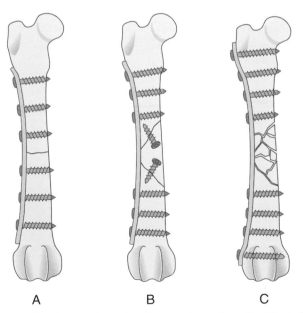

A　　　　　　B　　　　　　C

Figure 7-5 Functions of a bone plate. **A,** Compression plate. **B,** Neutralization plate. **C,** Buttress plate. (From Fossum TW: *Small animal surgery*, ed 3, St. Louis, MO, 2007, Mosby, by permission.)

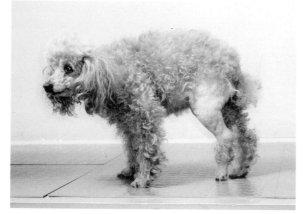

Figure 7-6 Poodle with rupture of the cranial cruciate ligament. The affected limb is held with the stifle in a flexed position and the paw off the floor. This is typical of (acute) stifle injuries. (From Millis D, Levine D: *Canine rehabilitation and physical therapy*, ed 2, St. Louis, MO, 2014, Saunders.)

a traumatic injury to the ligament. An occult degenerative process that may be present in the former group of animals predisposes the ligament to atraumatic rupture. In both groups, rupture of the opposite cruciate ligament often occurs within a year after injury to the first ligament. Approximately 50% of dogs with ligament rupture also demonstrate meniscal injury.

Treatment of this type of injury involves removal of the damaged tissue and stabilization of the joint. Many repair techniques have been reported; the choice of technique is usually based on the size of the dog, the activity level required by the animal, and the skill of the surgeon.

CLINICAL SIGNS

- Middle-aged, obese animals or highly active, athletic animals are commonly affected.
- Injury occurs infrequently in cats.
- Animal demonstrates non–weight bearing on rear leg or appears to be in pain when affected leg is used.
- Tibia usually rotates internally when the animal tries to bear weight.
- If the injury is recent, the joint may show effusion (swelling).
- Generally, the problem is acute in onset.

DIAGNOSIS

- Demonstration of a positive *cranial drawer movement*: (The tibia abnormally slides forward with respect to the femoral condyles.) The animal may need to be sedated to demonstrate this instability.
- Tibial compression test: The tibia moves forward with respect to the femur when the hock is flexed in the proper manner.
- Radiographs may show cranial displacement of the tibial plateau or a bony avulsion at the tibial attachment of the ligament.

TREATMENT

- Many methods of treatment can be found in the literature. The most successful techniques involve surgical stabilization of the stifle joint. In all cases, damaged tissue must be removed from the joint before stabilization.

Extraarticular Stabilization Techniques

- These techniques are most successful in animals weighing less than 15 kg.
- Suture material is placed around the caudal fabellae and through a tunnel in the tibial crest to stabilize the joint.
- Imbrication of the joint capsule and the lateral and medial muscle fascia is performed to "tighten" the joint.

Intraarticular Stabilization Technique

- "Over-the-top" patellar tendon graft uses a strip of the patellar tendon to replace the cranial cruciate ligament.
- Tibial plateau leveling osteotomy prevents the tibia from moving forward against the pull of the hamstring muscles.
- The surgical techniques mentioned, among others, can be found in most veterinary orthopedic surgical texts. No matter which technique is chosen, the goal is always the same—to stabilize the joint and prevent the development of DJD.

INFORMATION FOR CLIENTS

- The pet requires restricted exercise for the first 3 to 4 weeks after surgery. Restricted exercise means cage rest with leash walking for elimination.

- You may gradually increase exercise between 4 and 8 weeks after surgery.
- Your pet may return to full exercise between 8 and 12 weeks after surgery.
- The opposite cruciate frequently ruptures within 1 year after the first rupture.
- Weight reduction will benefit the obese animal.
- Even if surgical stabilization is performed, the animal will have some degenerative changes in the joint (arthritis) as it ages. Your pet may require treatment with antiinflammatory medication if lameness and pain occur.

Patellar Luxations

Patellar luxations occur frequently in dogs and occasionally in cats. They may be divided into several classes:
- Medial luxation: toy, miniature, large breeds
- Lateral luxation: toy, miniature breeds
- Medial traumatic luxations: any breed
- Lateral luxation: large, giant breeds

Medial Luxation of Toy, Miniature, and Large Breeds

Medial luxations of toy, miniature, and large breeds occur early in life and are not related to trauma. They are often called *congenital* because they are usually the result of anatomic deformities. Approximately 75% to 80% of patellar luxations are medial displacements. Anatomic derangements that predispose an animal to medial luxations include medial bowing of the distal third of the femur, shallow trochlear sulcus and a poorly developed medial ridge, medial torsion of the tibial tubercle, or medial bowing of the proximal tibia. Over time, these derangements put added stress on the cranial cruciate ligaments, predisposing 15% to 20% of these ligaments to rupture.

Surgery is required to correct these problems. The technique chosen will depend on the degree of displacement and the degree of rotation present.

CLINICAL SIGNS

- Neonates or young puppies with abnormal hind limb function should be examined.
- Young to mature animals with abnormal or intermittent gait problems are predisposed to this condition.

- Older animals with sudden rear leg lameness are predisposed to this condition.

Lateral Luxation in Toy and Miniature Breeds

Lateral luxation is seen later in life as the soft tissues in the stifle begin to break down. The lateral deviations produce more functional disruption than the medial luxations.

CLINICAL SIGNS

- Acute development of lameness often associated with trauma or strenuous exercise is commonly seen.
- Knock-kneed stance is seen in some cases.
- If lameness is bilateral, the animal may be unable to stand.

Combined Medial and Lateral Luxations or Medial Luxations from Trauma

Combined medial and lateral luxations or medial luxations from trauma occur infrequently in small animals.

Lateral Luxation in Large and Giant Breeds

Lateral luxation is seen in the same breeds that are affected by hip dysplasia. Abnormal conformation at the hip results in a medial rotation of the femur and lateral displacement of the patella.

CLINICAL SIGNS

- Lateral luxation is usually bilateral.
- Animals affected are frequently between 5 and 6 months of age.
- Cow-hocked (external tibial rotation) gait is a clinical sign.
- Foot twists laterally when weight bearing.

DIAGNOSIS

- Palpation is used to test the ability to luxate the patella while the knee is flexed.
- Radiographs indicate anatomic deformity and patellar displacement.

TREATMENT

- Surgical correction is the treatment of choice. Methods range from mild soft tissue techniques to bone reconstruction. Usually, both knees are corrected at the same time.

Soft Tissue Techniques
- Overlap of lateral or medial retinaculum
- Fascia lata overlap
- Patellar and tibial antirotational sutures
- Quadriceps release

Bone Reconstruction
- Trochleoplasty
- Transposition of the tibial tubercle
- Osteotomy or arthrodesis (joint fusion)

Goal
- The goal of all surgical correction is to stabilize the stifle and return the patella to its functional position within the joint (and to keep it there). Combinations of several techniques may be required in some animals to achieve stability.

INFORMATION FOR CLIENTS

- After surgery, limit exercise for 2 to 3 weeks; prevent jumping in particular.
- A support bandage may be placed on the knee for 10 to 14 days to protect the surgical site. It should be kept dry.
- Aspirin or other antiinflammatory drugs can be administered for pain.
- Physiotherapy such as swimming or passive flexion–extension of the joint (20–30 times four times daily) can be of benefit in animals that are reluctant to bear weight on the leg.
- The animal will probably have some degenerative changes in the joint later in life.

Hip Dysplasia

Dysplasia is one of the most prevalent disorders of the canine hip, although it is rarely seen in animals weighing less than 11 to 12 kg. However, it has been reported in the occasional toy or small breed dog. The disease is complex, and the following factors have been identified as contributing to the development of hip dysplasia:
- Genetic predisposition (polygenic)
- Environment and dietary factors
- A disparity between muscle mass and the developing skeletal system

- Failure of the soft tissues of the hip to maintain joint congruity between the surfaces of the hip joint, resulting in bony changes within the joint

Hip dysplasia is a dynamic process and is often defined as a congenital, bilateral DJD, or as hip laxity. Any view of the disease is only a point along the progression of symptoms. The disease can be separated into *acetabular hip dysplasia* and *femoral hip dysplasia*.

Acetabular Hip Dysplasia

Most cases of dysplasia are of the acetabular form. This type is characterized by excessive slope of the dorsal rim of the acetabulum and the changes that result. Failure of the femoral head to press correctly into the developing acetabular cup results in damage to the dorsal rim. Osteophyte formation and damage to the joint capsule result in an unstable, painful joint.

Femoral Hip Dysplasia

In femoral hip dysplasia, the femoral neck is shortened, decreasing the coverage by the acetabular rim and disrupting the congruity of the joint surfaces. In some cases, the femur may be rotated. The joint lacks support from the acetabulum, which leads to osteophyte formation and joint capsule damage with joint instability.

CLINICAL SIGNS

- Clinical signs may vary with the age of the patient.
- Young dogs between 5 and 8 months of age and mature animals with chronic disease are predisposed to femoral hip dysplasia.
- Difficulty in rising and stiffness that diminishes as the animal warms up on exercise are commonly seen.
- Pain is elicited on palpation of the dorsal pelvic area or over the hip joint.
- In older dogs, lameness, a waddling gait, and atrophy of the thigh muscles may be seen.
- Young dogs that are severely affected may be reluctant to stand or move.

DIAGNOSIS

- Radiographic confirmation of the disease is essential (Fig. 7-7). The technician is referred to current radiology texts for positioning techniques.

- The Orthopedic Foundation for Animals (OFA) has established seven grades of dysplasia:
  - Excellent—nearly perfect conformation
  - Good—normal for age and breed
  - Fair—less than ideal but within normal limits
  - Near normal—borderline conformation
  - Mild dysplasia—minimal deviation with slight flattened femoral head and subluxation
  - Moderate dysplasia—shallow acetabulum, flattened femoral head, poor joint congruency
  - Severe dysplasia—complete dislocation of the hip with flattening of the acetabulum and femoral head

- For OFA certification, dogs should be radiographed after reaching 2 years of age. Any dog with clinical signs should be radiographed under anesthesia or sedation.

TREATMENT

Conservative

- Moderate exercise
- Weight control
- Antiinflammatory medications:
  - Rimadyl (Carprofen): twice a day
  - Aspirin (buffered): twice a day
  - Prednisone: daily, decreasing to level that keeps animal comfortable

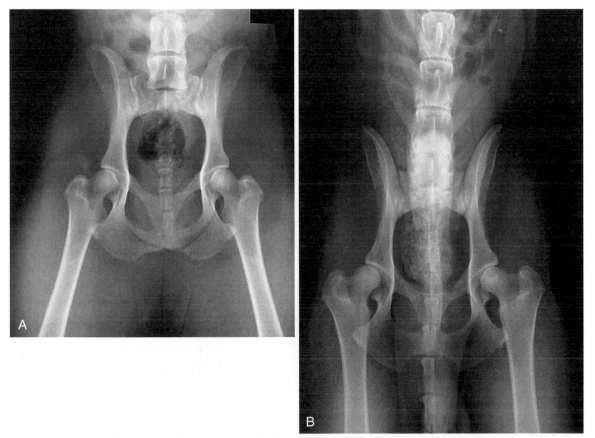

Figure 7-7 Examples of hip dysplasia in the dog. Note the lack of congruity at the hip joint. (From Kealy JK, McAllister H, Graham JP: *Diagnostic radiology and ultrasonography of the dog and cat*, ed. 5, St. Louis, MO, 2011, Saunders.)

Continued

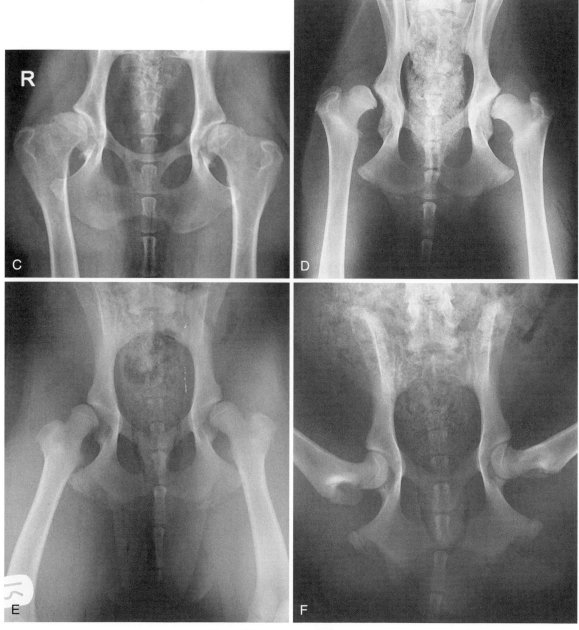

Figure 7-7, cont'd

- Nutriceuticals:
  - Polysulfated glycosaminoglycan (Adequan)
  - Glucosamine chondroitin sulfate (Cosequin)

Surgical

- Femoral head ostectomy (FHO) (Fig. 7-8): Removal of the femoral head decreases pain that results from physical contact between the bone surface of the femur and the acetabulum. Removal allows formation of a "false joint" from surrounding soft tissue. Vigorous exercise is required after surgery to increase muscle strength and limb function. Swimming, walking, or running should be adequate to build muscle strength. Short periods of exercise (5–10 minutes three times a day) can gradually be lengthened (10 minutes four times a day) as the animal gains strength. Nonsteroidal antiinflammatory drugs (NSAIDs) can be used during rehabilitation. The limb that undergoes surgery may be slightly shorter than the opposite leg, and occasional lameness may be seen, especially in larger dogs. This is not the suggested treatment for athletic dogs that require complete return to normal joint function. It may take up to 1 year before optimal function returns to the limb.
- Total hip replacement (Fig. 7-9): This is the most effective way to give the patient a functional, nonpainful joint. The procedure replaces the femoral head and neck together with the acetabular cup. A cobalt chrome shaft and head are implanted into the femoral shaft and placed into an artificial acetabular cup. The advantages of this surgical procedure are as follows:
  - Dogs achieve near-normal hindlimb function approximately 95% of the time.
  - Patients achieve full range of motion in the joint and are free of pain.
  - Patients have a quick return to function.
- Pelvic osteotomy: A triple osteotomy of the pelvis allows rotation of the dorsal acetabular rim to provide increased coverage to the femoral head. Although technically difficult, the surgery provides for good return of function with minimal osteoarthritis.

INFORMATION FOR CLIENTS

- Dogs intended for breeding should have their hips radiographed after 2 years of age.
- Signs of dysplasia may develop early in the dog's life.

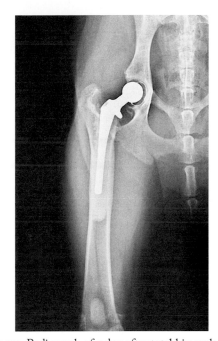

Figure 7-9 Radiograph of a dog after total hip replacement. Note the radiopaque cement mantel surrounding the femoral and acetabular prostheses. (From Fossum TW: *Small animal surgery*, ed 3, St. Louis, MO, 2007, Mosby, by permission.)

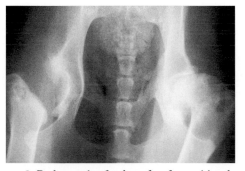

Figure 7-8 Radiograph of a dog after femoral head ostectomy. Note complete removal of the femoral neck. (From Fossum TW: *Small animal surgery*, ed 3, St. Louis, MO, 2007, Mosby, by permission.)

- This is a progressive disease, and degeneration of the joint continues throughout the life of the pet.
- Weight loss and moderate exercise can reduce the pain felt by the animal.
- Puppies born to hip dysplasia-free parents *may* experience development of dysplasia.
- Surgery is the only cure for the disease.
- Hip dysplasia is usually not seen in cats or small-breed dogs.

Legg–Calve–Perthes Disease (Avascular Necrosis)

Legg–Calve–Perthes disease involves a noninflammatory aseptic necrosis of the femoral head and neck and is primarily a disease of small-breed dogs. Although the exact cause is unknown, some vascular compression together with hormone activity has been suggested.

In affected dogs, the femoral head and neck undergo necrosis and deformation. The articular cartilage cracks and collapses because of the collapse of subchondral bone. The result of these changes is pain and loss of joint congruity. Toy breeds and terriers are most commonly affected.

CLINICAL SIGNS

- Young dogs between 5 and 8 months of age are predisposed to Legg–Calve–Perthes disease.
- Irritability and chewing at the hip or flank area are seen.
- Pain is a clinical sign.
- Atrophy of the muscles of the hip is noticeable.
- A gradual onset of lameness occurs.

DIAGNOSIS

- Radiographic signs include decreased bone density in the femoral head and neck area, flattened femoral head, and osteophytes in the joint (Fig. 7-10).

TREATMENT

- Excision arthroplasty removes the femoral head and neck. Postoperative treatment requires early, active use of the limb. As early as 2 weeks after surgery, animals should be encouraged to swim or run. Return to pain-free function may occur as early as 30 days after surgery.

INFORMATION FOR CLIENTS

- Animals may have both hips involved.
- A genetic predisposition for the disease may exist.
- Animals require frequent physical therapy during recovery (exercise and passive range-of-motion exercises).
- If disease has developed in both hips, the surgeries on each side are usually performed 8 to 10 weeks apart, depending on the surgeon's preference.

Osteochondrosis Dissecans

Osteochondrosis refers to the degeneration or aseptic necrosis of bone and cartilage followed by reossification. If the condition results in a dissecting cartilage flap with inflammatory joint changes, it is termed *osteochondrosis dissecans* (Fig. 7-11). The underlying defect in this disease is one of endochondral ossification. Failure of the lower layers of physeal or articular cartilage to mature into bone results in thickened cartilage that is prone to injury. If lack of ossification occurs at the physis, problems such as nonunited anconeal process or retained cartilage cores can occur. If it occurs at the articular surface, OCD may occur. The disease is seen in several joints (shoulder, stifle, hock, and elbow). OCD of the scapulohumeral joint (shoulder) is most commonly seen. Failure of the articular cartilage to become cemented to underlying bone, together with constant trauma during exercise, results in the formation of a nonhealing cartilage flap. The presence of this flap produces lameness and osteoarthrosis.

CLINICAL SIGNS

- Lameness in large-breed dogs (3–18 months of age)

DIAGNOSIS

- Radiographs show the cartilage flap with or without joint mice (loose cartilage pieces).

TREATMENT

- Rest and weight control in early stages
- If lame, surgical removal of the flap, mice, or both

INFORMATION FOR CLIENTS

- A return to normal function occurs almost immediately after surgery.

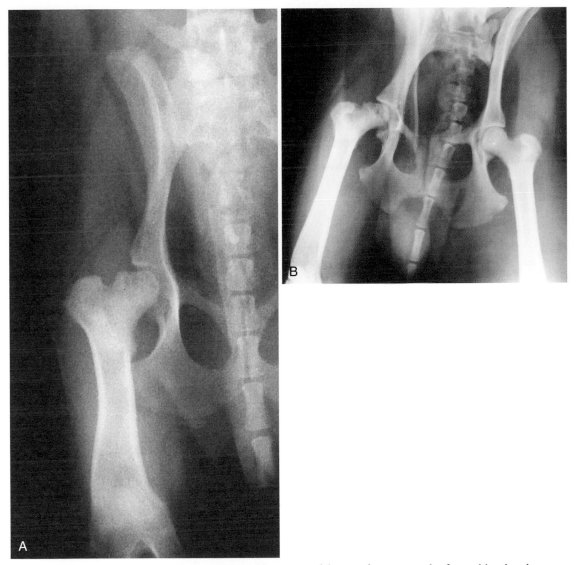

Figure 7-10 Legg–Calve–Perthes disease: Note areas of decreased opacity in the femoral head and the loss of the rounded contour of the femoral head. (From Kealy JK, McAllister H, Graham JP: *Diagnostic radiology and ultrasonography of the dog and cat*, ed 5, St. Louis, MO, 2011, Saunders.)

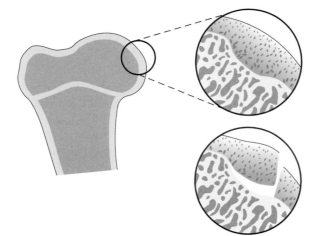

Figure 7-11 Failure of endochondral ossification leads to cartilage thickening. Loss of chondrocytes deep in the cartilage layer produces a cleft and causes development of vertical fissures in the cartilage. These fissures eventually communicate with the joint, forming a cartilage flap. (From Fossum TW: *Small animal surgery*, ed 3, St. Louis, MO, 2007, Mosby, by permission.)

- This is normally a disease of large-breed dogs.
- This disease may have a hereditary component.

Panosteitis (Endosteosis, Eosinophilic Panosteitis)

Panosteitis is a common disease that causes intermittent lameness in medium- and large-breed dogs. The average age of onset is 6 to 8 months. The lameness is usually acute, is not associated with trauma, and may appear to the owner to shift from leg to leg. Male dogs are more commonly affected (66% of cases), with the German Shepherd breed being overrepresented.

The cause of panosteitis is unknown, but some causes may include viral infection, genetic predisposition, metabolic disease, and allergic or hormonal excess. Viral infection is thought to be the most likely cause. The disease affects medullary bone marrow and endosteal bone, resulting in degeneration of medullary marrow and thickening of endosteal bone. Long bones such as the ulna, humerus, radius, femur, and tibia are most commonly involved.

Panosteitis is self-limiting, and virtually all affected dogs return to normal within 1 year. During bouts of pain and lameness, analgesics and NSAIDs can be administered to make the animal more comfortable.

CLINICAL SIGNS

- Intermittent lameness shifting from leg to leg
- Anorexia
- Fever
- Weight loss
- Reluctance to move

DIAGNOSIS

- Pain elicited on deep palpation of long bone
- Radiology: gray, hazy, patchy areas of increased radiodensity in the medullary cavity of long bone (Fig. 7-12).

TREATMENT

- Analgesics and antiinflammatory drugs for pain:
  - Aspirin: orally every 8 hours
  - Rimadyl (Carprofen): orally twice a day
  - Phenylbutazone: orally three times a day, then tapered (800 mg/day maximum dose)

INFORMATION FOR CLIENTS

- Panosteitis is self-limiting and usually leaves no permanent damage.
- Drugs such as aspirin and phenylbutazone can cause gastric upset and ulceration in the dog. Report any vomiting of blood, blood in the stool, or lack of appetite.
- Flare-up of the disease is common, so animals may appear cured only to relapse. The disease is seldom seen in animals older than 2 years.

Luxations

Luxations of the hip are fairly common secondary to trauma in small animals. All luxations involve tearing of the joint capsule and round ligament. Specific signs vary, depending on the location of the femoral head with respect to the acetabulum.

- *Craniodorsal*—the most common type. The leg appears shortened; the stifle rotates outward, and the hock rotates inward.
- *Craniocaudal*—rare. The stifle rotates inward and the hock outward.
- *Ventral*—rare. The affected limb appears longer.

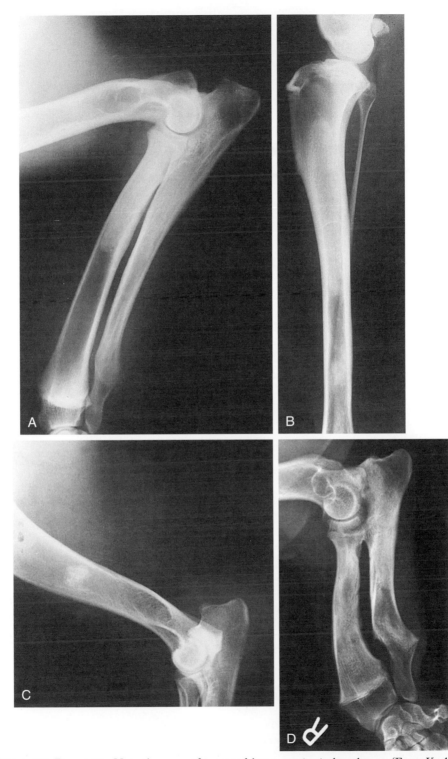

Figure 7-12 Panosteitis. Note the areas of increased bone opacity in long bones. (From Kealy JK, McAllister H, Graham JP: *Diagnostic radiology and ultrasonography of the dog and cat*, ed 5, St. Louis, MO, 2011, Saunders.)

CLINICAL SIGNS

- History of trauma
- Acute lameness, non–weight bearing
- Possible swelling over the hip joint or in area dorsal to hip joint

DIAGNOSIS

- Radiographs can rule out other diseases such as femoral neck fractures, acetabular fractures, or Legg–Calve–Perthes disease. The presence of fractures or bone chips indicates a need for open surgical reduction of the dislocation.

TREATMENT

- Closed reduction (requires anesthesia): The femoral head is manually rotated and replaced back into the acetabulum using traction.
- Open reduction: The femoral head is surgically replaced into the acetabulum and the soft tissue structures are used to secure the reduction. The limb should be supported in an Ehmer sling for a minimum of 7 to 10 days; exercise should be limited for 3 weeks after removal of the sling.

INFORMATION FOR CLIENTS

- The prognosis will depend on the stability of the reduced joint and the amount of soft tissue injury.
- Varying degrees of osteoarthritis may develop after traumatic luxation.
- An FHO should be considered if the hip does not remain reduced.

⬤ TECH ALERT

Luxations of other joints occur as a result of trauma. The goal of treatment is to return the joint to normal position and function. This is usually accomplished in a manner similar to that for the hip.

Myopathies

Myopathies are diseases that affect muscle. Although many types of myopathies exist, the most commonly seen include *inflammatory myopathy*, *immune-mediated myopathy*, and *acquired myopathy*.

Inflammatory Myopathies

Bacterial myositis, a rarely occurring disease in dogs and cats, typically occurs after a bite wound, trauma, or with contamination after surgical procedures. The most commonly involved microorganisms are *Staphylococcus* and *Clostridia* spp. Treatment should be based on culture and sensitivity results.

Protozoal myositis occurs when cysts are formed within the muscles of *Toxoplasmosis*-positive cats. Rupture of these cysts or immune response to their presence results in clinical signs of muscle *hyperesthesia*.

Immune-Mediated Myopathies

Polymyositis is an immune-mediated disease of muscles that affects dogs and cats. Middle-aged, large-breed dogs are most commonly affected. Weakness that gets worse with exercise, hyperesthesia on palpation, fever, and depression may all be signs of muscle involvement. Some dogs may have megaesophagus. Muscle atrophy may be seen with chronic cases. Diagnosis is most readily obtained through muscle biopsy; treatment involves prednisone (2.2 mg/kg daily).

Masticatory muscle myositis, also known as *atrophic myositis* or *eosinophilic myositis*, involves the muscles of mastication in the dog. These muscles contain a special type of fiber (type 2M) that has antigenic properties possibly shared with bacteria. Infections elsewhere in the body may incite an immune response that affects these muscle fibers. The masticatory muscles initially become swollen and painful. With chronic involvement, the muscles atrophy and fibrose. Glucocorticoids are the treatment of choice.

Acquired Myopathies

Feline polymyopathy occurs in cats of all ages and breeds in both sexes. Hypokalemia results in cervical ventriflexion, periodic weakness, and muscle pain. These symptoms may occur concurrently with renal disease. Treatment involves supplementation of potassium and adjustment of diet.

CLINICAL SIGNS

- Muscle weakness, pain, swelling, or atrophy

DIAGNOSIS

- Clinical signs
- Muscle biopsy

- Serum chemistries (creatine kinase level may be increased)

TREATMENT

- Appropriate antibiotics, if bacterial; antiprotozoal drugs, if parasite related
- Glucocorticoids: daily (may be needed long term in some cases)

INFORMATION FOR CLIENTS

- Most animals show improvement with treatment.
- Treatment may be required for the life of the animal.
- Early intervention improves the prognosis.

Tumors of Bone

The diagnosis of bone cancer is devastating to the animal, the owner, and the veterinarian. A high incidence rate of bone cancer exists in pet animals, especially dogs. The onset of the disease is often acute, and the progression of signs rapid.

Approximately 8000 cases of bone cancer are seen in dogs each year. Of these, 85% to 90% involve osteosarcoma, a primary bone neoplasm. As with most cancers, the cause of osteosarcoma is unknown. Studies suggest that a derangement of growth or differentiation of new bone at the metaphyses of long bones may result in tumor formation. The most common bones affected are the distal radius, proximal humerus, distal femur, and proximal tibia. The disease is most commonly seen in large-breed male dogs about 7 years of age. Most of these tumors show microscopic spread by the time they are diagnosed. Ninety percent of all animals diagnosed with bone cancer die despite treatment.

Primary bone cancer in cats is less common. As many as 90% of bone cancers seen in cats are osteosarcomas. Survival rates after amputation appear to be somewhat better than those for dogs.

CLINICAL SIGNS

- Lameness
- Weight loss
- Pain, especially over the affected bone
- Swelling in the affected limb

DIAGNOSIS

- Radiographs show mixed osteolysis, proliferation of bone, and periosteal reaction.
- Biopsy is required for diagnosis.
- Thoracic radiographs should be taken to rule out metastatic tumors.

TREATMENT

- Amputation of affected limb is required.
- Follow-up treatment with cisplatin or carboplatin may increase survival time.
- Radiation therapy can be provided for pain control.
- No recommended drug therapies exist for cats.

INFORMATION FOR CLIENTS

- Bone cancer is a fatal disease.
- Survival times of up to 12 months may be achieved with aggressive treatment.
- Biopsy of the tumor is necessary to confirm the tumor type.
- Amputation is required to remove the primary tumor; however, it will not prevent metastatic tumor cells occurring elsewhere in the body.
- Drug therapy is expensive, and patients require laboratory monitoring to avoid bone marrow or renal toxicities from the treatment.

REVIEW QUESTIONS

1. What type of support bandage provides good protection for a long bone fracture while radiographs are being taken?
   a. Robert Jones bandage
   b. Spica splint bandage
   c. Velpeau bandage
   d. Ehmer sling
2. Sudden hyperextension of the stifle joint in middle-aged, obese dogs can result in rupture of the:
   a. Patellar tendon
   b. Medial collateral ligament
   c. Anterior cruciate ligament
   d. Lateral collateral ligament

3. For OFA certification, dogs should be radiographed after reaching the age of:
   a. 6 months
   b. 1 year
   c. 2 years
   d. 3 years
4. Hip dysplasia is not a progressive, degenerative joint disease (DJD).
   a. True
   b. False
5. OCD lesions are most commonly seen in large-breed dogs in the:
   a. Coxofemoral joint
   b. Scapulohumeral joint
   c. Carpus
   d. Tarsus
6. What is the most frequently seen primary bone tumor in pet animals?
   a. Squamous cell carcinoma
   b. Fibrosarcoma
   c. Osteosarcoma
   d. Chondrosarcoma
7. Which of the following is a true statement?
   a. Most patellar luxations seen early in life are medial luxations.
   b. Most patellar luxations seen late in older dogs are medial luxations.
   c. Most patellar luxations seen in large-breed dogs are medial luxations.
   d. Most patellar luxations are traumatic in nature.

8. Which of the following statements is false?
   a. There is a genetic predisposition to hip dysplasia.
   b. An environmental factor is related to the development of hip dysplasia.
   c. No relationship exists between excessive growth and the development of hip dysplasia.
   d. There is a dietary component to the development of hip dysplasia.
9. Casts or splints may not prevent rotation or overriding of fractured long bones and may result in delayed healing.
   a. True
   b. False
10. Which of the following statements is false?
    a. Some degree of arthritis may develop in any traumatic joint injury.
    b. Physical therapy is needed for injured joints to return to function.
    c. Orthopedic injuries usually require analgesia after surgery.
    d. Hip dysplasia cannot develop in puppies born to female dogs without hip dysplasia.
11. Mary has a large breed dog and has been told by the breeder to give him supplements of calcium-rich vitamins for fast growth. Is this a good idea?
12. What advice would you give a client to avoid musculoskeletal injuries in their pet?

Answers found on page 552.

Diseases of the Nervous System

LEARNING OBJECTIVES

When you have completed this chapter, you will be able to:
1. Describe the arrangement of the nervous system.
2. Relate the dysfunctions of various portions of the nervous system to diseases seen in companion animals.
3. Discuss symptoms and treatments of neuronal disease with clients.

The nervous system can be divided into two primary divisions: (1) the *central nervous system* (CNS), composed of the brain and the spinal cord, and (2) the *peripheral nervous system* (PNS), composed of the cranial nerves and the peripheral nerves that connect the outside sensory world to the brain.

The functional cell of both systems is the *neuron*, whose job is to transmit electrical impulses to and from the brain. Pathology anywhere within the transmission system results in interruption of messages and clinical neurologic symptoms. The individual symptoms vary, depending on the location of the lesion. For the purpose of this chapter, diseases are divided into those of the brain, the spinal cord, and the PNS.

Anatomy and Physiology of the Nervous System

The Neuron

The functional cell of the nervous system is the neuron, a large, kite-shaped cell consisting of multiple input fibers (dendrites) and one output fiber (the axon). Neurons never touch each other; impulses are transmitted from one to another via chemical mediators such as acetylcholine or epinephrine. The axons of neurons may be covered by a lipid coating, called *myelin*, or they may be uncoated and unmyelinated. Myelinated nerve fibers conduct impulses rapidly while unmyelinated fibers are much slower. These fibers make up the white and gray matter of the nervous system. It is the network of these neurons that make up both the CNS and the PNS.

The Brain

The brain is composed of gray and white matter tracts that connect the higher centers of the cerebral cortex to the spinal cord and the peripheral nerves. The tracts decussate in the brain stem as they exit the foramen magnum, the right side of the brain controlling the left side of the body, and vice versa. The higher centers of the brain involved in the more sophisticated levels of intelligence involve multiple centers of neurons and nerve tracts throughout the many areas of the brain.

Brain Disorders

Trauma

In small-animal medicine, traumatic brain injuries are encountered frequently. The injuries generally have an acute clinical onset resulting from a traumatic experience (e.g., being hit by an automobile, having the head caught in a closing door, or falling). Injury to the brain from trauma can result from direct injury to the nervous tissues (primary event) or from secondary events, which intensify or worsen the neurologic damage and produce systemic derangements. *Primary* events may produce disruption of fiber tracts, which cannot be repaired, or reparable cell damage, which is reversible. *Secondary* events such as increased intracranial pressure (ICP), edema, hypoxia, and seizures occur as a result of the primary trauma. Increased ICP is caused by both edema and hemorrhage in or around the brain. Because the brain is encased in a nonflexible shell of bone (the skull), herniation of nervous tissue (primarily the brainstem) through the foramen magnum results. Treatment of head trauma involves preventing or decreasing the secondary effects of trauma.

CLINICAL SIGNS

- History of trauma to the head
- Seizures
- Blood in ears, nose, oral cavity
- Ocular hemorrhage
- Loss of consciousness or a decrease in responses to external stimuli
- Signs of shock, cardiac arrhythmias, altered respiratory patterns, coma

DIAGNOSIS

- History and physical examination
- Serum chemistries to rule out metabolic problems
- Clinical rating scale for prognosis of trauma (Table 8-1)

TREATMENT

- Correct any metabolic derangements.
- Provide oxygen through a mask or nasal cannula.
- Elevate the head.
- Administer osmotic agents to decrease cerebral edema:
  - Mannitol (20%): intravenous slow bolus

TABLE 8-1   Clinical Rating Scale for Evaluation of Craniocerebral Trauma

Criteria	Score*
Motor activity	
Normal gait, normal reflexes	6
Hemiparesis, tetraparesis, or decorticate activity	5
Recumbent with intermittent extensor rigidity	4
Recumbent with constant extensor rigidity	3
Recumbent with intermittent extensor rigidity or opisthotonos	2
Recumbent, hypotonic with depressed-absent spinal reflexes	1
Brainstem reflexes	
Normal PLR and OVRs	6
Slow PLR and normal to reduced OVRs	5
Bilateral or unresponsive miosis and normal-to-reduced OVRs	4
Pinpoint pupils and reduced-to-absent OVRs	3
Unilateral or unresponsive mydriasis and reduced-to-absent OVRs	2
Bilateral or unresponsive mydriasis and reduced-to-absent OVRs	1
Level of consciousness	
Occasionally alert and responsive	6
Depressed or delirious, but capable of response to stimulus	5
Obtunded or stuporous, but responds to visual stimuli	4
Obtunded or stuporous, but responds to auditory stimuli	3
Obtunded or stuporous, but responds to noxious stimuli	2
Comatose and unresponsive to noxious stimuli	1

*Prognosis: grave for 3–8 total score; poor to guarded for 9–14 total score; and good for 15–18 total score.
PLR, Pupillary light reflex; *OVR,* oculovestibular reflex.
From Fenner WR: Diseases of the brain. In: Ettinger SJ, Feldman EC, editors: *Textbook of veterinary internal medicine,* ed 5, Philadelphia, 2000, Saunders, by permission.

- Diuretics: furosemide intravenously (IV) every 4 hours
- Antiseizure medication, if needed:
  - Diazepam: divided into three or four doses
  - Phenobarbital: IV or intramuscularly (IM) twice a day
- Corticosteroids: prednisolone sodium succinate IV

INFORMATION FOR CLIENTS

- Some brain damage is irreversible. If the animal survives, it may never return to "normal."
- In general, animals in a coma for longer than 48 hours do not survive.
- Deteriorating signs represent a worsening of the animal's condition.

Idiopathic Vestibular Disease

Idiopathic vestibular disease is an acute disorder of both dogs (middle-aged) and cats. In cats, the disease is seen most frequently during the late spring, summer, and early fall.

Clinical signs involve loss of balance, nystagmus, disorientation, and ataxia. Many animals experience nausea early in the course of the disease. Animals stabilize rapidly, and clinical signs usually resolve in 3 to 6 weeks.

CLINICAL SIGNS

- Incapacitating loss of balance
- Nystagmus
- Disorientation
- Ataxia
- Vomiting
- Anorexia

DIAGNOSIS

- Clinical signs
- Blood work to rule out other diseases involving the nervous system
- Otic examination to rule out inner ear problem

TREATMENT

- Treatment is usually not recommended and does not alter the course of the disease.
- Supportive therapy and force feeding should be implemented.
- Confine the animal to prevent injury from falling.

TECH ALERT

Steroids and antibiotics are used routinely to cover possible causes not found by physical examination and laboratory work.

Neoplasia

An enlarging tumor within the brain produces tissue compression, replaces healthy neuronal tissue causing clinical signs that are *progressive*, or both. Primary brain tumors are typically singular, but metastatic tumors or secondary brain tumors may be solitary or multiple in occurrence. Most tumors are metastatic by the time the animal is examined. The disease is typically seen in older animals.

CLINICAL SIGNS

- Signs reflect tumor location
- Seizures (typically increasing in frequency and severity)
- Endocrine derangements
- Presence or absence of vestibular signs
- Tremor, ataxia

DIAGNOSIS

- Systematic screening for primary tumors in other organs
- Blood work: complete blood cell count (CBC) and serum chemistries
- Radiography
- Cerebrospinal fluid (CSF) tap results show increased pressure, increased albumin, and usually normal white blood cell (WBC) count.
- Ophthalmic examination indicates optic nerve edema.
- Computed tomography (CT) or magnetic resonance imaging (MRI) provides the best chance of locating the lesion.

TREATMENT

Treatment of the Tumor
- Surgical removal for superficial singular lesions (newer techniques may make deeper removal a possibility in the future)
- Radiation therapy
- Chemotherapy (lymphomas respond well, others are less responsive)

Treatment of Clinical Signs
- Antiseizure medication: phenobarbital orally (PO) two to three times a day
- Corticosteroids: prednisone twice a day or q12h

INFORMATION FOR CLIENTS

- Unless the tumor can be removed surgically, medication will not cure the condition.
- Symptoms will gradually become more severe as the tumor grows in size.

Idiopathic Epilepsy

Idiopathic epilepsy is a syndrome characterized by repeated episodes of seizures for which no demonstrated cause exists. The diagnosis is one of exclusion.

Idiopathic epilepsy is predominantly a disease in German Shepherds, Miniature and Toy Poodles, Saint Bernards, Cocker Spaniels, Beagles, Irish Setters, Golden Retrievers, and some mixed breeds. Seizures usually begin between 1 and 3 years of age. Affected animals may exhibit a short aura during which the animal may act abnormally. It may hide, seek companionship, vocalize, or exhibit other abnormal behaviors. Seizures are usually generalized in nature, lasting anywhere from 1 to 2 minutes. After the seizure, the animal is usually disoriented and occasionally blind. Seizures may occur singly or in clusters and may recur at fairly regular intervals. In some animals, inciting events such as excitement or estrus have been shown to precipitate seizure activity. Although the cause of idiopathic epilepsy is unknown, a hereditary basis has been suggested.

CLINICAL SIGNS

- Seizures, often occurring at regular intervals
- Young animals typically affected
- Normal behavior between seizures

DIAGNOSIS

- CBC and serum chemistries to rule out hypocalcemia, hypoglycemia, infection, hepatic encephalopathy, lead poisoning
- Radiography to rule out head trauma or hydrocephalus
- CT or MRI to rule out space-occupying lesions in the brain

TREATMENT

- Treatment should be directed at primary disease if one can be found.
- Initiate treatment if seizure frequency is more than once per month.

- Control seizure activity with phenobarbital (q12h).
- If seizures occur and phenobarbital concentration is adequate, add potassium bromide (KBr) 22 mg/kg once daily with food.

⦿ TECH ALERT

Phenobarbital takes 7 to 10 days to reach steady-state serum concentration in the body. If the animal continues to experience seizures after this period, measure serum phenobarbital concentration 2 hours before and after dosing. If less than 20 micrograms per milliliter (mcg/mL), slowly increase the dose by 10% to 20% until the concentration reaches 20 to 30 mcg/mL.

Status Epilepticus

Animals prone to seizures may exhibit status epilepticus, which is a medical emergency. Continual seizures for a prolonged period (>5–10 minutes) can lead to irreversible coma and death if not treated aggressively. Owners should be advised to seek emergency assistance if this situation develops.

CLINICAL SIGNS

- Prolonged, uninterrupted seizure activity

DIAGNOSIS

- History and clinical signs

TREATMENT

Immediate Treatment

- Diazepam: 2 mg IV (5-kg dog or cat); 5 mg IV (10-kg dog); 10 mg IV (20-kg dog). Can repeat two to three times over several minutes.
- Administer sodium pentobarbital IV to effect (not to exceed 15 mg/kg).
- Establish an airway, and give oxygen.
- Place an intravenous catheter and start fluids to provide vascular access (TKO [to keep open]).
- Check blood glucose and calcium concentrations; correct, if necessary. Perform serum chemistries to rule out metabolic causes of seizure.
- Monitor body temperature. If greater than 105°F, give a cool bath.
- If cerebral edema is suspected, give mannitol IV and prednisolone sodium succinate 10 to 30 mg/kg IV.

Maintenance Therapy

- Phenobarbital: IV or intramuscularly (IM) q12h
- Initiate oral therapy, if possible

INFORMATION FOR CLIENTS

- Epilepsy is an incurable disease.
- Even with treatment, animals may have seizures. The goal of treatment is to decrease the frequency and severity of the seizures.
- Spaying or neutering the animal will prevent any hormonal influence on seizure activity.
- Medication will probably be required for the life of the pet. Missing doses or abruptly stopping medication will precipitate a seizure.
- Most animals with seizures can live a fairly normal life.
- Periodic monitoring of serum anticonvulsant concentration is required.
- Animals that remain seizure free for 6 to 9 months may have their medication dose slowly decreased until it may eventually be discontinued (in consultation with the veterinarian).

Anatomy of the Spinal Cord

When looking at a cross-section of the spinal cord, one might be reminded of a butterfly. The two dorsal horns collect sensory information from the peripheral nerves, and the two ventral horns transmit motor impulses to the periphery. The nerve fibers that connect the dorsal and ventral horns, called *interneurons*, complete what is known as a *reflex arc*. The outermost layers of the spinal cord are composed of white matter tracts that carry information to the higher centers of the CNS. The innermost layers are gray matter tracts. Information travels in both direction in the spinal cord, and disruption of this "neural highway" can have grave significance for the patient (Fig. 8-1).

Spinal Cord Dysfunction

Just like the brain, the spinal cord is protected by a bony housing, the vertebral column. The spinal cord is located within the spinal canal, dorsal to the vertebral bodies. Between each of the vertebral bodies is a cushion known as the *intervertebral* disk. These disks

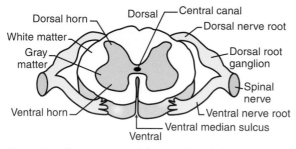

Figure 8-1 Cross-section of the spinal cord. (From Colville T, Bassert JM: *Clinical anatomy and physiology for veterinary technicians*, ed 2, St. Louis, MO, 2008, Mosby.)

are composed of an outer fibrous layer, the *annulus fibrosus*, and an inner gel-like nucleus, the *nucleus pulposus*. Their presence allows a larger range of motion in the vertebral column and prevents the vertebral bodies from rubbing against each other (Fig. 8-2).

Intervertebral Disk Disease

By far, one of the most common disorders involving the spinal cord of small animals is intervertebral disk disease. Disk protrusions can occur in all breeds of

dog and occasionally in cats. It has been reported that 75% to 100% of all disks in chondrodystrophic breeds have undergone degenerative changes by 1 year of age. Disk protrusion or extrusion occurs most commonly in the cervical, caudal thoracic, and lumbar spine. Two types of herniations have been reported. Type 1 (common in younger dogs) involves acute rupture of the annulus fibrosus and extrusion of the nucleus pulposus up into the spinal canal. In type 2 herniation (common in older [>5 years] large-breed dogs), the extrusion occurs over a longer period, producing less acute and less severe clinical signs. The severity of spinal cord injury depends on the speed at which the disk material is deposited into the spinal canal, the degree of compression, and the duration of compression. Clinical signs may be related to the location of the lesion (Fig. 8-3).

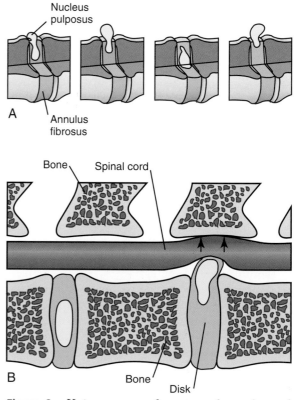

Figure 8-3 Various stages of a ruptured annulus and extruded nucleus, which may be degenerated, fibrotic, or even calcified.

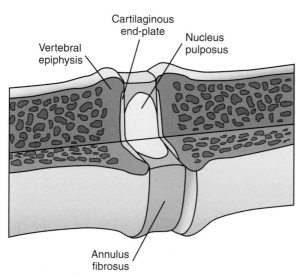

Figure 8-2 The intervertebral disk is an elastic cushion between the adjacent vertebrae. This is a view of an intervertebral disk space showing relations of the disk to the cartilaginous end plates and epiphyses of the vertebrae.

CLINICAL SIGNS

- Apparent pain; presence or absence of motor or sensory deficits
- Acute onset (type 1 usually)
- Paresis or paralysis that may be unilateral or bilateral
- Decreased panniculus reflex one to two vertebral spaces caudal to the actual lesion
- Altered deep pain response

DIAGNOSIS

- Age, breed, clinical signs, and history
- Complete neurologic examination
- Radiography requires anesthesia for proper positioning. Narrowed disk spaces at the location of the lesion may be seen (C7-T1, T9-10, L7-S1 are normally narrow)
- Myelogram is required for definitive location of the lesion

TREATMENT

Type 1

- Medical treatment is recommended for animals with pain, with or without mild neurologic deficits:
  - Strict confinement for a minimum of 2 weeks (cage rest)
  - Corticosteroids injected for 1 to 2 days to decrease edema and inflammation
- Intensive nursing care: These animals require soft padding in the cage; some may require indwelling urinary catheters or expression of the bladder; some may need to be turned frequently to prevent pressure sores; and all animals should receive proper nutrition to promote healing.
- Surgical treatment should be reserved for animals with multiple episodes, ataxia, paresis or paralysis, and absence of deep pain:
  - Fenestration, hemilaminectomy
  - Decompression should be performed as soon as possible to prevent further damage to the spinal cord.

Type 2

- Because of the slow progression of spinal compression accompanied by degeneration of spinal

tissue, these dogs may improve initially with cortisone therapy; however, surgery may fail to improve spinal function.

INFORMATION FOR CLIENTS

- Prevent excess weight gain in breeds prone to disk disease.
- Avoid having the animal stand on the hind legs or in any other position that strains the back.
- The prognosis for animals that lack deep pain for greater than 24 hours is poor.
- Animals that lack deep pain for less than 24 hours have a guarded to poor prognosis.
- The prognosis for animals having or regaining deep pain after surgery is fair to good.
- Approximately 40% of animals treated medically had recurrence of disease with more severe signs.
- Animals with paresis or paralysis require intensive nursing care. They may need extensive home care while they are recovering.
- Severe damage to the spinal cord currently is not reparable.

Trauma

Acute spinal cord injuries of the dog and cat usually result from motor vehicle accidents, gunshot wounds, or fights. The spinal cord trauma is sudden in onset and may be related to the velocity of cord compression, the degree of compression, and the duration of the compressive force. Signs of injury are typically nonprogressive, although they may worsen over the first 48 hours before stabilization. Injury may occur at a single or multiple levels within the spinal cord.

Blunt trauma to the spinal cord causes tissue injury through both "direct" and "indirect" mechanisms. Direct effects are due to primary disruption of neural pathways within the cord. Indirect effects are less well understood and include edema, hemorrhage, ischemia, lactic acidosis, inflammation, and neuronophagia by WBCs. It appears that mechanical deformation of any type can trigger these secondary events within the spinal cord. Autodissolution of the cord may be seen as early as 24 hours after injury.

CLINICAL SIGNS

- History of trauma (affected animals usually have serious injury to other organ systems)
- Presence of the Schiff–Sherrington sign: rigid hypertonicity of front legs, hypotonicity of the rear legs, normal reflexes, and pain perception caused by the release of inhibitory pathways along the spinal cord from L1-L7
- Lack of panniculus reflex caudal to lesion
- Paresis or paralysis

DIAGNOSIS

- Complete neurologic examination to localize the lesion
- Radiography

● TECH ALERT

To prevent additional damage, limit manipulation of the spinal column while performing radiography. Remember that the vertebral column may return to a normal position after trauma, hiding the original compressive event. A myelogram may be necessary to locate the actual sites of cord injury.

TREATMENT

Medical Treatment

- Corticosteroids:
  - Dexamethasone: IV
  - Prednisolone sodium succinate (SoluDelta Cortef): divided every 8 hours
- Mannitol: IV
- Dimethylsulfoxide (40%): IV
- Treat other life-threatening injuries with intravenous fluids, oxygen; monitor heart rhythms and urine production
- Strict confinement for 6 to 8 weeks for mild fractures or dislocation (showing few clinical signs)

Surgical Treatment

- Treatment should be instituted within 2 hours of trauma, if possible. Surgical treatment should be considered in cases of severe paresis or paralysis, myelographic evidence of continuing cord compression, or worsening clinical signs.
- Laminectomy should be performed at all sites of cord compression.
- Stabilization of vertebral column fractures or subluxations must be performed.
- Removal of all bone fragments or disk material from the spinal canal must be accomplished.
- A durotomy may be required to further relieve cord pressure.
- Complete confinement for a minimum of 2 weeks after surgery.

Nursing Care

- Daily physical therapy: padded resting surface to decrease the formation of ulcers over pressure points
- Bladder expression or maintenance of an indwelling catheter

INFORMATION FOR CLIENTS

- Treatment of these cases can be costly and often requires referral to a specialist.
- The animal will require extensive nursing care.
- Even in the best of circumstances, some residual neurologic deficit may remain.
- The prognosis for spinal cord trauma will depend on the neurologic examination results. Absence of deep pain for more than 24 hours has a poor prognosis. Worsening of clinical signs is another indicator of a poor outcome. Recovery time may extend to months in some cases.
- Keep pets confined or on a leash to avoid the possibility of traumatic injury to the spinal cord.

Cervical Spinal Cord Diseases

Atlantoaxial Subluxation (Atlantoaxial Instability)

Atlantoaxial subluxation is seen most frequently in young (<1 year) toy and miniature breeds of dogs and occasionally in other breeds. Spinal cord trauma occurs when the cranial portion of the axis is displaced into the spinal column. This displacement may occur as a result of congenital or developmental abnormalities, trauma, or a combination of both. Speculation continues that the mechanism is similar to that of femoral head necrosis (Legg–Calve–Perthes disease) seen in these breeds.

CLINICAL SIGNS

- Reluctance to be patted on the head
- Neck pain
- Presence or absence of tetraparesis or tetraplegia
- Sudden death due to respiratory paralysis

DIAGNOSIS

- Radiographs: Lateral projection with the neck in slight ventriflexion (Fig. 8-4). Care must be taken

to avoid further spinal cord damage when positioning the animal. Other congenital abnormalities of the cervical vertebrae may be present.

🔘 TECH ALERT

Avoid anesthesia if possible when obtaining radiographs of these animals. The decrease in muscle tone during anesthesia may result in further subluxation and spinal cord damage.

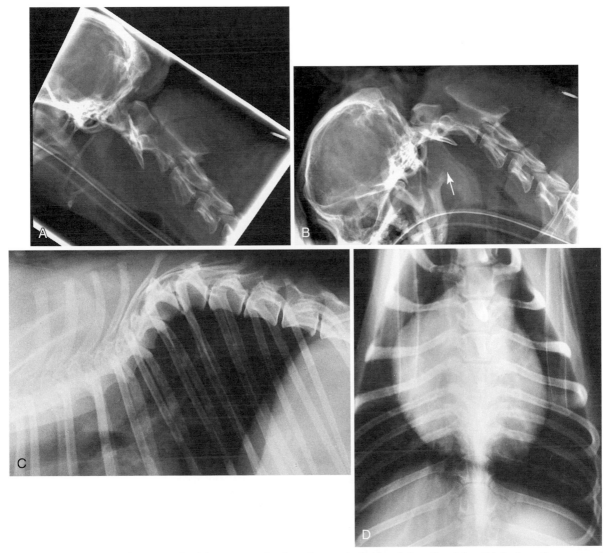

Figure 8-4 Atlantoaxial subluxation in the dog; the axis is displaced dorsally with mild flexion of the neck. (From Kealy JK, McAllister H, Graham JP: *Diagnostic radiology and ultrasonography of the dog and cat*, ed 5, St. Louis, MO, 2011, Saunders.)

TREATMENT

Medical

- Splint neck in extension with strict cage confinement for 6 weeks.
- Treat as for other spinal cord traumas.

Surgical

- Stabilization, decompression, or both are necessary if the animal has neurologic deficits or neck pain unresponsive to medical treatment.
  - Dorsal—Stainless steel wire is used to attach the dorsal process of the axis to the arch of the atlas. *Note:* Surgery may further damage the cord during positioning and placement of the suture material.
  - Ventral—Bone grafts and cross-pinning technique are accomplished to fuse the axis to the atlas. A neck brace is placed for 2 to 4 weeks after surgery.
  - Hemilaminectomy is performed to relieve spinal cord compression.

INFORMATION FOR CLIENTS

- Prognosis is fair to good for animals with mild signs.
- Affected animals should not be used for breeding because this condition may be hereditary.

Cervical Spondylomyelopathy (Wobbler Syndrome)

Cervical spinal cord compression as a result of caudal vertebral (C5-C7) malformation or misarticulation occurs in large-breed dogs, predominantly Great Danes (males) and Doberman Pinschers.

The onset of clinical signs occurs before 1 year of age in the Great Dane and after 2 years of age in the Doberman. Signs are normally progressive and involve hindlimb ataxia (a wobbly gait). Pelvic limbs may cross each other, abduct widely, or tend to collapse. The animal may drag its toes, producing abrasions on the dorsal surface or wearing of the nails dorsally. Proprioception will be abnormal. Some animals will have similar lesions in the thoracic limbs. Neurologic examination will be abnormal when testing postural reactions, hopping, and proprioception.

CLINICAL SIGNS

- History of progressive pelvic limb ataxia
- Abnormal wearing of the dorsal surface of the rear paws, nails, or both
- Swinging or wobbly gait in the rear limbs
- Gait worse on rising
- Similar signs in front limbs
- Presence or absence of atrophy of scapular muscles
- Rigid flexion of neck without neck pain

DIAGNOSIS

- CBC and serum chemistries should be performed to rule out hypothyroidism or other metabolic defects.
- Radiographs may indicate malalignment or "slipping" of the vertebrae or may indicate remodeling, new bone formation, and narrowing of the spinal canal. Myelography is essential to locate the regions of compression.
- CT and MRI are excellent diagnostic tools, if available.

TREATMENT

- Without treatment, the prognosis is poor.

Medical
- Antiinflammatory doses of cortisone
- Neck brace
- Cage confinement

Surgical

⬤ TECH ALERT

Before undertaking surgery, consider the high potential for morbidity and postsurgical complications.

- Decompression of the spinal cord by laminectomy or ventral slot procedures
- Stabilization of vertebral column:
  - Use wire and lag screws dorsally.
  - Use ventral approach with spinal fusion and an orthopedic implant to maintain distraction during healing.

INFORMATION FOR CLIENTS

- Overall, the prognosis for these dogs is guarded.
- This is most likely a hereditary defect.
- Dogs with multiple levels of compression have a less favorable prognosis than those with a single level of compression.
- Surgery is risky and costly, and some animals may experience development of other areas of compression after surgery.

Degenerative Myelopathy

Degenerative myelopathy is a disease seen primarily in the German Shepherd and German Shepherd mixed breed dogs. Other breeds may include Collies, Siberian Huskies, Labrador Retrievers, and Kerry Blue Terriers. The disease may have a genetic basis; however, evidence to support a hereditary susceptibility is lacking. Although the exact cause is unknown, it has been suggested that the disease may result from an autoimmune response to an antigen in the nervous system.

The lesion consists of a diffuse degeneration of white matter in both the ascending and descending tracts in all segments of the spinal cord. The lesion is most extensive in the thoracic region. The affected dog is usually an older animal (>5 years) with a 5- to 6-month history of progressive ataxia and paresis in the rear limbs. Loss of proprioception is often the first indication of a problem. Owners often report that the animal "falls down" when attempting to defecate. Muscle wasting may occur from disuse in the caudal thoracic and lumbosacral areas. Symptoms slowly progress until the animal is unable to support weight with the rear limbs.

CLINICAL SIGNS

- Slowly progressive hindlimb paresis and ataxia
- Muscle atrophy

DIAGNOSIS

Neurologic Examination

- Lesion in the region of T3-L3
- Decreased or absent proprioception and placing reactions
- Increased to normal patellar reflexes
- Lack of pain

- Normal sphincter tone
- Normal panniculus reflex

Radiographs

- Radiographs may show dural ossification or narrowed disk spaces but will be normal in most cases.

Cerebrospinal Fluid

- CSF may show increased protein concentrations from the lumbar subarachnoid space.

TREATMENT

- No treatment exists for this disease. The symptoms will slowly progress until the dog becomes nonambulatory. Corticosteroids will not improve the symptoms.

INFORMATION FOR CLIENTS

- Degenerative myelopathy is a progressive, incurable disease.
- This disease is not hip dysplasia. It involves a degeneration of the spinal nerves that is irreversible.
- When the dog can no longer support weight, it is time to consider euthanasia.

Discospondylitis (Vertebral Osteomyelitis)

Discospondylitis results when bacteria or fungi become implanted in the bones of the vertebral column. Implantation may occur through hematogenous routes, from penetrating wounds, paravertebral abscess or infection, surgery on the vertebral column, or migrating grass awns. Grass awns are sharp pieces of plant material that migrate through the skin into the spinal bone, causing infection. Discospondylitis is seen in both cats and dogs, with large and giant breeds being more commonly affected.

Hematogenous spread is probably the most common cause of discospondylitis. Urinary tract infections, bacterial endocarditis, and sites of dental extraction can all be routes for bacterial infection. Organisms typically cultured from lesions include *Brucella canis*, *Staphylococcus* spp., *Streptococcus canis*, *Escherichia coli*, *Corynebacterium* spp., *Proteus* spp., *Pasteurella* spp., *Aspergillus*, and *Mycobacterium*.

Clinical signs of the disease are often nonspecific. If bony proliferation or granulation tissue impinges on the spinal cord, neurologic signs may develop.

CLINICAL SIGNS

- Weight loss
- Fever of unknown origin
- Depression
- Reluctance to exercise
- Spinal pain
- Hyperesthesia over the lesion(s)
- Presence or absence of neurologic signs

DIAGNOSIS

- Radiographs may show destruction or lysis of bony end plates adjacent to the lesions, osteophyte formation, and collapse of the intervertebral disk space.
- Complete blood count may show increased WBC count.
- CSF may be normal or have increased protein concentration and WBC count.
- Myelography demonstrates areas of spinal compression.
- Aerobic, anaerobic, and fungal cultures of blood, CSF, and urine should be taken.
- *Brucella canis* slide agglutination test should be performed.
- Surgical biopsy and tissue culture are diagnostic.

TREATMENT

- Long-term antibiotic therapy based on culture and sensitivity results or the following:
  - Cephalosporins (Cephalothin and Cephalexin): PO every 12 hours
  - Clindamycin: IV, IM, PO q12h
  - Enrofloxacin: PO every 12 hours
  - Chloramphenicol: PO, IV, IM, SQ every 8 hours
- Continue treatment for at least 6 weeks. It may be necessary to treat for up to 6 months.
- If positive for *Brucella canis* infection:
  - Neuter or spay the animal.
  - Treat with tetracycline and streptomycin.

⦿ TECH ALERT

Brucellosis can be infectious to humans. Use care when handling body fluids or aborted tissue.

- Animals with discospondylitis are painful.
- Use care when handling and provide analgesics for the pain.

INFORMATION FOR CLIENTS

- *Brucella canis* infection is contagious to humans through urine or in aborted fetal fluids and tissue.
- The prognosis for this disease is guarded.
- Treatment for this disease is costly and long term.
- Periodic reevaluation of radiographs (every 2–3 weeks) may be needed to follow treatment response.

Ischemic Myelopathy Caused by Fibrocartilaginous Embolism

Ischemic myelopathy caused by fibrocartilaginous embolism most commonly occurs in large breed and giant breed dogs between the ages of 1 and 9 years. It has been reported in cats and smaller breeds of dogs, but less frequently. Ischemic myelopathy results from necrosis of the spinal cord gray and white fiber tracts when fibrocartilaginous emboli obstruct the veins and arteries in both the leptomeninges and the cord parenchyma. The pathogenesis of the emboli is unknown.

Affected dogs may have a history of mild-to-moderate exercise before the development of clinical signs. The onset of symptoms is always acute, and neurologic deficit may be severe, depending on the location of the insult. Symptoms at first may appear progressive but usually stabilize after the first 12 hours. Deficits are usually bilateral and may be asymmetric. Horner syndrome can be seen if the cervical spine is involved. An embolism in the lumbosacral spinal cord usually produces lower motor neuron signs in the rear limbs, the anal and urinary sphincters, and the tail.

CLINICAL SIGNS

- Large breed and giant breed dogs are predisposed to this condition
- Acute onset of neurologic signs
- Lack of acute spinal pain associated with neurologic signs
- Paresis or spastic paralysis of limbs
- Reluctance to move, inability to rise

DIAGNOSIS

- Rule out other causes of myelopathy.
- Radiographs are usually within normal limits.
- CBC is within normal limits.
- CSF is usually within normal limits.
- Myelogram may show mild edema of the cord up to 24 hours after injury.

TREATMENT

- Administer corticosteroids in the same dose as for spinal shock.
- Provide good nursing care to prevent injury to affected structures, limit pressure sores, and so forth.
- Most animals recover within a few months.

INFORMATION FOR CLIENTS

- The prognosis for this disease is guarded to good.
- Most animals will recover, but it may take months to regain normal function.
- Extensive nursing care may be required to keep the patient comfortable and prevent further injury.

The Peripheral Nervous System

Peripheral nerve disorders are represented clinically by a group of signs known as *neuropathic syndrome.* The syndrome is commonly associated with trauma to the peripheral, or sometimes the cranial, nerves. Signs of this syndrome include reduced or absent muscle tone, weakness (paresis), or paralysis of the limb or facial muscles followed in 1 to 2 weeks by neurogenic muscular atrophy.

Peripheral neuropathies may involve a single nerve (such as the peroneal, radial, or facial nerve) or multiple nerves (as in polyradiculoneuritis), and the cause of the neuropathy is often unknown.

Deafness

Deafness in animals may be of central origin, resulting from damage to the CNS and auditory pathways, or peripheral, resulting from cochlear abnormalities. Conductive deafness, usually a result of chronic otitis, rupture of the tympanic membrane, or damage to the middle ear, is common in animals.

Neural deafness can be hereditary or congenital, related to drug therapy, or a normal aging change. Deafness appears to be hereditary in Bull Terriers,

Dobermans, Rottweilers, Pointers, blue-eyed white cats, Dalmatians, Australian Heelers, English Setters, Catahoula, and Australian Shepherds. Animals with congenital deafness suffer from partial or total agenesis of the hearing organ, the organ of Corti, the spiral ganglion, and the cochlear nuclei. Drugs that commonly result in ototoxicity include the aminoglycosides (e.g., gentamicin, streptomycin, kanamycin), topical polymyxin B, chloramphenicol, and chlorhexidine with cetrimide.

Hearing impairment is normal in aging pets and is usually related to atrophy of nerve ganglia or cochlear hair cells.

CLINICAL SIGNS

- Lack of response to auditory stimuli
- Excessive sleeping
- Breed that is prone to deafness

DIAGNOSIS

- Partial loss of hearing and even unilateral complete loss of hearing is difficult to establish on clinical examination of dogs and cats.
- Inability to arouse a sleeping patient with a loud noise (banging a pot, using an air horn, etc.) is diagnostic.
- Behavior evaluation: Stimulate the animal with various sounds from different directions; evaluate the response.
- Physical examination of the external ear canals and the tympanic membrane may assist in reaching a diagnosis.

Electrodiagnostic

- Electrodiagnostic testing usually requires referral to a specialty clinic. Testing may be costly.
- Tympanometry: A probe is inserted into the ear canal, and it seals the canal. Sound and pressure changes are delivered through the probe. Tympanic membrane compliance measurements allow the specialist to determine whether the ossicles, the tympanic membrane, or both are abnormal.
- Acoustic reflex testing: Delivery of increasing sound pressure levels to the ear evokes the *acoustic reflex* (muscles of the middle ear contract to dampen sound response and prevent damage). If the reflex is present, the auditory system is probably intact.

- Auditory-evoked responses: Cochlear function may be assessed by measuring brain electrical responses to air-conducted clicks either from a probe placed in the external ear canal or from a bone vibrator placed firmly against the mastoid process of the temporal bone. This is especially effective in detecting hereditary and senile deafness. Puppies and kittens should be at least 6 weeks of age for this test to be valid.

TREATMENT

- No treatment is available in most cases. Loss of hearing is permanent.
- Hearing aids are available for animals. Many animals will not tolerate a hearing aid in the ear canal. Because hearing aids are expensive, owners are advised to experiment with foam rubber earplugs in the animal's ear canal before spending money on an actual hearing aid. If the animal will not tolerate the earplugs, it will not tolerate the hearing aid.

INFORMATION FOR CLIENTS

- Hearing loss is permanent. These animals are at risk for injury in their environment, especially in traffic. They may bite when startled.
- If the deafness is hereditary, do not breed the animal.
- Animals can be taught to respond to hand signals rather than voice commands.
- These animals should never be off their leashes when outside.
- Keep animals' ears clean and free of infection to avoid damage to the middle and inner ear. It will help to maintain the hearing they have.
- Hearing aids do exist for dogs; however, they are expensive, and many animals will not tolerate them in the ear canal.

Metabolic Neuropathy

Cases of polyneuropathy have been reported in dogs and cats with diabetes mellitus, in dogs with hyperadrenocorticism, and in dogs with hypothyroidism. Clinical signs are variable from progressive weakness to muscle atrophy and depressed spinal reflexes. Paresis, paralysis, or both may occur. Hypothyroid dogs show signs related to the cranial nerves, including head tilt, facial paralysis, strabismus, nystagmus, and circling. Good control of the underlying disease is required to limit neurologic damage.

CLINICAL SIGNS

- Varied

DIAGNOSIS

- The underlying disease process can be diagnosed through biochemical testing.
- Rule out other causes of neuropathy.

TREATMENT

- Correct the underlying disease process.

INFORMATION FOR CLIENTS

- The underlying disease process must be controlled with proper medication and frequent reevaluation.
- Treatment for the underlying disease may be lifelong in your pet.

Laryngeal Paralysis

Hereditary, acquired, and idiopathic laryngeal paralysis occur in dogs and cats. The hereditary form is seen in the Bouvier des Flandres and in young Siberian Huskies.

Acquired laryngeal paralysis can occur from lead poisoning, rabies, trauma, and inflammatory infiltrates of the vagus nerve. All persons should take care when examining any animal with suspected laryngeal paralysis because rabies is increasing in incidence in many parts of the United States.

The idiopathic form of laryngeal paralysis has been reported in middle-aged to old large and giant breed dogs. Castrated male dogs and cats appear to be more frequently affected compared with female and non-neutered animals.

CLINICAL SIGNS

- Hereditary: 4 to 6 months of age
- Acquired: 1.5 to 13 years of age
- Inspiratory stridor
- Respiratory distress
- Loss of endurance
- Voice change
- Dyspnea
- Cyanosis
- Complete respiratory collapse

DIAGNOSIS

- Laryngoscopy will show laryngeal abductor dysfunction.

TREATMENT

Surgical

- Arytenoidectomy
- Arytenoid lateralization
- Removal of the vocal folds

INFORMATION FOR CLIENTS

- The prognosis is guarded to good.
- Do not breed animals that acquire hereditary laryngeal paralysis.

Megaesophagus

The neurologic disease megaesophagus involves a lack of effective esophageal peristalsis, resulting in dilation of the esophagus and regurgitation of undigested food. The congenital form makes up about 25% of all cases and is common in Great Danes, German Shepherds, Irish Setters, Newfoundlands, Shar-Peis, and Greyhounds. The inherited form is seen in wire-haired Fox Terriers and Miniature Schnauzers.

The congenital form of megaesophagus usually becomes evident around weaning time when puppies begin eating solid foods. Chronic regurgitation of undigested food, weight loss, respiratory signs, and pneumonias are seen clinically.

Acquired megaesophagus may occur in animals of any age. Approximately 50% of these cases are idiopathic in nature, whereas 25% may actually be the result of focal myasthenia gravis or Addison disease. The appearance of symptoms may be linked to a variety of causes such as metabolic neuromuscular disease, distemper, tick paralysis, lead poisoning, laryngeal paralysis–polyneuropathy complex, and polymyositis.

The prognosis for megaesophagus is guarded to poor. Management techniques such as elevated feeding of high-calorie diets appear to decrease clinical signs. Feeding regimens vary. It has been suggested that liquid diets be used exclusively (easier for food to enter the stomach by gravity flow), whereas other studies recommend small meatballs of canned food to stimulate what little peristalsis exists. The goal of management is to decrease the frequency of regurgitation, prevent overdistension of the esophagus, and provide adequate nutrition for the patient.

Several small meals should be fed during the day. Gastrostomy tubes can be placed long term if solid meals are not well tolerated by the patient.

CLINICAL SIGNS

- Regurgitation of undigested food
- Respiratory signs: cough, dyspnea, drooling, pneumonia
- Lack of growth or weight loss

DIAGNOSIS

- Radiographic evidence of a dilated esophagus to the level of the diaphragm (Fig. 8-5):
  - *Barium meal*: mix barium with canned food; feed mixture and radiograph.
  - *Fluoroscopy* is performed with barium swallow.

● TECH ALERT

Animals with a dilated esophagus full of barium are at risk for aspiration pneumonia. Keep the animal in a vertical position for 5 to 10 minutes after the procedure.

- Rule out metabolic causes with serum chemistries, complete physical examination, CBC, and so on.

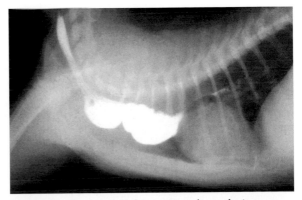

Figure 8-5 Persistent right aortic arch producing megaesophagus in a 3-month old kitten. (From Washabau RJ, Day MJ: *Canine and feline gastroenterology*, ed 1, St. Louis, MO, 2012, Saunders.)

TREATMENT

- Provide elevated feeding platform. If the animal will tolerate its use, a Bailey chair may increase the ease of feeding
- Provide liquid or soft diet high in caloric density.
- Give several small feedings daily.
- Treat any underlying metabolic disorders.

INFORMATION FOR CLIENTS

- The prognosis for this disease is guarded to poor.
- Treatment aims to decrease clinical signs and prevent the development of aspiration pneumonia. No cure for this disease exists.

Tick Paralysis

In the United States, the common dog tick *Dermacentor variabilis* and the Rocky Mountain wood tick *Dermacentor andersoni* are most often involved in a flaccid, afebrile, ascending motor paralysis. Cats appear to be resistant to tick paralysis.

The female tick produces a salivary neurotoxin that interferes with acetylcholine concentrations at the neuromuscular junction. The onset of clinical signs is gradual, beginning as incoordination in the pelvic limbs. Altered voice and dysphasia may be seen. Within 24 to 72 hours, dogs become recumbent. Reflexes are lost while sensation remains. Death may occur because of respiratory paralysis.

Recovery usually occurs within 1 to 3 days after removal of all ticks on the animal. Animals with respiratory involvement may need to be ventilated until signs subside.

CLINICAL SIGNS

- Gradual development of hind-limb incoordination that progresses to a flaccid ascending paralysis
- The presence of ticks on the dog

DIAGNOSIS

- Rule out other causes of neuromuscular disease.

TREATMENT

- Remove all ticks from the animal (manually or with a dip).
- Oral cythioate (Proban) can be used to remove hidden ticks (3.3–6.6 mg/kg PO).
- Supportive care is required.

Coonhound Paralysis or Polyradiculoneuritis

Coonhound paralysis (CHP) has generated intense interest because of its resemblance to Guillain-Barré syndrome in humans. Like the human syndrome, CHP may have an immunologic pathogenesis. However, the exact agent has not yet been isolated. Many, but not all, cases of CHP involve a raccoon bite before the development of clinical signs. Recent reports indicate that raccoon saliva contains the etiologic factor for CHP and that only certain susceptible dogs are at risk for acquiring CHP. Pathologic findings include segmental demyelination together with degeneration of myelin and axons, especially in the ventral nerve roots.

The disease can affect adult dogs of any breed and either sex. Clinical signs usually appear within 7 to 14 days after exposure to the raccoon, although some dogs experience development of the disease without exposure to a raccoon bite. Weakness begins in the hindlimbs with paralysis progressing rapidly to a flaccid, systemic tetraplegia. Some dogs may be more severely affected. In severely affected animals, spinal reflexes may be absent, and loss of voice, labored breathing, and an inability to lift the head may occur. These animals may die of respiratory paralysis. Paralysis may last 2 to 3 months, but the prognosis is generally good for most cases.

CLINICAL SIGNS

- Recent exposure to a raccoon or other nonspecific antigen stimulation
- Ascending, flaccid paralysis
- Alert, afebrile animal

DIAGNOSIS

- Clinical signs (lower motor neuron)
- History of some antigenic stimulation
- All other metabolic or infectious causes ruled out

TREATMENT

- Treatment consists of supportive nursing care.
- Corticosteroids in antiinflammatory doses have been used clinically.
- Support respirations, if necessary.

INFORMATION FOR CLIENTS

- Animals can develop this condition without exposure to raccoons.
- Affected animals may require long-term nursing care.
- Some animals may regain total function, whereas severely affected animals may not.

Facial Nerve Paralysis

Idiopathic, acute facial nerve paralysis has been reported in adult dogs and cats (>5 years). The cause of this condition is unknown. Cocker Spaniels, Pembroke Welsh Corgis, Boxers, English Setters, and domestic longhaired cats appear to be predisposed to facial nerve paralysis.

Biopsies of affected facial nerves show degeneration of myelinated fibers. The prognosis for complete recovery is guarded.

CLINICAL SIGNS

- Ear droop
- Lip paralysis
- Sialosis
- Deviation of the nose
- Collection of food in the paralyzed side of the mouth
- Absence of menace and palpebral reflex

DIAGNOSIS

- Electrodiagnostic testing of facial nerves
- Clinical signs of acute facial paralysis without signs of trauma

TREATMENT

- Corticosteroids can be provided; however, efficacy is unknown.
- Artificial tears to affected eye help to prevent corneal dryness.
- Keep the oral cavity clear of food.

INFORMATION FOR CLIENTS

- The cause of facial nerve paralysis is unknown.
- Complete recovery does not usually occur.
- Animals may experience development of keratoconjunctivitis sicca because of damage to the nerves that pass to the lacrimal gland.
- Affected animals may require lifelong maintenance care.

REVIEW QUESTIONS

1. Which of the following is a false statement concerning intervertebral disk disease?
   a. The severity of spinal cord injury depends on the speed at which disk material is deposited into the spinal canal.
   b. The severity of spinal cord injury depends on the degree of spinal cord compression.
   c. The severity of the spinal cord injury is related to the weight of the animal.
   d. The severity of the spinal cord injury is related to the duration of compression.
2. What percentage of intervertebral disks is estimated to be degenerative in a chondrodystrophic breed by 1 year of age?
   a. 30%
   b. 5%
   c. 45%
   d. 75%
3. In the absence of deep pain following a spinal cord injury for greater than 48 hours, the prognosis is:
   a. Poor
   b. Guarded
   c. Good
   d. Excellent
4. Cervical spondylomyelopathy (Wobbler syndrome) is seen primarily in:
   a. Golden Retrievers
   b. Toy Poodles
   c. Dobermans
   d. Cocker Spaniels
5. Until proven otherwise, animals with alteration of voice or laryngeal paralysis should be suspected of:
   a. Brucellosis
   b. Leptospirosis
   c. Rabies
   d. Aspergillosis
6. Which of the following diseases does not include the sign of ascending flaccid paralysis?
   a. CHP
   b. Tick paralysis
   c. Embolic ischemic myelopathy

7. Which of the following is *not* included in the treatment for tick paralysis?
   a. Manual removal of all the ticks on the animal
   b. Supportive care
   c. Chemical products for tick removal
   d. Antibiotics
8. Which of the following would not be a cause of megaesophagus in the dog?
   a. Congenital disease
   b. Lead poisoning
   c. Metabolic dysfunction
   d. Atlantoaxial subluxation
9. Phenobarbital takes _____ days to reach an adequate concentration in the blood. Until this time animals may continue to exhibit seizure activity.
   a. 2–3
   b. 7–10
   c. 21–30
   d. 18–24

10. Which of the following diagnostic examinations would be of least value in determining a cause for seizures in an older animal?
    a. CBC, serum chemistries
    b. Ophthalmic examination
    c. CSF evaluation
    d. MRI
    e. Radiography

Answers found on page 552.

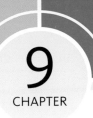

Pansystemic Diseases

9

CHAPTER

KEY TERMS

Effusion
Hyperkeratosis
Hyphema
Immunocompetence
Mucopurulent

Oocysts
Panleukopenia
Pansystemic
Polymerase Chain Reaction

Peritonitis
Perivasculitis
Pyogranulomatous
Tachyzoites

OUTLINE

Feline Panleukopenia (Feline Distemper)
Feline Infectious Peritonitis
Feline Leukemia Virus
Feline Immunodeficiency Virus
Toxoplasmosis
Rabies (Feline and Canine)
Canine Distemper

Canine Parvovirus
Rickettsioses
 Rocky Mountain Spotted Fever
 Canine Monocytic Ehrlichiosis
 Canine Granulocytic Ehrlichiosis
Lyme Disease (Borreliosis)

LEARNING OBJECTIVES

When you have completed this chapter, you will be able to:
1. Relate the specific cause of disease with the pansystemic clinical signs seen in dogs and cats.
2. Initiate the proper safety methods to prevent spread of these transmissible or infectious diseases within the clinic.

3. Discuss with clients the necessity of an effective vaccination program.
4. Explain how environment and husbandry conditions affect the health of the young or immunosuppressed older pet.

Pansystemic diseases include those that involve multiple body systems in addition to the primary target organ. The causes of these diseases may be viral, bacterial, or parasitic, and secondary infections are common. Box 9-1 lists some of the most commonly seen pansystemic diseases of dogs and cats.

Feline Panleukopenia (Feline Distemper)

Feline panleukopenia is caused by a deoxyribonucleic acid (DNA) virus of the family Parvoviridae, which is closely related antigenically to the canine parvovirus

163

BOX 9-1   Common Pansystemic Diseases

Feline
- Feline leukemia
- Feline immunodeficiency virus
- Feline infectious peritonitis
- Feline panleukopenia
- Toxoplasmosis

Canine
- Canine distemper
- Canine rabies
- Canine parvovirus
- Ehrlichiosis
- Lyme disease

(CPV), type 2. The disease is primarily one of young, unvaccinated cats and feral animals. Transmission is by direct contact or from a contaminated environment. The virus shed into the environment may remain infectious for years.

Feline parvovirus multiplies within actively dividing cells of the neonatal brain, bone marrow, and lymphoid tissue, and in the intestinal lymphoid tissue, causing destruction of the cells with release of a large number of virions. The incubation period is usually 4 to 5 days. Signs may be peracute, acute, subacute, or subclinical.

CLINICAL SIGNS
- Fever
- Depression
- Vomiting
- Fetid diarrhea
- Dehydration; may appear to be thirsty but will not drink
- Anorexia
- Fetal death, spontaneous abortion, or reabsorption in the pregnant queen
- Cerebellar or retinal defects in neonates

DIAGNOSIS
- Complete blood cell count (CBC): moderate to severe panleukopenia
- Positive result using SNAPtest for CPV (IDEXX)
- Serum antibody titers
- Viral isolation is difficult
- PCR for detection of viral DNA in fecal samples

● TECH ALERT

Isolate the cats with CPV infection from other animals. All body secretions contain the virus.

TREATMENT

Aggressive Supportive Therapy
- Maintain hydration and electrolyte balance.
- Force-feed after vomiting is controlled.
- Broad-spectrum antibiotics are required.

INFORMATION FOR CLIENTS
- Cats that survive the infection acquire a lifelong immunity.
- To prevent disease, kittens should be vaccinated between 8 and 10 weeks of age, and then again after 12 to 14 weeks. Yearly boosters have typically been recommended for all cats; however, new information indicates that current vaccine immunity may last up to 3 years.
- See Box 9-2.

Feline Infectious Peritonitis

Feline infectious peritonitis (FIP) is primarily a disease of catteries and multicat households. FIP does not occur without exposure to feline coronavirus. In catteries, 8% to 90% of cats have antibodies to feline coronaviruses (mostly feline enteric coronavirus [FECV]), and these cats shed the virus intermittently. FECV is highly contagious through feces as well as urine and saliva. Current thinking is that this virus may mutate to feline infectious peritonitis

BOX 9-2   A Clinical History of Canine Parvovirus

In the early 1980s, canine parvovirus made its swift and devastating appearance. Hundreds of pets, both pure-bred and mixed-breed dogs, were lost to the disease. Some veterinarians begin to vaccinate dogs weekly with the feline panleukopenia vaccine, hoping to avoid infection in their client's pets and in their own pets. Guess what happened! It worked in many cases, and until the parvovirus vaccine became readily available, it was the best and only way to protect dogs from a fatal parvovirus infection.

(FIPV) within some infected cats. FIPV then enters the macrophages, spreading throughout the body. Affected cats develop clinical signs related to granuloma formation in the target organs (central nervous system (CNS), eyes, vessels, and other organs).

FIPV and FECV are difficult to differentiate with current testing procedures. Enzyme-linked immunosorbent assay (ELISA) and immunofluorescence assays are nonspecific for FIPV. Because the gene mutation that converts FECV to FIP often involves a small number of gene sites, even the polymerase chain reaction (PCR) test cannot distinguish the two viruses. Immunofluorescence staining of tissue macrophages may be of use in confirming a diagnosis of FIP in those cats without effusion.

FIP occurs in two forms: (1) the effusive or "wet" form (75%) and (2) the noneffusive or "dry" form. About 45% of cats that have the dry form will have ocular or neurologic lesions. In the effusive form, perivasculitis results in the accumulation of a protein-rich fluid in the thoracic and/or abdominal cavity, the scrotum, the pericardial cavity, and the renal subcapsular space. The inflammatory process may also involve the liver and the pancreas. The clinical progression is more rapid than with the dry form.

Signs of noneffusive FIP are less clear. The pyogranulomatous lesions may be found anywhere in the body, especially the eyes and the neurologic system. Clinical signs may include ataxia, seizures, behavioral changes, paresis, hyperesthesia, or all of these. Ocular signs include iritis, retinitis, uveitis, hyphema, corneal edema, retinal hemorrhage, and retinal detachment.

CLINICAL SIGNS

Wet Form
- Ascites, pleural effusion
- Anorexia
- Depression
- Weight loss
- Dehydration
- May or may not be febrile

Dry Form
- Fever of unknown origin
- Anorexia
- Depression
- Weight loss

- Ocular lesions
- Neurologic signs
- Enlarged kidneys (uncommon)

DIAGNOSIS
- Clinical signs
- Other diseases ruled out
- Cytology and chemical analysis of abdominal and pleural fluid show the following:
  - Viscous, clear to yellow fluid
  - Less than 20,000 nucleated cells/μl
  - Protein-rich (>3.5 grams per deciliter (g/dL)
  - Albumin/globulin ratio >0.81
- High antibody titers may be *suggestive* of FIP

TREATMENT

Supportive
- Aspiration of pleural or abdominal fluids to make the cat more comfortable
- Steroids (daily), immunosuppressive drugs such as cyclophosphamide
- Broad-spectrum antibiotics

Immunotherapy
- ImmunoRegulin
- Ribavirin and adenine arabinoside inhibit FIPV in cell culture, but in a recent clinical trial, cats treated with ribavirin exhibited more severe symptoms and had a shorter survival time compared with cats treated with traditional therapies

Prevention
- Isolate pregnant queens 2 weeks before giving birth.
- Remove weaning kittens from queens by 5 weeks of age.
- Vaccinate seronegative cats with Primucell FIP (Pfizer), an intranasal vaccine, at 16 weeks of age. This drug provides effective protection against FIP but is ineffective in cats already exposed to FECV.

INFORMATION FOR CLIENTS
- Virtually every cat with a confirmed diagnosis of FIP will die from the disease.
- The virus is inactivated in the environment by most household disinfectants.

- Diagnosis of this disease can be difficult and may require a series of expensive tests to rule out other possibilities.

Feline Leukemia Virus

Feline leukemia is caused by a retrovirus that is associated with both neoplastic and nonneoplastic (immunosuppressive) diseases. Both vertical and horizontal transmissions occur. The virus is unstable in the environment; therefore, close contact between cats is required for infection to occur. The virus can be isolated from saliva, urine, tears, and milk, and it can be spread through fighting, grooming, or exposure to contaminated food bowls, food, water, or litter pans. Transplacental and transmammary transmission does occur. The outcome of exposure to the virus is variable and depends on several host factors: age or sex, immunocompetence, concurrent disease, viral strain, dose, and the duration of exposure.

Exposed cats may experience development of the following conditions: (1) a *regressive* infection (cats become aviremic after a transient infection), (2) a *progressive* infection (cats maintain persistent viremia) or (3) an *active* infection with clinical signs. Clinical signs associated with feline leukemia virus (FeLV) include anemia, anorexia, depression, weight loss, nervous system disease, and secondary infections. Vomiting and diarrhea may be seen if the gastrointestinal tract is involved.

Lymphoma is the most common FeLV-associated neoplastic disease. Tumors can occur in the thymus, the alimentary tract, or various lymph nodes throughout the body.

Treatment is primarily supportive, and prevention is through vaccination and limited contact with infected cats. All cats should be tested for FeLV using the standard peripheral-blood ELISA test before vaccination. If positive, cats should undergo an immunofluorescent antibody (IFA) test or be retested by ELISA in 3 to 4 months. Cats with recurring positive results will usually be positive for life and should be isolated from all other nonvaccinated cats. Many may remain in good health for prolonged periods if not stressed.

CLINICAL SIGNS

- Fever
- Anorexia
- Weight loss
- Anemia
- Secondary infections
- Vomiting and diarrhea
- Spontaneous abortion
- Renal disease
- Tumors of lymphoid origin
- Neurologic signs

DIAGNOSIS

- FeLV positive on ELISA test
- CBC: nonregenerative anemia
- IFA: positive
- Clinical signs of recurring infections

TREATMENT

Husbandry

- FeLV-positive cats should be isolated from all other cats.
- FeLV-positive cats should be kept indoors.
- FeLV-positive cats should be vaccinated for other feline diseases and rabies on a routine schedule.
- Eliminate stress in affected cats.

Medical

- No cure currently exists for FeLV; however, drug therapy may alleviate symptoms
- Immunomodulator drugs:
  - Acemannan (Veterinary Product Labs, Phoenix, AZ): orally (PO), subcutaneously (SQ) daily, or intraperitoneally (IP) once a week for 6 weeks
  - Propionibacterium acnes (ImmunoRegulin): intravenously (IV) 1 to 2 times weekly
  - Human recombinant interferon: every 24 hours PO for 7 days, repeated every other week
- Antiviral drugs:
  - Azidothymidine (AZT; Zidovudine): PO every 12 hours
  - 9-(2-phosphomethoxyethyl) adenine (PMEA): SQ every 12 hours
- Broad-spectrum antibiotics to control secondary infections
- Appetite stimulants:
  - Oxazepam (Serax, Zoetis, Madison, N.J.): PO
  - Diazepam (Valium, Roche Pharmaceutical; San Francisco, CA): IV
- Chemotherapy for solid tumors

INFORMATION FOR CLIENTS

- An FeLV-positive cat that is otherwise healthy need not be euthanized.
- If your cat is positive for FeLV, you should do the following:
  - Keep the animal indoors.
  - Isolate the cat from all other cats.
  - Keep up with vaccinations.
  - See your veterinarian if any signs of disease develop.

Feline Immunodeficiency Virus

Feline immunodeficiency virus (FIV), or feline acquired immunodeficiency syndrome (AIDS) is a lentivirus associated with an immunodeficiency disease in domestic cats, which is morphologically and biochemically similar to HIV but is antigenically distinct. FIV is highly species specific, growing only in feline-derived cells. Most infections are acquired by horizontal transmission among adult cats. Male, sexually intact cats living outdoors are at greatest risk for acquiring FIV infection. Fighting and bite wounds appear to be the major route of transmission. Little or no sexual transmission occurs in cats. Neonatal kittens may become infected by contact with infected queens, although plasma antibodies against FIV may be passed to kittens in colostrum when nursing. Because the ELISA test for FIV detects antibodies, kittens should not be diagnosed using these tests until after 6 months of age.

Clinical signs of FIV involve chronic, unresponsive infections (gingivitis, stomatitis, and skin, ear, respiratory tract infections, or all of these), anemia, ocular and neurologic signs, and weight loss. Chronic fever and cachexia are common findings. Cats may remain asymptomatic for long periods after infection or may suffer from recurring bouts of illness interspersed with periods of relatively good health. Cats infected with FIV are at increased risk for development of chronic renal insufficiency.

Prevention of infection is by limiting exposure to outdoor cats. Spaying and neutering outdoor cats can limit exposure by decreasing aggressive behaviors. A vaccine for FIV currently is available. Cats receiving this vaccine may test positive for FIV at a later date.

CLINICAL SIGNS

- History of recurrent bouts of illnesses
- Cachexia, anorexia
- Gingivitis, stomatitis
- Chronic, nonresponsive ear or skin infections
- Chronic upper respiratory infections
- Diarrhea
- Vomiting
- Neurologic disorders
- Ocular disease (anterior uveitis, glaucoma)
- Pale mucous membranes
- Chronic fever

DIAGNOSIS

- Clinical history
- Positive ELISA test (blood)
- CBC: anemia, lymphopenia

TREATMENT

Husbandry
- Keep infected cats indoors.
- Isolate affected cats if aggressive toward other cats in the household
- Transmission from fomites or casual contact is unlikely.

Medical
- No cure currently exists for FIV; however, drug therapy may alleviate symptoms

- Immunomodulator drugs:
  - Acemannan (VPL, Phonex, AZ): PO, SQ daily, or IP weekly for 6 weeks
  - ImmunoRegulin (Immunovet): intravenously (IV) 1 to 2 times weekly
  - Interferon-α (Intron-A, Schering-Plough, Kenilworth, N.J.): 30 international units per cat (IU/cat) PO every 24 hours for 5 days on alternate weeks
- Antiviral therapy: AZT (Retrovir, Glaxo-Wellcome, Research Triangle Park, N. C.): PO every 12 hours; if anemia develops, stop medication until CBC returns to normal, and then restart at previous dose and increase to original dose over 1 to 2 weeks

Surgical
- Whole-mouth extraction of teeth may be necessary in cats with chronic stomatitis and gingivitis.

INFORMATION FOR CLIENTS
- FIV poses *no* health hazard for humans.
- Infected cats may survive for prolonged periods before experiencing advanced stages of the disease.
- For cats with severe gingivitis and stomatitis, tooth extraction may be the best course of treatment. Cats are able to eat well even after whole-mouth extractions.
- Keeping your pet indoors will prevent infection.
- Keeping an infected cat free from stress and concurrent disease is *extremely* important.
- A vaccine is available for this disease; however, cats that receive the vaccine may test positive for FIV on later examinations. Owners should be aware of this.

Toxoplasmosis

Toxoplasmosis is caused by *Toxoplasma gondii*, an intracellular coccidian parasite with worldwide distribution. The feline is the only definitive host, but other warm-blooded animals, including humans, can serve as intermediate hosts. Exposure to *Toxoplasma* is common; an estimated 30% to 60% of adult humans are seropositive for exposure (Fig. 9-1).

Transmission can occur by three routes: (1) eating contaminated meat from an intermediate host, (2) fecal-oral route, and (3) transplacental route. In

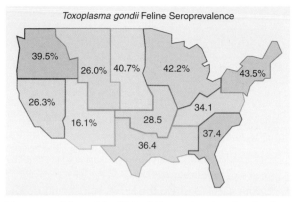

Figure 9-1 Map of the United States showing the distribution of *Toxoplasma gondii* antibody test results in cats. (From Ettinger SJ, Feldman EC: *Textbook of veterinary internal medicine*, ed 7, St. Louis, MO, 2010, Saunders.)

carnivores, ingestion of infected intermediate hosts is responsible for most infections.

Once sporulated oocysts are ingested, tachyzoites form and invade any tissue in the body. Clinical signs of disease are related to the tissue involved. The disease may be especially severe in immunocompromised animals or in very young animals. In cats, the two tissues most commonly involved are the lung and the eyes, whereas in dogs, the gastrointestinal, neurologic, and the respiratory systems are commonly infected. However, *Toxoplasma* infections are rare in the dog.

After infection, the cat sheds oocysts in its feces for 1 to 2 weeks. Because of this limited shedding of organisms, exposure to these infective oocysts is probably not an important source of infection for humans and other cats. Ingestion of uncooked or undercooked meat is most likely the main route of infection in both cats and humans. Therefore, prevention of infection involves eliminating hunting and feeding of raw meat to the cat, cooking all meat properly before feeding, and following good hygiene practices when handling cat feces.

Humans who are immunosuppressed should avoid contact with infected cats. Congenital infection in the first or second trimester can result in serious birth defects. Although infected cats are unlikely to pose a major threat to most pregnant women, the following steps may be taken to prevent infection:
- Avoid feeding raw meat to cats.
- Keep cats indoors.

- Have someone else clean the litter box daily. Rinse litter box weekly with hot water.
- Avoid the use of immunosuppressive drugs in the seropositive cat.
- Have yourself checked for antibody before becoming pregnant.
- Avoid acquiring a new cat during pregnancy.
- Wash hands thoroughly and wear gloves when gardening.
- Cook all meat properly.
- *Do not panic.* Speak with your doctor and veterinarian when you determine you are pregnant. You should not have to give away your pets.

CLINICAL SIGNS

Signs will depend on the organs involved.
- Anorexia
- Lethargy
- Fever
- Weight loss
- Diarrhea
- Vomiting
- Icterus
- Respiratory disease
- Lameness
- Pancreatic disease
- Anterior uveitis
- Glaucoma
- CNS disease
- Sudden death

DIAGNOSIS

⦿ TECH ALERT

Antemortem diagnosis is difficult because of the presence of antibodies found in the general population and the lack of long-term shedding of oocysts in the infected cat.

- CBC: nonspecific, variable changes
- Serum chemistries:
- Increases in alanine aminotransferase (ALT), alkaline phosphatase (ALP), and total bilirubin may occur.
- Creatine kinase concentration is often increased.
- Thoracic radiographs may show diffuse lesions with or without pleural effusion.

- ELISA test should be available to test for *Toxoplasma* species–specific immunoglobulin G (IgG), IgM, and antigen-containing immune complexes. The PCR test is available for diagnosis of ocular or CNS infections (Colorado State University Diagnostic Laboratory, Pueblo, CO).
- Paired titers with a fourfold increase are required for a presumptive diagnosis IgM >1:256 and increased IgG).

TREATMENT

- Clindamycin is the drug of choice for treatment: PO, IM divided into two doses daily for 2 to 3 weeks.
- Trimethoprim with sulfonamide combination and azithromycin have also been useful.

INFORMATION FOR CLIENTS

- See earlier section outlining advice to pregnant women. *Do not panic.*

Rabies (Feline and Canine)

Although rabies technically is not a pansystemic disease, it has been included in this chapter because exposure of veterinary technicians and veterinarians often occurs during the examination of animals with vague and seemingly unrelated symptoms. Examples include the cat or dog with hypersalivation (which could indicate dental disease, foreign body), the pet with rear-leg paralysis (possible trauma, tick paralysis, disk disease), and the wild or exotic pet that is listless or "just not doing right." People often have no idea that their pet or the animal they have just rescued from the woods may be infected with the rabies virus.

Rabies is a viral-induced neurologic disease of warm-blooded animals. It has a worldwide distribution. In the United States, raccoons, bats, skunks, foxes, and coyotes serve as the major wild animal hosts for the disease. The virus is spread through the saliva of the infected animal and may enter the body through a bite, open wound, or mucous membranes. Aerosol transmission has been documented. The incubation time from exposure to the onset of clinical disease is usually 3 to 8 weeks, but it may be longer in some cases. During this time, the virus enters the nerve endings around the bite or wound and ascends the nerve to the brain, where it multiplies in the neurons. It then travels along nerves to the salivary glands, where it appears in the saliva.

Rabies is characterized by three stages: (1) the prodromal stage, (2) the excitative (furious) stage, and (3) the paralytic stage. The prodromal stage is characterized by changes in behavior (wild animals become friendly, nocturnal animals come out during the day, dogs and cats become fearful or apprehensive); it is during this stage that people are at the greatest risk for exposure. During the excitative phase, the animal may appear hyperreactive. They may attack unprovoked or attack inanimate objects. Some may appear to be in a stupor ("dumb" rabies). The first two stages are followed by the paralytic stage in which the animal experiences an ascending paralysis of the hind limb eventually leading to respiratory paralysis and death. These three stages may be completed in less than 1 week.

The technician should be alert to the early symptoms of rabies to prevent accidental exposure. Always get a vaccination history and wear gloves when examining the oral cavity of an animal. Avoid handling wildlife brought in by clients, and take precautions with domestically raised skunks and raccoons. Rabies has no cure and is almost always a fatal disease. Protect yourself from exposure by following these guidelines:

- Obtain preexposure prophylaxis (vaccines are available).
- Wear gloves when examining any animal's oral cavity and during necropsy procedures.
- Promote vaccination of all dogs, cats, and horses.
- Advise clients to leave wildlife in the wild.
- Assume rabies is a possibility in all animals with neurologic symptoms or voice changes.

CLINICAL SIGNS

- Behavioral changes
- Difficulty swallowing
- Hypersalivation
- Extruded penis
- Hindlimb ataxia
- Depression, stupor

DIAGNOSIS

- Postmortem examination of brain tissue is definitive.
- Positive fluorescent antibody (FA) test for virus in the brain and brainstem. No antemortem test is available.

TREATMENT

- No treatment currently exists. If rabies is suspected, the animal should be euthanized. Exposed staff should receive postexposure treatment. Vaccinated animals exposed to a rabid animal should be revaccinated and observed for 90 days. Unvaccinated animals exposed to rabies should be euthanized or kept under *strict* isolation for 6 months. Rules for quarantine may vary with location.

INFORMATION FOR CLIENTS

- Well-vaccinated pets create a buffer zone against human infection.
- Never handle wild animals that appear tame or friendly.
- Avoid promoting visitations by raccoons and skunks by covering garbage cans and not leaving food out for them.
- Diagnosis requires intact brain tissue. Avoid injuring the brain when euthanizing the animal.
- If your pet bites a person, it must be quarantined for 10 days at your expense. This quarantine may be at a veterinary clinic or humane shelter. Animals that show no signs of disease after 10 days are considered to have been uninfected at the time of the bite. *The quarantine is to protect humans, not your pet.*

Canine Distemper

Canine viral distemper (CVD) is a highly contagious viral disease of dogs and other carnivores. The incidence of disease is greatest in dogs 3 to 6 months of age. Canine distemper virus is a paramyxovirus that is relatively labile in the environment. Most routine cleaning agents, disinfectants, and heat will readily destroy the virus.

CVD is transmitted through aerosolization of body secretions. Several strains of the virus exist, and they vary in virulence from mild to fatal. The hallmark of infection is immunosuppression followed by the development of secondary infections. Clinical signs usually associated with distemper are related to the presence of the secondary infections, although encephalitis and other neurologic signs may be caused by the direct effect of the virus on neurons.

A diagnosis of distemper is usually based on clinical signs in an unvaccinated animal, but FA testing is available. The only treatment is supportive. The fatality rate may be as high as 90%, depending on the strain involved. A good vaccination program is the best prevention.

CLINICAL SIGNS

- Fever
- Cough
- Mucopurulent nasal and ocular discharge
- Pneumonia
- Anorexia
- Vomiting
- Diarrhea
- Dehydration
- Abdominal pustules
- Hyperkeratosis of foot pads
- "Chewing gum" seizures (clonus)
- Muscle twitching
- Ataxia, circling, blindness

DIAGNOSIS

- Physical examination and history
- Serology: rising titers in paired serum samples
- FA test to detect the virus in epithelial cells collected from the conjunctiva or other mucous membranes

TREATMENT

- Antibiotics, fluids, nutrition, and vitamins are supportive measures.
- No specific treatment for the virus is available.
- No specific treatment for the clonus is available.

INFORMATION FOR CLIENTS

- A good vaccination program for all dogs is the only prevention.
- The prognosis is guarded, especially if neurologic signs are present.
- CDV is the most common cause of seizures in dogs younger than 6 months.
- Neurologic signs may appear weeks to years after the actual infection with CDV.

Canine Parvovirus

CPV is a common cause of infectious enteritis in the dog (Fig. 9-2). The disease is caused by a single-stranded,

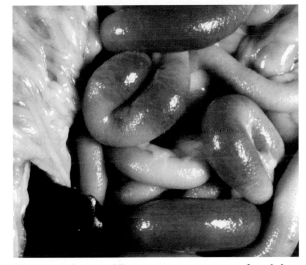

Figure 9-2 Intestinal lesions in a parvovirus infected dog. (Courtesy Veterinary Pathology, University of Georgia, Athens, GA. IN Greene C: *Infectious diseases of the dog and cat*, ed 3, St Louis, 2006, Elsevier)

nonenveloped DNA virus and is closely related to the virus that causes feline panleukopenia. The virus is one of the most resistant viruses known, often surviving for years in contaminated environments. The virus was first isolated in 1978 and was associated with an outbreak of hemorrhagic gastroenteritis with a high mortality. Parvovirus is primarily a disease of young puppies that lack sufficient antibody protection. The virus is spread via feces and transmission is by the fecal-oral route. The virus invades rapidly, dividing cells of the lymphoid system, the intestinal tract, bone marrow, and the myocardium (in utero or shortly after birth). Factors such as age, stress, genetics, and concurrent intestinal parasitism influence the severity of the disease. Dobermans and Rottweilers have a greater likelihood of severe disease than most other breeds.

Animals infected with parvovirus may become febrile and lethargic, followed several days later by anorexia, depression, vomiting, and bloody, foul-smelling diarrhea. These animals quickly become dehydrated. Viral invasion of the bone marrow and lymph system produces a profound lymphopenia and neutropenia in severely infected dogs (white blood cell [WBC] counts may be <2000). Puppies can become hypoglycemic and hypokalemic from lack of nutritional intake. Secondary sepsis may occur together with possible intestinal intussusceptions.

Diagnosis is by fecal ELISA test for the parvovirus antigen (CITE, IDEXX). Treatment consists of aggressive supportive therapy including intravenous fluids, antibiotics, antiemetics, antiinflammatory agents, and colony-stimulating factor (Nupogen, Amgen). Vaccination is the best preventive measure. Clients should avoid exposing their pets to other animals until their pets have established firm immunity (usually between 18 and 22 weeks of age, before the last parvo booster is given). Yearly boosters are recommended for most animals. In high-risk breeds, a booster every 6 months may be required. It appears that several new strains of the virus have emerged and that disease caused by these strains may be more severe. They may also not be prevented by current vaccines.

CLINICAL SIGNS

- Young puppy or older, unvaccinated dog

⦿ TECH ALERT

The disease has been seen in older vaccinated animals and in animals whose owners purchased vaccines from livestock stores or through catalogues.

- Depression
- Lethargy
- Anorexia
- Vomiting
- Bloody diarrhea
- Dehydration
- Fever

DIAGNOSIS

- Positive fecal ELISA test; PCR is available commercially
- CBC: Marked lymphopenia and neutropenia—increased packed cell volume (PCV)—lymphopenia is seen in less than 50% of the clinically ill dogs.
- Serum chemistries (not specific for CPV):
  - Hypoglycemia
  - Hyponatremia
  - Metabolic acidosis
  - Hypokalemia
- Fecal examination to rule out intestinal parasites
- Serology: High titer (1:10,000) for CPV

TREATMENT

⦿ TECH ALERT

Animals with CPV are highly infectious and should be handled in isolation.

Supportive

- Intravenous fluids: crystalloids are the fluids of choice
- Potassium chloride added: 8 milliequivalents per 500 milliters (mEq/500 ml) fluid
- Dextrose added as needed: 5% solution

⦿ TECH ALERT

Avoid subcutaneous fluids because animals with CPV are prone to infections from repeated injections through the skin. Also, maintain good asepsis of catheter sites, changing catheters every 48 to 72 hours, if possible. Keep bandages dry and clean.

- Antibiotics:
  - Ampicillin: IV, SQ every 6 to 8 hours
  - Amikacin: SQ every 8 hours
  - Gentamicin: SQ every 6 to 8 hours

⦿ TECH ALERT

Avoid fluoroquinolones in young animals because these agents damage cartilage.

- Antiemetics:
  - Reglan (Metoclopramide): IV, SQ every 6 to 8 hours
  - Nonsteroidal antiinflammatory drugs (NSAIDs) for pain—use only in well-hydrated patients
- Colony-stimulating factors (CSFs) promote maturation and release of specific cells from bone marrow (may not be of value)
  - RhG-CSF/filgastrim (Neupogen, Amgen): SQ every 24 hours
- Nutrition: partial parenteral nutrition until the patient remains 24 hours without vomiting

Prevention

- Vaccinate puppies beginning at 6 to 8 weeks of age with boosters every 3 to 4 weeks until 16 weeks of age. Revaccinate high-risk breeds at 22 weeks of age. Rebooster all dogs yearly. (Fecal parvo antigen tests may be weakly positive for 5 to 15 days after vaccination.)

INFORMATION FOR CLIENTS

- Make sure you have your new puppy vaccinated on a proper schedule. Consult your veterinarian.
- Many puppies can survive parvovirus infection with proper treatment. Some clinics report 80% to 90% success rates.
- Treatment may be expensive and require hospital stay of several weeks.
- Other dogs in the house may become infected if not adequately vaccinated.
- The virus can survive long term in the environment.
- Keep puppies free of intestinal parasites. Intestinal parasites appear to predispose dogs to parvovirus infection.

⊙ **TECH ALERT**

Tips for technicians dealing with parvovirus:
- Isolate all animals suspected of parvovirus infection until a diagnosis is confirmed. These animals should not be seen in the examination area used for well-patient examinations. Take animals suspected of infection directly to the isolation ward.
- All waste and bedding of infected animals should be disposed of directly from the isolation area.
- Wear protective clothing and shoe covers when treating these animals in isolation. Do not wear these clothes into the rest of the clinic.
- Affected animals require intensive care to keep clean and dry. Frequent cleaning of vomit and bloody diarrhea is unpleasant for the staff, but these substances must not be allowed to accumulate in an area. Secondary infections to wet skin and catheter sites can develop if patients are not cleaned frequently.
- Do not allow these puppies to become overhydrated. Carefully monitor fluid intake.

Rickettsioses

Rickettsiae are small, gram-negative, obligate, intracellular bacterial organisms. Of the three known families, two (*Rickettsiae* and *Ehrlichiae*) are pathogens of dogs. Both these organisms are tick-borne pathogens, with infection occurring through the saliva during feeding by the tick. Distribution and seasonal occurrence of these diseases are related to the life cycle of the corresponding tick. Transmission of the organism requires attachment of the tick to the host for 5 to 20 hours.

Rocky Mountain Spotted Fever

The causative agent of Rocky Mountain spotted fever disease, *Rickettsia rickettsii*, induces vascular endothelial injury. The disease is spread by the ticks *Dermacentor variabilis* and *Dermacentor andersoni*. The transmitted rickettsiae replicate in vascular endothelial cells, causing inflammation, necrosis, and increased vascular permeability. Clinical signs are related to the areas of inflammation. The pulmonary, CNS, myocardial, ocular, renal, and musculoskeletal systems may be involved.

Clinical signs of edema, hypotension, shock, conduction abnormalities, heart blocks or arrhythmia, seizures, coma, pulmonary edema, retinal hemorrhages, and acute renal failure may be seen in infected dogs. These signs are vague and may mimic other infectious and noninfectious diseases. Diagnosis requires a direct immunofluorescent test for *R. rickettsii* in the skin or tissue biopsy.

Tetracycline and doxycycline are the treatments of choice; rapid improvement is seen after initiation of therapy. Owners should be educated as to the risks of tick exposure and the possibility of human infection through the environment.

CLINICAL SIGNS

- Fever
- Anorexia
- Depression
- Mucopurulent ocular discharge
- Tachypnea
- Coughing
- Vomiting and diarrhea
- Muscle pain
- CNS signs
- Severe weight loss
- Retinal hemorrhages
- Scrotal edema

⊙ **TECH ALERT**

Rocky Mountain spotted fever usually appears in the spring and summer months.

DIAGNOSIS

- Direct immunofluorescent test of tissue biopsy
- Indirect immunofluorescent test showing a four-fold increase in serum titers
- History of tick exposure
- CBC:
  - Anemia
  - Leukopenia to leukocytosis
  - Thrombocytopenia
- Serum chemistry:
  - Increased ALT
  - Increased ALP
  - Hypoproteinemia
  - Hypocalcemia
  - Hyponatremia

● TECH ALERT

Blood from patients with Rocky Mountain spotted fever may be infectious to persons handling it. Avoid contact by wearing protective clothing. Avoid blood from the tick as well.

TREATMENT

- Tetracycline: three times a day for two weeks
- Doxycycline: for two weeks
- Monitoring fluid intake carefully to avoid exacerbation of the edema already present

INFORMATION FOR CLIENTS

- If you develop signs of an upper respiratory tract infection, fever, headache, myalgia, or abdominal pain, see your doctor.
- Supportive care is important for infected animals and should be performed under careful veterinary supervision.
- Antibiotics only reduce the number of organisms; the animal must have a good immune response to eliminate them.
- Control of tick infestation is the best way to prevent the disease. Keep pets out of heavily infested areas, and remove ticks quickly.

Canine Monocytic Ehrlichiosis

The rickettsial disease canine monocytic ehrlichiosis is caused by *Ehrlichia canis*, whose vector tick is *Rhipicephalus sanguineus*, the brown dog tick.

Although diagnosed primarily in the southeastern and southwestern United States, the disease first gained attention as a devastating disease of military working dogs in Vietnam. After infection, *E. canis* causes acute, subclinical, and chronic disease phases. The acute stage lasts between 2 and 4 weeks, during which time the organism multiplies within circulating mononuclear cells and cells of the spleen and liver. Infected mononuclear cells are transported to other organs such as lungs, kidneys, and meninges. A resulting vasculitis and subendothelial tissue infection develops. The subclinical phase appears 6 to 9 weeks after infection. Dogs may not show clinical signs during this period before progressing to the chronic phase. During the chronic phase, bone marrow is suppressed, resulting in thrombocytopenia, nonregenerative anemia, and pancytopenia. Some dogs with chronic disease will experience development of glomerulonephritis.

Diagnosis is by indirect immunofluorescent antibody technique, ELISA testing, or Western blot analysis. Finding morula within monocytes cytologically can also be diagnostic. Tetracycline or doxycycline is the treatment of choice, and the prognosis is generally good.

CLINICAL SIGNS

Acute Phase

- Lymphadenopathy
- Anemia
- Depression
- Anorexia
- Fever
- Weight loss
- Ocular and nasal discharge
- Dyspnea
- Edema (extremities and scrotum)

Subclinical Phase

- Few clinical signs
- CNS symptoms

Chronic Phase

- Severe weight loss
- Debilitation
- Anterior uveitis
- Retinal hemorrhage
- CNS signs

- Secondary bacterial infections
- Bleeding tendencies

DIAGNOSIS

- Positive indirect immunofluorescent antibody test, ELISA test (IDEXX), PCR
- CBC:
  - Pancytopenia (25% of patients)
  - Nonregenerative anemia
  - Thrombocytopenia
- Serum chemistry: hyperglobulinemia

TREATMENT

- Tetracycline: three times a day for 14 days
- Doxycycline: every 14 days
- Supportive care will be required for some animals:
  - Intravenous fluid therapy
  - Blood transfusions
  - Anabolic steroids
- For recurrent infections, tetracycline daily for long term

⬤ TECH ALERT

Infection with *E. canis* produces no long-term immunity. Antibodies to *E. canis* have been found in humans with monocytic ehrlichiosis. Take care when handling ticks or serum or tissue from infected dogs.

Canine Granulocytic Ehrlichiosis

Two forms of canine granulocytic ehrlichiosis (GE) exist: (1) canine GE caused by *Ehrlichia ewingii* and (2) canine GE caused by *Ehrlichia equi*. Dogs infected by *E. ewingii* present with acute polyarthritis and inflammatory joint disease. This syndrome is linked to the tick *Amblyomma americanum* as its vector, and it is not seasonal. Dogs infected with *E. equi* present with nonspecific signs of severe lethargy and anorexia. This disease is seasonal and corresponds to the peak feeding season of the vector *Ixodes dammini*, the deer tick.

CLINICAL SIGNS

Ehrlichia Ewingii

- Sudden onset of fever
- Lethargy
- Anorexia
- Lameness
- Muscular stiffness

Ehrlichia Equi

- Acute onset of fever
- Severe, often debilitating lethargy
- Anorexia

DIAGNOSIS

E. Ewingii

- CBC:
  - Mild, nonregenerative anemia
  - Thrombocytopenia
  - Monocytosis
  - Eosinophilia
  - Morulae in neutrophils (1%–9%)
- Serum chemistries: increased ALT
- Positive *E. canis* test

E. Equi

- CBC:
  - Thrombocytopenia
  - Lymphopenia
- Serum chemistries:
  - Increased ALP (100%)
  - Increased amylase (50%)
  - Hypoalbuminemia
- Urine: proteinuria
- Positive *E. canis* test

TREATMENT

- Tetracycline: three times a day every 14 days
- Doxycycline: every 12 hours for 7 to 10 days
- Supportive care, if required

INFORMATION FOR CLIENTS

- Ticks present a disease threat for pets and humans.
- The prognosis for these syndromes is good.
- Clinical signs should improve within 48 hours from the start of treatment.
- Check pets frequently for ticks, and remove the ticks when found.
- Avoid tick-infested areas. Do not expose yourself to the blood from the tick.

Lyme Disease (Borreliosis)

Lyme borreliosis is a complex, multiorgan disorder caused by the spirochete *Borrelia burgdorferi*. The spirochete is passed to the host animal or human through the bite of a tick in the genus *Ixodes*. Ticks must remain attached to the host for a minimum of 48 hours for infection to occur. Although the disease is worldwide in distribution, it is endemic in most of the northeastern states, with approximately 90% of all cases occurring in New York, New Jersey, Connecticut, and Pennsylvania.

Symptoms include dermatologic, arthritic, cardiac, and neurologic abnormalities. Some animals may experience development of a severe nephritis (possibly in Labrador Retrievers). Signs may appear months after the tick bite and may be vague and nonspecific, making diagnosis difficult. Animals that spend time outdoors in tick-infested areas are at greatest risk for infection.

Diagnosis is based on clinical signs and a positive ELISA or antibody titer. (It may be difficult to evaluate titers when dogs have been vaccinated.) Investigation of the molecular structure of the *Borrelia* organism has shown that a region of the amino acid sequence, labeled the IR6 region, is common in human and canine infections with *B. burgdorferi*. Serology tests looking for the region named C6 are available and specific for Lyme disease in the dog. These newer tests will distinguish vaccinated from infected animals. Doxycycline is the drug of choice for the treatment of borreliosis. Antibiotic therapy may *not* eliminate the organism from the infected animal, and some animals may be permanently infected, which leads to chronic cases with flare-ups.

CLINICAL SIGNS

- Fever
- Anorexia
- Lethargy
- Lymphadenopathy
- Episodic lameness
- Presence or absence of myocardial abnormalities
- Rash around the tick bite
- Nephritis (especially in Labrador Retrievers)

DIAGNOSIS

- No specific hematologic or biochemical changes have been noted except where specific organ systems are involved.
- Synovial fluid: suppurative polyarthritis (increased numbers of nucleated cells)

- Antibody titers greater than 64 may indicate infection
- Positive ELISA test: SNAP 3Dx or 4Dx anti C-6 antibody test (IDEXX)

TREATMENT

- Doxycycline: PO every 24 hours for 21 to 28 days
- Antiinflammatory drugs for pain:
  - Aspirin: PO every 8 hours
  - Prednisolone: daily

PREVENTION

- Vaccination of seronegative dogs is recommended in endemic areas (LymeVax, Ft. Dodge, IA); vaccination of seropositive dogs or dogs not in endemic areas is not recommended
- Tick control

⬤ TECH ALERT

No antibiotic is 100% effective in eliminating the organism.

INFORMATION FOR CLIENTS

- Animal infection should alert owners to the possibility of human infection from ticks in the environment.
- Infected animals may have relapses of symptoms even after treatment.
- Vaccination of dogs already exposed to *B. burgdorferi* is ineffective.
- Avoid exposure to environments where high concentrations of ticks might be found.
- Use a tick collar or other means of tick repellent for animals traveling to infested areas.

REVIEW QUESTIONS

1. Which of the following is a correct statement?
   a. Feline infectious peritonitis (FIP) virus and feline coronavirus are difficult to differentiate with current testing.
   b. A limited number of cats will have antibodies against feline coronavirus.
   c. The majority of cats with FIP will have the effusive, or "wet," form.
   d. An effective FIP vaccine is available.

2. The feline immunodeficiency virus (FIV) virus is primarily spread between cats via _____
   a. Fecal contamination
   b. Fomite contamination
   c. Fighting and bite wounds
   d. Flea transmission
3. Feline Leukemia Virus (FeLV) is stable in the environment, lasting up to 6 weeks.
   a. True
   b. False
4. Which of the following animals is the definitive host for *T. gondii*?
   a. Raccoon
   b. Opossum
   c. Cat
   d. Deer tick
5. Canine parvovirus (CPV) is resistant and may remain viable in the environment for up to _____.
   a. 6 weeks
   b. 1 year
   c. 3 weeks
   d. Several years
6. Patients with parvovirus and white blood cell counts less than 2000 usually have a _____ prognosis.
   a. Good
   b. Poor
   c. Excellent
   d. Fair
7. Which of the following antibiotics should be avoided in young animals?
   a. Ampicillin
   b. Enrofloxacin (Baytril)
   c. Gentamicin
   d. Amoxicillin and clavulanate (Clavamox)
8. *E. canis* infections can be diagnosed by finding the organisms in the _____.
   a. Red blood cells
   b. White blood cells
   c. Feces
   d. Serum
9. To transmit *B. burgdorferi*, how long must a tick remain attached to the host?
   a. Longer than 48 hours
   b. No longer than 12 hours
   c. Longer than 3 days
   d. No longer than 1 hour

10. Which of the following might not be a sign of rabies in an animal?
    a. Vomiting
    b. Difficulty swallowing
    c. Changes in voice
    d. Ataxia
    e. Hyperreactivity
11. Primarily in what season is idiopathic vestibular disease seen?
    a. Winter
    b. Fall
    c. Summer
12. Rigid hypertonicity of the front legs and hypotonicity of the rear limbs is known as:
    a. Necrotizing neurologic syndrome
    b. Marphan syndrome
    c. Schiff-Sherrington syndrome
13. Myelinated nerve fibers carry impulses _____ compared with unmyelinated fibers.
    a. Faster
    b. Slower
14. Kittens should be at least _____ of age before testing for FIV.
    a. 12 months
    b. 4 months
    c. 2 months
    d. 6 months
15. This is the most commonly seen form of FIP.
    a. Wet
    b. Dry
16. Why do you think Lyme disease vaccine is not included in the core canine vaccines?
17. Current thinking is that once infected with FeLV a cat may remain infected with the virus.
    a. True
    b. False
18. What advice would you give owners concerning a young cat with a positive FeLV test?

Answers found on page 552.

Diseases of the Reproductive System

Agalactia: absence of milk secretion

Anasarca: extreme generalized edema of the skin

Androgen: any substance that promotes masculinization

Cryptorchid: an animal with one or more retained testicles

Endometritis: Inflammation of the endometrial tissue of the uterus

Galactostasis: presence of excessive amounts of breast milk leading to inflammatory response

Gynecomastia: enlargement of breast tissue in males

Hyperplasia: increase in the number of cells

Myelosuppression: suppression of the bone marrow

Ovarohysterectomy: surgical removal of the ovaries and uterus (spay)

Pedunculated: elongated stalk of tissue

OUTLINE

Diseases of the Female Reproductive System
  Vaginitis
  Pseudopregnancy
  Eclampsia
  Pyometra
  Pregnancy Disorders
  Dystocia
  Inappropriate Maternal Behavior
  Lactation Disorders
Diseases of the Male Reproductive System
  Prostatic Disease
  Benign Prostatic Hyperplasia

Prostatitis
Prostatic Abscessation
Prostatic Neoplasia
Priapism and Paraphemosis
Neoplasia of the Genital System and Mammary Glands
  Testicular Tumors
  Penile, Preputial, Scrotal Tumors
  Tumors of the Female Genital Tract
  Mammary Gland Tumors

LEARNING OBJECTIVES

When you have completed this chapter, you will be able to:

1. Explain to clients the health reasons for ovariohysterectomy or castration of their pets.
2. Recognize the problem areas in the reproductive system of the male and female and relate them to the clinical symptoms.
3. Advise clients on pregnancy-related problems.

The female reproductive system consists of two ovaries and the female duct system, including the oviducts, uterus, cervix, vagina, and vulva (Fig. 10-1). The primary functions of this system are to provide eggs for fertilization and to protect the developing embryo during pregnancy. All of these structures are composed of tissue that is sensitive to hormones produced by the female.

Hormones such as estrogen and progesterone act on the reproductive system to prepare it for pregnancy and to maintain pregnancy. When the response to these hormones is abnormal, disease can result. Although not technically a part of the female reproductive system, the mammary glands are also reactive to hormonal abnormalities, and diseases involving them are frequently seen in small-animal practice.

The male reproductive system consists of two testicles and the male duct system, including the urethra, prostate gland, and penis (Fig. 10-2). Other structures often involved in disease processes are the scrotum and the prepuce. The main hormonal influence in the male reproductive system is testosterone, although abnormal estrogen levels can also affect the male reproductive system.

Diseases that involve the reproductive system are frequently seen in veterinary practice. These include vaginal disorders, uterine disorders, pregnancy disorders, lactation disorders, disease of the prostate, and neoplasia of the genital system and mammary glands.

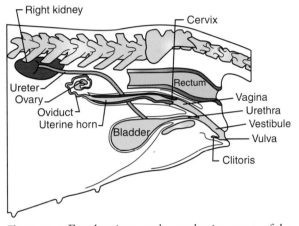

Figure 10-1 Female urinary and reproductive organs of the bitch (lateral view). (From Colville T, Bassert JM: *Clinical anatomy and physiology for veterinary technicians*, St. Louis, MO, 2008, Mosby, by permission.)

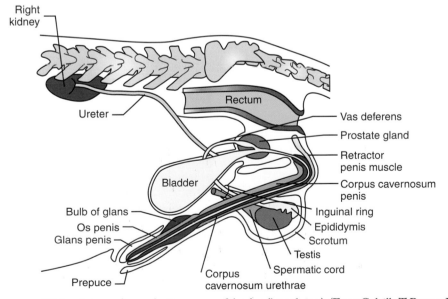

Figure 10-2 Male urinary and reproductive organs of the dog (lateral view). (From Colville T, Bassert JM: *Clinical anatomy and physiology for veterinary technicians*, St. Louis, MO, 2008, Mosby, by permission.)

Diseases of the Female Reproductive System

Vaginitis

Vaginitis is a fairly common occurrence in prepuberal bitches. The most common sign of juvenile (puppy) vaginitis is vulvar discharge. This condition responds well to systemic antibiotic therapy and usually resolves after the first estrous cycle. Adult vaginitis can be the result of a variety of factors. Anatomic abnormalities, bacterial infection, traumatic injuries, or chemical irritation may all result in vaginal inflammation. Viral vaginitis also occurs in conjunction with canine herpesvirus infections.

Pseudopregnancy

Pseudopregnancy is an exaggeration of the normal hormonal changes that occur during the estrous cycle in the nonpregnant bitch. Clinical signs can be related to decreasing levels of progesterone and increasing levels of prolactin. Dogs undergoing pseudopregnancy may exhibit weight gain, mammary gland enlargement, lactation, and a mucoid vaginal discharge. These dogs may carry around stuffed toys and demonstrate increased mothering behavior.

Signs of the pseudopregnancy usually develop 6 to 12 weeks after estrus and may last 1 to 3 weeks. Signs are usually self-limiting. Therapy, when necessary, is usually aimed at decreasing milk production. Therapeutic methods including mild water restriction, diuretics, and preventing oral stimulation by the bitch can be used. Ovariohysterectomy is the only permanent cure for those dogs that exhibit this problem.

> ### ◉ TECH ALERT
>
> Avoid the use of phenothiazine tranquilizers in these animals because they may increase prolactin secretion.

Eclampsia

Eclampsia is a problem seen in heavily lactating females. The disease is commonly seen within 2 to 3 weeks after whelping. Heavy lactation demands on the mother often accompanied by a diet deficient in calcium may result in hypocalcemia. Clinical signs include nervousness, salivation, stiff gait, ataxia and seizures. Treatment must be initiated soon after the first signs of problems occur. Slow intravenous (IV) administration of 10% or 20% calcium gluconate should result in remission of clinical signs. It is important to monitor the heart rate via a stethoscope or an electrocardiogram (ECG) while administering the IV calcium solution. If bradycardia or arrhythmias occur, the infusion should be stopped. Oral calcium supplements may be started after clinical signs regress while serum calcium levels are monitored to assure they remain normal throughout lactation. This problem tends to recur with subsequent pregnancies, so it may not be a good idea to use affected dogs for breeding. In some cases, eclampsia may be avoided with good prenatal nutrition and calcium supplementation.

Pyometra

Pyometra is also frequently seen in small-animal medicine. Increasing levels of progesterone after ovulation result in hyperplasia and hypertrophy of the endometrial glands of the uterus. Inappropriate response results in cystic endometrial hyperplasia with accumulation of fluid within the uterine lumen (Fig. 10-3). Progesterone also produces a decrease in myometrial contractions and predisposes the uterus to secondary bacterial infection (pyometra). The most common microorganism isolated in pyometra is *Escherichia coli*, although *Staphylococcus* spp., *Streptococcus*

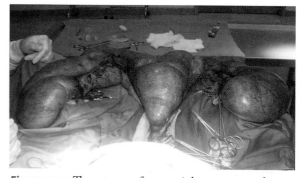

Figure 10-3 The uterus, after ovariohysterectomy, from a 3-year-old mongrel bitch with a closed cervix pyometra. Medroxyprogesterone acetate was administered for 2 consecutive years before the pyometra diagnosis. (From Ettinger SJ, Feldman EC: *Textbook of veterinary internal medicine*, ed 7, St. Louis, MO, 2010, Saunders.)

spp., *Klebsiella*, *Pasteurella*, *Proteus*, and *Moraxella* have also been implicated.

The development of pyometra appears to be the final stage of a continuum beginning with endometrial hyperplasia and progressing through cystic endometrial hyperplasia and endometritis. Animals presented for treatment tend to be middle-aged or older, within 60 days of their last estrous cycle.

CLINICAL SIGNS

- Vulvar discharge
- Abdominal enlargement
- Vomiting
- Lethargy
- Polyuria or polydipsia
- Dehydration
- Azotemia

DIAGNOSIS

- Radiology indicates an enlarged uterus (must rule out pregnancy).
- Ultrasound examination can distinguish between fluid and pregnancy.
- Complete blood cell count (CBC) shows leukocytosis, neutrophilia with a left shift, and dehydration. A nonregenerative anemia may be seen.
- Serum chemistry may show the following:
  - Increased alkaline phosphatase levels
  - Increased serum protein level
  - Increased blood urea nitrogen
- Vaginal cytology shows degenerative neutrophils, endometrial cells, and bacteria.
- Culture and sensitivity should be performed if medical treatment is to be attempted or if the animal is systemically ill.

TREATMENT

- Ovariohysterectomy is the preferred treatment for pyometra.
- Dehydration and azotemia must be corrected before surgery.
- If the animal is used for breeding, owners may elect medical treatment:
  - Prostaglandin $F_2\alpha$ (Lutylase): 0.1 to 0.25 mg/kg subcutaneously (SQ) one to two times daily for 3 to 5 days or until the uterus is empty. Side effects seen with prostaglandin infection

usually resolve within 60 minutes of injection (e.g., sweating, panting, salivation, vomiting or defecation, urination).
- Systemic broad-spectrum antibiotics should be given until culture results come back from the laboratory.

INFORMATION FOR CLIENTS

- Ovariohysterectomy (spaying) of the female prevents this disease.
- Early and aggressive treatment is important.
- The treatment of choice for pyometra is ovariohysterectomy (even in older dogs and cats).
- Approximately 26% to 40% of bitches have a recurrence of pyometra within 1 year of medical treatment.
- Medical treatment is more successful when the cervix is open and draining.
- In bitches with pyometra, 5% to 8% mortality rate is associated with ovariohysterectomy.

Pregnancy Disorders

Disorders of pregnancy include fetal death and abortion or reabsorption, dystocia, inappropriate maternal behavior, mastitis, and puerperal tetany. Although other problems are associated with pregnancy and parturition, these are the most commonly seen problems in small-animal medicine. The normal gestation period for dogs and cats is between 62 and 65 days. Fetuses may be palpated about 25 to 36 days after breeding in dogs, and 21 to 28 days in cats. Fetal skeletal mineralization can be detected radiographically at 45 days of gestation. Ultrasonography provides information on the status of the fetuses after about 20 days. It is difficult to determine the number of fetuses, especially in large litters.

Fetal deaths early in gestation result in reabsorption with no expulsion of uterine contents. Owners may report that the animal has "failed to conceive" after what they consider a successful breeding. Organisms such as *Brucella canis*, canine herpesvirus, feline infectious peritonitis, feline leukemia virus (FeLV) and panleukopenia may produce fetal death or abortion.

Dystocia can be defined as difficulty in delivery of fetuses through the birth canal. The causes of dystocia are divided into fetal factors, maternal factors, and combinations of both. Fetal factors include large fetuses (large puppy or kitten, fetal anasarca, or hydrocephalus) and abnormal positioning (transverse presentation). Breech presentation is *not* an abnormality in the bitch or in the queen. Maternal factors include a narrowed birth canal (developmental or trauma related) and uterine inertia (lack of coordinated contractions or exhaustion of the uterine musculature from prolonged contractions).

Dystocia

CLINICAL SIGNS

- A bitch or queen has been in labor longer than 4 hours without producing a fetus.
- A green vaginal discharge develops during parturition.
- More than 1 hour has elapsed between births.

DIAGNOSIS

- Physical examination with digital palpation of vagina
- Radiography to evaluate fetal position, size, and number
- Ultrasonography to evaluate fetal viability and distress

TREATMENT

- Manual manipulation: a fetus lodged in the vaginal canal can be manually dislodged through careful manipulation.
- Oxytocin 1.1 to 2.2 international units per kilogram (IU/kg) can be used to correct secondary inertia.
- If medical treatment fails to correct the situation, a cesarean section is recommended.

INFORMATION FOR CLIENTS

- Owners should prepare a whelping box for the animal, and make sure the animal is comfortable sleeping in that box before whelping.
- Nutrition of the pregnant animal is important, with increased demands being placed on the mother as the litter develops.
- During the birthing process, owners should be advised to closely supervise the animal but not

hover around, creating stress for the mother. Children and other pets should be kept out of the area.
- If labor and delivery are not progressing steadily, veterinary help should be obtained.
- Owners can predict parturition by monitoring the rectal temperature of the animal. Rectal temperature usually declines below 100°F 24 hours before the beginning of labor.
- After a cesarean section, owners may have to support the neonates until the mother is fully recovered.
- Ovariohysterectomy can be performed at the same time as the cesarean section in animals not used for breeding.

Inappropriate Maternal Behavior

Appropriate maternal behavior is important to the survival and development of neonates. Nursing, retrieving, grooming, and protecting are all considered normal behavior. The dam should demonstrate caution when moving about the whelping box; she should lie quietly while the neonates nurse. Because puppies and kittens do not have the ability to thermoregulate their body temperature during the first few weeks of life, the mother is responsible for keeping them warm. Grooming is important to stimulate cardiovascular and respiratory function, to stimulate elimination, and to remove waste material from the coat. Some dams, however, display increased protective behavior or fear-induced behaviors. Some cannibalize their litters. When these inappropriate behaviors occur, it is the responsibility of the owner to intervene and protect the health and well-being of the neonates.

CLINICAL SIGNS

- The mother is restless (will not stay in the box with the puppies or kittens).
- Neonates are constantly crying.
- The mother is actively attacking and killing her young. Owners may not directly see such acts; however, the number of neonates will be seen to decrease.

DIAGNOSIS

- Observation of mother

TREATMENT

- Tranquilization of the mother:
  - Acepromazine: low doses orally (PO) or SQ to calm the mother
  - Diazepam: PO for dogs and cats to calm them

INFORMATION FOR CLIENTS

- Do not use affected bitches for breeding.
- Do not leave puppies or kittens unattended with an affected bitch.

Lactation Disorders

The mammary gland achieves its maximum growth and development during pregnancy. The decline in progesterone levels before parturition results in the synthesis of enzymes that permit lactogenesis. Oxytocin released in response to suckling increases milk letdown within the gland. *Agalactia*, lack of milk production, can result from stress, malnutrition, premature parturition, or infection.

Galactostasis, or milk stasis, may result in painful engorgement of the mammary glands, and *mastitis*, a septic inflammation of the mammary gland, occurs in pets. Mastitis is probably seen more commonly in the bitch and the queen compared with the other two problems. Mastitis may be acute or chronic, and it may involve one or more of the mammary glands.

CLINICAL SIGNS

- Mammary discomfort
- Discolored milk
- Fever
- Reluctance to allow nursing
- Abscessed glands

TREATMENT

- Prescribe broad-spectrum systemic antibiotic:
  - Cephalexin: PO every 8 hours
  - Amoxicillin and clavulanate (Clavamox): PO every 8 to 12 hours
- Administer warm compresses; then milk the affected glands.
- Protect the affected gland(s) from trauma.

INFORMATION FOR CLIENTS

- Mastitis may recur in subsequent lactations.

- Prophylactic use of antibiotics is not advocated.
- Puppies and kittens should not be allowed to nurse from affected glands but can continue to use the noninfected teats.

Male Reproductive Disease

Prostatic Diseases

Although both dogs and cats have prostate glands, prostatic disease is much more common in dogs. The canine prostate gland is the only accessory sex gland in the dog. The gland is located just caudal to the bladder, encircling the proximal urethra at the neck of the bladder. The size and position of the gland changes with the age of the dog so that the gland is mostly abdominal in the animal that is older than 5 years. The purpose of the prostate gland is to produce fluid as a transport and support medium for sperm during ejaculation.

The prostate increases in size and weight as the dog matures. Dogs castrated before maturity have normal prostatic growth totally inhibited. When adult dogs are castrated, the prostate undergoes involution.

Clinical diseases associated with the prostate include benign hyperplasia, cysts, prostatitis, abscessation, and neoplasia. Clinical signs of prostatic disease are similar regardless of the cause. Accurate diagnosis depends on thorough physical examination, laboratory evaluation, and biopsy.

Benign Prostatic Hyperplasia

Benign prostatic hyperplasia is an aging change that occurs in dogs as early as 2.5 years of age. The condition is associated with an altered androgen–estrogen ratio and requires the presence of the testes. Although the size increases with hyperplasia, secretory function decreases. Blood supply to the gland increases, and the gland tends to bleed easily. Most dogs exhibit no clinical signs.

CLINICAL SIGNS

- May be asymptomatic
- Tenesmus
- Prostate palpates symmetrically (enlarged and nonpainful)

DIAGNOSIS

- A physical examination is recommended.
- Biopsy provides the only accurate diagnosis.

TREATMENT

- Castration results in a 70% decrease in size of the gland within 7 to 14 days
- Low-dose estrogen therapy: diethylstilbestrol 0.2 to 1 mg/day for 5 days; potential side effects must be considered when selecting estrogen therapy (bone marrow suppression)
- Flutamide (not approved for veterinary use and is expensive)
- Megestrol acetate: daily for 4 weeks (*not* approved for use in male dogs)

INFORMATION FOR CLIENTS

- Early castration prevents benign prostatic hyperplasia.
- Castration, even in the older animal, alleviates this condition.
- Drug therapy results in temporary improvement, but the condition will recur when drug therapy is discontinued.

Prostatitis

The prostate gland is predisposed to bacterial infection through the urinary system as well as direct infection of the gland itself (Fig. 10-4). *E. coli* is the most frequently isolated bacterial organism involved in canine prostatitis. Other gram-negative microorganisms such as *Proteus*, *Klebsiella*, *Pseudomonas*, *Streptococcus*, *Staphylococcus*, and *B. canis*, have also been found to cause this disease. Bacterial prostatitis may be acute or chronic, and it affects sexually mature male dogs.

CLINICAL SIGNS

Acute Prostatitis

- Anorexia
- Fever
- Lethargy
- Stiff gait in the rear limbs
- Caudal abdominal pain

Chronic Prostatitis

- May be asymptomatic
- History of chronic, periodic urinary tract infections

DIAGNOSIS

- Urinalysis: urine shows blood, increased white blood cell (WBC) count, and the presence of bacteria
- Physical examination
- Urine culture

TREATMENT

- Antibiotic therapy should be instituted for 28 days (acute form). (For the chronic form, use same antibiotic therapy regimen for at least 6 weeks.) The choice of antibiotic should be based on culture and sensitivity results and may be started IV if the animal is in serious condition:
  - Enrofloxacin: every 12 hours
  - Trimethoprim/sulfonamide: q12 hours
  - Erythromycin: every 8 hours
  - Chloramphenicol: every 8 hours
  - Ciprofloxacin: every 12 hours
- Castration may be beneficial.
- Prostatectomy, a difficult surgery with serious postsurgical side effects, may be considered.

INFORMATION FOR CLIENTS

- Long-term antibiotic therapy is essential to control prostatitis.

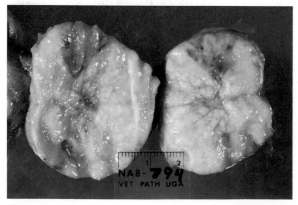

Figure 10-4 Purulent prostatitis in the dog. (From Greene C: *Infectious diseases of the dog and cat*, ed 3, St. Louis, MO, 2006, Elsevier.)

- Prolonged use of antibiotics requires monitoring with prostatic fluid cultures and examinations to ensure that toxic side effects do not develop.
- Castration may be beneficial.

Prostatic Abscessation

Prostatic abscessation is a serious form of bacterial prostatitis in which pockets of purulent exudate develop within the gland. The disease may present with systemic signs.

CLINICAL SIGNS

- Tenesmus
- Urethral discharge
- Lethargy
- Pain
- Vomiting
- Hematuria
- Fever
- Depression

DIAGNOSIS

- History and physical examination
- CBC and serum chemistries
- Leukocytosis or normal WBC count
- Liver enzymes may be elevated
- Hypoglycemia
- Hypokalemia
- Prostatic aspiration—hemorrhagic, purulent, septic

TREATMENT

- Surgical drainage is the treatment of choice
- Castration
- Antibiotic therapy
- Intravenous fluid therapy (in cases of sepsis or peritonitis)

INFORMATION FOR CLIENTS

- Prostatic abscessation care is expensive, and the disease is difficult to treat.
- Survival rate is approximately 50% after 1 year.

Prostatic Neoplasia

Prostatic neoplasia is uncommon in dogs but has been seen in cats. It can develop in both intact and neutered males. All neoplasms that affect the prostate are malignant. Clinical signs are similar to other prostatic diseases. Treatment is unrewarding, and a cure is unlikely.

Priapism and Paraphimosis

Priapism is occassionally seen in dogs. It is usually a problem for the owner, who is embarrassed by the inappropriate erection, but it can also be painful to the dog. Excessive parasympathetic stimulation or possible impairment of venous drainage from the penis may result in priapism. A delay in treatment may result in necrosis of the penis, requiring amputation of the penis.

Paraphimosis is the inability of the dog to retract the penis into the preputial sheath. Causes include self-mutilation, constriction by a hair ring, fracture of the os penis, strangulation with a rubber band or string, and trauma. Drying of the tissue, necrosis, and tissue contamination occur the longer the penis remains extruded. Treatment of acute cases involves sedation, removal of any causative agents, immersing the tissue into a cold hypertonic glucose solution to reduce swelling, and gentle cleaning of the penile tissue. Replacement of the penis within the scrotum is followed by placement of a purse-string suture. Chronic cases or those not responding to treatment will require surgery.

Neoplasia of the Genital System and Mammary Glands

Tumors of the male genital tract include those of the testicles, prostate, penis, prepuce, and scrotum.

Testicular Tumors

Approximately 5% to 15% of all tumors seen in male dogs are testicular tumors. Cryptorchid dogs and those with inguinal hernias are at greatest risk for testicular tumors; tumor development is twice as common in testicles retained in the inguinal canal as those within the abdomen. These tumors are usually seen in older, intact male dogs (9–12 years of age). Testicular tumors are uncommon in cats.

CLINICAL SIGNS

- Older, intact male dogs (9–12 years of age) are predisposed to this condition.
- Nonpainful testicular enlargement may be seen.
- Feminization (bilateral nonpruritic alopecia, hyperpigmentation in the inguinal region, gynecomastia,

nonregenerative anemia, and thrombocytopenia) occurs in approximately 25% to 50% of dogs with Sertoli cell tumors.
- Enlarged lymph nodes may be seen in some animals (10%–20%).

DIAGNOSIS
- Clinical signs

TREATMENT
- Castration is the treatment of choice for testicular tumors.
- If adjunct treatment is required, chemotherapy and radiation therapy may be used.
- Whole blood transfusion should be performed if the animal is myelosuppressed.

INFORMATION FOR CLIENTS
- Castration of male dogs at an early age prevents this disease.
- Dogs with myelosuppression from excess estrogen levels may need whole blood transfusion.

Penile, Preputial, and Scrotal Tumors

Penile tumors are rare in cats and dogs. The most commonly seen neoplasia involving the penis and the prepuce is the transmissible venereal tumor (TVT). This tumor occurs only in dogs. It is most commonly seen in temperate climates and in areas that have large free-roaming dog populations. It is spread during sexual contact and can be transmitted through licking and sniffing.

CLINICAL SIGNS
- Penile, preputial, and scrotal tumors are found on sexually intact male dogs.
- Cauliflower-like masses appear at the base of the penis or on the lining of the prepuce; they are seen on the vulva in the female (tumors are friable and bleed easily).
- Lesions may also be seen on the face and the rectum.

DIAGNOSIS
- Cytology: Imprint smears show large, round-to-oval cells with abundant pale cytoplasm containing many vacuoles; the nuclei contain frequent mitotic figures and visible nucleoli.

TREATMENT
- TVTs are immunogenic and may spontaneously regress with adequate tumor stimulation.
- Chemotherapy: Vincristine therapy (IV once a week) cures more than 90% of cases. Treatment should continue for 2 weeks after resolution of the tumor (generally four to six treatments).
- Surgical removal of small, localized lesions is recommended.

Tumors of the Female Genital Tract

Tumors of the female genital tract include ovarian tumors, uterine and cervical tumors, vaginal and vulval neoplasia, and tumors of the mammary glands. Tumors of the ovaries and uterus are uncommon in both dogs and cats. Surgical removal of these tumors is the treatment of choice. Vaginal and vulvar tumors are the most common tumors of the female genital tract in dogs. They are uncommon in cats.

CLINICAL SIGNS
- A pedunculated mass protruding from the vulva may be seen.
- Perineal swelling, vaginal discharge, dysuria, or constipation may be seen.

DIAGNOSIS
- Clinical signs

TREATMENT
- Surgical removal with ovariohysterectomy prevents recurrence.

INFORMATION FOR CLIENTS
- Most of these tumors are benign.
- The prognosis is good for this tumor.

Mammary Gland Tumors

Tumors of the mammary gland are the most common tumor of female dogs, representing approximately 50% of all tumors of female dogs. They are the third most common tumors of female cats. These are usually tumors of older animals. The tumors are hormone dependent in dogs but less so in cats. The risk for mammary tumor is 0.5% for bitches spayed before their first estrus, 8% for those spayed after one estrous cycle, and 26% for bitches spayed after two or more cycles. The risk in cats is similar for spayed and non-spayed female cats.

Approximately 50% of canine mammary tumors are benign. In cats, only 10% to 20% are benign. Tumors may be singular or multiple, occurring in any of the glands.

Malignant and benign tumors may occur simultaneously. Both tumor types may occur as firm, well-demarcated lesions, so it is impossible to distinguish malignant lesions from benign lesions on the basis of appearance. Rapid growth, local tissue invasion, and ulceration are usually hallmarks of malignant tumors. In dogs and cats, tumor size is probably the best prognostic indicator, whereas factors such as age of the patient, tumor numbers, and tumor location have less prognostic value.

CLINICAL SIGNS

- A firm nodule is palpable in the mammary chain or gland.
- Surrounding tissue may be involved; lymph nodes in the region may be enlarged.

DIAGNOSIS

- Physical examination
- CBC, serum chemistries, and thoracic radiographs, which should be evaluated before surgery

TREATMENT

- Any accepted method of surgical removal may be used. The surgeon should choose the simplest procedure that removes the entire tumor.
- Chemotherapy may have minimal antitumor activity in both dogs and cats
- Adjunct chemotherapy may be used together with surgery. Doxorubicin or dactinomycin may be used in dogs; doxorubicin and cyclophosphamide may be used in cats (doxorubicin 30 mg/m^2 IV every 21 days; dactinomycin 0.7 mg/m^2 every 21 days; cyclophosphamide 100 mg/m^2 PO once daily on days 3, 4, 5, 6 after doxorubicin).

INFORMATION FOR CLIENTS

- Veterinarians cannot distinguish benign tumors from malignant ones without biopsies. Surgical removal is advised for all mammary tumors, followed by histology.

- In cats with tumors smaller than 2 cm, survival times of up to 3 years have been reported; larger masses usually result in shorter survival times.
- About 80% to 90% of all feline mammary tumors are malignant, whereas only 50% of canine tumors are malignant.
- In animals, chemotherapy is not curative for this type of tumor.
- Although ovariohysterectomy has not been proved to increase survival, it is recommended because 50% to 60% of canine mammary tumors have estrogen receptors on their cells that may increase the recurrence of tumors.

REVIEW QUESTIONS

1. It is often difficult to determine by visual inspection whether a mammary gland tumor is malignant.
   a. True
   b. False
2. Feline mammary gland tumors have a lower incidence of malignancy compared with those in dogs.
   a. True
   b. False
3. What is the treatment of choice for male dogs with prostatic hypertrophy?
   a. High-dose estrogen therapy
   b. Castration
   c. Antibiotic therapy
   d. Prostatic drainage
4. The normal gestation period for dogs and cats is between _____.
   a. 62 and 65 days
   b. 35 and 40 days
   c. 12 and 14 weeks
   d. 6 and 7 weeks
5. Older bitches with pyometra often present for symptoms similar to those seen in kidney failure.
   a. True
   b. False
6. A bitch or queen in active labor for longer than _____ hours without delivering a fetus should be examined.
   a. 8
   b. 2
   c. 6
   d. 4

7. The best way to prevent male reproductive system problems such as prostatic abscesses or testicular tumors is to _____.
   a. Remove the prostate
   b. Castrate the animal at an early age
   c. Prevent mating
   d. Use hormone therapy

8. Female dogs receiving an ovariohysterectomy before their first heat cycle will develop fewer mammary tumors later in life than those dogs that are spayed later in life.
   a. True
   b. False

9. Breech births are not uncommon in dogs and cats.
   a. True
   b. False

10. The choice of antibiotic for treatment of a prostatic abscess should be based on:
    a. Blood cultures
    b. Semen cultures
    c. Culture and sensitivity of prostatic fluid
    d. Urine culture and sensitivity

Answers found on page 552.

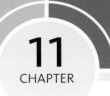

Diseases of the Respiratory System

Antibody: a Y-shaped protein produced by B-cells as part of the immune system

Antigen: a substance that evokes the production of antibodies

Antitussive: effective against coughs

Empyema: pus in the pleural space

Fistula: an abnormal connection or passageway between two epithelium-lined organs or vessels

Hemoptysis: coughing up blood or bloody sputum from the airways

Hyaline: substance with a glass-like appearance

Mesothelioma: cancer that develops from the mesothelial tissue layer

Mucopurulent: containing mucous and pus

Nasopharynx: airway passage in the back of the throat leading to the trachea

Olfactory: having to do with the sense of smell

Oropharynx: The area of the pharynx leading to the esophagus

Paroxysmal: a sudden attack or recurrence of a disease

Stertorous: heavy snoring or gasping sound

Thoracocentesis: surgical puncture of the chest wall

Thoracostomy: incision of the chest wall with maintenance of the opening for drainage.

When you have completed this chapter, you will be able to:
1. Review the anatomy of the respiratory system.
2. Recognize the difference between the upper and lower respiratory diseases.
3. Discuss with owners the prescribed medications and treatments commonly used for respiratory diseases in the small-animal clinic.
4. Recommend vaccination to owners as a way to prevent some of the viral and bacterial respiratory diseases.

All of the cells within an animal's body require oxygen for metabolism. When glucose is burned (in the cell) with oxygen, the by-products are energy, water, and carbon dioxide. Carbon dioxide, a waste product, must be eliminated from the body, whereas water and energy are used to maintain all of the life processes. The respiratory system transports oxygen to the bloodstream and removes carbon dioxide. Malfunction of this system affects all functions in the living animal.

We can arbitrarily divide the respiratory system into the *upper respiratory tract* (nasal cavity, sinuses, nasopharynx, and larynx; Fig. 11-1) and the *lower respiratory tract* (trachea, bronchi, lungs, and pleural cavity; Fig. 11-2).

Anatomy of the Respiratory Tract

The respiratory tract begins at the nostril, the passageway into the nose. The nose serves several purposes: 1) It warms air entering the respiratory system; (2) it moisturizes the entering air; 3) the hair and mucosa serve to protect the rest of the system from air-borne particulate matter such as pollen and dust; and 4) the mucosal surface of the nasal chonchae serve as home to the olfactory organs necessary for the sense of smell. A cartilage septum separates the left side from the right side. The nasal passage opens caudally into the naso-pharynx. This is the location of the epiglottis, the fleshy flap that covers the opening to the trachea known as the *glottis*. The vocal folds are

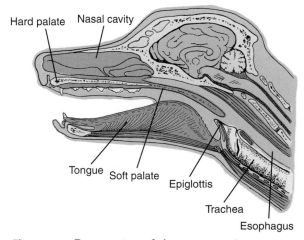

Figure 11-1 Cross-section of the upper respiratory tract of the dog. (From McBride DF: *Learning veterinary terminology*, ed 2, St. Louis, MO, 2002, Mosby, by permission.)

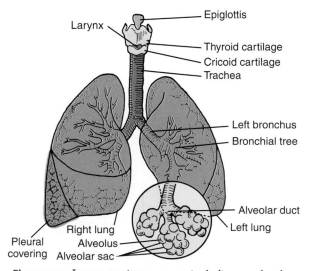

Figure 11-2 Lower respiratory tract, including an alveolus. (From McBride DF: *Learning veterinary terminology*, ed 2, St. Louis, MO, 2002, Mosby, by permission.)

located here as well. The trachea acts as the passageway through which air is moved from the outside of the animal to the inside of the lungs. In dogs and cats, the trachea is made up of incomplete hyaline cartilage rings separated by soft connective tissue. The ends of each hyaline ring are closed by a strap of muscle completing the circle.

The trachea bifurcates just before the heart into the left and right mainstem bronchi. The bronchi continue to split into smaller and smaller airways containing less and less cartilage. Finally, the bronchi end at the alveoli, the air sacs of the lung. It is here that gas exchange occurs. The alveolus is lined with a single cell layer of squamous epithelium with a basement membrane. It makes up half of the *respiratory membrane*. The capillary that serves that alveolus provides the next two layers of that membrane. In the alveolus oxygen diffuses across the respiratory membrane into the capillary whereas carbon dioxide diffuses in the opposite direction, from the blood to the alveolus. As the chest expands and contracts during *breathing*, air is drawn into the respiratory system and is pushed out into the surroundings.

Anything that alters the ability of the animal to move air into and out of the lungs or that interferes with gas diffusion at the alveolus, will have serious effects on all the organ systems of the body.

Vaccine Recommendations

It is no longer the belief that one vaccine protocol fits all cats or dogs. The current vaccine protocols promote vaccination based on environmental conditions in which the animal lives. Vaccine councils have made recommendations for "core vaccines" based on the possibility of infection. For example, most house cats that do not go outside have a low possibility of infection whereas outdoor cats would have a high possibility and would require additional vaccines. Box 11-1 lists the core vaccines for cats and dogs.

Diseases of the Upper Respiratory Tract

Diseases of the upper respiratory system include rhinitis, nasal tumors, epistaxis, sinusitis, tonsillitis, and laryngitis. Although upper airway disease is

---

BOX 11-1   Core Vaccines for Cats and Dogs

Vaccines included in the feline core vaccines are:
Feline viral rhinotracheitis *
Calicivirus *
Panleukopenia
Rabies *

For outdoor cats, feline leukemia, feline immunodeficiency virus, *Chlamydophila felis*, and *Bordetella* vaccines may be given. Vaccines not usually recommended for routine use in cats include vaccines for feline infectious peritonitis and *Giardia*.

Canine vaccine councils have recommended the following "core" vaccines for most house dogs:
Distemper *
Parvovirus
Adenovirus-2
Rabies *

Non–core vaccines for dogs that may be needed include:
Bordetella and parainfluenza *
Leptospirosis
Lyme disease
Rattlesnake toxoid

*These diseases have respiratory signs.

---

not nearly as common in dogs and cats as it is in humans, it is still seen clinically and causes concern in owners.

Rhinitis

CLINICAL SIGNS

- Serous, mucoid, or mucopurulent nasal discharge
- Sneezing, pawing at nose
- Coughing or gagging
- Encrustation on nares
- Rarely presents as single disease (usually appears as sequela to other respiratory infections)

DIAGNOSIS

- Clinical signs
- Culture and sensitivity results may show *Staphylococcus* strains

TREATMENT

- Clean the nares gently, and apply a soothing ointment.

- Administer systemic antibiotics if necessary.
- Administer vasoconstrictive drugs in combination with antihistamines to clear the nasal cavity.
  - Phenylephrine (Neo-Synephrine) drops: place drops in each nostril three to four times daily
  - Ephedrine: orally (PO) every 8 to 12 hours

Nasal Tumors

CLINICAL SIGNS

- Unilateral mucoid nasal discharge unresponsive to therapy
- Nasal hemorrhage
- Sneezing (uncommon)

DIAGNOSIS

- Radiographs to locate the mass, computed tomography (CT) and magnetic resonance imaging (MRI) can also be used
- Endoscopy
- Biopsy

TREATMENT

- Surgical removal (surgery is usually only palliative)
- Masses usually recur

Epistaxis

- Bleeding from the nose may be caused by systemic diseases and not primarily respiratory disease or may be caused by trauma, fungal infection, bacterial infection, or tumors.

CLINICAL SIGNS

- Bleeding from the nares (may be unilateral or bilateral)
- Usually associated with trauma, foreign objects, or tumors

DIAGNOSIS

- Fresh blood from the nasal cavity

TREATMENT

- Locate the exact site of bleeding in the nasal cavity
- Stop the bleeding:
  - Vasoconstrictive drugs instilled into the nasal cavity

- Apply pressure to the area if possible
- Vitamin K therapy (if coagulation is a problem)

Sinusitis

Sinusitis usually involves the frontal or maxillary sinus in dogs and manifests as a collection of pus in the area, resulting in swelling over the sinus. The most common cause of this problem in dogs is tooth root abscess.

CLINICAL SIGNS

- Swelling under the eye on the side of the bad tooth
- Unilateral nasal discharge

DIAGNOSIS

- Examination of the nasal and oral cavity
- Radiographs to determine resorption of bone
- Culture and sensitivity of all fistula tracts

TREATMENT

- Antibiotics (based on culture and sensitivity results)
- Removal of the infected tooth to promote drainage
- Flushing of fistula tracts with antiseptic solution

Tonsillitis

Tonsils are the "sentinels" of the respiratory tract, providing lymphoid protection to the lower respiratory system pathway. When invaded by infectious agents, the tonsils hypertrophy, resulting in difficulty swallowing and sore throats. Neoplasia involving the tonsils is fairly common in domestic animals.

CLINICAL SIGNS

- Anorexia
- Increased salivation
- Pain on opening the mouth

DIAGNOSIS

- Visual examination shows inflamed, swollen tonsils.
- Tonsils may be coated with mucus or pus or have abscesses on the surface.

TREATMENT

- Systemic antibiotics
- Soft or liquid diet

- Medication for pain relief: nonsteroidal antiinflammatory drugs (NSAIDS) PO (by mouth) every 8 to 12 hours (dogs); every other day (cats)
- Surgical removal in cases of chronic infection or neoplasia

Laryngitis

Although the most common cause of laryngitis is excessive barking, howling, or meowing, infection from high in the respiratory tract can spread to the larynx, causing the loss of voice.

CLINICAL SIGNS

- Loss of voice or alteration in quality of voice
- Cough
- Increased concentration of mucus in the back of the throat

> ⬤ **TECH ALERT**
>
> Handle all animals with a history of voice change with care. Rabies can also cause a change in vocal quality.

DIAGNOSIS

- History
- Physical examination: red, inflamed throat

TREATMENT

- Restrict barking or meowing
- Antibiotics (if infection is part of symptoms)
- Antiinflammatory medication: glucocorticoids daily; taper dose after 7 days

INFORMATION FOR CLIENTS

- Upper airway diseases are usually self-limiting.
- Tumors of the nasal cavity and tonsils are most commonly squamous cell carcinomas.
- In most cases, treatment is aimed at making the animal more comfortable. In cases of infection, antibiotics may be required for several weeks.

Diseases of the Lower Respiratory Tract

Diseases that involve the lower respiratory tract are of more serious clinical significance than those of the upper airways (Fig. 11-3). Examples of lower airway

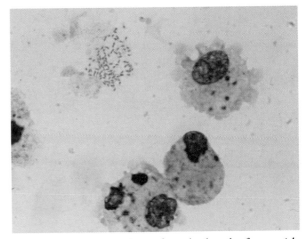

Figure 11-3 Cytology of an endotracheal wash of a cat with *Bordetella bronchiseptica*. (Courtesy University of Georgia, Athens, GA. IN Greene C: *Infectious diseases of the dog and cat*, ed 3, St Louis, 2006, Elsevier)

diseases include tracheobronchitis, tracheal collapse, feline asthma, feline viral respiratory infections, pneumonia, heartworm disease (feline), neoplasia, pulmonary edema, and hemothorax or pneumothorax.

Infectious Canine Tracheobronchitis (Kennel Cough)

Infectious canine tracheobronchitis syndrome involves a collection of agents including viruses, bacteria, mycoplasmas, fungi, and parasites. Some of the most commonly incriminated agents are canine parainfluenza virus, canine adenovirus, canine herpesvirus, reovirus, *Bordetella bronchiseptica*, mycoplasma, and occasionally the canine distemper virus. Tracheobronchitis is contagious and is commonly seen where groups of dogs congregate (kennels, shelters, and boarding facilities).

CLINICAL SIGNS

- A history of exposure to other animals at a kennel, hospital, grooming facility, or dog show
- A dry, hacking, paroxysmal cough (except for cough, a normal, healthy-looking animal)

DIAGNOSIS

- Clinical signs and history
- Cough on tracheal palpation in an otherwise healthy dog

TREATMENT

- Administration of antibiotics if any deeper respiratory involvement is found or if animal is febrile (choice based on culture and sensitivity results)
- Glucocorticoids may be useful in decreasing the severity of the cough
- Trimeprazine with prednisolone (Temaril-P): every 12 hours
- Prednisone, prednisolone: twice a day for 5 to 7 days, followed by tapered dose
- Antitussives:
  - Hycodan (5 mg hydrocodone bitartrate): PO two to four times a day
  - Codeine: every 6 to 8 hours
  - Butorphanol tartrate (Torbutrol): every 6 to 12 hours
- Bronchial dilators:
  - Aminophylline: PO q8h
  - Terbutaline (Brethine): PO every 8 to 12 hours

INFORMATION FOR CLIENTS

- Infectious canine tracheobronchitis is a self-limiting disease. It can take 2 to 3 weeks to resolve.
- Treatment is aimed at making the animal (and often the owner) more comfortable.
- Vaccination with an injectable vaccine should be obtained 2 to 3 weeks before boarding or possible exposure to the disease. Intranasal vaccine can be given closer to the time of exposure. Vaccination significantly reduces the severity of the disease.

Feline *Bordetella* Infection

B. bronchiseptica organisms colonize the ciliated respiratory mucosa, a tissue normally designed to eliminate foreign material from the respiratory tract. The resulting damage and loss of tracheal lining cells is thought to contribute to the clinical symptoms and spread of the disease. After colonization of the tracheal cells, the organism releases toxins that are responsible for local and systemic inflammatory damage. The disease is usually self-limiting in cats; however, severe bronchopneumonias and fatalities have been seen in young kittens.

CLINICAL SIGNS

- Fever
- Sneezing
- Nasal discharge
- Submandibular lymphadenopathy
- Coughing and rales

⬤ TECH ALERT

Many of the signs of *B. bronchiseptica* infection look exactly like those of respiratory viral infections.

DIAGNOSIS

- Culture from oropharyngeal swabs

TREATMENT

- The disease is usually self-limiting.
- Antibiotics may be of value:
  - Tetracycline PO or doxycycline PO

PREVENTION

- Elimination of stress
- Good hygiene
- Good nutrition
- Isolation of sick cats
- Vaccination of cats

INFORMATION FOR CLIENTS

- This respiratory disease looks similar to those caused by feline herpes viruses and feline caliciviruses.
- The disease is usually self-limiting.
- Vaccination of cats in multicat households or catteries should be considered.
- Cats with this disease are infective to other cats.

Collapsing Trachea

The cause of collapsing trachea is not entirely known; however, a reduction in the glycoprotein and glycosaminoglycan content of the hyaline cartilage of the tracheal rings is a constant finding in dogs affected by this syndrome. This syndrome is frequently seen in middle to old age, in obese toy and miniature breeds, but can also be seen in young animals (Yorkies seem to be over-represented). The defect involves tracheal rings that lose their ability to remain firm, subsequently collapsing during respiration. Although it is a progressive disease, many animals can be managed medically for years before surgical management is considered.

CLINICAL SIGNS

- History of paroxysmal cough (harsh, dry, "goose honk" cough)
- Cough often worse on exercise or excitement or when pulling on the collar
- Often concurrent signs of heart disease

DIAGNOSIS

- Tracheal palpation elicits a "goose honk" cough.
- All other physical examination parameters may be normal.
- Radiography on static views may or may not show an alteration in the contour of the trachea. Dorsoventral (DV) and lateral views (both inspiratory and expiratory) are necessary to see this condition.
- Bronchoscopy demonstrates the actual ring collapsing when the animal breathes.
- Ultrasonography provides real-time pictures of collapse.
- Fluoroscopy shows collapse on respirations.
- Rule out all other causes of cough.

TREATMENT

Symptomatic

- Treatment to slow breathing in acute cases:
  - Acepromazine: intravenously (IV), intramuscularly (IM), subcutaneously (SQ)
  - Oxygen therapy (mask) or intubation
  - Dexamethasone: IV
  - Butorphanol: IV, IM, SQ every 6 to 12 hours
- Treatment to slow breathing in chronic cases:
  - *Antitussives*:
    Hycodan (5 mg hydrocodone bitartrate): PO two to three times a day
    Butorphanol: PO every 12 hours
  - *Glucocorticoids*:
    Prednisolone: PO every 12 hours; taper dose after 7 to 10 days
  - *Bronchial dilators* (bronchial dilators act to decrease intrathoracic pressures during expiration, thereby decreasing the collapse of the tracheal membrane):
    Theophylline: PO every 12 hours
    Terbutaline (Brethine, Ciba): PO every 8 to 12 hours

Surgical

- Keep the trachea open with the insertion of external prosthetic supports. For collapse involving only the cervical trachea, external artificial rings can be placed to hold the trachea open. For intrathoracic collapse a mesh stent is the most common choice.
- Surgical correction involves a number of possible complications, making the procedure somewhat unrewarding. Placement of the stents does not affect the progression of the disease.

INFORMATION FOR CLIENTS

- Once this condition develops, it requires lifelong management.
- Treatment is aimed at reducing inflammation in the airway and making the animal more comfortable.
- Management techniques that help include the following:
  - Aggressive weight reduction
  - Decreased exposure to inhaled irritants such as cigarette smoke
  - Use of a harness instead of a collar for restraint
  - Aggressive treatment of respiratory infections
  - Monitoring and treatment of congestive heart failure if it develops

Feline Asthma

Feline asthma, as in human asthma, is a disease characterized by spontaneous bronchoconstriction, airway inflammation, and airway hyperreactivity. Clinical signs of feline asthma include coughing, wheezing, and labored breathing, usually of acute onset.

In affected cats, airway epithelium may hypertrophy, goblet cells and submucosal glands may produce excessive amounts of mucus, and the bronchial mucosa may become infiltrated with inflammatory cells. All of these changes result in decreased air flow. A 50% decrease in the lumen of the airway results in a sixteenfold decrease in the amount of air moving through the system.

It would seem that chronic airway inflammation plays an important role in feline asthma. Decreasing inflammation in the airways and improving air flow are the primary goals of treatment.

CLINICAL SIGNS

- Acute onset of labored breathing (condition may become chronic)
- Cough (may be chronic)
- Wheeze
- Lethargy

DIAGNOSIS

- No physical examination findings are diagnostic for feline asthma. Time of year or exposure to certain environments may provide a clue to the allergen.
- Clinical signs and history help establish diagnosis.
- Radiographs may show signs of diffuse prominent bronchial markings consistent with airway inflammation (often described as "doughnuts").
- Rule out other possibilities such as feline heartworm disease, hair balls, pneumonia, cancer, or lung trauma.

TREATMENT

Acute Onset: Establish an IV Catheter Using Minimal Restraint of the Cat

- Terbutaline IV; dose may be repeated up to 6 times a day until breathing improves
- A short acting steroid: prednisilone sodium succinate or dexamethasone.
- Nasal oxygen; oxygen-rich cage environment, if available
- Nebulization with albuterol

Chronic Disease

- Manage airway inflammation with high-dose, long-term corticosteroid therapy:
  - Prednisone: PO every 12 hours for 10 to 14 days, then slowly taper over 2 to 3 months
  - DepoMedrol: IM every 2 to 4 weeks (if unable to dose orally)
- Bronchodilators:
  - Terbutaline (Brethine): SQ, IM every 12 hours; or PO every 12 hours

- Cyproheptadine: PO every 12 hours (used in cats not responding to the maximum doses of terbutaline and corticosteroids)
- Oxygen therapy

INFORMATION FOR CLIENTS

- The prognosis for cats with asthma is variable.
- If allergens can be determined and exposure decreased before permanent damage occurs, most cats do well.
- Most cats with asthma require periodic medication. Cats with chronic asthma may require continuous medication.
- Aggressive treatment at the veterinary hospital is needed for acute bouts of respiratory distress.
- A cure is usually not possible.

Feline Heartworm Disease

Heartworm infection in cats is less common than in dogs (about 5% to 20% of canine prevalence). Clinical symptoms of the disease in cats, however, are often more severe than in dogs, although the worm burden is usually small (Table 11-1). This disease is seen in 38 of the 50 states, mostly along coastal areas and the Mississippi River Valley. The disease is spread via mosquitos. After taking a blood meal from an infected dog, the microfilaria (immature larva) develop further in the salivary glands of the mosquito and are then transferred to the next animal when the mosquito feeds. The larvae spend about 6 months migrating within the body, finally reaching the bloodstream and the pulmonary artery where the adult worms live. It is the presence of the adult worms in the pulmonary artery that results in many of the clinical symptoms.

Clinical signs in cats are often different from those seen in dogs. Cough and dyspnea are hallmark signs. In many cats, adult worms never develop and yet greater than 50% of infected cats will exhibit clinical signs of pulmonary disease. Antigen-positive cats will almost always have adult worms in the pulmonary artery but antibody-positive cats typically have no adult worms. The standard enzyme-linked immunosorbent assay antigen tests are of little value, missing as many as 50% of natural infections. Male cats (aged 4–6 years) were once thought to be predisposed to this condition but there actually appears to be no sex predilection.

TABLE 11-1   Feline Heartworm Disease Versus Canine Heartworm Disease

	Dog	Cat
Biology of *Dilofilaria immitis*		
Microfilaremia	30%–80% of infected dogs	Rare, transient
Number of adult worms	>50 common	1–3 common
Ectopic migration	Rare	More common
Adult lifespan	Approximately 5 yr	Approximately 2 yr
Clinical Signs of Heartworm Disease		
No signs	Most common	Most common
Respiratory signs	Common	Common
Vomiting	Unusual	Fairly common
Exercise intolerance	Common	Rare
Ascites	Common	Rare
Sudden death	Rare	More common
Radiographic Findings		
Enlarged pulmonary arteries	Characteristic	Characteristic
Blunting or tortuosity	Common	Occasional
Infiltrates in lung	Possible	Possible
Right-sided heart enlargement	Occasional	Rare
Pulmonary artery "knob"	Characteristic	Not seen

CLINICAL SIGNS

- Cough
- Dyspnea
- Weight loss, anorexia
- Vomiting
- Lethargy

Acute or Peracute Presenting Signs

- Salivation
- Tachycardia
- Dyspnea
- Hemoptysis, cough
- Central nervous system (CNS) signs
- Sudden death (uncommon)

DIAGNOSIS

Laboratory

- Microfilarial tests: Cats are usually microfilaria negative or have too small a number of organisms to be detected.
- Antigen tests: Cats typically have low worm burdens (one to two worms) that are missed by these tests.
- Antibody tests: A negative test is 100% specific; a positive test indicates the following:
  - Infection
  - Past exposure
  - Ectopic infection

Radiography

- Radiographs may show enlarged caudal pulmonary arteries (1.6 times the width of the ninth rib at the ninth intercostal space).

Echocardiography

- An experienced echocardiography technician can detect linear foreign bodies in the pulmonary artery or right ventricle.

TREATMENT

- The use of adulticide in cats is *not recommended* because most infections are self-limiting.

Supportive Care

- Cage rest and confinement
- Cortisone PO to reduce inflammation

PREVENTION

- Ivermectin (Heartgard, Merial, Duluth, GA.): PO every 30 days
- Milbemycin: 2000 micrograms per kilogram (mcg/kg)
- Revolution: a monthly spot-on preparation

INFORMATION FOR CLIENTS

- Feline heartworm disease is a self-limiting disease in cats (elimination of most adult worms occurs within 2 to 4 years).
- Both outdoor and indoor cats are at risk for infection but cats are less likely to be bitten by mosquitos than are dogs.
- Cats living in areas where heartworm disease is prevalent should be on monthly prevention.

Feline Viral Respiratory Infections (Feline Viral Rhinotracheitis, Calicivirus)

Even though vaccines are readily available, feline respiratory diseases caused by viral agents continue to be a problem in house cats, in multicat facilities, and in feral cats. The two viral agents responsible for most respiratory problems are feline herpesvirus (FHV) and feline calicivirus (FCV).

Feline Herpesvirus (Feline Viral Rhinotracheitis)

Feline viral rhinotracheitis (FVR) is a highly contagious upper respiratory disease of cats, with a high morbidity and moderate mortality rate, and it may be extremely severe in young kittens. Infections occur year-round in both vaccinated and unvaccinated cats, with clinical symptoms being more severe in the unvaccinated population. Transmission of the virus is via aerosolization (sneezing) and by direct cat-to-cat contact. Queens may transmit the disease to their kittens during grooming. The virus is not hardy and is usually inactivated in the environment within 18 to 24 hours. Cats usually shed the virus for up to 3 weeks after infection; food dishes, clothing, bedding, and toys can act as fomites for spread of the disease.

CLINICAL SIGNS

- Acute onset of sneezing
- Conjunctivitis (usually severe), purulent rhinitis
- Fever
- Depression
- Anorexia
- Ulcerated nasal planum
- Excessive salivation
- Abortion in pregnant queens
- Corneal ulcers

DIAGNOSIS

- Clinical signs
- Direct immunofluorescence testing of nasal smears

TREATMENT

Supportive

- Give fluids (IV, SQ) to correct dehydration.
- Administer broad-spectrum antibiotics.
- Decongestants, vaporization, antihistamines can be administered.
- Nursing care: Clean eyes and nose several times daily.
- Increase the environmental temperature.
- Force-feed or provide a food with a noticeable odor (cats that cannot smell their food tend not to eat). In addition, warming the food may improve the taste to the cat.
- In general, avoid cortisone as an antiinflammatory.
- Decrease stress on the animal.

Antiviral

- Use the following topically for ocular infections:
  - Idoxuridine (Stoxil)
  - Vidarabine (Vira-A)
  - Trifluridine (Viroptic) 1%

PREVENTION

- A good vaccination program prevents FVR.

INFORMATION FOR CLIENTS

- FVR is a highly contagious disease.
- Vaccinated cats may show mild clinical signs of infection.
- You can transmit this disease to other cats by contact with your hands and clothes.
- Warming food or using an odoriferous type of cat food may improve appetite in sick cats.
- Disinfectants kill feline herpesvirus type 1 viruses.
- This disease is infectious only to cats.

Feline Calicivirus

Like FVR, FCV infection produces an acute, highly contagious upper respiratory tract disease in cats (Fig. 11-4). Ulcerative stomatitis is seen frequently with FCV in upper respiratory tract disorders but is not routinely seen with FVR infections. The calicivirus is resistant to disinfectants and can remain active in the environment for several days. The morbidity of the disease is high, but mortality is low. Clinical signs can appear year-round and are most severe in kittens 2 to 6 months of age. Transmission occurs through direct contact with infected cats.

CLINICAL SIGNS

- Fever
- Serous ocular or nasal discharge
- Mild conjunctivitis
- Oral ulcers with increased salivation
- Pneumonia
- Acute arthritis in kittens (limping kitten syndrome)
- Diarrhea

DIAGNOSIS

- Clinical signs
- Viral isolation

TREATMENT

Supportive Care
- Good nursing care
- Broad-spectrum antibiotics

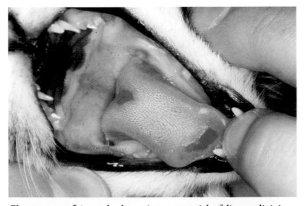

Figure 11-4 Lingual ulcers in a cat with feline calicivirus infection. (From Gaskell RM, Radford AD, Dawson S: Feline infectious respiratory disease, p. 588. IN Chandler EA, Gaskell CJ, Gaskell RM (eds): *Feline medicine and therapeutics*, ed. 3, Oxford, 2004, Blackwell Publishing.)

- Force-feeding, if ulcers prevent cat from eating
- Oxygen therapy (if dyspneic)
- Disinfect environment using bleach

PREVENTION

- A good vaccination program is important.

INFORMATION FOR CLIENTS

- FCV is highly contagious.
- Clinical signs usually last 5 to 7 days.
- Oral ulcers can last 7 to 10 days and require no special treatment.
- Cats that salivate profusely can become dehydrated and may require fluid therapy.
- Force-feeding may be necessary.
- Vaccination is effective in preventing the disease.

Virulent Systemic Calicivirus Infection

This acute, severe systemic disease of cats, also known as *hemorrhagic calicivirus*, has emerged within the last decade. Signs include acute respiratory disease, vasculitis, facial and limb edema, cutaneous ulceration, multisystem organ failure, and disseminated intravascular coagulation (DIC). This form of calicivirus infection is not prevented by the usually used feline herpes-1 vaccine. Newer vaccines are available that do protect against the hemorrhagic strain of the virus. Since the few outbreaks of this form of the disease have been in shelter-housed cats, the vaccine is not currently recommended for routine use in house cats.

Pleural Effusion

Pleural effusion, the build-up of fluid within the pleural space, results in respiratory distress for the patient. Several diseases are associated with pleural effusion.

Congestive heart failure, especially right-sided failure, represents a principal cause of pleural effusion in both canine and feline patients. As systemic venous hypertension increases, significant amounts of the straw-colored transudate accumulate within the pleural space, causing respiratory difficulty.

Any intrathoracic neoplasia can result in pleural effusion through obstruction of lymphatics, inflammation, hemorrhage, or obstruction of venous drainage. It is common to find effusion associated with mediastinal masses (lymphoma), mesotheliomas of the pleura, or metastatic carcinomas. (Primary pulmonary tumors are uncommon in pets.)

Empyema, or purulent exudative pleural effusion, may occur secondary to trauma, foreign body, or pulmonary infection. It may be idiopathic in dogs.

Chylothorax is the condition defined by the accumulation of chylous fluid in the pleural space. *Chyle* is a term used to describe lymphatic fluid arising from the intestine and containing a high concentration of fat. Any disease that increases systemic venous pressure may result in chylothorax (malignancy, pancreatitis, trauma, infection, parasites, and idiopathic disorders). Breed or age predisposition for the formation of chylothorax has not been documented; however, Afghans and oriental breeds of cats appear to have a predisposition to this condition. Older cats are more likely to experience development of chylothorax than younger cats.

All pleural effusions produce similar clinical symptoms of respiratory distress, dyspnea, cough, and circulatory compromise. Diagnosis is made from physical examination findings, thoracocentesis, cytology, culture and sensitivity, and radiographic findings. See Table 11-2 for a classification of pleural effusions.

CLINICAL SIGNS

- Dyspnea
- May have cough, fever, pleural pain

DIAGNOSIS

Thoracic Radiographs (signs of Pleural Effusion)
- Unilateral or bilateral fluid accumulation (usually bilateral) is seen (fluid is visible if there is >50 mL in small animals and >100 mL in large dogs).
- Increased radiopacity is seen on lateral projection in the ventral portion of the thorax with a

TABLE 11-2   Guidelines for Characterizing Effusions Other than Hemorrhagic Effusions

Finding	CATEGORY		
	Transudate	Modified Transudate	Exudate
Total protein (g/dL)	<2.5	>2.5	>2.5
Nucleated cell count (cells/μL)	<1000	<1000	>5000
	<5000 (horse)	<5000 (horse)	>10,000 (horse)
Predominant nucleated cell type	Mesothelial or macrophage	Mesothelial or macrophage	Neutrophil
	Horse: up to 60% may be nondegenerate neutrophils	Horse: up to 60% may be nondegenerate neutrophils	
	COMMON CAUSES		
	Portal hypertension secondary to hepatic insufficiency or portal vein hypoplasia	Right-sided heart failure Impaired venous flow between origin of hepatic vein and right atrium of the heart	Inflammation: septic Inflammation: nonseptic— feline infectious peritonitis irritant: urine, bile, chyle, foreign body
	Space-occupying mass Severe hypoalbuminemia (serum albumin < ~ 1.5g/dL)	Space-occupying mass Horse: intestinal disorder	Space-occupying mass Horse: intestinal disorder

From Meyer DJ, Harvey JW: *Veterinary laboratory medicine: interpretation and diagnosis*, ed 3, St. Louis, MO, 2004, Saunders, by permission.

scalloped appearance caused by the presence of fluid between lobes of the lung (Fig. 11-5).
- DV or ventrodorsal projection shows the following:
  - Retraction of lung borders from the thoracic wall
  - Blunting of costophrenic angles
  - Partial to total obliteration of the cardiac borders
  - Widened mediastinum

⬤ TECH ALERT

Use extreme care when restraining any animal with pleural effusion.

Thoracocentesis Technique
- Prepare and block the skin and the subcutaneous tissues over the seventh or eighth intercostal space, just above the costochondral junction. Use a small needle and 2% lidocaine (Fig. 11-6).
- Insert the chosen device with syringe through the prepared space (a butterfly catheter works well).

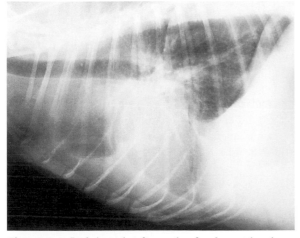

Figure 11-5 Left lateral radiograph of a dog with a large volume of fluid in the pleural space. The cardiac silhouette is partially obscured by surrounding fluid, there are interlobar fissures, and the overall radiopacity of the thorax is increased. In addition, there is an area of radiopacity just dorsal to the sternum, the margins of which are scalloped because of fluid accumulation in the ventral thorax. (From Thrall DE: *Textbook of veterinary diagnostic radiology*, ed 5, St. Louis, MO, 2007, Saunders, by permission.)

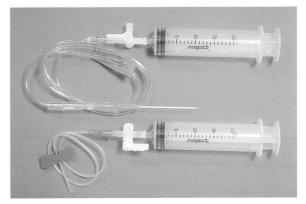

Figure 11-6 A small-gauge butterfly needle (*bottom*) or an over-the-needle catheter attached to extension tubing (*top*) and a three-way stopcock and syringe are used for needle thoracocentesis. (From Fossum TW: *Small animal surgery*, ed 3, St. Louis, MO, 2007, Mosby, by permission.)

- Avoid the intercostal artery along the caudal portion of the rib.
- Using gentle suction, remove the fluid.
- Send samples to the laboratory for cytology, specific gravity, pH, protein concentration, packed cell volume, and total and differential white blood cell count.

TREATMENT
- Treatment depends on the pathology responsible for the effusion.

Congestive Heart Failure
- Treat the underlying disease and use therapeutic thoracocentesis (if needed) to relieve dyspnea.

Neoplasia
- Therapeutic thoracocentesis
- Chemotherapy
- Pleurodesis

Pyothorax
- Tube thoracostomy with continual drainage. Chest tubes can be placed on both sides of the chest if necessary.
- Antibiotic therapy based on culture and sensitivity results
- Long-term treatment (at least 3 months)

- Good choices for initial treatment include the following:
  - Ampicillin: IV, IM, SQ every 6 to 8 hours
  - Clindamycin: IM, SQ, PO every 12 hours
  - Chloramphenicol: IM, SQ, IV every 6 to 8 hours

INFORMATION FOR CLIENTS

- Whether pleural drainage is required depends on the animal and type of effusion.
- Unless the primary disease is treated, the effusion will return.
- Treatment can be long term and expensive.
- Periodic reevaluation of the patient is required.

Fungal Diseases

Most fungal disease results from the inhalation of fungal spores or from wound contamination. The fungi, found as inhabitants of the animal's environment, damage the host cells by releasing enzymes. They kill, digest, and invade surrounding cells. Some fungi produce toxins. Mycotic diseases are found worldwide, but in North America they are endemic along the eastern seaboard, the Great Lakes regions, and the river valleys of the Mississippi, Ohio, and the St. Lawrence waterways (Fig. 11-7).

Inhalation is the common route of infection, and pulmonary symptoms occur with most fungal

infections. Treatment is often prolonged, and relapses are frequent. Fungal infections may disseminate to other organ systems; in these cases, the prognosis is usually guarded to grave. Commonly seen fungal diseases of animals include blastomycosis, coccidioidomycosis, histoplasmosis, and aspergillosis.

Blastomycosis

Blastomyces dermatitidis is the dimorphic fungus responsible for blastomycosis in dogs and cats. The mycelial phase of the organism is found in soil and laboratory cultures, but the yeast form is the phase found in the tissues. States having the highest incidence of canine blastomycosis are Kentucky, Illinois, Tennessee, Mississippi, Indiana, Iowa, Ohio, Arkansas, and North Carolina, with some cases occurring in north and south central Texas.

Three clinical forms of the disease exist: primary pulmonary infection, disseminated disease, and local cutaneous infections. Inhalation is the primary route of infection, although wound contamination also occurs. The incubation period is 5 to 12 weeks. The disease is more prevalent in dogs than in cats.

CLINICAL SIGNS

- Anorexia
- Depression
- Weight loss
- Fever (>103°F)
- Cough, dyspnea
- Ocular, nasal discharge
- Wound exudates (serosanguinous to purulent)
- Lymphadenopathy
- CNS signs

DIAGNOSIS

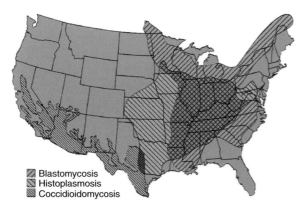

Blastomycosis
Histoplasmosis
Coccidioidomycosis

Figure 11-7 Areas in the United States endemic for blastomycosis, coccidioidomycosis, and histoplasmosis. (From Ettinger SJ, Feldman EC: *Textbook of veterinary internal medicine*, ed 6, St. Louis, MO, 2005, Saunders, by permission.)

> ◯ **TECH ALERT**
>
> Lack of appropriate response to antibiotic and corticosteroid therapy should alert the clinician to the possibility of fungal infection.

- Complete blood cell count (CBC) and blood chemistry results yield nonspecific signs of chronic disease.
- Hypercalcemia is seen in some dogs.

- Cytology: Aspirates or impression smears yield a definitive diagnosis in most cases. The presence of thick-walled budding yeast is typical for *Blastomyces* (Fig. 11-8).
- Radiology shows generalized diffuse, nodular interstitial pattern. Osseous lesions are seen in the epiphyseal area of long bones.
- Serology testing is available.

TREATMENT

- Amphotericin B is the most effective medication for blastomycosis; it can be administered intravenously, subconjunctivally, topically, or intraperitoneally; side effects include anorexia, nausea, vomiting, chills, seizures, fever, anemia, cardiac arrest, and renal impairment.
  - *Slow-drip therapy*: amphotericin B added to 500 to 1000 mL 5% dextrose and given over a 3- to 6-hour period one to three times weekly
  - *Bolus therapy*: amphotericin B added to 20 to 50 mL 5% dextrose and administered as intravenous bolus one to three times weekly
- Ketoconazole: daily PO for 60 days (33% cure rate)
- Itraconazole: PO every 24 hours (long term)

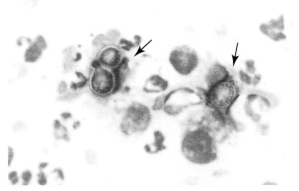

Figure 11-8 Pyogranulomatous inflammation from a dog with blastomycosis. A *Blastomyces dermatitidis* organism (*arrow*) is in the center of the field. Neutrophils, macrophages, and an inflammatory giant cell are present. (From Cowell RL, Tyler RD, Meinkoth JH, DeNicola DB: *Diagnostic cytology and hematology of the dog and cat*, ed 3, St. Louis, MO, 2008, Mosby, by permission.)

INFORMATION FOR CLIENTS

- In most cases, blastomycosis is *not* transmitted from animals to humans; however, owners should use caution when handling animals with draining lesions.
- Owners share the same environment as the pet and are likely to be exposed to the same type of fungal spores.
- The prognosis for the pet depends on the stage of the disease and the sex of the pet. Female animals have a higher survival rate.
- Relapses are common, and treatment may require long-term management.
- The drugs required to treat blastomycosis are expensive.

Coccidioidomycosis

Coccidioides immitis is a dimorphic soil fungus found in semiarid areas with sandy soils and mild winters (California, Nevada, Utah, Arizona, New Mexico, and Texas).

Clinical signs of infection may not appear for weeks to years after exposure to the fungal spores. Young, male dogs are most likely to be infected.

CLINICAL SIGNS

- Mild, nonproductive cough
- Low-grade fever
- Anorexia
- Weight loss
- Weakness and depression if systemic
- Lameness, soft-tissue swelling, and pain if bone involvement
- Lymphadenopathy may or may not be present
- Myocarditis may or may not be present
- Skin lesions
- Signs of CNS involvement

DIAGNOSIS

- CBC or blood chemistry results show nonspecific signs of chronic disease.
- Cytology/biopsy may show thick, double-walled spherical bodies (Fig. 11-9).
- Radiology shows a wide range of parenchymal changes in the lung.
- Serology testing is available.
- Titers greater than 1:16 to 1:32 indicate active disease.

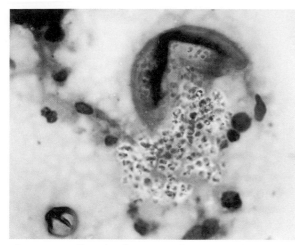

Figure 11-9 Coccidioidomycosis. Large, poorly staining round bodies are the spherules of coccidioidomycosis. (From Cowell RL, Tyler RD, Meinkoth JH, DeNicola DB: *Diagnostic cytology and hematology of the dog and cat,* ed 3, St. Louis, MO, 2008, Mosby, by permission.)

TREATMENT

- Ketoconazole: PO twice a day (dogs)
- Itraconazole: PO one to two times a day (dogs)
- Treatment may be required for 6 to 12 months

INFORMATION FOR CLIENTS

- No known risk for animal-to-human transmission exists; however, use caution when treating animals with draining lesions.
- Response to treatment usually is good, but relapses are common.
- Lifelong treatment may be necessary to keep the pet in remission.
- Medications are expensive.

Histoplasmosis

Histoplasma capsulatum, a dimorphic soil fungus, is endemic in 31 of the 48 continental states (most common in Ohio, Missouri, and the Mississippi River Valley). The fungus has also been associated with bird and bat droppings. Clinical histoplasmosis is as common in cats as in dogs. Inhalation is the prime source of infection with a 12- to 16-day incubation period. The gastrointestinal (GI) tract may also be susceptible to *Histoplasma* infection.

CLINICAL SIGNS

Feline: Pulmonary Signs
- Weight loss
- Fever
- Anorexia
- Pale mucous membranes
- May or may not show dyspnea
- Hepatomegaly
- Peripheral lymphadenopathy
- May or may not show ocular lesions

Canine: Gastrointestinal Signs
- Weight loss
- Diarrhea (large bowel)
- Dyspnea
- Cough
- Pale mucous membranes
- Low-grade fever

DIAGNOSIS

- CBC: Results demonstrate normocytic, normochromic, nonregenerative anemia. Occasionally organisms are seen in neutrophils or monocytes.
- Blood chemistry results are usually normal.
- Cytology or histopathology: Small, round intracellular bodies surrounded by a light halo are seen (Fig. 11-10).
- Radiology: Diffuse or linear pulmonary interstitial patterns (thorax) are seen.
- GI tract radiography may indicate ascites.
- Serology is also available (results are often false negative).

TREATMENT

- Ketoconazole: PO one to two times a day for 3 months
- Itraconazole: PO one to two times a day (dogs and cats)

INFORMATION FOR CLIENTS

- Prognosis is fair to good for the pulmonary form, but guarded to grave for the systemic form.

Cryptococcosis

Cryptococcus neoformans is a budding yeast surrounded by a mucoid capsule. Inhalation is the primary means of entry into the body, and immunosuppressed

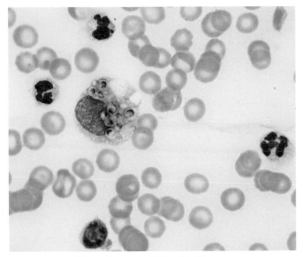

Figure 11-10 Histoplasmosis. Mixed inflammatory response surrounding large central macrophage, which contains *Histoplasma* organisms. (From Raskin RE, Meyer DJ: *Canine and feline cytology*, ed 2, St. Louis, MO, 2010, Saunders.)

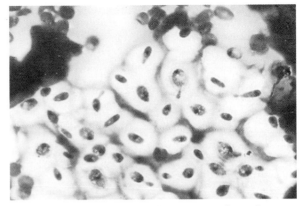

Figure 11-11 *Cryptococcus neoformans* is a spherical, yeast-like organism that frequently has a thick, clear-staining mucoid capsule. (From Cowell RL, Tyler RD, Meinkoth JH, DeNicola DB: *Diagnostic cytology and hematology of the dog and cat*, ed 3, St. Louis, MO, 2008, Mosby, by permission.)

animals are more likely to become infected than healthy animals. Organisms commonly grow in avian excreta, especially pigeon droppings.

CLINICAL SIGNS

Feline (the Most Common Systemic Mycosis in the Cat)
- Nasal cavity and sinus lesions
- Chronic nasal discharge
- Nasal granulomas
- Lymphadenopathy
- May or may not show CNS involvement (seen in 25% of cases)
- Eye lesions (may or may not be seen)
- Low-grade fever, malaise
- Weight loss, anorexia

Canine (Less Common Than in Cats)
- Mostly CNS lesions (vestibular dysfunction)
- Skin lesions in about 25% of cases

DIAGNOSIS
- Cytology of aspirates, impression smears, or cerebrospinal fluid (Fig. 11-11)
- Antigen test available commercially

TREATMENT
- Amphotericin B: IV three times weekly with 5-flucytosine
- 5-Flucytosine: PO every 12 to 24 hours
- Ketoconazole: every 12 to 24 hours
- Itraconazole: PO every 24 hours
- Minimum treatment time is 2 months

INFORMATION FOR CLIENTS
- The prognosis is fair to good unless there is CNS involvement, which worsens the prognosis.
- No known health hazard to humans exists.

Aspergillosis

Aspergillus fumigatus can be found throughout the world in decaying vegetation, sewage sludge, compost piles, and moldy seeds and grains. Inhalation is the most common route of infection, and the nasal cavity is the predominant location of lesions in the dog. Cases of systemic infections have been reported, although they are uncommon.

CLINICAL SIGNS

Feline Aspergillosis (uncommon)
- May be immunocompromised with feline leukemia virus

- Abnormal lung, GI, liver, spleen, and renal (sometimes) functions
- Lethargy, fever
- Weight loss, anorexia

Canine Aspergillosis: Localized Infection
- Young to middle-aged dogs
- Chronic nasal discharge, usually unilateral
- Sneezing
- Stertorous breathing
- Facial pain

Canine Aspergillosis: Generalized Infection
- Predominantly seen in German Shepherds 1 to 7 years of age
- Weight loss, anorexia
- Fever
- Lameness, back pain, paresis, paralysis
- Ocular signs

DIAGNOSIS

- Radiology shows loss of nasal turbinates, increased lucency, punctate erosions of the frontal bones. Starts unilaterally.
- Biopsy or endoscopy shows yellow-green to gray-black fungal plaques on nasal mucosa. Hyphae are seen on biopsy with hematoxylin and eosin stain (Fig. 11-12).

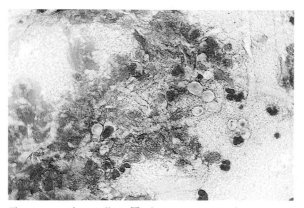

Figure 11-12 Aspergillosis. The long, narrow, angular, negative-stained organism with narrow stained central region is compatible with fungal cause, probably caused by *Aspergillus* spp. (From Raskin RE, Meyer DJ: *Canine and feline cytology*, ed 2, St. Louis, MO, 2010, Saunders.)

TREATMENT
- Topical clotrimazole: 1 g clotrimazole in 100 mL polyethylene glycol, instilled twice daily through indwelling nasal catheters (surgically placed) or in continuous contact therapy for 1 hour.

INFORMATION FOR CLIENTS
- Localized disease has a fair prognosis, but disseminated disease carries a grave prognosis.
- There is no known health risk to humans handling *Aspergillus*-infected animals.
- *Aspergillus* tends to be an opportunistic fungus; infected animals may have a concurrent immunodeficiency problem.

Pulmonary Neoplasms

Although primary lung tumors are relatively uncommon in dogs and cats, the lungs can be affected by primary neoplasms, metastatic neoplasms, lymphoma, and neoplasms from surrounding tissues.

The incidence of primary neoplasms in dogs and cats appears to be increasing, although they are still uncommon. Most of the primary tumors seen are adenocarcinomas (70%–80%), although squamous cell carcinomas, anaplastic carcinomas, fibrosarcomas, osteosarcomas, chondrosarcomas, and benign adenomas are seen occasionally. Pulmonary neoplasms are seen most often in dogs 9 to 12 years old. Primary tumors may metastasize to regional lymph nodes, long bones, heart, brain, eye, and mediastinal lymph nodes.

Metastatic disease is common in pet animals. Primary tumors involving the thyroid gland and the mammary gland typically metastasize to the lungs, although *any* tumor has the potential to result in metastatic disease. Although primary lymphoma of the lung has not been reported in pet animals, dogs with multicentric lymphoma frequently have lung involvement.

The prognosis for pulmonary neoplasia depends on the degree of tissue involvement, metastasis of lesions, and lymph node involvement. Surgery is the treatment of choice for tumors that are resectable.

CLINICAL SIGNS
Primary Neoplasia
- Cough (usually nonproductive)
- Exercise intolerance

- Weight loss, poor condition
- Dysphagia, vomiting
- Anorexia

Metastatic Neoplasms

- Evidence of a primary tumor at site other than the lung
- All clinical signs as for primary tumor
- Any signs associated with the organ system involved in the primary tumor

DIAGNOSIS

Thoracic Radiographs

- Thoracic radiographs do not provide a *definitive* diagnosis—lesions of abscesses, parasitic disease, fungal infections, and bacterial infections may look similar radiographically.
- Radiographs may miss lesions smaller than 5 mm.
- Two lateral views should be taken (a left and right); to confirm diagnosis, more than one radiologist should read the films.

Biopsy or Cytology

- Biopsy and cytology can be performed transthoracically, transbronchially, or surgically.
- Histology provides the *definitive* diagnosis.
- Ultrasound or fluoroscopic guided biopsy can be performed; however, the chances for complications increase (nonrepresentative sample, hemothorax or pneumothorax).

TREATMENT

- Surgical excision is the treatment of choice.
- Lobectomy is usually required for solitary tumors.
- Chemotherapy may reduce the size and effect of the lesion but may not result in increased survival time.

Metastatic Tumors

- Surgical removal of the primary tumor is required.
- Chemotherapy should be based on the sensitivity of the primary tumor (although metastatic tumors may have sensitivities different from those of the primary tumor).
- Many tumors are untreatable by the time they are diagnosed.

INFORMATION FOR CLIENTS

- The prognosis for these animals is guarded to grave.
- By the time these tumors are diagnosed, they are usually in advanced stages.
- Chemotherapy may help to reduce clinical symptoms produced by the tumor.

REVIEW QUESTIONS

1. Which of the following diagnostic procedures might be of use in diagnosing nasal tumors or masses? (There may be more than one answer.)
   a. Serum chemistry
   b. Radiograph
   c. Endoscopy
   d. Computed tomography or magnetic resonance imaging
2. Which of the following bacteria plays a part in infectious canine tracheobronchitis?
   a. *Brucella*
   b. *Bordetella*
   c. *Borrelia*
3. The life span of the adult *Dilofilaria immitis* in the cat is approximately.
   a. 5 years
   b. 10 years
   c. 2 years
   d. 3 years
4. Which of the following signs of heartworm infection in the cat is not commonly seen in the heartworm-infected dog?
   a. Coughing
   b. Vomiting
   c. No sign of disease
5. The feline herpesvirus responsible for feline viral rhinotracheitis (FVR) is hardy and will remain in the environment for years.
   a. True
   b. False
6. Technicians can transmit respiratory viruses to uninfected cats by contact with hands and clothes.
   a. True
   b. False

7. Which of the following are characteristics of a transudate? (There may be more than one answer.)
   a. High total protein
   b. Low nucleated cell count
   c. Low total protein
   d. High nucleated cell count
8. The preferred spot for thoracocentesis is the _____ space.
   a. Fifth intercostal
   b. Third intercostal
   c. Seventh intercostal
   d. Tenth intercostal
9. The most common systemic mycotic disease in cats is caused by:
   a. *Aspergillus*
   b. *Cryptococcus*
   c. *Coccidioides*
   d. *Blastomyces*

10. A 5-year-old dog has an exudative, serosanguinous wound that is nonresponsive to antibiotics and corticosteroid therapy. This should alert the clinician to the possibility of this type of problem.
    a. Fungal
    b. Neoplastic
    c. Viral
    d. Bacterial
11. The systemic signs of feline *Bordetella* infection are caused by:
    a. Toxins released by *Bordetella bronchiseptica* bacteria
    b. The presence of virus particles carried in macrophages
    c. Pulmonary edema caused by the presence of lung abscesses
    d. Pericarditis related to the presence of viral particles

Answers found on page 552.

Diseases of the Urinary System

LEARNING OBJECTIVES

When you have completed this chapter, you will be able to:

1. Explain the anatomy of the urinary system and the functions it performs.
2. Describe how bacterial and viral infections can occur and how these may lead to the formation of stones.
3. Identify the most commonly seen canine bladder stones.
4. Explain the benefits of castration as it relates to prostate disease in the male dog.
5. Discuss the cause of urinary incontinence in spayed female dogs.

Anatomy of the Urinary System

Anatomically, the urinary system is composed of the *kidneys, ureters, bladder,* and *urethra* (Fig. 12-1). The main job of the urinary system is waste removal, although it is also instrumental in red blood cell (RBC) production, the regulation of water and electrolyte balances, and control of blood pressure. The system is a blood plasma balancer. It processes blood plasma by adjusting the water and electrolyte content, removes waste materials not needed by the body, and returns those necessary substances to the systemic circulation.

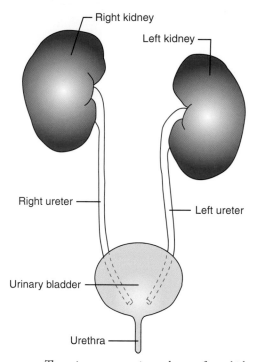

Figure 12-1 The urinary system is made up of two kidneys, two ureters, one urinary bladder, and one urethra. (From Colville T, Bassert JM: *Clinical anatomy and physiology for veterinary technicians*, St. Louis, MO, 2008, Mosby, by permission.)

It also regulates the pH of the plasma. The final product is urine, which is stored for elimination.

The kidneys are located in the retroperitoneal space along the vertebral column from T13-L3. Internally, the kidney is divided structurally into the cortex (the outer region) and the *medulla* (the inner region) (Fig. 12-2). The "filtration units," or *glomeruli*, are concentrated in the cortical region, whereas the "concentration or exchange tubules," or *nephron loops*, are found in the medulla (Fig. 12-3). Blood enters the kidney and is filtered through the capillaries of the glomerulus. Glomerular capillaries are unique in that they contain pores that selectively allow certain substances to pass through them. Blood filtration depends on blood pressure and the dilation or constriction of the glomerular vessels. When vascular fluid volume decreases or blood pressure drops, the filtration in the glomerulus decreases and urine production stops. The nephron loop concentrates the filtrate and reabsorbs vital nutrients. Needed substances such as glucose, amino acids, and bicarbonate are 100% reabsorbed in the proximal convoluted tubules of the nephron loop. As the filtrate passes through the loop it is diluted, concentrated, has its pH altered, exchanges sodium, hydrogen, and potassium and is subject to the action of the hormones antidiuretic hormone (ADH) and aldosterone. Finally, *urine* passes into the ureters and then on to the bladder for storage before elimination.

Clinical disease may result when any portion of this system fails to function properly. Failure of the renal system can be divided into three types: (1) pre-renal, (2) renal, and (3) post-renal. The most commonly seen clinical problems involving the urinary system include cystitis, cystic calculi, urinary obstruction, acute and chronic renal failure (CRF), and incontinence.

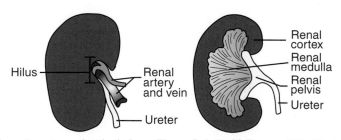

Figure 12-2 Frontal section of right kidney. (From Colville T, Bassert JM: *Clinical anatomy and physiology for veterinary technicians*, St. Louis, MO, 2008, Mosby, by permission.)

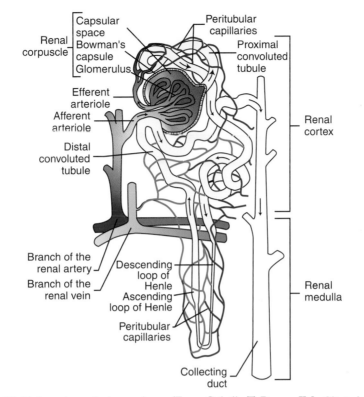

Figure 12-3 Fluid flow through the nephron. (From Colville T, Bassert JM: *Clinical anatomy and physiology for veterinary technicians*, St. Louis, MO, 2008, Mosby, by permission.)

Cystitis

Feline Cystitis (Idiopathic [Interstitial] Cystitis)

Feline cystitis (idiopathic cystitis) is a nonmalignant inflammatory condition, previously known as *feline urologic syndrome* or *feline lower urinary tract disease*, which occurs frequently in cats. At Ohio State University, in a study of 132 cats examined for symptoms of irritative voiding (dysuria, hematuria, and pollakiuria), 61% were found to have idiopathic cystitis. The cause for this disease is unknown, although a virus may be the causative agent. The disease can be divided into two forms: (1) ulcerative and (2) nonulcerative, or (1) obstructive and (2) nonobstructive. Most cats will have the nonulcerative form. The disease appears to be self-limiting in most cats, with clinical signs subsiding within 1 week to 10 days. *Any* treatment appears to help because of the self-limiting nature of the cystitis.

Cats with undocumented bacteriuria should not be treated with antibiotics. Needless antibiotic treatment only results in an increased number of antibiotic-resistant organisms.

Change of diet may be the most beneficial treatment, especially if it results in dilute urine without an increase in urine pH. If possible, cats should be fed canned food or have water added to dry food.

Cats should be given places to hide; toys and scratching poles allow cats to exercise normal play behavior and reduce stress, which has been shown to help in the treatment of this disorder.

Use of analgesics such as buprenorphine, butorphanol, or fentanyl patches is advocated to reduce pain and decrease clinical symptoms. A dose just sufficient to calm the cat is given orally once daily at bedtime. Antiinflammatories such as carprofen may also be useful. Liver enzymes should be monitored while the cat is receiving these medications.

TECH ALERT

Avoid the use of indwelling urine catheters in these cats. If using a catheter to obtain a urine sample, make sure it is done as aseptically as possible.

CLINICAL SIGNS

- Hematuria (frank blood or a pink urine)
- Dysuria (pain on urination)
- Inappropriate urination (e.g., floors, sinks, bathtub)
- More frequent urination (small volumes)

DIAGNOSIS

- Urinalysis: Both dipstick and sediment examination should be performed to rule out bacterial cause or systemic disease.
- Urine culture is negative.
- Radiographic contrast studies may indicate irregular mucosal lining and thickened bladder wall, or radiographs may be normal.

TREATMENT

- Avoid unnecessary use of antibiotics unless urinalysis indicates a bacterial cause.
- Change diet to produce dilute urine.
- Provide analgesics to relieve clinical signs and ease discomfort.
- Antiinflammatory medications should be used with caution. (There have been *no* positive clinical effects seen in controlled studies.)
- Administer propantheline orally (PO) every 72 hours to relieve incontinence until the condition resolves.

INFORMATION for CLIENTS

- This disease is self-limiting.
- This may be a recurring problem.
- There is no definitive cure.
- Reduction of stress in the cat's environment helps prevent recurrence.
- It may be difficult to change the diet. Be creative and patient.

Canine Cystitis (Bacterial Cystitis)

Although bacterial urinary tract infection accounts for only 1% to 3% of all feline cystitis, it is the most common cause of cystitis in the dog. The urinary tract is normally sterile (free of bacteria) and resistant to infection. Natural defense mechanisms such as frequent voiding of urine, urethral and ureteral peristalsis, glycosaminoglycans in the surface mucosal layer, pH, and constituents of the urine assist in preventing the invasion of bacteria into lower urinary tract structures.

Urinary tract infections are most commonly the result of ascending migration of bacteria up the urethra. The blood-borne route does not seem of much importance in animal infections. The motility of some bacteria such as *Escherichia coli* and *Proteus* spp. may assist in this migration. Once in the bladder, the microorganisms must adhere and colonize the mucosal lining. Bacteria that may be nonpathogenic in the healthy animal may be virulent in hosts with altered immunity.

CLINICAL SIGNS

- Increased frequency of urination
- Hematuria
- Dysuria
- Cloudy urine, abnormal odor
- Frequent licking of the urethral area

DIAGNOSIS

- Urinalysis: Dipstick and sediment examination show increased white blood cell (WBC) counts and bacteria.
- Urine culture and sensitivity: Collect by cystocentesis and culture within 30 minutes for best results. This should *always* be done.

TREATMENT

Preventive

- Avoid unnecessary use of indwelling urinary catheters.
- Use a closed system when using indwelling urinary catheters (Fig. 12-4).
- Avoid trauma to the urinary tract during surgical procedures.
- Select the least expensive, least toxic, most effective antibiotic to start treatment. Because of frequency of urination, it is recommended to dose the drug every 8 hours when possible. Treatment should be of sufficient duration to eliminate the bacteria.
- Treatment for acute infections should be for 10 to 14 days. Chronic or relapsing infections require 4 to 6 weeks of treatment.

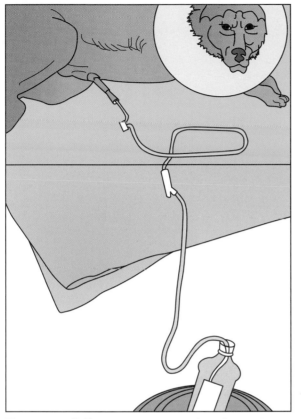

Figure 12-4 Collection apparatus in place for continuous urine drainage. Note that collection container is below the level of animal's urinary bladder.

Antibiotics

- Choice should be based on culture and sensitivity results.
- Empiric choice of antibiotics: Drug should attain effective concentrations in the urine and tissue. Some good choices include the following:
  - Ampicillin: PO every 8 hours
  - Amoxicillin trihydrate (clavulanate potassium): PO every 8 hours
  - Trimethoprim-sulfonamide: PO every 12 hours
  - Cephalexin: PO every 8 to 12 hours
  - Enrofloxacin: PO every 12 hours

INFORMATION FOR CLIENTS

- Most uncomplicated urinary tract infections resolve without treatment.

- If antibiotics are needed, make sure you give them as directed and for the prescribed period to avoid creating resistance to the drug.
- Relapses are common (many relapses are due to inadequate treatment).
- The prostate may be the source of recurring infections in male dogs.
- Repeat cultures during treatment to follow progress.

Feline Uroliths and Urethral Plugs

A detailed description of feline uroliths is beyond the scope of this text. Students are referred to veterinary medical texts for more information.

"Plugged" cats are a frequent occurrence in the small-animal hospital. The inability to pass urine may have serious and even fatal consequences. Two common causes of urethral obstruction in cats are uroliths and urethral plugs. These terms should not be used synonymously because they are physically distinct from one another. *Uroliths* are polycrystalline concretions composed of minerals with a small amount of matrix. *Urethral plugs* consist of small amounts of minerals in a large amount of matrix. This section discusses each of these as they affect urinary tract disease in cats.

Feline Uroliths

A number of different minerals can be found in feline uroliths (Fig. 12-5). These include the following:

- Struvite (approximately 60%)
- Calcium oxalate (27%)
- Ammonium urate (5.5%)
- Cystine
- Mixed mineral

Uroliths, also called *bladder stones*, may be located anywhere in the urinary tract. Some are radiopaque and are easily diagnosed by radiographs (e.g., calcium oxalate, urates, and struvites), whereas others are radiolucent and require double-contrast cystography to be seen.

In most cases, the cause of urolith formation cannot be determined, although studies show that diets high in magnesium produce struvite uroliths experimentally in cats. Obese, older cats (>2 years)

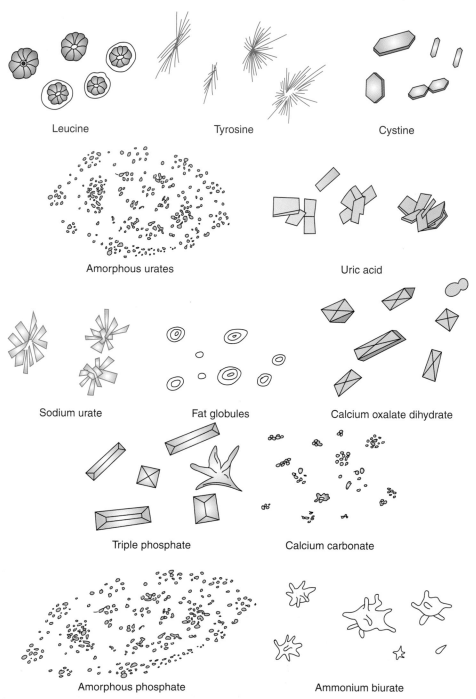

Figure 12-5 Various types of crystals that may be found in urine. (From Hendrix CM, Sirois M: *Laboratory procedures for veterinary technicians*, ed 5, St. Louis, MO, 2007, Mosby, by permission.)

appear to be predisposed to urolith formation. There appears to be no breed predisposition for struvite uroliths; however, Burmese, Himalayan, and Persian breeds have a greater prevalence of calcium oxalate uroliths. Cats that form uroliths typically have concentrated urine with altered pH (either too alkaline or too acidic). Cats with uroliths may be asymptomatic or may present with signs of lower urinary tract disease or urethral obstruction. Spontaneous reabsorption of uroliths has been documented.

Uroliths that remain in the bladder can damage the bladder lining, resulting in secondary bacterial infections and hematuria. Small uroliths that become lodged in the outflow tract present a special problem. As urine flow out of the bladder stops, the bladder distends with urine. This results in a backup of urine through the ureter and into the kidney, virtually halting renal filtration and urine production. The cat becomes azotemic within 24 hours, and clinical signs relating to this begin to be evident at this time. If the obstruction to urine flow is not relieved within 3 to 6 days, the cat will die.

This section focuses on struvite uroliths because they are the most commonly seen type. Refer to medical texts for treatment of other types of uroliths.

CLINICAL SIGNS
- Signs depend on the degree of trauma and whether urinary obstruction is present.
- Some cats with bladder or renal uroliths may be asymptomatic. However, clinical signs include the following:
  - Hematuria
  - Dysuria
  - Urinating in strange places
  - Straining to pass urine (owners may report the cat is constipated)
  - Vomiting
  - Collapse, death

DIAGNOSIS
- Radiology may show uroliths on routine films.
- If there is a strong suspicion, a double-contrast study should be done.
- Ultrasonography locates the position of uroliths in the urinary tract.

- An analysis of the uroliths is critical for proper treatment.
- Small uroliths may be collected by catheter while obtaining a urine sample.

TREATMENT
Medical
- Struvite uroliths can be treated by inducing their dissolution. By feeding a diet that reduces urine pH to 6 to 6.3 and that is low in magnesium (Prescription Diet Feline s/d), uroliths will dissolve. This type of diet may also prevent the recurrence of these uroliths.
- Dissolution is usually completed in 4 to 8 weeks. Animals should be examined radiographically every 2 to 4 weeks to monitor the dissolution process. Continue the diet for 1 month after all uroliths have disappeared.
- Antibiotic treatment helps prevent secondary bacterial infections that may occur in traumatized tissues.

Surgical
- Consider surgery for uroliths that do not resolve with diet.
- Postsurgical radiographs should be taken to ensure that all uroliths have been removed.

TREATMENT (FOR OBSTRUCTIVE UROLITHS)
Medical
- Uroliths must be retrograded back into the bladder or removed from the urethra. Using a well-lubricated, open-end feline catheter, which has been atraumatically inserted in the urethra (under sterile technique), and a saline or lactated Ringer solution, gently propel the urolith back toward the bladder. This reestablishes urine flow and allows time for further medical management (Fig. 12-6).
- Dietary dissolution: Diets low in magnesium, which promote a urine pH of 6 to 6.3, are recommended for dissolution of struvite uroliths (Prescription Diet Feline s/d). Dissolution may take 4 to 8 weeks. Follow progress with radiographs taken every 2 to 4 weeks. Continue diet for 1 month after uroliths disappear from the radiographs.
- Antibiotics should be used to prevent secondary bacterial infections in the already traumatized

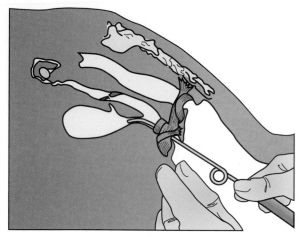

Figure 12-6 Introducing a urethral catheter into a female cat.

urinary tract. Choice may be empirical or based on culture and sensitivity results.
- Monitor the animal's urine flow daily, because reobstruction may occur.
- Monitor the ECG and potassium levels in cats that have been obstructed for several days.
- Post-obstruction diuresis can occur in some cats—monitor the fluid input and urine output carefully in these cats to prevent dehydration.

Surgical
- Surgery (perineal urethrostomy with or without cystotomy) should be performed if uroliths cannot be removed from the urethra or dissolution does not occur. Owners should be advised of the risks associated with perineal urethrostomies (increased bladder infections, strictures). A cystotomy may be needed to remove the uroliths in the bladder.

INFORMATION FOR CLIENTS
- If the uroliths do not dissolve, surgery is required.
- Feed the cat the prescription diet exclusively. *Avoid giving treats or table food!*
- Medical treatment requires periodic monitoring by radiography and urinalysis.
- Canned food provides more dietary water, and hence more dilute urine.
- Antibiotics may be needed for the long term in certain cats.

- Long-term effects from a perineal urethrostomy may include a greater susceptibility to bacterial cystitis and strictures.
- A veterinarian should examine the cat that seems "constipated" as soon as possible.

Feline Urethral Plugs

The same factors associated with the formation of uroliths are risk factors identified in urethral plug formation in the cat. Plugs contain varying quantities of minerals in proportion to large amounts of matrix. The matrix is a mucoprotein associated with a local host defense mechanism in the urinary tract. Plugs may also contain RBCs, WBCs, epithelial cells, bacteria, and spermatozoa.

CLINICAL SIGNS
- Straining to urinate; cat may be crying or just spending excessive time in the litter box (seen more frequently in male cats)
- Vomiting
- Dehydration
- Collapse (subsequent death within 3 to 6 days)

DIAGNOSIS
- Diagnosis is the same as for other causes of urethral obstruction.
- Bladder is enlarged and firm on palpation.
- There is a history of straining or no urine production.
- Radiographs show enlarged bladder.
- Serum chemistries demonstrate increases in blood urea nitrogen (BUN), creatinine, potassium, phosphate, and calcium. (Levels measured depend on length of time urine flow has been obstructed.)
- Manual restraint alone or in combination with anesthetics may be used. Propofol, isoflurane, or short-acting barbiturates may be used.

TREATMENT
- Stepwise attempt to relieve the obstruction is recommended:
  - Gently massage the urethra, using the thumb and forefinger, to break up the plug. (This technique is rarely successful.)
  - Gently attempt to compress the bladder to force the plug out of the urethra. (This technique almost never works when used alone.)

- Back-flush the urethra with sterile saline or lactated Ringer solution.
- Periodically reevaluate the patency of the urethra because reobstruction may occur.
- Avoid the use of indwelling catheters because they further traumatize the bladder and urethra and provide an introductory route for ascending bacterial infections. If these must be used, make sure that you use a soft, nontraumatic catheter that is connected to a closed, sterile drainage system (see Fig. 12-4).
- Surgery: Perineal urethrostomy may be attempted if the obstruction cannot be removed.

⊙ TECH ALERT

Reestablish urethral patency!

⊙ TECH ALERT

If anesthetic drugs are used, remember that doses less than those recommended are required in azotemic cats.

⊙ TECH ALERT

Exercise caution with these techniques. You can easily rupture a distended bladder.

Cystocentesis, when properly performed, reduces the back pressure on the plug in the urethra, allowing it to be hydropulsed into the bladder. Cystocentesis also provides the technician with a sample suitable for urinalysis and culture and sensitivity.

Urolithiasis (Canine)

A small incidence of urolithiasis occurs in the dog. Several studies indicate a prevalence of less than 1%. In the dog, the most common type of urolith is composed of magnesium ammonium phosphate, whereas calcium oxalate, urate, cystine, and calcium phosphate uroliths occur less frequently (see Fig. 12-5).

Uroliths form in urine supersaturated with specific substances (minerals). Many researchers think that minerals precipitate from the urine after formation of a crystal nidus or center. Once the nidus has formed,

mineral continues to be deposited around it forming a "stone" or urolith. This process may be complete in as little as a few days to as long as several weeks.

After formation, uroliths may pass out of the urinary tract, continue to grow in the tract, dissolve, or become inactive. The sequelae of those that remain within the urinary tract can include dysuria, infection, partial or complete obstruction, and polyp formation.

Urinary tract infection is common in dogs with urolithiasis. Uroliths mechanically disrupt the mucosal lining of the tract, opening it to bacterial colonization and partially disrupting bladder emptying. Small uroliths can become lodged in the penile urethra of the male dog, and slightly larger ones can block the female urethra. Complete obstruction to urine outflow can quickly result in destruction of renal parenchyma and uremia.

Common Types of Canine Uroliths

Struvite (Magnesium Ammonium Phosphate)

No specific breed predilection for struvite uroliths has been demonstrated; however, approximately 80% of dogs with struvite uroliths are female between the ages of 3 and 8 years. Alkaline urine, urease-producing bacteria, and dietary minerals facilitate the formation of this type of urolith. These stones are radiopaque, smooth or speculated and are often pyramidal in shape. Stones larger than 10 cm are almost always struvite.

Treatment includes long-term antibiotics (until radiography demonstrates absence of uroliths); urine acidification using dietary management and dietary restriction of urea, phosphorus, and magnesium (s/d diet). Use of the prescription s/d diet results in the dissolution of struvite uroliths within approximately 1 to 3 months. Dietary modification and long-term use of prophylactic antibiotics may prevent recurrence.

Calcium Oxalate

Calcium oxalate uroliths occur primarily in male dogs between the ages of 5 and 12 years. Veterinarians are seeing an increase in the number of cases involving this type of urolith because of the frequent use of medical protocols to dissolve struvite, urate, and cystine uroliths. The increased rate of oxalate uroliths may also be related to diets high in animal protein.

Hypercalcemia is a significant finding in dogs with calcium oxalate uroliths. Studies of dogs that experience development of calcium oxalate crystals also show the presence of a structural abnormality in the urine protein, *nephrocalcin*, which is necessary for inhibition of calcium oxalate crystal growth.

These stones are radiopaque, have sharp projections and may be mulberry shaped. Commonly there are multiple small stones in the bladder.

Currently, surgical removal is the only means of removing calcium oxalate uroliths. Prevention should be aimed at reducing serum calcium levels, reducing dietary calcium and oxalate (milk products), and restricting dietary sodium. Diets such as Hill's Prescription u/d, which are moderately protein restricted (and low in calcium, sodium, and oxalate), are available. Other choices include Hill's Prescription Canine w/d and k/d diets.

Urates (Ammonium Urates and Others)

Uric acid is one of several biologic products of purine nucleotide metabolism. Ammonium urate is a salt of this acid and accounts for most of the purine uroliths in the dog.

Dalmatian dogs are predisposed to urate uroliths. The hepatic and renal metabolic pathways in this breed result in a secretion of excess uric acid from the kidneys (two to four times that found in non-Dalmatian breeds). This excess predisposes the breed to urate uroliths. Other breeds with an increased incidence include the English Bulldog, Miniature Schnauzer, Shih Tzus, and Yorkshire Terriers. Most of the dogs affected are male between the ages of 3 and 6 years. Research suggests that prolonged use of severely restricted protein diets in non-Dalmatian dogs may be responsible for urate urolith formation. These are radiolucent stones that are smooth and often yellow-green in color.

Treatment includes use of dietary management to dissolve the uroliths (Hill's Prescription Diet u/d), Waltham s/o Lower Urinary Tract Support Diet, allopurinol (15 mg/kg every 12 hours) to decrease uric acid production, alkalinization of the urine with sodium bicarbonate or potassium citrate (pH 7.0), and control of concurrent bacterial infection in the urinary tract.

CLINICAL SIGNS (STRUVITE UROLITHS)

- Dysuria
- Hematuria

DIAGNOSIS

- Urinalysis will show crystalluria, hematuria, increased protein, and increased numbers of bacteria.
- Radiography can be used to verify the number, location, and size of uroliths. Double-contrast studies can be used to visualize some uroliths (urates). Radiography may miss uroliths smaller than 3 mm.
- Serum chemistry may indicate metabolic abnormalities underlying urolith formation.
- Stone analysis is important for formulating treatment plans; commercial laboratories are available for stone analysis, or one can "guesstimate" the stone type based on several criteria (Table 12-1).

TREATMENT

Medical

- Treatment must be aimed at decreasing urine saturation, increasing the solubility of crystalline material in the urine, and increasing urine volume:
  - Change diet to decrease solids in the urine.
  - Promote acid urine.
  - Induce diuresis.
- Provide antibiotics for infection.

Surgical

- Remove uroliths not manageable with medical treatment or in patients with severe infections.
- The cause of urolith formation must be addressed medically.

Nonsurgical

- A catheter can be used to remove small uroliths.
- Urohydropulsion, or digital pressure on the bladder of an anesthetized dog, may propulse small stones through the urethra.

INFORMATION FOR CLIENTS

- A special diet may be needed throughout the dog's life.
- Table scraps and treats should be limited.
- Long-term antibiotics may be necessary to control the urinary tract infection.

TABLE 12-1 Predicting Mineral Composition of Uroliths

	PREDICTORS					PREDICTORS				
Mineral Type	Urine Ph	Crystal Appearance	Urine Culture	Radiographic Density	Radiographic Contour	Serum Abnormalities	Breed Predisposition	Sex Predisposition	Common Ages	
Magnesium ammonium phosphate	Neutral to alkaline	4 to 6 sided colorless prisms	Urease-producing bacteria (*Staphylococcus, Proteus, Enterococcus, Mycoplasma*)	+ to ++++	Smooth, round, or faceted; may assume shape of bladder or urethra	None	Miniature Schnauzer, Bichon Frise, Cocker Spaniel	Females (>80%)	2-8 yr or younger	
Calcium oxalate	Acid to neutral	Dihydrate salt, colorless envelope or octahedral shape; monohydrate salt-spindles or dumbbell shape	Negative	++ to ++++	Rough or speculated (dehydrate salt); small, smooth, round (monohydrate salt); sometimes jackstone	Occasional hypercalcemia	Miniature Schnauzer, Lhasa Apso, Yorkshire Terrier, Miniature Poodle, Shih Tzu, Bichon Frise	Males (>70%)	5-12 yr	
Urate	Acid to neutral	Yellow-brown amorphous shapes or sphericals (ammonium urate)	Negative	+ to ++	Smooth, round, or oval	Low urea nitrogen and serum albumin in dogs with hepatic portal systemic shunts	Dalmatian, English Bulldog, Miniature Schnauzer, Yorkshire Terrier	Males (>85%)	1-4 yr	
Calcium phosphate	Alkaline to neutral (brushite forms in acidic urine)	Amorphous, or long, thin prisms	Negative	++ to ++++	Smooth, round, or faceted	Occasional hypercalcemia	Yorkshire Terrier, Miniature Schnauzer, Cocker Spaniel	Males (>60%)	7-11 yr	
Cystine	Acid to neutral	Flat, colorless, hexagonal plates	Negative	+ to ++	Smooth to slightly irregular, round to oval	None	English Bulldog, Dachshund, Basset Hound	Males (>90%)	1-8 yr	
Silica	Acid to neutral	None observed	Negative	++ to ++++	Round center with radial spokelike projections (jackstone)	None	German Shepherd, Golden Retriever, Labrador Retriever, Miniature Schnauzer	Males (>90%)	9 yr	

+, Low radiographic density; ++, moderate radiographic density; +++, high radiographic density; ++++, high radiographic density (opaque); −, radiolucent (not visible).
From Ettinger SJ, Feldman EC: *Textbook of veterinary internal medicine*, ed 5, Philadelphia, PA, 2000, Saunders, by permission.

- Uroliths may recur at any time.
- Follow-up laboratory tests and radiography are required to monitor medical dissolution of uroliths.

Renal Failure

Renal failure is one of the most commonly seen diseases in veterinary medicine. The unique structure of the kidney and its job of filtration and waste management within the body predispose the kidney to numerous insults throughout the life of the animal. Approximately 20% of the total cardiac output passes through the kidney at any time. The content of this blood is filtered through the glomerular capillary membrane, removing small molecules, electrolytes, drugs, and other materials. These substances become the glomerular filtrate, which enters the proximal convoluted tubule, the nephron loop, and the distal convoluted tubule before leaving the kidney by way of the collecting duct, the renal pelvis, and the ureter. The tubules reabsorb water and other substances necessary to maintain bodily functions. Waste materials are excreted. The resulting product, urine, leaves the kidney to be stored in the bladder for elimination from the body. A reduction in blood flow to the nephron (hypoperfusion) or damage to the nephron unit itself may result in renal failure. Renal failure may be *acute* or *chronic*. In both types of failure, the nephron unit is damaged and glomerular filtration declines, resulting in *azotemia*, a buildup of toxins within the body. The azotemia produces the clinical symptoms of renal failure.

Acute Renal Failure

Acute renal failure refers to an *abrupt* decrease in glomerular filtration, causing azotemia. This is usually the result of hypoperfusion or nephrotoxic injury to the kidney, which causes damage to the proximal convoluted tubular cells or those of the ascending nephron loop. Nephrotoxic drugs such as the aminoglycosides (gentamicin, streptomycin, amikacin), cephalosporins (cephalexin, cephalothin), the sulfonamides (Albon, Di-Trim, Primor), chemotherapeutic agents, antifungal medications, some analgesics (acetaminophen), and anesthetics (methoxyflurane [Metofane]) may produce acute renal failure if used for prolonged periods or at high doses. The most common nontherapeutic agents

that produce renal damage include ethylene glycol (antifreeze), heavy metals, and hemoglobin. Infections, immune-mediated diseases, and hypercalcemia have also been implicated as causes of acute renal failure in both humans and animals.

Nephrotoxic injury may affect any portion of the nephron; when one section is damaged, the entire unit is lost. Destroyed nephrons cannot be replaced by the body, but other nephron units have the ability to hypertrophy (enlarge) in an attempt to maintain normal renal function. Acute renal failure occurs in three distinct phases: (1) induction—the time from the initial insult until decreased renal function is apparent; (2) maintenance—the period during which renal tubular damage occurs; and (3) recovery—the time during which renal function improves, existing nephrons hypertrophy and compensate for those damaged, and tubular repair occurs (when possible).

Risk factors for acute renal failure include disorders that affect renal perfusion (shock, hypovolemia, hypotension, dehydration), electrolyte (potassium, calcium, sodium) disturbances, administration of nephrotoxic drugs, systemic diseases, and increased age. Technicians should be alert to these risk factors when monitoring animals under anesthesia, animals with trauma, and older animals with systemic diseases. Every effort should be made to normalize blood flow through the kidney and avoid prolonged periods of hypotension, hypovolemia, or both. Careful monitoring of pulse quality, hydration status, packed cell volume, total solids, and body weight make it possible to observe early changes that may suggest the development of acute renal failure. Early intervention may prevent permanent damage to the kidneys.

Signs of acute renal failure are often nonspecific. Patients may present with a variety of symptoms, but a thorough history would pinpoint a recent ischemic episode or toxin exposure. The kidneys are enlarged and painful on palpation, and the patient may be exhibiting signs of azotemia such as anorexia, vomiting, diarrhea, and weakness. Laboratory tests indicate active urine sediment, normal to increased hematocrit, acidosis, and normal to increased potassium levels. BUN and creatinine levels may be increased. Patients may be oliguric (passing decreased amounts of urine) or polyuric (passing increased amounts of urine).

Treatment is aimed at restoring renal hemodynamics, relieving any tubular obstruction, discontinuing any potentially nephrotoxic drugs, and promoting cellular repair. Intravenous fluid therapy (with isotonic saline being the initial fluid of choice) is the hallmark of therapy for acute renal failure. Correction of acid–base imbalances and control of hyperphosphatemia, hyperkalemia, and gastroenteritis is also necessary. Although treatment may not restore renal function to previous levels, it will improve the clinical picture, make the animal feel better, and give the kidney time to heal.

The prognosis for acute renal failure in veterinary patients is guarded and is related to the severity of the azotemia. Animals with nephrotoxic injuries have a slightly better prognosis than those with hypoperfusion injury. Older animals have a less favorable prognosis compared with younger animals.

Great care should be taken to protect animals at risk for development of acute renal failure. With careful monitoring, early recognition, and aggressive therapy, renal damage can be kept to a minimum in many animals.

CLINICAL SIGNS

- Oliguria, polyuria
- Fever (if infectious)
- Kidneys painful on palpation
- Vomiting and diarrhea
- Anorexia
- Dehydration

DIAGNOSIS

- Physical examination
- History of ischemic episode or toxin exposure
- Urinalysis—active sediment, casts
- Blood chemistries—increased packed cell volume; increased BUN and creatinine levels; increased potassium, phosphorus, acidosis

TREATMENT

- Dietary modifications: diets especially designed for renal disease
- Intravenous fluid therapy—initial choice is isotonic saline

- Discontinue potentially nephrotoxic drugs
- Intestinal protectants:
  - Metoclopramide: intravenously (IV), intramuscularly (IM), PO every 6 to 8 hours
  - Cimetidine: IV every 8 to 12 hours
  - Sucralfate: PO every 6 to 8 hours
- Phosphate binders, if necessary: Maalox, Amphojel
- Sodium bicarbonate—body weight (in kg) $\times$ 0.3 $\times$ base deficit (mEq/L) = mEq of bicarbonate; give half IV slowly over 15 to 30 minutes
- Diuretics:
  - Dopamine: IV
  - Furosemide: IV every 8 hours
  - Mannitol (20%): IV slowly over 15 to 20 minutes

INFORMATION FOR CLIENTS

- Although renal function may be improved with treatment, it may never return to completely normal levels.
- The prognosis for this disease is guarded.
- The underlying condition responsible for the acute renal failure may require long-term management.
- Care must be taken to avoid events that would precipitate further damage to the kidneys. Appropriate diet and water access must be assured for these pets.

Chronic Renal Failure

CRF is a common disease of older pets. It represents an irreversible and progressive decline in renal function caused by destruction of the nephron units. The course of the disease may be months to years, with clinical signs appearing when nephron loss reaches levels that result in the development of azotemia. The incidence of disease is higher in older animals (dogs >8 years, cats >10 years), but it can be seen in animals of any age. CRF may be congenital, familial, or acquired in origin. Cats appear to be more affected than dogs, with an increased frequency of disease seen in Maine Coon, Abyssinian, Siamese, Russian Blue, and Burmese breeds. Whatever the cause, the irreversible destruction of the nephron results in uremia and its related clinical symptoms.

One of the most frequently seen signs of uremia is gastrointestinal upset—anorexia, weight loss, vomiting, diarrhea, constipation, and stomatitis (oral ulceration).

Unfortunately, owners do not often associate these signs with renal disease, and pets go undiagnosed until symptoms become severe.

As the kidneys lose their ability to concentrate urine, signs of polydipsia, polyuria, and nocturia may develop. This loss of concentrating ability is the result of impairment of (ADH) response, disruption of the countercurrent mechanism and renal tubular epithelium, together with the increased solute load passing through the remaining nephrons.

Other signs of CRF include arterial hypertension, nervous system dysfunction (dullness, lethargy, tremors, seizures), scleral injection, retinal lesions, and acute blindness. An increased tendency for bruising may also be seen. Most animals with moderate to advanced CRF are anemic because of a decreased level of the hormone erythropoietin, which is produced by the kidney. The severity and progression of the anemia correlate well with the degree of renal failure. Metabolic imbalances also produce hyperphosphatemia (decreased excretion), hypokalemia (increased secretion, especially in cats), proteinuria, and metabolic acidosis.

Therapy should be individualized on the basis of an animal's needs. Owners should be informed that the loss of renal function is permanent and progressive. The prognosis for CRF is poor. Treatment is aimed at correcting metabolic imbalances and minimizing clinical symptoms. General goals of treatment are to decrease the dietary protein intake while maintaining adequate caloric intake, provide relief of nausea and vomiting through the use of H_2-receptor antagonists such as cimetidine or ranitidine, correct the hypokalemia with oral potassium therapy, and avoid dehydration by giving subcutaneous or intravenous fluids. Phosphorous binding agents such as aluminum hydroxide (Amphojel) may be used to control hyperphosphatemia.

In cases in which systemic hypertension is compromising kidney function, therapy with angiotensen-converting enzyme (ACE) inhibitors (enalapril), β-adrenergic antagonists (propranolol), or calcium channel blockers (diltiazem) may improve renal function. Loop diuretics (furosemide) may be used to reduce blood pressure by reducing body fluid loads.

Epoetin (Epogen), a replacement erythropoietin, may be given to correct the anemia. Some clinicians have suggested using calcitriol to decrease parathyroid hormone levels and thereby normalize calcium and phosphorus balance, but studies indicate that the risks of using calcitriol outweigh the benefits, and its use is no longer suggested in CRF.

It should be stressed to owners that all these treatments only *limit* or *slow* the progression of this disease. The condition is fatal.

CLINICAL SIGNS

- Dullness, lethargy
- Weakness
- Weight loss
- Anorexia
- Vomiting, diarrhea (constipation in cats) or both
- Polyuria or polydipsia
- Gait disturbances: cervical ventriflexion in cats
- Sudden blindness

DIAGNOSIS

- Acidosis
- Anemia
- Increases in BUN, creatinine
- Hyperphosphatemia
- Hypercalcemia or hypocalcemia
- Hypokalemia
- Proteinuria

TREATMENT

- Treatment should be aimed at supportive care and correction of imbalances (dehydration, electrolytes, metabolic acidosis, gastrointestinal symptoms)
- Provide fluids IV or SQ for dehydration: suggested fluids include a mixture of two parts D_5W (5% dextrose in water) and one part lactated Ringer solution (by volume) supplemented with potassium, as needed; owners can be instructed in how to give subcutaneous fluids at home (two to three times weekly or as needed to maintain hydration)
- Potassium gluconate (Tumil-K or Kaon Elixir): daily
- Phosphorous binders: aluminum hydroxide PO once to three times a day with meals
- Calcium carbonate (for hypocalcemia): PO daily

- Sodium bicarbonate: every 8 to 12 hours (A solution can be prepared that contains 80 mg/mL by adding one third of an 8-ounce box of sodium bicarbonate to 1 quart of water.); store in the refrigerator and give PO
- Cimetidine: PO, IM, IV three to four times a day
- Ranitidine: PO twice a day
- Sucralfate: 0.5 to 1 tablet (dogs); 0.25 to 0.5 tablet PO every 8 hours (cats)
- ACE inhibitors
- Enalapril: PO every 12 to 24 hours
- Calcium channel blockers
- Diltiazem: PO every 8 to 12 hours (dogs); PO every 8 to 12 hours (cats)
- α-Adrenergic antagonist
- Propranolol: PO two to three times a day (dogs); PO two to three times a day (cats)
- Diuretics
- Furosemide: PO every 8 to 12 hours
- Hormones
- Epoetin: SQ three times weekly
- Calcitriol: PO once daily (no longer recommended)
- Vitamin B supplements

Diets lower in protein and sodium have been suggested to slow the progression of CRF; however, studies have shown patients may benefit from diets low in protein and phosphate, with the addition of omega-3 fatty acids, potassium, and antioxidants. If the BUN values are greater than 75 mg/dL, then protein restriction is suggested to reduce nonrenal toxicities.

INFORMATION FOR CLIENTS

- CRF is a progressive, irreversible disease.
- Treatment is aimed at *slowing* the progression and relieving clinical symptoms.
- Treatment with subcutaneous fluids at home is required to maintain the pet's hydration. You will be instructed in how to give the fluids.
- You can improve the palatability of renal diets by warming foods and adding tasty liquids such as tuna oil, clam juice, or broth. You should limit foods that contain high levels of salt.
- Eventually, your pet will experience a decrease in its quality of life. You may have to consider euthanasia.

Urinary Incontinence

Urinary incontinence is frequently reported by clients, especially when older pets are involved. Urinary incontinence can be defined as the loss of voluntary control of micturition. It occurs for a variety of reasons, and treatment should be based on an accurate diagnosis. In dogs and cats, urethral closure is not accomplished by a single anatomic sphincter, but is primarily the result of smooth muscle tone along the entire urethra in female dogs and along the proximal fourth of the urethra in male dogs. When the urethral closure pressure is greater than the bladder pressure, urine remains stored in the bladder until voluntary urination occurs. When bladder pressure increases above urethral closure pressure, incontinence occurs. Other types of incontinence include neurogenic incontinence, nonneurogenic incontinence, paradoxical incontinence, and miscellaneous incontinence.

Neurogenic incontinence may be seen in animals with spinal cord disease or trauma. Intervertebral disk disease, vertebral fractures, inflammation, or neoplasia of the spinal cord may disrupt normal neural function to this region of the urinary system, resulting in a paralytic bladder. In these animals, the bladder overdistends with urine, increasing intravesical urine pressure and resulting in dribbling of urine.

Nonneurogenic causes of incontinence include congenital abnormalities such as ectopic ureters, patient urachus (seen in younger animals), endocrine imbalances after ovariohysterectomy (estrogen deficiency), urethral sphincter mechanism (degenerative changes, urinary surgery), and hypercontractile bladder.

Paradoxic incontinence occurs in patients with partial obstruction of the urethra. This situation is encountered most frequently in male dogs. The bladder becomes overdistended with urine, which cannot pass because of some type of obstruction, increasing the intravesical pressure above that of the urethra and causing incontinence.

Miscellaneous causes can include primary diseases of the bladder, which result in replacement of normal bladder wall smooth muscle tissue with fibrous or neoplastic tissue. Classification of urinary incontinence is shown in Table 12-2.

TABLE 12-2   Classification of Urinary Incontinence

Type	Normal Micturition	Involuntary Dribbling of Urine	Overdistended Bladder	Small, Contracted Bladder	Ability to Catheterize Bladder
Neurogenic	Absent	Present	Present	Absent	Easy
Nonneurogenic	Present	Present	Absent	Absent	Easy
Paradoxic	Absent	Present	Present	Absent	Difficult
Miscellaneous	Absent	Present	Absent	Present	Variable

From Osbome CA, Low DG, Finco DR: *Canine and feline urology*, Philadelphia, PA, 1972, Saunders, by permission.

CLINICAL SIGNS

- Owner reports urine leakage when the pet is sleeping or exercising.
- Perineal area of pet is always wet.
- Signs of concurrent urinary tract disease are present.
- Older spayed female dogs and noncastrated male dogs are predisposed to this condition.

DIAGNOSIS

- Urinalysis
- Radiology or cystography
- Serum chemistries to rule out polyuria from endocrine disease

TREATMENT

- Treatment should be based on determination of a specific cause.

Endocrine Imbalance in Spayed Female Dogs
- Diethylstilbestrol: once daily by mouth for 3 to 5 days, weekly

Urethral Sphincter Hypotonus
- Phenylpropanolamine (Propagest, Prop-in): PO every 8 hours
- Propagest may be used with testosterone in male dogs with incontinence.

TECH ALERT

Avoid use of phenylpropanolamine in animals with glaucoma, hypertension, diabetes mellitus, and prostatic hypertrophy.

Hypercontractile Bladder
- Propantheline (Pro-Banthine, Roberts): PO every 8 to 12 hours (dogs); PO every 24 to 72 hours (cats)
- Oxybutynin (Ditropan): PO every 8 to 12 hours (small dogs, cats); PO every 12 hours (large dogs)

TECH ALERT

Side effects from anticholinergic medications include sedation, ileus, vomiting, constipation, dry mouth, dry eyes, and tachycardia. Their use is contraindicated in patients with glaucoma.

INFORMATION FOR CLIENTS

- A complete physical and laboratory workup is needed to diagnose the specific cause of your pet's incontinence.
- Medication doses may need to be adjusted to achieve success in stopping the incontinence.
- Drugs used to treat incontinence cannot be used in pets that have other health problems such as glaucoma, diabetes mellitus, hyperthyroidism, or cardiac disease.
- If the incontinence is due to trauma or inflammation, it may correct itself with time.
- If the incontinence is due to paralytic bladder, you may need to catheterize your pet several times daily or manually express the bladder to prevent overfilling.

Disease of the Prostate

The prostate is the only accessory sex gland in the male dog. It is an oval, bi-lobed gland that surrounds the urethra on the pelvic floor. The gland constantly produces prostatic secretions which flow into the urethra and represent a major contribution to the male's ejaculate. The gland enlarges throughout the life of the dog in response to the presence of androgens. Therefore, prostatic disease is a problem found only in noncastrated male dogs.

Benign Prostatic Hyperplasia

This problem occurs in noncastrated male dogs. The disease is common in male dogs over 5 years of age. As the prostate hypertrophies it puts pressure on the prostatic urethra which results in obstruction to urine flow and, in advanced stages, compresses the colon making defecation more difficult. Palpation of the prostate reveals bilateral, symmetrical enlargement that is non-painful. The enlarged prostate is at an increased risk for infection or cyst formation.

Therapy is aimed at reducing the size of the prostate to alleviate clinical signs of the disease. Castration will result in a rapid decrease in the size of the prostate (75% decrease in 3 months).

CLINICAL SIGNS

- Difficult defecation
- Difficulty in urinating—multiple attempts with small volumes
- Hematuria, dysuria
- Serosanguinous discharge from the penis not related to urination

DIAGNOSIS

- Rectal palpation
- Radiography shows enlarged prostate; ultrasonography may demonstrate cysts or abscesses
- Prostatic biopsy

TREATMENT

- Castration is the ideal treatment for this condition.
- In dogs used for breeding the condition may be treated with medications that "chemically castrate" the dog. This castration is reversible.
  - Finasteride (Proscar, Merck)
  - Osaterone acetate (Ypozane, Virbac)
  - Gestagens (synthetic progesterones)
  - Estrogens
  - GnRH (gonadrophin-releasing hormone)

- Antibiotics use is based on culture and sensitivity testing of the prostatic fluid.

INFORMATION FOR CLIENTS

- Castration of the male dog will prevent or treat BPH entirely, no matter the age of the animal.
- Prostatic neoplasia can occur in the noncastrated male.

REVIEW QUESTIONS

1. Urine removed from the bladder by cystocentesis should contain _____ microorganisms.
   a. 0–100/hpf
   b. 200–500/hpf
   c. No
   d. 500–1000/hpf
2. Long-term antibiotic therapy for cystitis should be based on:
   a. Culture and sensitivity results
   b. Finding bacteria on sediment examination
   c. Resolution of clinical signs
   d. Absence of bacteria in posttreatment urine sediments
   e. All of the above
3. Urethral plugs are made largely of _____.
   a. Small concretions of minerals and large amounts of matrix
   b. Large concretions of minerals and small amounts of matrix
   c. White cells with a large amount of matrix
4. The two most common types of uroliths seen in the dog are:
   a. Urates
   b. Calcium oxalate
   c. Magnesium ammonium phosphate
   d. Cystine
5. Which of the following uroliths is not radiopaque?
   a. Cystine
   b. Calcium oxalate
   c. Magnesium ammonium phosphate
   d. Urate
6. Which of the following drugs is nephrotoxic?
   a. Amikacin
   b. Aspirin
   c. Amoxicillin
   d. Enrofloxacin (Baytril)

7. In cats that present with the gait disturbance of cervical ventriflexion, which electrolyte needs to be checked?
   a. Sodium
   b. Potassium
   c. Calcium
   d. Magnesium

8. Older surgical veterinary patients should be provided intravenous fluids during surgery to prevent _____, which can cause acute renal failure.
   a. Dehydration
   b. Hypotension
   c. Electrolyte disturbances
   d. All of the above

9. Which of the following laboratory values can be increased because of diet?
   a. Blood urea nitrogen
   b. Creatinine
   c. Alanine aminotransferase
   d. Alkaline phosphatase

10. Urethral closure in the female dog is primarily related to:
   a. The external urethral sphincter
   b. The internal urethral sphincter
   c. The smooth muscle surrounding the entire urethra
   d. The smooth muscle surrounding the proximal half of the urethra

11. A bladder stone is 15 cm in diameter. It is most likely a _____ stone.
   a. Urate
   b. Oxalate
   c. Purine
   d. Struvite

12. Diets high in animal protein may predispose the dog to what type of bladder stone?
   a. Urate
   b. Oxalate
   c. Struvite
   d. Purine

13. The fluid of choice for acute renal failure patients is _____.
   a. Lactated Ringers
   b. Half-strength saline
   c. Normal saline
   d. Ringers

Answers found on page 553.

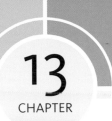

13
CHAPTER

Overview of Ferrets, Rodents, and Rabbits

LEARNING OBJECTIVES

When you have completed this chapter, you will be able to:
1. Recognize commonly kept pocket pets and breeds of rabbits.
2. Discuss husbandry of these pets with new owners.
3. Handle these pets in the exam room with more confidence.

The Ferret

The name *ferret* can be loosely translated to mean "mouse-killing, smelly, thief" (*Mustela putorius furo*), and, surely, these small bundles of energy and play are smelly. Yet they make good pets for adults and families without small children. Ferrets are generally clean, quiet, and playful, and they love interacting with humans. They have been used for many purposes other than as pets: They hunt rabbits and rodents; they run cable through pipes; they have been used in biomedical research; and more frequently, they have become house pets. The popularity of ferrets has increased in the past few decades, and although it is illegal in many states to keep them as pets, they make a good alternative pet for those unable to have a dog, cat, or other mammal.

Anatomy

Ferrets have long bodies with short legs, allowing them to get into and out of tight tubular spaces. Their spine is very flexible. Male ferrets are usually about twice the size of female ferrets. Ferrets are monogastric animals whose organ arrangement is similar to that of the cat. The coat of the ferret is soft and exists in many color variations (at least 30 colors are recognized). They molt in the spring and fall as their weight changes (increase in the fall and decrease in the summer). Molting can be related to season and to ovulation. The skin should have a smooth appearance. Ferrets have no sweat glands, but they do have active sebaceous glands that produce the characteristic body odor. Ferrets have well-developed anal glands that produce a serous yellow liquid with a powerful odor. As with skunks, ferrets that are threatened or frightened may expel the contents of these glands over a long distance (and usually the technician or veterinarian treating them). Removal of these glands (descenting) will help alleviate much, but not all, of the odor of the ferret.

Ferrets have good special senses and can see well in low light. They have nonretractable claws that need to be trimmed periodically. All the other organ systems are similar to those of the cat.

Behavior

Ferrets are predators, and even today their behaviors mimic those of their ancestors. They are able to live in communal groups and to interact well with humans. They engage in play, territory marking, and hunting behaviors throughout life. Play can become aggressive if not curtailed. Ferrets may scream, a noise that is quite loud and disturbing, when playing. They also love to burrow in soft materials, including carpet, furniture, and litter boxes. This can be quite destructive. They love to explore tunnel-like areas and prefer having an enclosed sleeping place. Ferrets can be taught to use a litter box, and they will never soil their sleeping quarters. They can also get into trouble by chewing on rubber items such as electric cords, toys, appliances, and rubber bands, causing intestinal upsets or obstructions. It is not uncommon for them to escape through small holes in the environment.

Housing

A ferret's environment must be "ferret proofed" before the addition of a pet. Because most ferrets do not adapt well to continuous caging, the entire play area must be made safe. This usually means closing any small holes that might provide escape, removing all rubber objects, covering the bottom of all furniture pieces to prevent burrowing, and providing a secluded area for sleeping. Ferrets can be housed in wire or wooden cages if these provide adequate ventilation. If kept outdoors, they must be protected from the sun and extreme temperatures, because they have little ability to regulate their body temperatures and can become heat stressed. Toys for ferrets include boxes, bags, plastic pipes, sleeping bags, dryer vent tubing, and burrowing pits. Owners should avoid providing any toys that contain latex rubber. Ferrets will use a litter box, but the walls of the box should be high enough to catch the urine deposited when the ferret backs up to the corner. Pelleted litter usually works better than clay or clumping litter. It is suggested that owners provide several boxes placed around the house instead of one centrally located box.

Nutrition

Ferrets are strict carnivores designed to eat whole prey. Their digestive tracts cannot handle carbohydrates and fiber well. The most common diet for pet ferrets is dry kibble. The diet should contain 30% to 35% protein (high-quality meat source) and about 15% to 20% fat. Many prepared dog and cat chows contain too much carbohydrate and plant protein, which can lead to health problems. A limited amount of soft, fresh meat or eggs can be added to the dry diet if desired. Because ferrets love sweets and will develop dietary preferences early in life, owners should be discouraged from feeding fruits, raisins, or other sweet foods to their ferrets. All ferrets should have access to clean, fresh water at all times.

The Ferret as a Patient

Most pet ferrets are accustomed to being handled and will not present a problem to the veterinarian or clinic staff; however, one should always inquire about the animal's temperament before the examination. Ferrets will bite without warning, unlike most dogs and cats. They may be scruffed by the loose skin on the neck and suspended with all four legs off the ground (Fig. 13-1), or they may be restrained much like a cat on the table for routine procedures. If the procedure is likely to be painful (e.g., drawing blood), the ferret should be scruffed and held at the hips. All ferrets should be vaccinated against rabies and canine distemper (IMRAB 3 [Merial] and Fervac-D [United

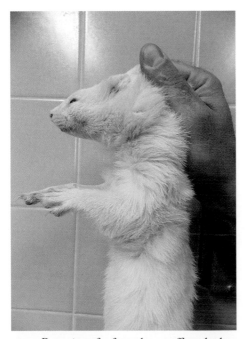

Figure 13-1 Restraint of a ferret by scruffing the loose skin on the back of the neck. (From Quesenberry KE, Carpenter JW: *Ferrets, rabbits, and rodents*, ed 3, St. Louis, MO, 2012, Saunders, by permission.)

Vaccines] or PureVax [Merial]). Anaphylactic vaccine reactions are not uncommon in ferrets, especially from the distemper vaccine, and diphenhydramine, epinephrine, or corticosteroids should be used if a reaction occurs.

Rodents

Many homes have rodents, however they are not pests, but are pets. Pocket pets (mice, rats, gerbils, hamsters) are fairly inexpensive, easy to care for, and easy to handle for both children and adults. Veterinary care for these pets has lagged behind their popularity because many veterinarians are not familiar with their diseases and have not gained the confidence to handle them. Several examples in the literature refer to veterinary staff learning the "rodent etiquette" required to be successful with this population of pet owners.

"Rodent Etiquette" or "How to Make Your Rodent Pets Feel at Home in Your Clinic"

Just like humans who do not get enough sleep, rodents can become irritable if they are disturbed during their normal hours of rest. Hamsters and rats are nocturnal and sleep during the day when most veterinary clinics see patients. Gerbils and mice can be active during both the day and night. By trying to schedule the patient's appointment at a time they would normally be awake, the veterinary staff may find a happier patient, one that is less likely to bite or become aggressive.

Owners should be instructed to bring the animal to the clinic in its cage and not to clean the cage before the appointment. In this way the veterinarian can assess the care being provided to the pet and the environment in which the pet lives. Many times, these clues can help to determine the problem.

It might be best to avoid making rodent appointments when the waiting room is filled with cats or other natural predators. Try to schedule them when the room will be quiet and calm. A checklist would be helpful to enable the technician or receptionist to get a complete medical history from the owner before being seen by the veterinarian. It is important to also obtain an accurate weight for all small patients because it will be essential in determining the dose of medication needed for treatment.

Rodents Commonly Kept as Pets

Rats and Mice

Mice, and especially domesticated rats, make good pets; however, they may produce severe allergic reactions in some people. Because of their resemblance to the wild pest species, many people shy away from handling rats and mice. These pets have a limited life span, which may present a problem for the owners. Rats may live 2 to 3 years and mice an even shorter time. The best diet for pet rats is a laboratory chow designed specifically for rats, together with limited amounts of grains, vegetables, and fruits. Owners typically overfeed rats on junk food, resulting in obese, obnoxious pets that beg for food. Rats can be housed in a variety of cages, some with condos and luxury furniture for the comfort of the occupant. Whatever type of cage is used, it must have good ventilation because rats urinate frequently and the ammonia buildup in poorly ventilated cages can affect the health of the animal. Rats respond well at normal room temperatures but should not be left to roam the house unattended.

Hamsters

The Syrian or golden hamster is a desert-dwelling animal from Syria. These hamsters are commonly kept in plastic hamster-habit-trail cages equipped with little wheels, water bottles, and cedar shavings that are totally foreign to the animal. It is little wonder that they often become ill. Habitat-related diseases are a problem for hamsters; poor air circulation, the presence of volatile oils in bedding, and owners that keep cages too clean can all present a problem to the pet hamster. Hamsters need to stash food around their cage to feel secure. During the night, they retrieve the food and eat. Owners who constantly clean cages and remove the stored food upset the hamster and force the pet to store his food in his cheek pouches, which often become impacted. Hamsters are also susceptible to stress of poor nutrition and overhandling. Their diet should consist of a good rodent chow supplemented with grains and some plant material. They should have access to fresh water at all times, although they may drink little. In the wild, hamsters burrow to regulate body temperature and for protection; something they cannot do in plastic houses. It is not uncommon for hamster mothers to cannibalize their young when stressed.

Gerbils

Gerbils are tunnel-dwelling rodents from Mongolia. They are usually housed in a manner similar to hamsters, unfortunately. When stressed, as with handling, gerbils may experience a seizure without provocation. Gerbils do not make good pets for young children but are suitable for older children. Gerbils are active and agile, climbing and burrowing in their cages. Because gerbils are usually territorial, they should be kept singularly in their habitat. If picked up incorrectly by the tail, gerbils may slough their tail skin.

General Husbandry Information

Housing for rodents must be easy to clean, and provide good ventilation and easy access to the pet. Access to fresh water must be available at all times; water bottles can be mounted to the side of the cage. Exercise is important for these pets. Exercise wheels, tunnels, mazes, and hamster balls can provide the opportunity for both play and exercise.

Many commercially available units are designed as playgrounds for rodent pets. Pine-shaving bedding is frequently used for small rodents, but cedar shavings should be avoided; the volatile oils can be toxic to the rodent. Recycled paper products, compressed straw, citrus litter, or hardwood shavings may also be used. Sandboxes should be provided for gerbils for their bathing pleasure.

Nutrition

Because obesity is a problem common to all rodent species, a proper diet is essential for maintaining these animals. Seed diets commonly fed to these pets are high in fat and low in calcium and should not be fed as the main diet. Pelleted diets containing vitamins and minerals are available commercially for all species. Any diet should consist of a minimum of 16% protein and 4% to 5% fat. Sunflower seeds and other grains can be offered as treats.

General Anatomy and Physiology of Rodents

The word *rodent* is derived from the Latin word *rodere*, which means "to gnaw." Rodents have the dental formula 2 (incisor (I)1/1, canine (C) 0/0, molar (M) 3/3). The four incisors are open-rooted and grow continuously.

Behind the eye is the Harderian gland, which produces a secretion rich in lipid and porphyrin used to lubricate the eye and also to moderate behavior. The porphyrins produce a reddish coloration to the tears and can stain the face and feet when spread by grooming.

Most rodents are prone to heat stress because they have no sweat glands and must depend on their ears and tails for dissipation of heat.

All rodents are monogastric and herbivorous or omnivorous. They are also coprophagic; their stools contain nutrients such as B vitamins and fats. Most are unable to vomit or regurgitate.

Most rodents are spontaneous ovulators and are polyestrous. Gerbils require little water and produce a small volume of concentrated urine. Both sexes have a distinct, orangish oval area of alopecia on the midventral abdomen called a *ventral marking gland*, which is composed of sebaceous glands that are controlled by hormones. The musky secretions are often used for territorial scent marking.

Hamsters have large cheek pouches used for storing food, bedding, and often their young. The dark brown patches on the flanks are glands that play a role in scent marking and breeding. Hamsters can hibernate when temperatures drop to less than 40°F. Female hamsters are typically bigger than male hamsters.

Male mice are much larger than female mice. Male mice exhibit intermale aggression and should be housed separately unless raised together.

Handling

Proper handling is important to avoid injury to the rodent and to reduce stress. They may be scruffed by the skin on the back of the neck while resting the body against the palm of your hand (Fig. 13-2). Hamsters and gerbils have a reputation as biters, and they do not tolerate excessive restraint. When unthreatened, they can easily be picked up or scruffed. One should avoid using the tail for restraint because serious injury to the tail may occur. The tail of the mouse or rat may be used to initially grab the animal if one grabs the base of the tail and not the tail itself. They may then be scruffed. Unruly animals may be

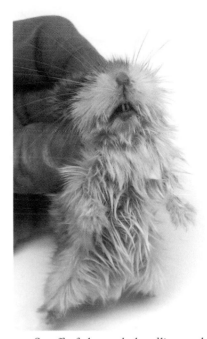

Figure 13-2 Scruff-of-the-neck handling technique in a hamster. (Courtesy of Angela Lennox, DVM. IN Quesenberry KE, Carpenter JW: *Ferrets, rabbits, and rodents*, ed 3, St Louis, 2012, Saunders, by permission)

placed into a stockinette or wrapped using a small towel.

TECH ALERT

Rodents bite! Avoid startling them, and protect your fingers when handling them.

The Rabbit

Since the Middle Ages rabbits have been kept for food and fur. Today, they are often kept as pets, living as members of the family. That they are quiet, clean, and easy to handle makes rabbits the ideal pet for those unable to own a dog or a cat. However, rabbits are not dogs and cats, and they require special husbandry to survive and flourish.

Rabbit Breeds

Rabbits are usually grouped by size (dwarf, standards, and giants) or by ear orientation (lop-ear or erect).

Box 13-1 provides information on the different breeds of rabbits that make good pets.

Housing

Most pet rabbits will be housed in a cage of some kind. Adult rabbits should be housed individually in sturdy wire cages that are easy to clean and are protected from predators and weather. The size of the cage depends on the size of the rabbit; large rabbits require a minimum of 5 square feet of cage floor space, whereas small rabbits need only 3 square feet. Cages should be at least 14 inches high.

Rabbits may be housed either inside or outside. They are sensitive to high temperatures and should be housed indoors if the temperature is higher than 85°F. Outdoor housing requires a shaded area and perhaps a fan if the ambient outdoor temperatures are to be increased.

If the cage has wire floors, a solid platform should be provided for resting and to prevent injury to the hocks of the rabbit. Hay can be added for warmth as the weather becomes cooler.

Rabbits kept indoors can be litter trained. Compressed paper products make the best litter for indoor litter boxes. Bedding in the indoor cage should be changed frequently to prevent ammonia buildup. Metal dog crates, rabbit cages with plastic bottoms and wire tops, or plywood cages can be used indoors where weather is not a factor.

Nutrition

Rabbits require a diet high in fiber for normal digestion. Pellets that contain 20% to 30% fiber together with high-fiber hay (Timothy or grass hay) are convenient for most rabbits. Fresh fruits and vegetables in small amounts can also be fed to rabbits. Fresh water should be available at all times.

Restraint

Rabbits are delicate animals. Only 8% of their body weight is from bone. Their powerful hindquarters are adapted for jumping, and improper restraint can result in fractures of the spine and injury to the person performing the restraint. Gloves should not be used when restraining rabbits because they do not allow for adequate control of a frightened animal. *Never* grab a rabbit by the ears for restraint. A towel or nonslip mat should be placed on the table, and the rabbit should be wrapped in a towel, like a burrito. Rabbits can be scruffed by the back of the neck and carried for short distances as long as the rear quarters are supported with the other hand. Rabbits may be placed on their back for examination; stroking the abdomen will relax and calm the animal. Failure to support the rear quarters of a struggling animal can cause severe damage to the spine and large scratches on the technician's abdomen or chest.

Coprophagia

Rabbits are monogastric herbivores. They are also coprophagic—that is, they eat their own feces. Two types of feces are passed in rabbits: the round, firm type and the soft, wet cecotrophs passed at night. "Night feces," as cecotrophs are called, are a source of vitamin B and protein for the rabbit and, as such, should be consumed by all normal rabbits. These soft feces are incorrectly thought to be diarrhea by some new owners.

Sex and the Average Rabbit

Rabbits mature from 4 to 5 months of age in small breeds and 9 to 12 months of age in larger breeds. Female rabbits (does) can induce their ovulation, with ovulation occurring 10 to 13 hours after breeding. Male rabbits (bucks) have two external testes in a hairless scrotum. Does have a V-shaped vagina that is easily visible. The gestation period is 30 to 33 days, and typical litter sizes are from 4 to 10 kits. Mothers will nurse the baby rabbits once or twice daily until weaning at about 6 to 8 weeks of age. The sex of young rabbits can usually be determined after they reach 14 weeks of age.

Medicating the Average Rabbit

The microflora of the rabbit's digestive tract are necessary for normal digestion. Many oral antibiotics reduce the number of helpful bacteria in the gut and can result in serious problems in the rabbit. For this reason, care should be used in the selection of oral antibiotics for treatment of disease in the pet rabbit.

REVIEW QUESTIONS

1. Ferrets have a poor ability to utilize what two groups of food sources?
2. Domestic ferrets should be vaccinated against what two diseases?
3. Which of the following substances represents a significant danger to the ferret if swallowed?
   a. Rubber products
   b. Compressed paper litter
   c. Dry kibble
   d. Hair
4. For dietary requirements, domestic ferrets are _____.
   a. Strict carnivores
   b. Strict vegetarians
   c. Obligate carnivores
   d. Obligate omnivores
5. When examining any small mammal, bird, or reptile, it is important to record an accurate _____.
   a. Weight
   b. Rectal temperature
   c. Heart rate
   d. Birth date

6. Which of the following could be useful in prolonging the life of the pet rodent? (Select all that apply.)
   a. Proper nutrition
   b. Breeding yearly
   c. Clean, fresh water
   d. Adequate ventilation in housing
   e. Yearly dental checkups
   f. Spaying or neutering
   g. Exercise
7. When being handled, what behavior is not uncommonly exhibited by some gerbils?
   a. Vomiting
   b. Urinating
   c. Going limp
   d. Onset of seizure
8. The pigment produced by the Harderian glands of the rat, located behind the eyes, is:
   a. Rhodopsin
   b. Porphyrin
   c. Melanin
   d. Bilirubin
9. In general, gerbils produce a _____ amount of urine daily.
   a. Large
   b. Small
10. The skeleton comprises _____ of a rabbit's total body weight?
    a. 15%
    b. 24%
    c. 8%
    d. 3%
11. Cecotrophs ingested by the rabbit contain large amounts of:
    a. Glycogen
    b. Volatile fatty acids
    c. Starch
    d. Vitamins
12. Young rabbits are usually weaned at _____ weeks of age.
    a. 14–16
    b. 3–5
    c. 18–20
    d. 6–8

13. Why are many oral antibiotics not recommended for use in the rabbit?
    a. The bacteria of the rabbit are not susceptible to most oral antibiotics.
    b. Most rabbit diseases are caused by viruses and not bacteria.
    c. Rabbits break down oral antibiotics before they can enter the circulation.
    d. The microflora in the rabbit gastrointestinal tract is sensitive to oral antibiotics.

14. Rabbits are _____ ovulators.
    a. Induced
    b. Seasonal

15. Rodent and rabbit teeth should be _____ twice yearly.
    a. Brushed by the owner
    b. Trimmed
    c. Professionally cleaned

Answers found on page 553.

Diseases of the Cardiovascular System

LEARNING OBJECTIVES

When you have completed this chapter, you will be able to:
1. Realize the need to examine the cardiovascular system even in the smallest of patients.
2. Discuss the prevention of heartworm disease with owners of ferrets.
3. Monitor treatment with cardiac drugs in the exotic patient.

The Ferret

Acquired heart disease is relatively common in middle-aged to older ferrets (>3 years of age), whereas there are few reports of congenital disease. Diagnosis is based on clinical signs, physical examination, radiography, ultrasonic examination, and electrocardiography (Fig. 14-1).

Cardiomyopathy

Cardiomyopathy, both dilated and hypertrophic, is reported in pet ferrets. The dilated form results in an enlarged left ventricle with systolic dysfunction, whereas the hypertrophic form produces a hypertrophy of the left ventricular wall resulting in decreased filling, a diastolic function.

CLINICAL SIGNS

- Lethargy
- Dyspnea
- Anorexia
- Weight loss
- Pale mucous membranes
- Tachycardia
- Hypothermia
- Weakness
- Presence or absence of pulmonary edema, pleural effusion, pericardial effusion

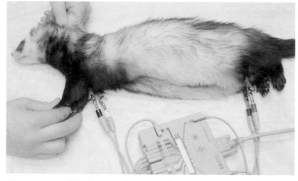

Figure 14-1 Technique for recording the electrocardiogram of the ferret. (From Quesenberry KE, Carpenter JW: *Ferrets, rabbits, and rodents*, ed 3, St. Louis, MO, 2012, Saunders, by permission.)

DIAGNOSIS

- Physical examination and history
- Radiography; enlarged cardiac silhouette
- Ultrasound; left ventricular dilation, presence or absence of mitral and tricuspid regurgitation (dilated form)
- Left ventricular diastolic and systolic dimensions are decreased, and left atrium may be enlarged (hypertrophic form)
- Electrocardiography: presence or absence ventricular premature contractions, atrial premature contractions, atrial or ventricular tachycardias, and atrial fibrillation

TREATMENT

Dilated Form

- Oxygen
- Diuretics (furosemide)
- Nitroglycerin
- Pleurocentesis

Long-term Therapy

- Diuretics (used at low doses)
- Angiotensin-converting enzyme (ACE) inhibitors to reduce afterload
- Digoxin
- Low-salt diet
- Animals should be monitored frequently using radiographs and serum chemistries with digoxin levels

Hypertrophic Form

- Oxygen
- β-Blockers (atenolol) or calcium channel blockers (diltiazem)
- Diuretics, if needed
- Animals should be monitored frequently using electrocardiogram (ECG), serum chemistries, and echocardiography

INFORMATION FOR CLIENTS

- Many ferrets with cardiomyopathy respond well to treatment.
- Life-long treatment and frequent monitoring will be necessary.
- These diseases may progress and worsen with time.

Valvular Heart Disease

Valvular heart disease is common in middle-aged to older ferrets, with mitral and tricuspid regurgitation being the most common cause. The systolic murmur of mitral regurgitation can be best heard over the left apical thorax, whereas tricuspid regurgitation can be best heard over the right sternal region of the thorax. Aortic regurgitation or aortic insufficiency may also occur.

CLINICAL SIGNS

- If present, clinical signs will be related to congestive heart failure
- Lethargy
- Weakness
- Dyspnea
- Weight loss
- Pale mucous membranes

DIAGNOSIS

- Physical examination and history
- Presence of an audible murmur
- Radiography: presence or absence of pulmonary edema; presence or absence of enlargement of the heart
- ECG: presence or absence of atrial arrhythmias
- Echocardiography: thickening of valves with ventricular and atrial enlargement; regurgitation can be identified
- Complete blood cell count (CBC) and serum chemistries to identify secondary disease processes such as renal failure

TREATMENT

- Recommended if congestive heart failure exists
- Digoxin
- ACE inhibitors
- Diuretics
- Oxygen, if needed

INFORMATION FOR CLIENTS

- The prognosis for ferrets with valvular disease is uncertain.
- The presence of other underlying diseases will complicate the situation.
- Life-long treatment and monitoring will be necessary.

Heartworm Disease

Ferrets living in areas of the country endemic to heartworms (*Dirofilaria immitis*) may be infected. The presence of as few as a single heartworm may produce clinical signs. Microfilaria may be found in as many as 50% to 60% of infected ferrets (Fig. 14-2). Clinical signs are usually related to right heart disease and are similar to those seen in cats.

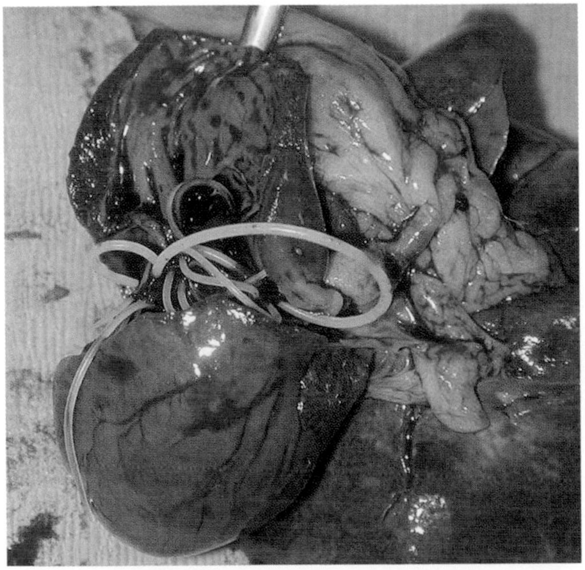

Figure 14-2 Heartworm (*Dirofilaria immitis*) disease in the ferret. (From Quesenberry KE, Carpenter JW: *Ferrets, rabbits, and rodents*, ed 3, St. Louis, MO, 2012, Saunders, by permission.)

CLINICAL SIGNS

- Coughing
- Lethargy
- Weakness
- Dyspnea
- Presence or absence of pleural effusion and ascites
- Hypothermia
- Sudden death

DIAGNOSIS

- Physical examination and history
- Radiographs: cardiac enlargement
- Presence or absence of pleural effusion, ascites, or both
- Echocardiography: will show linear parasites in the pulmonary artery, right ventricle, right atrium, or all
- Heartworm antigen testing

TREATMENT

- Depends on animal
- Symptomatic animal with microfilaria:
  - Ivermectin subcutaneously until clinical signs disappear and no microfilaria are present
  - Adulticide therapy: melarsomine (Immiticide) in two-stage protocol
- Diuretic, if needed
- Strict cage rest for 4 to 6 weeks after therapy
- Prevention can be accomplished using one-fourth of the smallest dose ivermectin tablet (Heartgard— either canine or feline)

⊙ TECH ALERT

Immiticide supplies are severely limited at the present time. It may be difficult to obtain the drug for the treatment of ferrets with heartworm disease. Heartworm prevention is not licensed for use in ferrets. Oral dosing with Ivermectin diluted in propylene glycol has been recommended in the literature, or Iverheart for cats has also been used.

INFORMATION FOR CLIENTS

- Ferrets are susceptible to heartworm disease. Preventions should be used in all ferrets living in parts of the country that have high incidence of heartworm disease.

- After treatment for heartworm disease, it is important that the ferret be cage rested for 4 to 6 weeks to allow the dying and dead worms to be safely reabsorbed by the body. This will help to avoid pulmonary emboli and further problems.

Rodents

Cardiovascular disease is seen in rodents, especially the hamster. Cardiomyopathy and atrial thrombosis occur in older hamsters (>1.5 years of age).

CLINICAL SIGNS

- Hyperpnea
- Tachycardia
- Cyanosis
- Lethargy
- Anorexia

DIAGNOSIS

- Physical examination and history
- Radiography
- Ultrasonography of the heart

TREATMENT

- Digoxin
- Diuretics
- ACE inhibitors
- Anticoagulants

INFORMATION FOR CLIENTS

- Most thromboses occur secondary to heart disease. They may occur in hamsters as young as 1 year of age, and the hamster may die within 1 week of diagnosis.
- Castration of male hamsters seems to increase the incidence of thrombosis.
- Dosages for cardiac drugs may be extrapolated from other species for hamsters, but you must closely observe the pet for response.

The Rabbit

The cardiovascular system of the rabbit is different from the feline and canine cardiovascular systems in several ways. First, the tricuspid valve has only two cusps. Second, and maybe most important, there is little collateral circulation for the coronary vessels, making the myocardium susceptible to ischemia. And third, the aortic nerve is regulated by baroreceptors, not chemoreceptors.

Cardiomyopathy is seen in pet rabbits, with the giant breeds being the most susceptible. The cause is unknown. Vitamin E deficiency, corona virus infection, and some bacterial infections can affect the heart muscle. Drugs such as the ketamine–xylazine combination and doxorubicin have been shown also to cause myocardial disease in the rabbit. Congenital heart disease, although not frequently seen, has also been reported in rabbits (ventricular septal defects). Mitral and tricuspid insufficiencies have been reported in pet rabbits as well. Arteriosclerosis of the aorta and other arteries is seen in almost all breeds of rabbits.

CLINICAL SIGNS

- Similar to those in other animals with myocardial disease
- Weight loss
- Exercise intolerance
- Dyspnea; pulmonary edema, pleural effusion
- Hepatomegaly
- Weakness

DIAGNOSIS

- Physical examination and history
- Radiography
- Echocardiography
- Electrocardiogram
- Culture and sensitivity if bacterial infection is suspected

TREATMENT

- Diuretic; furosemide intravenously or intramuscularly
- Oxygen cage
- ACE inhibitors: enalapril maleate or digoxin
- Nitroglycerin 2% ointment every 6 to 12 hours

INFORMATION FOR CLIENTS

- Handle any rabbit with breathing difficulty with care.
- The goal of therapy is to improve cardiac performance, not necessarily to cure the disease.
- Continued monitoring of the rabbit undergoing therapy will be necessary.

REVIEW QUESTIONS

1. Ferrets are not susceptible to heartworm disease, and therefore do not need to take preventive medication monthly.
   a. True
   b. False

2. What defect in the ferret's cardiac function is involved in hypertrophic cardiomyopathy?
   a. Enlargement of the ventricles
   b. Enlargement of the atria
   c. Thickening of the walls of the heart
   d. Thinning of the walls of the aorta

3. Most cases of thrombosis in the hamster occur secondary to _____ disease.
   a. Heart
   b. Lung
   c. Bone
   d. Renal

4. The main goal of treating heart disease in rabbits is to:
   a. Correct the defect
   b. Improve cardiac performance
   c. Decrease blood pressure

5. Mitral regurgitation is best heard over:
   a. Left apex
   b. Right apex
   c. Left base
   d. Right base

6. Microfilaria can always be found on ferret blood smears.
   a. True
   b. False

7. Drug doses for cardiac disease in rodents may be extrapolated from other species.
   a. True
   b. False

8. The rabbit tricuspid valve has _____ leaflets.
   a. 4
   b. 3
   c. 2

9. The rabbit myocardium is susceptible to myocardial ischemia because of _____.
   a. Lack of adequate collateral circulation
   b. Hypertension within the cardiac muscle
   c. Inadequate calcium levels within the cardiac muscle

Answers found on page 553.

Diseases of the Digestive System

LEARNING OBJECTIVES

When you have completed this chapter, you will be able to:
1. Discuss the pros and cons of owning a ferret as a pet.
2. Discuss the unique husbandry practices needed for ferret owners.
3. Explain the common diseases seen in pet ferrets and their treatment.

The Ferret

Digestive system disease in the ferret parallels those of dogs and cats. Dental diseases, diarrheas (infectious), gastrointestinal (GI) foreign bodies, neoplasia, and rectal disease are common occurrences in pet ferrets.

Dental Disease

Gingivitis and periodontal disease are common in older ferrets (Fig. 15-1). Animals fed moist or semi-moist diets or those high in sweets are most commonly affected. As in dogs and cats, as tartar accumulates on

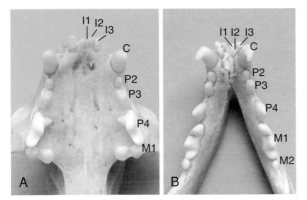

Figure 15-1 Dental formula for the ferret. (Courtesy of Vittorio Capello, DVM. IN Quesenberry KE, Carpenter JW: *Ferrets, rabbits, and rodents*, ed 3, St Louis, 2012, Saunders, by permission)

teeth, inflammation of periodontal tissues occurs, causing dysphagia and drooling.

CLINICAL SIGNS

- Discolored teeth with tartar accumulation
- Halitosis
- Presence or absence of loose or lost teeth
- Presence or absence of pain on chewing
- Presence or absence of drooling

DIAGNOSIS

- Physical examination and history
- Complete dental examination

TREATMENT

- Dental cleaning and extractions if necessary
- Prevention same as for cats and dogs

INFORMATION FOR CLIENTS

- Ferrets' teeth can be cleaned and brushed using products formulated for cats.
- Loose teeth should be extracted to prevent pain and further irritation to the surrounding tissue.

⊙ TECH ALERT

Ferrets have small oral cavities, and you will need to use a mouth speculum to properly examine the rear teeth.

Gastrointestinal Foreign Bodies

GI foreign bodies are common in ferrets. These animals are curious and love to chew, which puts them at risk for swallowing almost anything they can chew on, particularly items of latex rubber or sponge materials. Hairballs can also cause obstruction in older ferrets (Fig. 15-2).

CLINICAL SIGNS

- Lethargy
- Anorexia
- Diarrhea
- Vomiting (usually *not* reported by owner)
- Weakness: may be profound
- Slobbering, face rubbing

DIAGNOSIS

- Physical examination and history
- Radiography: ± ileus, gas distention, visible foreign body
- Complete blood cell count (CBC) and serum chemistries

TREATMENT

- Surgical removal
- Intravenous (IV) fluids
- Antibiotics
- Use of laxatives formulated for cats can prevent the accumulation of hair in older ferrets

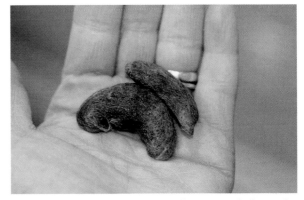

Figure 15-2 Tricobezoars surgically removed from the stomach of a ferret. (From Quesenberry KE, Carpenter JW: *Ferrets, rabbits, and rodents*, ed 3, St. Louis, MO, 2012, Saunders, by permission.)

INFORMATION FOR CLIENTS

- Avoid allowing ferrets unsupervised, free roam of the house.
- Do not give your pet ferrets soft, squeaky rubber toys.
- Routinely use a laxative formulated for cats to prevent hairball obstruction in older ferrets.

● TECH ALERT

Do not allow ferrets access to any rubber products; this may mean you need to watch them around tissue drains, catheter administration sets, and clinic toys.

Enteritis and Diarrhea

Most cases of enteritis and diarrhea may be related to bacterial or viral infections in the ferret. *Salmonella, Mycobacteria, Campylobacter,* rotavirus, canine distemper virus, and human flu virus may all be causes of diarrhea in the ferret. Epizootic catarrhal enteritis, a highly transmissible disease, is more common in older ferrets exposed to new or young ferrets that may be asymptomatic carriers. Inflammatory bowel disease does occur with some frequency in pet ferrets. Although the exact cause is unknown, it may be related to a hyperimmune response to dietary components.

CLINICAL SIGNS

- Diarrhea
- ± Dehydration
- ± Weight loss
- ± Upper respiratory disease (human flu virus)

DIAGNOSIS

- Physical examination and history
- Fecal to rule out parasites (fairly uncommon in pet ferrets)
- Stool culture and sensitivity
- ± Radiography to rule out foreign body
- CBC, serum chemistries
- Biopsy of affected bowel (inflammatory bowel disease)

TREATMENT

- Maintain hydration (subcutaneous [SQ], oral fluids)
- Antibiotics (per culture results or metronidazole and amoxicillin are good choices)
- Kaolin or pectin may be given orally to protect the intestines

- ± Cortisone for inflammatory bowel disease and epizootic catarrhal enteritis (ECE)
- Change diet to easily absorbable food: i/d, z/d

INFORMATION FOR CLIENTS

- Diagnosis of the exact cause of ferret diarrhea may be time consuming and require numerous tests.
- To avoid most cases of diarrhea, maintain routine diet, avoid foreign body ingestion, and do not allow the ferret access to garbage or other uncooked food sources.
- Avoid exposing your ferret to unvaccinated, young ferrets.

Wasting Disease in Ferrets

Helicobacter mustelae, proliferative bowel disease (PBD), and eosinophilic gastroenteritis can all cause diarrhea and wasting in ferrets. Most ferrets are exposed to *H. mustelae* as kits, becoming persistently infected but asymptomatic until later. Infection may result in mucous gland depletion in the stomach, followed by gastric ulceration or chronic gastritis. Stress is usually the underlying cause for development of clinical symptoms. PBD is caused by the bacterium *Lawsonia intracellularis.* Infection usually results in segments of the intestine becoming thickened by cellular infiltration of the intestinal wall (Fig. 15-3). This disease, primarily transmitted by the fecal–oral route, is most common in young, fast-growing juveniles; stress also plays a role in development of clinical symptoms.

CLINICAL SIGNS

- Diarrhea with or without blood and mucous
- Wasting, rapid and severe
- Vomiting or nausea, pawing at mouth
- Dehydration
- Lethargy
- Anorexia
- Presence or absence of Anemia

DIAGNOSIS

- Physical examination and history
- CBC, serum chemistries; hypoalbuminemia, anemia, with or without eosinophilia (10% to 35%)
- Radiography
- Stool culture and sensitivity
- Biopsy of affected tissue

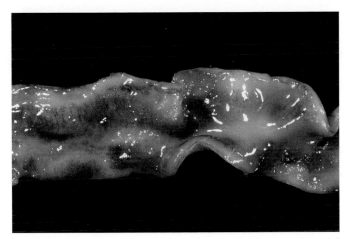

Figure 15-3 Thickened, hemorrhagic mucosa in the bowel of a ferret with proliferative enteritis. (From Quesenberry KE, Carpenter JW: *Ferrets, rabbits, and rodents*, ed 3, St. Louis, MO, 2012, Saunders, by permission.)

TREATMENT

- Antibiotics:
  - Chloramphenicol for PBD (bacteria only sensitive to chloramphenicol)
  - Metronidazole and ampicillin for *Helicobacter* infection
- Cimetidine or other histamine (H_2) blockers
- Corticosteroid therapy for eosinophilic gastroenteritis
- Bismuth subsalicylate
- Hypoallergic diet
- Ivermectin (for eosinophilic gastroenteritis)

Supportive Care
- IV or SQ fluids

INFORMATION FOR CLIENTS

- Avoid exposure of your pet ferret to young ferrets whose *Helicobacter* status is unknown.
- Sick ferrets may need to be tube fed and have SQ fluids administered frequently.
- It may take a long time for the ferret to recover, even with aggressive and persistent treatment.

Rodents

Digestive disturbances are frequent occurrences in rodents. Overgrowth of incisors is a common problem in rats, whereas enteritis or diarrhea is seen more commonly in gerbils and hamsters.

Overgrowth of Incisors

Incisors of rats grow constantly. If these teeth are not worn down by chewing, they can overgrow and cause digestive problems (Fig. 15-4).

CLINICAL SIGNS

- Anorexia
- ± Nasal discharge

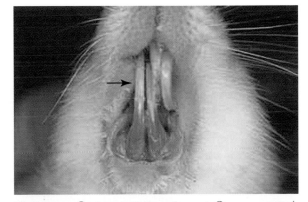

Figure 15-4 Overgrown incisors in a rat. Overgrown teeth can be cut with a high-speed drill. (Courtesy of Thomas M. Donnelly, DVM, BVSc, DAVLAM.)

- Overgrown incisors may prevent normal closure of the mouth

DIAGNOSIS

- Physical examination and history

TREATMENT

- May require sedation for proper trimming
- Use a high-speed dental drill for shortening teeth; avoid using nail trimmers because they will result in enamel damage to teeth
- Extraction may be needed if teeth are nonfunctional or seriously damaged
- ± Antibiotics if soft tissues are involved

⬤ TECH ALERT

The oral cavity of rodents is difficult to examine without sedation and a good oral speculum.

Sialodacryoadenitis in Rats

Inflammation of the cervical salivary glands occurs in rats, giving them the appearance of having the mumps. This highly contagious disease is the result of coronavirus infection.

CLINICAL SIGNS

- Rhinitis (initial symptom)
- Enlarged cervical lymph nodes
- Enlarged salivary glands and lacrimal glands
- ± Ocular lesions of conjunctivitis, keratitis, corneal ulceration

DIAGNOSIS

- Physical examination and history
- Other causes of infection ruled out
- Serology

TREATMENT

- No treatment is currently available. Clinical signs usually decrease within 30 days.

INFORMATION FOR CLIENTS

- This condition is highly contagious.
- Chronic eye lesions may result from the primary infection.

Enteropathy (Wet Tail, Proliferative Ileitis)

Diarrhea seen in young and mature hamsters is usually associated with bacterial infection. In young hamsters, the bacterium *Lawsonia intracellularis* is often the cause, whereas in mature hamsters and gerbils, *Clostridium piliforme* is the cause (Tyzzer disease).

CLINICAL SIGNS

- Severe diarrhea
- Dehydration
- Anorexia

DIAGNOSIS

- Physical examination and history of high mortality in the colony or recent antibiotic therapy with lincomycin, penicillin, or bacitracin
- Culture of the organism in feces

TREATMENT

- Replace fluid and electrolyte loss; IV, SQ, oral fluids
- Force-feed: Critical Care (Oxbow Pet Products, Murdock, NE) or slurry of rodent pellets combined with pureed vegetables and fruits
- Antibiotics: tetracycline, oxytetracycline, enrofloxacin, or trimethoprim with sulfa
- Intestinal protectants such as bismuth subsalicylate

INFORMATION FOR CLIENTS

- Reducing stress resulting from poor husbandry can prevent the development of Tyzzer disease in hamsters.
- The term *wet tail* is commonly used to refer to any diarrhea in hamsters, regardless of the cause.

The Rabbit

Rabbits are monogastric herbivores. They are also hindgut fermenters; that is, they can digest fiber in the cecum and produce energy. They require a diet high in fiber; many of the digestive problems seen in rabbits can be related directly to improper diets. The anatomy of the digestive tract is similar to that of the horse in that rabbits have a large cecum and a sacculated colon. Large indigestible fiber particles stimulate the intestinal tract motility, whereas the digestible nutrients are broken down and absorbed by specific areas of the GI tract. A population of microorganisms that lives in the cecum are able to break down the digestible portion of the diet, and some absorption of nutrients occurs directly from the cecum. Cecotrophs are formed from the remainder of the digestible material. These are full of nutrients and are passed to the outside to be re-eaten by the rabbit. Any disruption of dietary content, stress, dehydration, or disease can result in intestinal stasis and digestive upset.

Intestinal Stasis (Hairballs, Trichobezoars, "Wool Block")

The diagnosis of hairball obstruction in the rabbit is a common one. However, hair is not the problem; the main problem is the lack of intestinal motility which allows the hair to accumulate. Intestinal stasis may result from a number of causes: inappropriate diet (one high in carbohydrates and low in fiber), dehydration, stress, or painful conditions such as dental disease or the presence of foreign objects in the GI tract. It is normal to find hair in the stomach of the rabbit, mixed with stomach contents in a soft mass. As intestinal motility slows, this soft mass begins to dehydrate and become drier and firmer. The result is an impaction, which results in signs of clinical disease.

CLINICAL SIGNS

- Anorexia
- Dehydration
- Decrease or lack of feces
- Rabbits may chew on fiber in the environment in an attempt to replace necessary dietary fiber not provided
- Lethargy
- Death

DIAGNOSIS

- Physical signs and dietary history
- Radiography to confirm the presence of dehydrated material in the intestinal tract (Fig. 15-5)

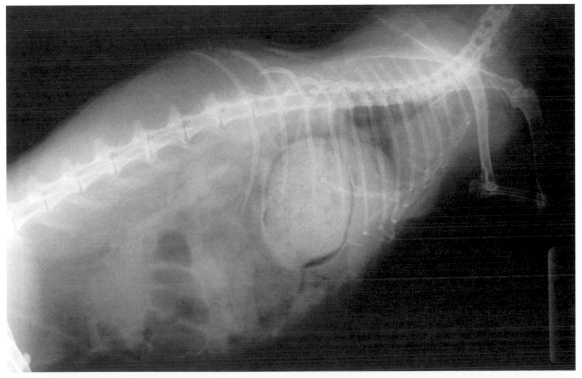

Figure 15-5 A trichobezoar in the stomach of a rabbit. (From Harcourt-Brown F: *Textbook of rabbit medicine*, Oxford, U.K., 2002, Butterworth-Heinemann, by permission.)

TREATMENT

- Rehydrate the patient—with both oral and IV fluids.
- If the animal is eating, give fresh, leafy greens.
- Administer drugs that stimulate gastric motility: cisapride, metoclopramide.
- Analgesia: Gas buildup in the intestines can be painful.
- Change the diet to include more fiber and moisture.
- *Note:* Enzymatic digestion of hairballs is of little use; the problem is GI stasis, not the hair in the intestines.

INFORMATION FOR CLIENTS

- Rabbits require a diet high in fiber and low in carbohydrates. Grass hay is a good source of fiber.
- Rabbits need exercise to stimulate normal bowel function. They also must have access to their "night feces" for proper nutrition.
- Signs of gastric stasis may appear gradually. You will need to monitor your animal's dietary consumption and fecal output carefully to catch the problem early.

Obesity

Obesity is a common problem in pet rabbits. Lack of exercise and excessive food together produce a fat rabbit. Fat rabbits, similar to overweight humans, dogs, cats, and horses, have more health problems compared to rabbits that maintain a normal weight.

CLINICAL SIGNS

- Abnormally large amounts of internal and external body fat
- Lethargy
- Inability to groom properly; matted and dirty hair, dandruff
- Pododermatitis, lameness from orthopedic problems, or both

DIAGNOSIS

- Physical examination and history of improper diet and exercise
- Radiographs show excessive internal and external body fat or joint abnormalities
- Serum chemistries may show elevation of liver function if fatty liver is present

TREATMENT

- Correct the diet: decrease the level of carbohydrates and increase the level of fiber in the diet.
- Increase exercise.

INFORMATION FOR CLIENTS

- It is easier to prevent obesity than to treat it.
- Make sure your rabbit is given a proper diet—high in fiber, low in carbohydrates—and make sure the rabbit has adequate room to exercise.
- Obesity will predispose your rabbit to other problems that can affect the quality of life for your pet.

Dental Disease

Pet rabbits are frequently seen in veterinary practice for dental problems. Many of these problems arise from poor husbandry practices, but others may be related to trauma, cancer, or genetic malformations of the jaw. The structure of the jaws in rabbits is similar to that in horses, with the lower dental arcade being narrower than the upper arcade. This predisposes the back teeth to uneven wear and overgrowth (Fig. 15-6 and Fig. 15-7). Incisors also become overgrown, which could result in mouth sores and decreased ability to eat.

CLINICAL SIGNS

- Inability to eat or dropping food from the mouth when chewing
- Reluctance to eat favorite "hard" foods
- Increased drooling (usually related to oral pain)
- Visible overgrown teeth
- Excessive tearing (overgrown teeth may block tear ducts)
- Progressive weight loss

DIAGNOSIS

- Complete oral examination (may require anesthesia)
- Dental radiography

TREATMENT

- Grind and polish overgrown teeth.
- Correct the diet: add more abrasive materials for the rabbit to gnaw on.
- Treat any oral lesions that arise from the malocclusion.
- Remove any malaligned teeth.

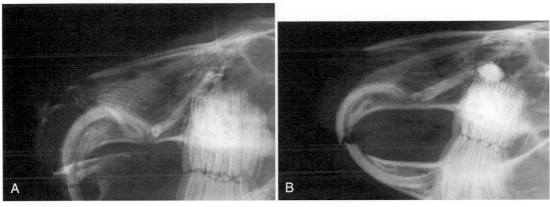

Figure 15-6 Rabbit dental arcade. Overgrown incisors are a common problem in domestic rabbits. (From Harcourt-Brown F: *Textbook of rabbit medicine*, Oxford, U.K., 2002, Butterworth-Heinemann, by permission.)

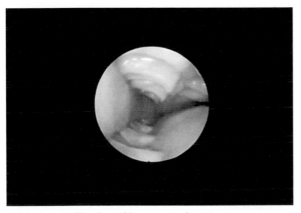

Figure 15-7 Cheek teeth examined using an otoscope. (From Harcourt-Brown F: *Textbook of rabbit medicine*, Oxford, U.K., 2002, Butterworth-Heinemann, by permission.)

INFORMATION FOR CLIENTS

- Rabbits need to chew. Give them hay cubes, soft wood, or other safe abrasive items that will help wear the teeth in a normal manner.
- Have your rabbit's teeth examined for abnormal wear two times yearly. Correct any problems at that time.

Soft Stools (Intermittent Diarrhea)

Rabbits not fed adequate amounts of fiber will often have intermittent soft stools. This is the result of diets high in carbohydrates, which alter the bacterial flora in the cecum and result in the production of soft, mushy feces. Inflammation of the cecum and parasites may also cause soft stools and should be investigated if the diet is proper.

CLINICAL SIGNS

- Both soft and normal stools present in the cage
- Fur around the rectum may be stained from soft feces
- ± Other signs of systemic disease

DIAGNOSIS

- Physical examination and dietary history
- Fecal sample to rule out parasites
- CBC to rule out inflammatory disease

TREATMENT

- Correct the diet: place the rabbit on a grass hay only diet until stools become normal.
- Remove any high-carbohydrate prepared foods from the diet permanently.
- Treat intestinal parasites, if found, with ivermectin.
- Correct underlying cause of cecal inflammation.

INFORMATION FOR CLIENTS

- Always make sure you are feeding your rabbit a properly balanced diet high in fiber.
- Periodic fecal examinations are necessary to keep your pet parasite-free (especially if your rabbit is frequently outside on grass).

Internal Parasites

Internal parasites found in rabbits include pinworms (*Passalurus ambiguous*) and coccidia (*Eimeria* spp.), cestodes (*Hymenolepis*), and trematodes (uncommon in house rabbits).

CLINICAL SIGNS

- Diarrhea
- Dehydration
- Weight loss
- Distended abdomen
- Death (*Eimeria stiedae*)
- No clinical symptoms (especially with pinworms)

DIAGNOSIS

- Physical examination
- Visible worms—especially pinworms found around the anus
- Fecal flotation
- Serum chemistries; liver dysfunction (if *E. stiedae* involved)

TREATMENT

- Anthelmintics
- Cage cleaning and disinfection
- Coccidiostats (sulfadimethoxine)
- Supportive care in severe cases (adequate hydration, warmth, caloric support)

INFORMATION FOR CLIENTS

- Rabbits should be examined for parasites soon after purchasing. Routine fecal examinations should allow your rabbit to remain parasite-free.
- *E. stiedae* can infect the liver and may cause the death of the animal. *E. stiedae* is difficult to distinguish from other more common *Eimeria* species.
- Keep the rabbit's environment clean, and keep exposure to feces of other animals to a minimum to prevent infection.

● TECH ALERT

Owners may be upset and nervous after finding pinworms on their pet rabbit. This parasite is species specific and not transmissible to humans.

Cecal Impaction

The cause of cecal impaction in the rabbit is unknown, but stress, dehydration, and the ingestion of small fiber particles that absorb water have all been implicated. Cecal impaction is difficult to treat and can best be avoided by proper feeding of grass hay and providing a low-stress environment with a constant supply of fresh drinking water.

CLINICAL SIGNS

- Sluggishness
- Gradual loss of appetite
- Weight loss
- Decreased fecal material
- Increased mucus in stool

DIAGNOSIS

- Physical examination and history
- The impacted cecum can often be palpated as a sausage-shaped mass in the ventral abdomen
- Radiography

TREATMENT

- Rehydration of the patient (oral, IV, and SQ fluids)
- Softening of GI tract contents (can use leafy green veggies, fruits)
- Cisapride or metoclopramide to stimulate motility
- Analgesics (carprofen is the suggested nonsteroidal antiinflammatory drug but may result in gastric ulceration)
- Dinoprost (as a last resort; experimentally this has been shown to result in rapid evacuation of the GI tract after administration)

INFORMATION FOR CLIENTS

- Cecal impaction can be avoided by feeding free-choice grass hay and providing constant access to clean water.
- Avoid using clay cat litter or other short-fiber particulate matter for bedding.

Mucoid Enteropathy

Although not commonly seen in pet rabbits, mucoid enteropathy is occasionally seen in young rabbits obtained from a pet store or breeder and in breeding does.

CLINICAL SIGNS

- Anorexia
- Abdominal distension
- Subnormal body temperatures
- Depression
- Crouched body stance
- "Sloshy gut sounds"
- Presence or absence of diarrhea or constipation
- Increased passage of mucus
- Teeth grinding (related to abdominal pain)
- Change in water consumption (may be increased or decreased)
- Presence or absence of cecal impaction

DIAGNOSIS

- Other causes such as parasitism, and bacterial or viral agents ruled out
- Radiography: cecal impaction, gas in cecum and small intestine, gastric distension

TREATMENT

- Similar to that for cecal impaction
- Fluids
- Increased fiber diet (grass hay)
- Fresh leafy greens
- Probiotic to reestablish intestinal bacteria
- Presence or absence of antibiotics

INFORMATION FOR CLIENTS

- The prognosis for mucoid enteropathy, even with treatment, is guarded to poor.
- This disease is usually progressive and fatal.

Hepatic Lipidosis

As in cats, anorexia in rabbits may result in hepatic lipidosis and liver failure. Rabbits produce glucose and lactates in cecotrophs from fermentation in the stomach. The cecotrophs also contain amylase and volatile fatty acids, which are reabsorbed in the intestinal tract from consumed cecotrophs. During periods of anorexia, glucose levels decline, and the cecal microflora decrease production of fatty acids. This stimulates lipolysis and the mobilization of fatty acids from adipose tissue. These must pass through the liver to be metabolized. The liver, unable to handle the excess of fatty acids, begins to accumulate fat in the hepatocytes, blocking or impairing metabolic pathways. The result, hepatic lipidosis, may lead to liver failure and death. Obese rabbits and rabbits on high-fat diets are at greatest risk for development of this disease.

CLINICAL SIGNS

- Prolonged anorexia
- Depression
- Dehydration
- As disease progresses, animal may become disorientated and ataxic

DIAGNOSIS

- Physical examination and history of prolonged anorexia
- Radiography: gastric hypomotility may be present
- CBC and serum chemistries: increases in liver enzymes

TREATMENT

- Nutritional support (tube-feed if necessary)
- Correct dehydration
- Treat intestinal hypomotility if present
- Presence or absence analgesics
- Questran; treat developing enterotoxemias

INFORMATION FOR CLIENTS

- Prevent the formation of hepatic lipidosis by making sure your rabbit is eating well.
- If the rabbit must be stressed by boarding, travel, or breeding, ensure adequate caloric intake to prevent a shift in metabolic pathways.
- Avoid obesity in your pet rabbit with proper nutrition and exercise.

REVIEW QUESTIONS

1. Infection with _____ bacteria can result in gastric ulceration and chronic gastritis in ferrets.
   a. *Helicobacter* spp.
   b. *Staphylococcus* spp.
   c. *Proteus* spp.
   d. *Streptococcus* spp.

2. Humans who have the flu should avoid handling ferrets.
   a. True
   b. False

3. What is another term for proliferative ileitis in the hamster?
   a. Tyzzer disease
   b. Wet tail
   c. Sialodacryoadenitis
   d. Chromodacryorrhea

4. Overgrowth of _____ presents the most problems to rats.
   a. Molars
   b. Canine
   c. Incisors
   d. Premolars

5. Hepatic lipidosis in the rabbit can be precipitated by _____.
   a. Prolonged anorexia
   b. Exposure to pesticides
   c. Drug therapy
   d. Eating a diet high in fiber

6. Cecotrophs ingested by the rabbit contain large amounts of:
   a. Glycogen
   b. Volatile fatty acids
   c. Starch
   d. Vitamins

7. The proper diet for a pet rabbit should include _____. (Select all that apply.)
   a. Grass hay
   b. Meat protein
   c. Animal fats
   d. Clean water
   e. Fresh vegetables
   f. Peanuts
   g. Alfalfa hay
   h. Commercial pellets

8. The formation of "trichobezoars" in rabbits is not a problem of ingested hair as much as a problem of _____.
   a. Anorexia
   b. Dietary intolerance
   c. Intestinal motility
   d. Increased exercise

9. Teeth grinding in rabbits is usually related to _____.
   a. Pain
   b. Dental tartar
   c. Diarrhea
   d. Hairballs

10. Rabbit pinworms can be a zoonotic problem.
    a. True
    b. False

Answers found on page 553.

Diseases of the Endocrine System

Cataract
Fasciculation

Gluconeogenesis
Gonadotropin

Nodulectomy

LEARNING OBJECTIVES

When you have completed this chapter, you will be able to:
1. Explain the genesis of endocrine problems in ferrets, rodents, and rabbits.

2. Discuss treatment options available to clients.

The Ferret

Endocrine disease is common in older ferrets. The organs affected include the pancreas and the adrenal glands. Estrogen excess is covered in Chapter 22.

Adrenal Disease

Adrenal gland disease (hyperplasia, adenoma, or adenocarcinoma) is the most common endocrine problem in older ferrets. Clinical signs include a progressive, symmetric, pruritic alopecia that begins in the rump area and spreads cranially and ventrally (Fig. 16-1). The disease affects both male and female ferrets, with female ferrets being overrepresented. It is estimated that about 70% of female ferrets with adrenal disease will also exhibit vulvar enlargement, and that male ferrets may experience urinary blockage from cystic tissue in the region of the prostate. Surgical treatment is

preferred but medical treatment is available, although the prognosis with medical treatment is unpredictable.

CLINICAL SIGNS

- Progressive alopecia
- Presence or absence of pruritus
- Presence or absence of enlarged vulva (female) or urinary dysuria or obstruction (male)

DIAGNOSIS

- Clinical signs and physical examination, history
- Complete blood cell count (CBC) and serum chemistries: may be normal or may show anemia or a pancytopenia in severe cases; chemistries usually normal
- Radiography: usually not helpful
- Ultrasonography: should detect enlarged adrenal gland(s)

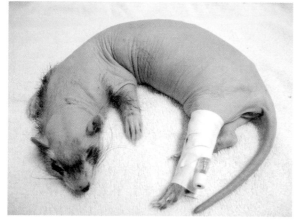

Figure 16-1 Hair loss seen in a ferret with adrenocortical tumor. (From Quesenberry KE, Carpenter JW: *Ferrets, rabbits, and rodents*, ed 2, St. Louis, MO, 2004, Saunders, by permission.)

- Computed tomography (CT) or magnetic resonance imaging (MRI)
- Serum concentrations of steroid hormones will show increased levels of estradiol, androstenedione, and 17-hydroxyprogesterone.
- Clinical Endocrinology Laboratory, University of Tennessee: best for diagnosis

TREATMENT
- Surgical removal of the diseased gland is treatment of choice
- Medical treatment for nonsurgical candidates*:
  - Treatments commonly used in dogs may be ineffective in ferrets. None of the medications listed in Box 16-1 are licensed for use in ferrets.

INFORMATION FOR CLIENTS
- Adrenal disease is a disease of older neutered ferrets.
- Surgical treatment will give the best chance for a favorable prognosis. This surgery is not routine and will require a surgical specialist.
- With medical treatment, results will be less satisfactory and relapses may occur if medication is discontinued.

---

*Medical treatment may be helpful in some ferrets but not all will respond favorably.

BOX 16-1   Medications Used in Dogs that are Ineffective in Ferrets

- Mitotane (Lysodren): rarely successful with adrenal tumors
- Flutamide (Eulexin): androgen receptor blocker
- Anastrozole (Arimidex®): aromatase inhibitor blocks conversion of testosterone to estrogen
- Bicalutamide (Casodex®): inhibits production of testosterone
- Leuprolide (Lupron): gonadotropin-releasing hormone analogs; decreases levels of both testosterone and estrogen

---

- Adrenal tumors may metastasize and cause other medical problems.

Pancreatic Islet Cell Tumors (Insulinomas)

Islet cell tumors in the pancreas are common in middle-aged to older ferrets. Most tumors in ferrets involve the β-islet cells, which produce insulin. These functional tumors trigger hormone release from the brain, and the normal feedback system which either increases insulin release or decreases it in relation to blood glucose levels becomes ineffective. Excessive levels of insulin produce decreasing levels of blood glucose concentrations over time (weeks to months).

CLINICAL SIGNS
- Hypoglycemia
- Weakness
- Lethargy
- Ataxia
- Seizures
- Coma
- Hypothermia
- Tachycardia
- Muscle fasciculations
- Irritability

DIAGNOSIS
- Physical examination and history of episodes of collapse or weakness
- CBC and serum chemistries
  - Hypoglycemia: blood glucose level less than 60 milligram per deciliter (mg/dL)

- Serum insulin levels: elevated
- Alanine aminotransferase (ALT) serum may be increased
- Radiography or ultrasonography: may locate a mass in the liver if metastasis has occurred.

TREATMENT

Medical

- Will not slow tumor growth
- Prednisone: used to increase blood glucose levels by inhibiting glucose uptake and increasing gluconeogenesis
- Diazoxide: inhibits insulin release and inhibits gluconeogenesis
- Dietary management: feed frequent small meals and avoid fasting; use high-protein food; and avoid sugars and carbohydrates

Surgical

- Not curative but may slow progression
- Nodulectomy or partial pancreatectomy

INFORMATION FOR CLIENTS

- Insulinomas in ferrets are usually malignant and can spread to the liver and other organs.
- Surgery should be performed by a surgical specialist.
- Many ferrets will still require medical management of hypoglycemia after surgery, and blood glucose levels must be checked every 2 to 3 months.
- Aggressive surgical treatment may result in hyperglycemia (diabetes mellitus) in the ferret. This may be a transient effect in some animals.

Rodents

Endocrine disease in rodents is not a common finding; however, several cases of hyperadrenocorticism (Cushing disease) have been reported in pet hamsters.

Hyperadrenocorticism (Cushing Disease)

CLINICAL SIGNS

- Polydipsia or polyuria
- Polyphagia

- Alopecia
- Hyperpigmentation

DIAGNOSIS

- Physical examination and history
- Increased plasma cortisol and alkaline phosphatase levels

TREATMENT

- o,p-DDD (mitotane) orally every 24 hours
- Metyrapone orally every 8-12 hours

INFORMATION FOR CLIENTS

- Treatment may not benefit all hamsters with Cushing disease.
- More information on endocrine disease is needed for the rodent species.

Diabetes Mellitus in Degus (Trumpet Tail Rats)

CLINICAL SIGNS

- Development of cataracts
- Polyuria or polydipsia
- Weight loss

DIAGNOSIS

- Physical examination and history
- Increased blood glucose level

TREATMENT

- None found in the literature for diabetic degus

REVIEW QUESTIONS

1. Which disease represents the most commonly seen endocrine disorder in domestic ferrets?
   a. Estrogen toxicity
   b. Insulinoma
   c. Adrenal disease
   d. Pituitary adenoma
2. Alopecia, hyperpigmentation, polyuria, polydipsia, and polyphagia in the hamster are typical signs of:
   a. Hypoadrenocorticism
   b. Hyperadrenocorticism
   c. Diabetes mellitus
   d. Insulinoma

3. Rats fed diets high in _____ can result in the formation of cataracts.
   a. Starch
   b. Sucrose
   c. Protein
   d. Lipids

4. Overgrowth of the rabbit's upper incisors may result in _____. (Check all that apply.)
   a. Blocked lacrimal ducts
   b. Epiphora
   c. Blepharitis
   d. Conjunctivitis

Answers found on page 553.

Diseases of the Eye

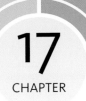

Blepharospasm
Chromodacryorrhea
Cyclophotocoagulation

Enucleation
Epiphora
Erythema

Glaucoma
Keratoconjunctivitis
Uveitis

LEARNING OBJECTIVES

When you have completed this chapter, you will be able to:
1. Explain the causes of many of the common eye problems seen in ferrets, rodents, and rabbits.
2. Discuss treatments for a variety of eye problems when asked by clients.
3. Recognize normal clinical signs of eye disease in ferrets, rodents, and rabbits.

The Ferret

Diseases of the eye in ferrets are similar to those in other species. The three most frequently seen disorders are (1) conjunctivitis, (2) cataract or lens luxations, and (3) retinal atrophy.

Conjunctivitis may have many causes—bacterial, viral (canine distemper virus or human influenza virus), or environmental (dust, debris, vapors). Cataract and lens luxations are believed to be inherited traits, and animals with these traits should not be used for breeding. Likewise, retinal atrophy may also be related to genetic causes or nutritional deficiencies (taurine). Typically, no treatment is suggested for these genetically based diseases.

Common Disorders of the Eye

CONJUNCTIVITS CLINICAL SIGNS

- Ocular discharge
- Red, swollen conjunctiva
- ± Blepharospasms

CATARACT/LENS LUXATIONS CLINICAL SIGNS

- Opacity of the pupil

RETINAL ATROPHY CLINICAL SIGNS

- Progressive loss of vision

DIAGNOSIS

- Physical examination and history
- Complete ocular examination
- Culture and sensitivity of ocular discharge

TREATMENT

- Ophthalmic antibiotic ointment based on culture or sensitivity
- Canine distemper is usually fatal in ferrets; no treatment is available
- No treatment for genetic dysfunction

Rodents

Cataracts

Cataracts occur in rats and mice as both inherited and congenital lesions and secondary to other diseases and trauma. Nutritionally induced cataracts are also seen in laboratory rats fed increased levels of sucrose, xylose, or galactose.

CLINICAL SIGNS

- Opacity of the lens in one or both eyes
- Usually will not impair vision

DIAGNOSIS

- Complete ophthalmologic examination

TREATMENT

- Correct diet if nutritional cause is suspected
- No treatment is available for most pet rats

INFORMATION FOR CLIENTS

- The occurrence of cataracts resulting in loss of vision in pet rats is unusual.

Epiphora, Conjunctivitis, and Chromodacryorrhea (Pigmented Tears)

Many rodents produce tears that contain the pigment porphyrin. These red-brown secretions are often mistaken for blood in the medial canthus and on the front paws of the animal. Both bacterial and viral diseases may be associated with conjunctivitis in rodents. Noninfectious causes include irritation from soiled bedding, malocclusion of overgrown incisors, and poor nutrition and hygiene. Stress can also result in an increase in pigmented tears.

CLINICAL SIGNS

- Overproduction of tears or lack of tear duct drainage
- Red, swollen conjunctival tissues
- ± Signs of systemic disease
- ± Signs of incisor overgrowth

DIAGNOSIS

- Physical examination and history; stress in a new home may increase incidence
- Exfoliative cytology of conjunctiva
- Flushing of lacrimal ducts
- Distinguish porphyrin from blood (porphyrin will fluoresce under ultraviolet light, blood will not)
- Culture and sensitivity of conjunctiva

TREATMENT

- Systemic antibiotics based on culture and sensitivity results
- Topical ophthalmic antibiotic ointments
- Improved hygiene and nutrition
- Correction of any underlying dental problems
- Decreasing stress in the environment

INFORMATION FOR CLIENTS

- Treatment for conjunctivitis may need to be based on laboratory findings, which may be expensive. Often therapy is started on the basis of previous experience with your pet or other similar cases.
- It is natural for many rodents to shed red tears.

⬤ TECH ALERT

Owners will report bleeding from the eyes when they see red tears. Even though the color may be normal, do not rule out disease as a cause of epiphora.

Periocular Dermatitis in Gerbils

CLINICAL SIGNS

- Erythema
- Crusting around eyes
- Alopecia around nares, forepaws, and facial areas

DIAGNOSIS

- Physical examination and history

TREATMENT

- Decrease ambient temperatures (will decrease excessive grooming)
- Gently cleanse secretions from affected areas
- Apply protective ophthalmic ointment to area
- Change bedding materials if they are irritants

Keratoconjunctivitis in Hamsters

Keratoconjunctivitis in hamsters is usually the result of environmental trauma and unsanitary bedding.

CLINICAL SIGNS

- Inflammation of cornea and conjunctiva

DIAGNOSIS

- Physical examination and history
- Complete ophthalmologic examination

TREATMENT

- Difficult because systemic antibiotic therapy may produce fatal enteritis in hamsters
- Topical ophthalmic ointments

The Rabbit

The eye of the rabbit is structurally similar to that of the dog and the cat but with a few exceptions. Important eye disorders of the rabbit include epiphora, conjunctivitis, uveitis, blepharospasms, and glaucoma.

Epiphora (Runny Eyes)

Runny eyes in the rabbit may be related to the overgrowth of the upper incisors, which results in blockage of the lacrimal (tear) duct. Other causes may be related to environmental conditions (dust, pollen, household fumes), disease of the cornea, entropion or ectropion, districhiasis (abnormal eyelash placement),

third eyelid disease, or foreign body obstruction of the tear duct. A thorough ophthalmic examination should provide a definite diagnosis.

CLINICAL SIGNS

- Excessive watering of the eyes
- Wet facial hair with staining
- ± Squinting, rubbing the eyes, mucous discharge, swelling, or redness

DIAGNOSIS

- Physical examination and history
- Complete ophthalmic examination
- Dental examination
- Culture and sensitivity
- Radiographs (facial)

TREATMENT

- Grind or cut overgrown incisor teeth if present
- Flush the lacrimal canal
- Apply topical ophthalmic antibiotic ointment based on culture results
- Correct abnormalities of eyelids or cilia
- ± Systemic antibiotics

Conjunctivitis and Blepharitis

Conjunctivitis and blepharitis, together with epiphora, are commonly seen in pet rabbits. Infectious causes that have been isolated include *Pasteurella multocida*, *Staphylococcus aureus*, *Pseudomonas* spp., *Treponema cuniculi* (rabbit syphilis), and *Chlamydia* organisms. Noninfectious causes such as trauma, dust, and eyelid disorders may also be causes of conjunctivitis and blepharitis.

CLINICAL SIGNS

- Excessive watering of the eyes
- Redness, swelling
- Squinting; sensitivity to light
- ± Uveitis (*Pasteurella*)
- ± Dry, crusty lesions on eyelids (*Treponema*)

DIAGNOSIS

- Physical examination and history
- Culture and sensitivity
- Cytology
- Viral isolation if a viral causative agent is suggested from intracytoplasmic inclusions

- Dark-field microscopy of perilesional scrapings if rabbit syphilis suspected (will see ulcerations of mucous membranes, eyelids with dry, crusty lesions over ulcerated skin)

TREATMENT

- Antibiotic ophthalmic ointment based on culture results
- Systemic antibiotics
- Clean-up of the environment

INFORMATION FOR CLIENTS

- It is important to accurately diagnose the cause of eye infections in rabbits before treatment.
- Eye problems should be seen by your veterinarian as soon as noticed to prevent permanent damage to the eye.

Glaucoma

Glaucoma (i.e., increased intraocular pressures) is a recessive trait in New Zealand White rabbits. Rabbits affected by this disease have increased intraocular pressures by about 3 to 6 months of age.

CLINICAL SIGNS

- Corneal edema
- Exposure keratitis
- Blindness

DIAGNOSIS

- Physical examination and history
- Age-related symptoms
- Measurement of increased intraocular pressures

TREATMENT

- Enucleation of the affected eye
- Laser cyclophotocoagulation
- Cyclocryotherapy

INFORMATION FOR CLIENTS

- Affected rabbits should not be used for breeding.
- Medical therapy of this disease is usually ineffective.
- Glaucoma can occur in other breeds as a result of trauma or infection. Enucleation is the treatment of choice for rabbits with glaucoma.

REVIEW QUESTIONS

1. Retinal atrophy is the result of nutritional or genetic defects. What is the most common clinical sign of retinal atrophy?
   a. Acute loss of vision
   b. Red, swollen eye
   c. Progressive loss of vision
   d. Opacity of the pupil
2. What pigment does the Harderian gland of the rat, located behind the eyes, produce?
   a. Rhodopsin
   b. Porphyrin
   c. Melanin
   d. Bilirubin
3. Rabbit syphilis may cause crusty eyelid lesions and is caused by:
   a. *Pasteurella* spp.
   b. *Pseudomonas* spp.
   c. *Treponema* spp.
   d. *Chlamydia* spp.
4. Hamster polyoma virus produces _____ in young hamsters.
   a. Bone tumors
   b. Skin tumors
   c. GI tumors
   d. Oral tumors

Answers found on page 553.

Hematologic and Immunologic Diseases

Hemopoietic   Oncology   Visceral
Malignancy   Remission

Ferrets   **Rodents**
   Lymphoma   Lymphoma (Hamsters)

When you have completed this chapter, you will be able to:

1. Recognize the usual causes of tumors in ferrets and rodents.

2. Explain why treatment may not be a good option for the pet.

Ferrets

Estrogen toxicosis and bone marrow suppression resulting in a life-threatening anemia are covered in Chapter 22.

Lymphoma

Lymphoma is the most common malignancy of the ferret. Several forms of lymphoma exist; the most frequent is the lymphocytic form, which involves the lymph nodes and spreads to visceral organs later in the disease. The lymphoblastic form, seen mostly in young ferrets, produces visceral neoplasms early on in the disease. Another form is a combination type, which is rarely seen.

CLINICAL SIGNS

- Enlarged peripheral lymph nodes
- Chronic lethargy
- Cycles of illness and recovery
- Anorexia
- Weight loss

DIAGNOSIS

- Clinical signs and history
- Needle aspirate of lymph node may suggest diagnosis
  - Mature, well-differentiated lymphocytes present with adult form
- Excisional biopsy of lymph nodes or organ biopsy
- Complete blood cell count (CBC) may show lymphocytosis
- Radiography or ultrasonography
- Cytology of any fluid (pleural or abdominal)

TREATMENT

- Available chemotherapy or multidrug protocols include the following:
  - Prednisone

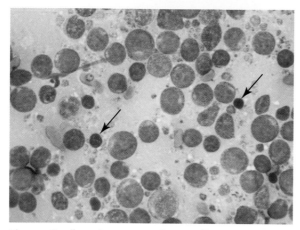

Figure 18-1 Lymphosarcoma: fine-needle aspirate from a ferret. (From Quesenberry KE, Carpenter JW: *Ferrets, rabbits, and rodents*, ed 3, St. Louis, MO, 2012, Saunders, by permission.)

- Vincristine
- Cyclophosphamide or L-asparaginase
- Doxorubicin
- Methotrexate
- Vincristine and cyclophosphamide and prednisone
- Dietary supplementation (high calorie)
- Fluids to maintain hydration

INFORMATION FOR CLIENTS

- The prognosis for this disease is poor. Many ferrets will not respond well to chemotherapy, with about 10% achieving complete remission.
- Treatment is expensive, time-consuming, and usually involves referral to a veterinary oncology specialist.

Rodents

Lymphoma (Hamsters)

Neoplasia (lymphoma) is a common finding in hamsters. In older hamsters, the lymphoma typically involves the hemopoietic system, thymus, spleen, liver, lymph nodes, and other sites. In younger hamsters, the disease involves skin tumors caused by the

hamster polyomavirus. Adult hamsters can also exhibit a third form of the disease, which involves cutaneous tissues.

CLINICAL SIGNS

- Swollen lymph nodes
- Dyspnea
- Weight loss
- Alopecia (with cutaneous lesions)
- Anorexia
- Lethargy
- Distended abdomen

DIAGNOSIS

- Physical examination and history
- Radiography
- Fine-needle aspiration or biopsy of the masses

TREATMENT

- Chemotherapy (extrapolate dosages from drugs used in other species)

INFORMATION FOR CLIENTS

- Treatment may be expensive and these drugs may be toxic to the patient.
- Euthanasia may be the best option.

REVIEW QUESTIONS

1. What is the most common malignancy in ferrets?
   a. Adenocarcinoma
   b. Lymphoma
   c. Squamous cell carcinoma
   d. Fibrosarcoma
2. What is a common neoplasm in hamsters?
   a. Fibrosarcoma
   b. Chondrosarcoma
   c. Lymphoma
   d. Squamous cell carcinoma
3. Fur mites of mice are transmitted by _____.
   a. Fomites in the cage
   b. Sexual transmission
   c. Direct contact with infected mice
4. The most common tumor in rats is _____.
   a. Fibroadenoma of the mammary gland
   b. Fibrosarcoma of the mammary gland
   c. Squamous cell carcinoma of the skin

5. Myxomycosis is seen mostly in this region of the country.
   a. Southern U.S.
   b. Western U.S.
   c. East coastal U.S.
   d. West coastal U.S.

6. If one were to see mice in the same cage all with normal skin but thinning hair, one might suspect:
   a. Barbering
   b. Fungal infection
   c. Fleas
   d. All of the above

Answers found on page 554.

19 CHAPTER

Diseases of the Integumentary System

LEARNING OBJECTIVES

When you have completed this chapter, you will be able to:
1. Recognize common parasites of skin in these species.
2. Be able to discuss treatments for these diseases with clients.
3. Explain how to prevent initial infestation or re-infestation of skin parasites in these species.

The Ferret

The normal hair coat of the ferret contains a thick, cream-colored undercoat with coarse guard hairs that determine the coat color. Numerous sebaceous glands give the coat a greasy feeling and produce a musky odor. Thinning of the coat occurs twice yearly in relation to photoperiods—increasing when daylight hours and temperature increase. Hair removed during the seasonal thinning periods may not regrow for several months.

The most common diseases affecting skin include adrenal disease, parasites, and occasionally neoplasia. Endocrine alopecia has been covered in Chapter 16.

Parasites

Fleas (*Ctenocephalides* spp. and *Pulex irritans*) and ear mites (*Otodectes cynotis*) are the most commonly seen parasites of pet ferrets, although if housed outdoors, ticks and *Cuterebra* may also be seen. Benign neoplasms also occur. Sarcoptic mange is uncommon in pet ferrets but has been seen.

CLINICAL SIGNS

- Pruritus with or without alopecia dorsally
- Dark brown, waxy discharge in the ears (ear mites)
- Head tilt (with severe infestations)

DIAGNOSIS

- Finding parasites on examination

TREATMENT

Fleas

- No flea treatments have been approved for ferrets. Care should be used if topical products manufactured for dogs and cats are used. Sprays should be applied to a cloth and rubbed onto the ferret. Avoid all products that contain organophosphates.
- New flea control products have been reported to be useful:
  - Lufenuron
  - Fipronil
  - Revolution
  - **Use of these products constitutes off-label usage.**

Ear Mites

- Cleaning ears to remove exudates
- Ivermectin given subcutaneously (SQ) every 2 weeks until mite free
- Topical preparations:
  - Thiabendazole neomycin or dexamethasone (Tresaderm)
  - 1% ivermectin diluted 1:10 in propylene glycol
  - Selamectin at cat dosage (off-label use)
- Treatment of the environment is required to prevent reinfestation

Bacterial Skin Disease

Bite wounds and punctures may result in the formation of abscesses in ferrets. Anal gland abscesses may also be seen in these animals.

CLINICAL SIGNS

- Swollen, fluctuant mass located at the site of trauma

DIAGNOSIS

- Gram stain of aspirated mass; most common organisms found include:
  - *Staphylococcus* spp.
  - *Streptococcus* spp.
  - *Corynebacterium* spp.
  - *Pasteurella* spp.
- Anaerobic and aerobic culture and sensitivity

TREATMENT

- Draining and flushing of abscess
- Systemic antibiotic based on culture and sensitivity

INFORMATION FOR CLIENTS

- Keep the abscess site open to allow drainage and to allow healing to proceed from the deeper levels to the surface.

Skin Neoplasia

Benign neoplasms of the skin are a common problem in ferrets. The most frequently involved lesions are mast cell tumors, basal cell tumors, and sebaceous cell tumors.

CLINICAL SIGNS

- Mass located in skin

DIAGNOSIS

- Biopsy of the mass

TREATMENT

- Surgical removal

INFORMATION FOR CLIENTS

- Most of these growths are benign (nonmalignant); however, some may recur after removal.
- Occasionally a skin mass will be malignant. Have all masses examined by your veterinarian!

Rodents

It has been estimated that about 25% of all problems seen in mice involve the integumentary system. These problems result from behavioral problems, poor husbandry, bacterial infections, and parasitic infestations. Mice live a highly structured social life. The dominant mouse "barbers" others in the group, chewing off whiskers and facial hair. Fighting wounds are also common when male mice are kept together. Mice mayget abrasions from rubbing against the cage and objects in the cage. Fur mites are seen in mice and result in overall thinning of the hair and pruritus. Lesions can become infected and ulcerated. Mice areprone to skin tumors (especially mammary gland adenocarcinomas and fibrosarcomas) or abscesses caused by *Staphylococcus*, *Pasteurella*, and *Streptococcus* bacteria.

Fur Mites

Three mite species commonly infect mice: *Myobia musculi*, *Myocoptes musculinus*, and *Radfordia affinis*. Mites are spread by direct contact between mice or from infected bedding. Mite infestation is less common in rats than in mice and treatment is the same for both animals.

CLINICAL SIGNS

- Generalized thinning of the hair
- Greasy coat
- ± Pruritus
- ± Secondary infections and ulcerations

DIAGNOSIS

- Identification of mites, nymphs, or eggs on hair shafts

TREATMENT

- Ivermectin SQ or orally (PO) twice at 10-day intervals
- Remove all bedding and clean cage thoroughly

INFORMATION FOR CLIENTS

- Have all new pets examined for mites before placing them in cages with other pets.
- Purchase new pets from reputable dealers.

Tumors

Mice are prone to mammary adenocarcinomas and fibrosarcomas. Most are malignant, and the prognosis is poor even with surgery. The most common tumor in rats is the fibroadenoma of the mammary gland.

Tumors become large and may occur in both male andfemale rats. These tumors are not malignant but do tend to recur.

CLINICAL SIGNS

- A firm swelling involving the mammary gland or subcutaneous tissue anywhere on the body
- Tumor usually ulcerated by the time it is examined

DIAGNOSIS

- Physical examination and history
- Cytology from fine-needle biopsy
- Biopsy after surgical removal

TREATMENT

- Surgical excision

INFORMATION FOR CLIENTS

- Even with surgical excision the prognosis for the mouse is poor.
- Recurrence of these tumors is common.
- Mammary tumors in rats are typically nonmalignant but tend to recur.

Impacted Cheek Pouches in Hamsters

Hamsters have large cheek pouches used to carry food, bedding, and their young. Food or other materials left in the pouches for long periods may become impacted.

CLINICAL SIGNS

- Large swellings on either side of the face
- ± Rubbing with front paws

DIAGNOSIS

- Physical examination and history
- Radiography

TREATMENT

- Gentle removal of the material with fine-tipped forceps (animal may require sedation)
- Correct predisposing conditions such as malocclusion and stress

INFORMATION FOR CLIENTS

- It is common for hamsters to place material into their cheek pouches. It usually does not cause any problem.

The Rabbit

Diseases of the integumentary system are common in rabbits.

Ulcerative Pododermatitis (Sore Hocks)

Ulcerative pododermatitis is frequently seen in heavy-bodied rabbits kept in wire mesh cages or on dirty floors. The condition involves the ventral metatarsal region of the leg and is usually secondary to constant trauma to the area. The round, ulcerated areas are well-circumscribed and often covered with a scab (Fig. 19-1). If the infection goes untreated, abscesses may develop and subsequent joint infections may occur, with arthritis being the final outcome.

CLINICAL SIGNS

- Obese rabbit
- Well-circumscribed, ulcerated lesions on the ventral surface of the metatarsals
- ± Lameness

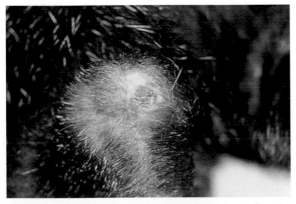

Figure 19-1 Advanced pododermatitis ("sore hocks") in the rabbit. (From Harcourt-Brown F: *Textbook of rabbit medicine*, Oxford, U.K., 2002, Butterworth-Heinemann, by permission.)

DIAGNOSIS

- Physical examination and history
- Culture and sensitivity of ulcerated sores
- ± Radiography to rule out arthritis of the joints

TREATMENT

- Reduce the weight of the rabbit.
- Improve the cage surfaces:
  - Compliant surfaces (surfaces that give as the rabbit walks on them)—for example, deep straw bedding, fake fur fabric, rubber pressure mats—may helpdistribute pressure.
  - Remove abrasive surface products such as carpet, vinyl, or plastic.
- Administer systemic antibiotics (depending on culture results).
- Provide antiinflammatory medication (steroids).
- Administer pain medication.
- Apply artificial skin preparations or bandage to prevent further damage

INFORMATION FOR CLIENTS

- Provide your rabbit with a cage surface that allows for compliance when the foot hits the ground. Avoid hard, unforgiving surfaces such as vinyl, plastic, concrete, carpet, or wood.
- Ensure that your rabbit does not become obese.
- Keep the rabbit's nails trimmed properly to allow the foot to rest flat on the surface.
- Preventing sore hocks is easier than curing it.

Abscesses

Abscesses in rabbits are similar to those in reptiles; they are caseous in nature and do not drain well. Treatment includes surgical excision or opening of the abscess with curettage; surgical drains are usually ineffective in removing pus. These abscesses are usually well walled off by a thick capsule, and infections do not become systemic. The most common cause of abscesses in rabbits is bite wounds and infections of tooth roots and tear ducts.

CLINICAL SIGNS

External Abscesses
- Firm, palpable mass anywhere on the body (facial more common site)
- ± Pain on palpation

Internal Abscesses
- May be difficult to find

DIAGNOSIS
- Physical examination and history
- Complete blood cell count (CBC) and serum chemistries
- Cytology or fine-needle biopsy
- Culture and sensitivity of contents and abscess wall (both aerobic and anaerobic)
- Radiography (for internal abscesses)

TREATMENT
- Surgical removal or curettage of the abscess
- Leaving the site open for several weeks for flushing to promote healing from the inside out
- Systemic antibiotics (oral or injectable)
- Pain medication if needed
- Ensuring that the environment of the rabbit is clean and that nutrition is adequate

INFORMATION FOR CLIENTS
- Rabbit abscesses have a high probability of reoccurrence.
- Have all lumps investigated as soon as possible by your veterinarian.
- Keep your rabbit's environment safe, and make sure you feed your pet a well-balanced diet to support the immune system.

Treponema cuniculi Infection

The spirochete *Treponema cuniculi* is transmitted by direct contact, usually during breeding or to offspring at birth. Lesions involve the vagina or the prepuce. The rabbit is the only natural host of this disease, which is commonly known as "rabbit syphilis."

CLINICAL SIGNS
- Edema with or without redness of the vaginal or preputial area
- Presence of macules, papules, pustules, scabs on the genitalia, eyelids, nose, and lips
- No other signs of systemic disease

DIAGNOSIS
- Physical examination and history

- Dark-field microscopy: presence of spiral-shaped bacteria on skin scrapings
- Serology positive for the organism

TREATMENT
- Systemic antibiotics (suggested treatment consists of three penicillin G benzathine–penicillin G procaine injections at 7-day intervals)

INFORMATION FOR CLIENTS
- Avoid purchasing young rabbits with this type of lesion.
- Avoid using infected rabbits for breeding.
- Most lesions will regress after several weeks.

Myxomatosis

Myxomatosis is an arthropod-transmitted viral disease which is primarily a problem for wild rabbits and domestic rabbits in the western United States. The virus has several strains, and symptoms of the disease range from mild to fatal.

CLINICAL SIGNS
- Palpebral edema, conjunctivitis
- Gelatinous subcutaneous swellings of the face, ears, and external genitalia

DIAGNOSIS
- Physical examination, history, clinical signs
- History of vector exposure
- Virus isolation (fluorescent antibody technique)
- Histopathology (swellings that contain undifferentiated mesenchymal cells)

TREATMENT
- No treatment for myxomatosis exists.

INFORMATION FOR CLIENTS
- Prevent myxomatosis by keeping rabbits in insect-proof enclosures and eliminating exposure to wild rabbits.

Shope Fibroma Virus

The Shope fibroma virus, a pox virus related to the virus that causes myxomatosis, can cause papillomas on the neck, shoulders, and abdomen of rabbits (seen in the midwestern United States).

CLINICAL SIGNS

- Begin as warts that develop as red, raised areas at the site of infection
- Warts become papillomas with rough, rounded surfaces
- Some may become malignant squamous cell carcinomas

DIAGNOSIS

- Physical examination, history, and clinical signs
- Histopathology

TREATMENT

- No treatment for Shope fibroma virus exists.

INFORMATION FOR CLIENTS

- Prevent this disease by raising rabbits in insect-proof enclosures.
- Prevent exposure to wild cotton-tailed rabbits.

Dermatophytosis (Fungal Infections)

Fungal infections are common in pet rabbits. *Microsporum canis*, *Microsporum gypseum*, and *Trichophyton schoenleinii* are common agents, but the most common ringworm of rabbits is caused by *Trichophyton mentagrophytes*. Lesions most often appear on the head, face, or forelimbs and are irregular, coin-shaped, alopecic areas surrounded by a ring of inflammation with crusting. The lesions are usually pruritic, and often pet owners will have similar lesions on their faces, arms, and hands from handling infected bunnies.

CLINICAL SIGNS

- Round, alopecic lesions on the face, forelimbs, head, and back
- Pruritic
- Lesions are crusty and have a ring of inflammation surrounding them

DIAGNOSIS

- Physical examination and history
- Fungal elements identified from skin scrapings (potassium hydroxide [KOH] slide)
- Positive dermatophyte culture
- Evidence of human exposure and infection

TREATMENT

- Clip all the affected hair.
- Bathe the animal with an iodine-based shampoo.
- Topical fungal preparations may be useful.
- Administer oral griseofulvin.
- Sanitize the environment by vacuuming and bydisinfection using a dilute bleach solution.

◉ TECH ALERT

Dermatophytosis is a zoonotic disease. Use care when handling and treating these patients.

INFORMATION FOR CLIENTS

- Fungal spores may live on and in furniture, bedding, and clothing for long periods. It is important to clean the environment to prevent further infection.
- Use care when handling infected rabbits. The disease can be transmitted to humans and other pets.
- Consult your physician if you suspect you have contracted this disease.

Parasites

Ear mites (*Psoroptes cuniculi*)

Ear mites frequently cause problems in pet rabbits. The lesions are found in the ear canal first but gradually extend upward as honey-colored crusty exudates covering a red, irritated, raw skin surface (Fig. 19-2). If allowed to continue unchecked, the infection may spread to the head and surrounding tissues.

CLINICAL SIGNS

- Dry, honey-colored crusts in ear canals
- Intensely pruritic
- Head-shaking, pain

DIAGNOSIS

- Physical examination and history
- Otoscopic examination and microscopic examination of exudates

TREATMENT

- Flushing the ear under anesthesia to remove debris
- Topical treatment with Tresaderm

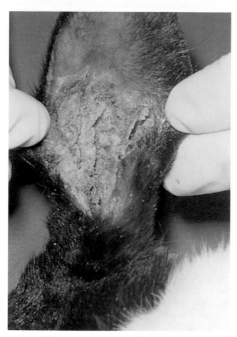

Figure 19-2 Ear mites in a domestic rabbit. (From Harcourt-Brown F: *Textbook of rabbit medicine*, Oxford, U.K., 2002, Butterworth-Heinemann, by permission.)

- Oral ivermectin repeated every 10 days until all mites are gone
- Treatment of the environment with an insecticide for 4 weeks to prevent spread or reinfection

INFORMATION FOR CLIENTS

- Check inside the ear canal of your pet rabbit frequently. If you find any exudates, have your rabbit examined by your veterinarian.
- The skin under the exudate may be raw and painful. Some rabbits will require oral antibiotics if a secondary bacterial infection is present.
- This infection is highly contagious to other rabbits.

Cheyletiella Parasitovorax

The fur mite *Cheyletiella parasitovorax* is commonly found on pet rabbits in certain geographic regions. It is called "walking dandruff," because the mites are large and visible to the naked eye.

CLINICAL SIGNS

- Thinning of the hair over the shoulders and back

- Red, oily, hairless patches over the back and head if untreated
- Mild-to-moderate pruritus

DIAGNOSIS

- Physical examination and history
- Finding the mite on the fur (cellophane tape method)

TREATMENT

- Bathing with an insecticide shampoo
- Oral ivermectin
- Treatment of the environment (female mite may live off the rabbit for several weeks)

INFORMATION FOR CLIENTS

- These mites are visible as small white flakes moving on the surface of the rabbit's hair.
- They are mildly contagious to humans and may produce a transient dermatitis.
- You must eliminate the mite from the rabbit and the environment to effect a cure.

Cuterebra (Warbles)

Cuterebra are frequently seen during the summer months in rabbits housed outdoors. Flies lay eggs around the rabbit hutch, and the larvae enter the host through the nasal or oral openings. The larvae develop, mature, and then drop out of the rabbit, pupate in the soil, and become flies the next warm season. Lesions develop during larval development and consist of swellings containing larva.

CLINICAL SIGNS

- Fistulated 2- to 3-cm swelling in the head area
- Larva often seen within the swelling or at the opening
- Lesions often moist around the opening and painful

DIAGNOSIS

- Physical examination, history, season
- Visualization of the larva in the fistulous opening

TREATMENT

- Open the mass to facilitate removal of the intact larva (may require anesthesia)
- Flush the wound well and treat with an appropriate topical antibiotic

◐ TECH ALERT

When removing the larva, take care not to rupture the cystic cavity or tear the larva, because an anaphylactic reaction may occur. Take care to remove the entire larva intact.

INFORMATION FOR CLIENTS

- Keeping rabbits in insect-proof housing will prevent infection with *Cuterebra*.
- *Do not* try to remove the larva using tweezers at home. A fatal anaphylactic reaction may result from rupture of the larva.

Fleas and Ticks

Fleas and ticks are found on domestic rabbits housed outdoors. Treatment is similar to that for dogs and cats: bathing with an approved insecticidal shampoo and treating the environment with any preparation suitable for cats.

Fur Plucking

Preparturient does will commonly pluck fur from the belly, dewlap, and sides of the body. They use this fur to line the nest before kindling. Diagnosis is made by eliminating other causes of fur plucking and by determining that the doe is pregnant. No treatment is necessary.

REVIEW QUESTIONS

1. Which of the following products is approved for use in flea control in the domestic ferret?
   a. Ivermectin
   b. Selamectin
   c. Pyrethrins
   d. All of the above
   e. None of the above

2. Which of the following species is the commonly seen fur mite of mice and rats?
   a. *Mallophaga* spp.
   b. *Cnemidocoptes* spp.
   c. *Radfordia* spp.
   d. *Lynxacarus* spp.

3. To treat impacted cheek pouches in the hamster _____.
   a. Gently remove impacted materials
   b. Lance and drain
   c. Do nothing; this is normal

4. What is the most common cause of ulcerative pododermatitis in heavy-bodied rabbits?
   a. Constant trauma to the area
   b. Parasitic infection of the skin
   c. Neurologic disease with abnormal gait
   d. Systemic bacterial infections

5. Spondylosis in the older rabbit may result in paralysis.
   a. True
   b. False

6. Which of the following surfaces would be best for the examination of the rabbit?
   a. Rubber mat on the exam table
   b. Bath towel on the exam table
   c. Stainless steel exam table

Answers found on page 554.

Diseases of the Musculoskeletal System

LEARNING OBJECTIVES

When you have completed this chapter, you will be able to:
1. Understand the need for proper restraint and handling of the rabbit during examination and treatment.

2. Discuss aging changes that occur in rabbits with respect to the vertebral column.

The Ferret

Diseases of the musculoskeletal system are not common in ferrets. They may suffer traumatic long-bone fractures or spinal injury from rough play or falls. Treatment is similar to those of dogs and cats.

Rodents

As with all small animals, fractures and dislocations from falls and rough handling do occur. Fractures can be treated as for avian and reptilian patients, using splints, casts, or lightweight internal fixation.

The Rabbit

Rabbits have a weak skeletal system that can be easily damaged with improper handling. Only about 8% of their body weight is made up by the skeleton (much less than in dogs and cats).

Trauma

Improper handling is a frequent cause of paralysis in the domestic rabbit. Damage may also occur as a result of falling or being jumped on by other rabbits while playing. Typically, the rabbit will kick or twist suddenly, causing fracture of the vertebral column with damage to the spinal cord (Fig. 20-1).

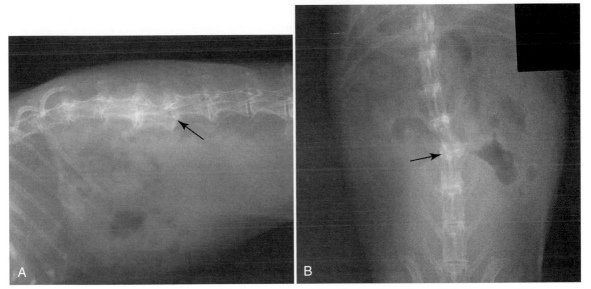

Figure 20-1 Radiograph of a spinal fracture in a rabbit. (From Quesenberry KE, Carpenter JW: *Ferrets, rabbits, and rodents*, ed 2, St. Louis, MO, 2011, Saunders, by permission.)

CLINICAL SIGNS

- Complete or partial paralysis immediately after injury
- ± Loss of bladder or bowel control, or both

DIAGNOSIS

- Physical examination and history
- Complete neurologic examination
- Radiography; ± myelogram

TREATMENT

- None, if spinal cord is severely damaged
- If mild to moderate contusion of the cord is present:
  - Antiinflammatory drugs
  - Cage confinement for 6 to 8 weeks

⦿ TECH ALERT

Always support the rear quarters of the rabbit when handling. Prevent sudden kicking or twisting by firmly holding the rabbit against your body or using the "bunny burrito" method of restraint by wrapping the animal in a blanket.

INFORMATION FOR CLIENTS

- Allowing your rabbit to exercise frequently will result in a stronger skeletal system and decrease the chance of a fractured spine or other bony injuries.
- Avoid overfeeding your rabbit. Obese rabbits are more prone to musculoskeletal diseases.

Spondylosis of the Lumbar Spine

Spondylosis of the lumbar spine is a fairly common disease of rabbits older than 4 years, especially in large and medium breeds. The bones of the lower vertebra develop spurs that eventually bridge to the adjacent vertebra, reducing the flexibility of the vertebral column. This disease is made worse by excess body weight and inadequate exercise.

CLINICAL SIGNS

- Decreased ability to run and jump (decreased flexibility)
- ± Pain on movement
- Difficulty grooming, using litter box
- Reluctance to move

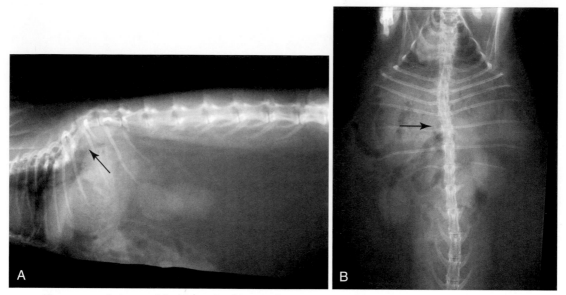

Figure 20-2 A 6-year-old rabbit with a history of progressive rear limb weakness. (From Quesenberry KE, Carpenter JW: *Ferrets, rabbits, and rodents*, ed 3, St. Louis, MO, 2012, Saunders, by permission.)

DIAGNOSIS

- Physical examination and history
- Radiography shows bony fusion of the spine (Fig. 20-2).

TREATMENT

- Pain medications
- Antiinflammatory drugs
- Gentle back massage over affected area
- Weight reduction
- Keeping animal groomed and clean

INFORMATION FOR CLIENTS

- Prevent or decrease the development of this condition by providing sufficient exercise and a well-balanced diet. Prevention of obesity is easier than weight reduction.
- This aging change occurs more frequently in female rabbits.

REVIEW QUESTION

1. What percentage of a rabbit's body weight does the skeleton comprise?
   a. 15%
   b. 24%
   c. 8%
   d. 3%

Answers found on page 554.

Diseases of the Nervous System

LEARNING OBJECTIVES

When you have completed this chapter, you will be able to:
1. Recognize signs of central nervous system (CNS) disease in these species.
2. Discuss medications used for treatment of CNS disease with the pet owners.

3. Exhibit awareness of the genetic seizure disorder in gerbils.

The Ferret

Primary neurologic disease is not common in the ferret. Most symptoms of (CNS) disease are the result of concurrent systemic disease processes such as hypoglycemia, cardiac disease, estrogen toxicosis, adrenal disease, or toxin ingestion. Intervertebral disk disease may be seen in the ferret.

Intervertebral Disk Disease

CLINICAL SIGNS

- Ataxia

- Posterior paresis
- Seizures

DIAGNOSIS

- Physical and neurologic examination
- Laboratory tests to rule in or rule out systemic diseases
- Complete blood cell count (CBC) or serum chemistries
- Radiography: whole-body ± myelogram, if disk problem
- Computed tomography (CT) or magnetic resonance imaging (MRI), if suspect central lesion in CNS

- Spinal tap, if infection is ruled out
- Electromyogram for peripheral nerve problems

TREATMENT

- Treat primary disease

Seizures

- Glucose for hypoglycemia
- Intravenous diazepam
- Prednisolone if cerebral edema suspected
- Oral phenobarbital for long-term management

INFORMATION FOR CLIENTS

- Nervous system signs are almost always a sign of some systemic disease. That disease must be first diagnosed to treat properly.
- Any CNS signs in a feral ferret (one found living free): suspect rabies and take precautions when handling.

Rodents

Up to 40% of all gerbils will experience seizures after the age of 2 months. This disorder is inherited and is the result of an enzyme deficiency in the brain. Seizures are usually short lived and leave no permanent damage. Some of these gerbils will have seizures when handled or stressed. Many gerbils will outgrow these seizures.

Seizures

CLINICAL SIGNS

- Development of seizures in a young gerbil, many when being handled

DIAGNOSIS

- Physical examination and history

TREATMENT

- No treatment is required.

INFORMATION FOR CLIENTS

- This defect is inherited.
- Many pets will outgrow this.
- Avoid using gerbils with seizure disorders for breeding.

The Rabbit

Neurologic signs are common in pet rabbits. Causes may be primary disease of the nervous system or secondary to some systemic problem. A complete physical and neurologic examination should be performed to diagnose the cause of the disorder.

Lameness

Abnormalities of gait can be seen by observing the rabbit move on a nonslip surface. The causes of lameness may include pododermatitis, fractures, dislocations, spinal disease, arthritis, neoplasia, bone abscesses, or hypertrophic osteopathy.

CLINICAL SIGNS

- Abnormal gait
- ± Pain on palpation
- ± Swollen joints
- ± Bony enlargements
- ± Fractures

DIAGNOSIS

- Complete history and physical examination
- Radiography
- CBC
- Culture and sensitivity if abscess is present
- Biopsy if tumor is present

TREATMENT

- Treatment will depend on the cause of lameness.

Encephalitozoonosis

Encephalitozoonosis is a disease of the CNS and is the result of infection by the microsporidian parasite *Encephalitozoon cuniculi*. This disease is widespread in rabbits and may result in granuloma formation in the kidney and the brain.

CLINICAL SIGNS

- ± Incontinence
- ± Polyuria or polydipsia
- Sudden deafness or strange behavior

Neurologic Signs in the Central Nervous System

- Vestibular disease (most common sign)
- Seizures

- Torticollis
- Ataxia
- Paralysis
- Sudden death

DIAGNOSIS

- Physical examination and clinical signs
- Radiography
- CBC

TREATMENT

- Albendazole or fenbendazole orally
- Corticosteroids: use is controversial because they may reduce clinical symptoms but immunosuppress the patient
- Oxytetracycline every 12 hours

INFORMATION FOR CLIENTS

- Treatment will depend on differentiating between *E. cuniculi* and *Pasteurella* as the cause of clinical symptoms.
- The prognosis is poor for rabbits that are unable to eat.
- Euthanasia may be the best option for animals with severe clinical signs.

Spinal Disease

Spinal disease in rabbits may occur for a variety of reasons. Congenital defects, nutritional deficiencies, degenerative disk disease, and trauma are among the most common causes. Spinal deformities may result in failure to groom, abnormal gaits, uneaten cecotrophs, and perianal dermatitis.

CLINICAL SIGNS

- Abnormal gait
- Inability to groom perineal region
- Reluctant to move
- Behavioral changes (pain related)
- ± Paralysis
- ± Urination problems

DIAGNOSIS

- Physical examination, history of trauma
- Radiography
- CBC, serum chemistry (calcium abnormalities)

TREATMENT

- Antiinflammatory medications (nonsteroidal anti-inflammatory drugs [NSAIDs])
- Treatment of fractures or spinal subluxations or disk disease is unrewarding in rabbits.

TECH ALERT

Always support the rear quarters of the rabbit when lifting or handling. Struggling by the rabbit may cause fractures to the vertebral column.

INFORMATION FOR CLIENTS

- Rabbits need adequate room to move around to prevent the development of spinal deformities.
- Make sure that children learn to pick up and carry rabbits correctly to prevent injury to the animals' back.

REVIEW QUESTIONS

1. When handled, it is not uncommon for some gerbils to exhibit:
   a. Vomiting
   b. Urinating
   c. Going limp
   d. Onset of seizures
2. The formation of granulomas in the kidney and brain of the rabbit is frequently a result of infection with:
   a. *Pasteurella multocida*
   b. *Staphylococcus aureus*
   c. *Encephalitozoon cuniculi*
   d. *Sarcocystis neurona*
3. Rabbits with *Encephalitozoon cuniculi* infection might present with: (Check all that apply)
   a. Vomiting
   b. Head-tilt
   c. Paralysis
   d. Lameness

Answers found on page 554.

22 CHAPTER

Diseases of the Reproductive System

Dysuria   Laparotomy   Serosanguinous

The Ferret
    Estrogen Toxicosis
    Reproductive Tumors
    Prostate Disease
Rodents
    Mammary Gland Tumors in Rats and Mice

The Rabbit
    Uterine Disease
    Pyometra and Endometritis
    Pseudopregnancy
    Mastitis
    Reproductive System Problems in the Male Rabbit

When you have completed this chapter, you will be able to:
1. Describe the common reproductive disorders of these species.

2. Discuss with owners the need to spay or neuter any pets not being used for breeding.

The Ferret

Estrogen Toxicosis

Estrogen toxicosis is perhaps the most well-known disease affecting the reproductive tract in ferrets. Because ferrets experience induced ovulation, estrous ferrets may maintain increased estrogen levels for long periods if not bred. Today this disease has almost been eliminated because of ovariohysterectomies performed before the female ferret reaches maturity.

CLINICAL SIGNS

• Anorexia
• Lethargy
• Weakness
• Pale mucous membranes
• Swollen vulva with a discharge (Fig. 22-1)
• ± Petechial hemorrhages
• Dorsally symmetric alopecia

DIAGNOSIS

• Clinical signs and history of unspayed female ferret
• Complete blood cell count (CBC): nonregenerative anemia, nucleated red blood cells, neutropenia, thrombocytopenia
• Bone marrow aspirate: confirmation of blood results

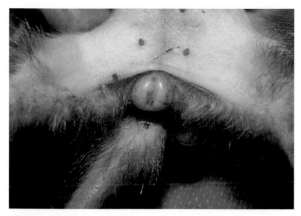

Figure 22-1 Enlarged vulva in a ferret with estrogen toxicosis. (From Quesenberry KE, Carpenter JW: *Ferrets, rabbits, and rodents*, ed 3, St. Louis, MO, 2012, Saunders, by permission.)

TREATMENT

- Breed or mechanically stimulate the female to ovulate.
- Ovariohysterectomy is the treatment of choice; these animals are poor surgical candidates because of thrombocytopenia. They may need transfusion before surgery.

Medical
- Gonadotropin-releasing hormone therapy
- Epogen
- Anabolic steroids

Prognosis Based on Original Packed Cell Volume
- Packed cell volume (PCV) greater than 25%: good
- PCV 15% to 25%: fair
- PCV less than 15%: poor

INFORMATION FOR CLIENTS

- Do not purchase an unspayed female ferret as a pet. If breeding ferrets, do not let a jill stay in estrous for longer than 2 to 4 weeks.

⬤ **TECH ALERT**

Advise owners of all young ferrets to have them spayed if they are intact. Most ferrets are spayed before entering the pet trade. Ferrets will remain in heat until bred because they are induced ovulators.

Tumors of the Reproductive Tract

Tumors of the female reproductive tract are common in unspayed female ferrets. Leiomyomas are the most common ovarian tumor recognized. In male ferrets, Sertoli cell tumors, seminomas, and interstitial cell tumors have been reported.

CLINICAL SIGNS
- Lethargy
- Depression
- Anorexia
- Persistent estrus (female)
- Dorsal alopecia (in male ferrets because of hyperestrogen levels from Sertoli cell tumors)

DIAGNOSIS
- Clinical signs and history
- Ultrasonography

TREATMENT
- Surgical removal; spay or castrate

INFORMATION FOR CLIENTS
- Spay or castrate all pet ferrets not used for breeding.

Prostatic Disease

Prostatic disease does occur in ferrets but usually in association with adrenal disease. It may result in urinary obstruction, which may lead to serious electrolyte disturbances.

CLINICAL SIGNS
- Dysuria
- Signs of adrenal dysfunction

DIAGNOSIS
- Radiography showing distended bladder, enlarged prostate
- Ultrasonography may differentiate cysts or abscesses from prostatomegaly
- Ultrasound-guided fine-needle aspiration

TREATMENT
- Resolve urinary obstruction: catheter placement
- Remove affected adrenal gland, if present
- Diazepam for smooth muscle relaxation
- Leuprolide (Lupron) to shrink prostatic tissue

Surgical

- Remove the diseased adrenal gland and drain prostatic abscesses or cysts.

INFORMATION FOR CLIENTS

- Failure to pass urine can lead to serious electrolyte disturbances. Contact your veterinary clinic if you notice lack of urine production or excessive straining to urinate in your male ferret.
- The adrenal disease must be treated together with the prostatic disease (see Chapter 16).

Rodents

Problems of the reproductive system in rodents include mammary gland tumors, pyometra, cannibalism, and cystic ovaries, although most of these are not common in pets.

Mammary Gland Tumors in Rats and Mice

Mammary gland fibroadenomas are common in rats. These tumors can develop in both male and female rats and can become large. Adenocarcinomas are also seen but represent only a small percentage of mammary tumors in rats. Most mammary tumors in mice are malignant and not amenable to surgery.

CLINICAL SIGNS

- Enlarged mammary glands (may be located anywhere from the neck of the rat to the inguinal area) (Fig. 22-2)

DIAGNOSIS

- Clinical signs, history, and physical examination
- Biopsy

TREATMENT

- Surgical removal

INFORMATION FOR CLIENTS

- Most mammary tumors of mice are malignant, and surgery is not an option.
- Mammary tumors in rats may recur in uninvolved glands or at the site of surgically removed tumors.

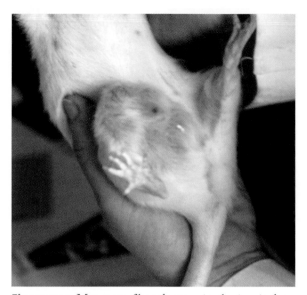

Figure 22-2 Mammary fibroadenoma in the inguinal region of a female rat. (From Quesenberry KE, Carpenter JW: *Ferrets, rabbits, and rodents*, ed 3, St. Louis, MO, 2012, Saunders, by permission.)

The Rabbit

The reproductive system of the rabbit is similar to those of other small mammals. Rabbits are induced ovulators; that is, they ovulate only after being bred and do not show signs of regular estrous cycles. Litter sizes vary with breeds; smaller breeds generally have smaller litters. Gestation is 30 to 32 days; thus multiple litters per year are possible. Female rabbits (does) make nests of hay or bedding and hair pulled from their abdomens. Most kitting is done in the early morning. The young rabbits are born blind and helpless. They will be nursed one to two times daily by the doe, which may leave the nest for the entire day. Rabbit milk is concentrated, containing about 14% to 15% protein, 10% to 12% fat, and 2% carbohydrates. Young rabbits should be weaned by about 25 days of age. The male rabbit has two testicles that are located externally on each side of the penis in hairless scrotal sacs. These testicles can be drawn back into the inguinal canals during times of illness or stress, as the inguinal rings in the rabbit remain open throughout life.

Uterine Disease

Uterine adenocarcinomas are the most common tumor of the reproductive tract in the female rabbit. These tumors may occur even in animals not used for breeding. The incidence of disease increases with the age of the rabbit. The Dutch type of rabbit is reported to be more susceptible to the disease. These tumors often involve multiple sites within the uterus and may be easily palpated in the later stages of the disease (Fig. 22-3). Metastasis is fairly common.

CLINICAL SIGNS

- History of reproductive problems in the 6 to 12 months before detection of the mass:
  - Decreased litter size
  - Stillborn litters
- Anemia
- Hematuria or serosanguinous vaginal discharge
- ± Cystic mammary glands
- Depression
- Anorexia
- Dyspnea if pulmonary metastasis occurs late in disease
- ± Ascites

DIAGNOSIS

- Physical examination and history
- Radiography or ultrasonography: abnormal uterus

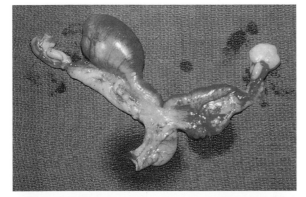

Figure 22-3 Tumor in the uterus of a female rabbit. (From Quesenberry KE, Carpenter JW: *Ferrets, rabbits, and rodents*, ed 2, St. Louis, MO, 2004, Saunders, by permission.)

TREATMENT

- If early in the disease, ovariohysterectomy may be performed.
- If metastasis has occurred, no treatment is effective.

INFORMATION FOR CLIENTS

- Prevention of uterine disease involves having the rabbit spayed (ovariohysterectomy) if it will not be used for breeding (between the ages of 6 and 12 months).
- The female rabbit should be examined a minimum of twice yearly to allow for early detection of the disease. This becomes more important as the rabbit ages past 4 years.

Pyometra and Endometritis

Postpartum bacterial infections of the uterus are seen in breeding rabbits. Microorganisms cultured from these pyometras include *Pasteurella multocida* and *Staphylococcus aureus*.

CLINICAL SIGNS

- Vaginal discharge
- Inability to rebreed
- Anorexia
- Lethargy
- Weakness
- Enlarged abdomen

DIAGNOSIS

- Physical examination and a history of recent kindling
- CBC and serum chemistries:
  - CBC: may be normal or show a slight leukocytosis
  - Serum chemistries: may show signs of renal failure
- Radiology or ultrasonography: enlarged, doughy uterus
- Culture and sensitivity of vaginal discharge

TREATMENT

- Ovariohysterectomy with a laparotomy recommended
- Intravenous fluids to correct dehydration and support the cardiovascular system

- Antibiotics (parenteral) based on culture and sensitivity

INFORMATION FOR CLIENTS

- Avoid this problem by having your pet rabbit spayed at an early age.

Pseudopregnancy

Pseudopregnancy (false pregnancy) is seen in pet rabbits even when they are not used for breeding. The condition usually lasts about 2 to 3 weeks and may include nesting behavior. Mammary development may occur early in the pseudopregnancy. The condition may lead to pyometra, and ovariohysterectomy is recommended for rabbits with this problem.

CLINICAL SIGNS

- Nest building, fur pulling
- Mammary development
- Doe may become territorial

DIAGNOSIS

- Clinical signs and physical examination

TREATMENT

- Ovariohysterectomy

INFORMATION FOR CLIENTS

- If you have more than one rabbit, they may be stimulating pseudopregnancy by mounting each other. You may need to house them separately to prevent this condition.
- This condition is usually self-limiting. If it is recurrent, have the doe spayed.

Mastitis

Mastitis can be seen in the lactating doe or during pseudopregnancy. Trauma to the glands from young nursing or from other does, poor sanitation, and heavy lactation all predispose the rabbit to infection.

CLINICAL SIGNS

- Fever
- Anorexia
- Lethargy
- Depression
- Increased thirst

- Hot, swollen, painful mammary glands
- Septicemia
- Death

DIAGNOSIS

- Physical examination and history of nursing
- Clinical signs
- Culture and sensitivity of the mammary gland (contents)
  - *Staphylococcus* spp. and *Streptococcus* spp. are the most common causes

TREATMENT

- Removal of all nursing kits; hand-feeding
- Antibiotics based on culture results
- Fluid therapy
- Application of hot packs to promote drainage
- Analgesia if pain is present

INFORMATION FOR CLIENTS

- Treatment of mastitis in the rabbit will require a lot of nursing care. Hot packing the glands, feeding the kits, and cleaning of the environment to prevent spread of the disease are all important.
- Do not attempt to foster the kits by using another doe; this may spread the infection to the new doe.

Reproductive Problems in the Male Rabbit

Reproductive problems in the male rabbit are not a common occurrence. They may include cryptorchidism, orchitis, epididymitis, and testicular neoplasms. Because male rabbits can become aggressive, they should be housed separately to prevent scrotal or testicular injuries when fighting.

REVIEW QUESTIONS

1. Domestic ferrets are _____ ovulators.
   a. Induced
   b. Seasonal
2. Which of the following clinical signs would not likely indicate estrogen toxicosis in the domestic ferret?
   a. Anemia
   b. Swollen vulva
   c. Bilateral alopecia
   d. Swollen lymph nodes

3. Mammary tumors in mice are usually benign and should be removed surgically.
   a. True
   b. False
4. What is the most common tumor of the reproductive tract in the female rabbit?
   a. Mastocytoma
   b. Lymphoma
   c. Adenocarcinoma
   d. Sarcoma
5. What anatomic difference is the reason for the castration of the male rabbit being done differently from that of the male dog and cat?
   a. Open inguinal rings
   b. Lack of external scrotum
   c. Presence of accessory testicles internally

6. Which of the following antibiotics would be the better treatment for mastitis in the rabbit?
   a. Gentomycin
   b. Streptomycin
   c. Amoxicillin
   d. Amikacin
7. Oral antibiotics should be avoided in rabbits because of their effect on GI flora.
   a. True
   b. False

Answers found on page 554.

Diseases of the Respiratory System

LEARNING OBJECTIVES

When you have completed this chapter, you will be able to:

1. Explain to clients the need for vaccination of all ferrets against canine distemper.
2. Become aware of the need for preoxygenation for patients with respiratory compromise.
3. Provide emergency treatment for rabbits presenting with signs of heatstroke.

The Ferret

There are only a few causes of respiratory disease in the ferret. Canine distemper virus and human flu virus may produce respiratory disease. Most pet ferrets today are routinely vaccinated against canine distemper, so this disease is not commonly seen.

Canine Distemper Viral Disease

Canine distemper viral disease is transmitted via aerosol exposure and should be suspected in any unvaccinated ferret with clinical signs (Fig. 23-1).

CLINICAL SIGNS

- Rash on the chin
- Swollen, crusty skin around the lips and chin
- Anorexia
- Depression
- Fever
- Photophobia
- Mucopurulent ocular and nasal discharge
- Hyperkeratosis of foot pads
- Vomiting and diarrhea (usually uncommon)
- Coughing

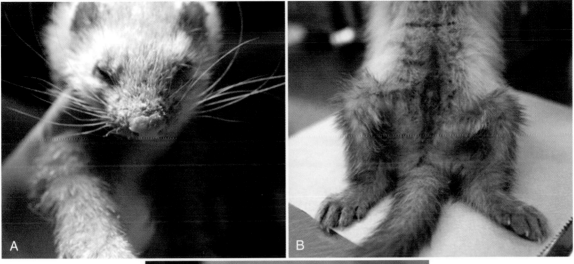

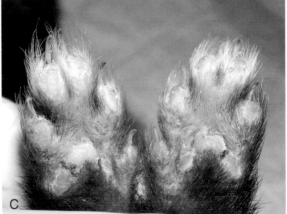

Figure 23-1 Young ferret with canine distemper viral disease. **A,** Encrusted eyes. **B,** Crusting around lips and chin. **C,** Hyperkeratosis of the footpads. (**A,** Courtesy of S. White. IN Miller WH, Griffin CE, Campbell KL: *Muller and Kirk's Small Animal Dermatology*, ed 7, St Louis, 2013, Mosby **B and C,** From Quesenberry KE, Carpenter JW: *Ferrets, rabbits, and rodents*, ed 3, St. Louis, MO, 2012, Saunders, by permission.)

- Neurologic signs (incoordination, torticollis, nystagmus)

DIAGNOSIS

- Physical examination and history of exposure in unvaccinated animal
- Complete blood cell count (CBC) (leukopenia)
- Serum titer (for canine distemper virus) will be positive in unvaccinated animal
- Fluorescent antibody test on conjunctival scrapings or blood smears will be positive in first few days of disease

TREATMENT

- No treatment of value currently exists. Supportive therapy is an option, but euthanasia is recommended as the only humane option.

INFORMATION FOR CLIENTS

- Canine distemper viral disease is a preventable disease. Have all pet ferrets vaccinated annually against canine distemper virus.
- The virus is relatively unstable in the environment, so cleaning and disinfecting may destroy it.
- The mortality rate for ferrets infected with this disease is nearly 100%. Euthanasia is recommended for those animals that exhibit clinical signs of disease.

⦿ TECH ALERT

Use only vaccines designated as safe for ferrets. Do not use feline distemper vaccines.

Human Influenza Virus

Ferrets are susceptible to human influenza virus. The virus is transmitted via aerosols and causes an upper respiratory disease in ferrets. It can be transmitted between ferrets and humans.

CLINICAL SIGNS

- Fever, followed by decreased temperature after 48 hours
- Sneezing
- Watering of the eyes
- Mucoid or mucopurulent nasal discharge
- Lethargy
- Anorexia

DIAGNOSIS

- Physical examination and history of exposure
- Increased serum antibody titer to virus
- Virus isolation from nasal secretions

TREATMENT

- The disease is self-limiting; its course in adult animals is about 7 to 14 days.
- Maintain hydration and nutrition with force-feeding if necessary.
- Administer cough suppressant or antihistamine to relieve nasal congestion and coughing (if present).
- Human antiviral drugs such as amantadine or zanamivir have been used with some success in experimental trials. Administer antibiotics for secondary infections.

INFORMATION FOR CLIENTS

- Prevent the spread of flu from humans to ferrets by not allowing your ferret to be handled by infected persons.
- Vaccination against flu is not usually recommended for ferrets because strains are relatively benign and change yearly.

Rodents

Rodents are frequently seen in veterinary practice for respiratory problems. Care should be taken when handling and collecting laboratory samples if the animal is dyspneic. The most common causes of respiratory diseases in mice are the Sendai virus and *Mycoplasma pulmonis*. Sendai viral infection is an acute respiratory infection with a high mortality rate in neonates and weanlings. Adult mice generally recover. *Mycoplasma* infection generally results in pneumonia, suppurative rhinitis, and sometimes otitis media. Antibiotic therapy will help eliminate the symptoms but not the disease.

Mice

Sendai Virus and *Mycoplasma pulmonis*

Rodents kept under sanitary conditions and fed a balanced diet have few problems with disease. However, when pneumonia does develop, Sendai virus and *Mycoplasma* are often the cause.

CLINICAL SIGNS

- "Chattering"
- Labored breathing
- Pneumonia
- Purulent nasal secretions
- ± Pulmonary abscesses

DIAGNOSIS

- Clinical signs and history
- Culture and sensitivity if specimen can be obtained without stress to patient
- Radiography

TREATMENT

- Antibiotics
  - Enrofloxacin
  - Doxycycline

Rats

Chronic respiratory disease is the most common multifactorial respiratory disease of rats. The major component of the disease is *Mycoplasma pulmonis*. Other respiratory pathogens in the rat include *Streptococcus pneumoniae* and *Corynebacterium kutscheri*, whereas many of the mouse pathogens play a minor or synergistic part in the disease process in rats.

Chronic Respiratory Disease

CLINICAL SIGNS

- Highly variable signs:
  - Snuffling
  - Nasal discharge
  - Polypnea
  - Weight loss
  - Ruffled coat
  - Head tilt
  - Red tears
- Signs that may become chronic
  - Otitis media
  - Cilio-stasis with increased airway secretions
  - Lung abscesses

DIAGNOSIS

- Clinical signs and history
- Culture and sensitivity if possible
- Radiography

TREATMENT

- Antibiotic therapy
  - Enrofloxacin
  - Doxycycline
- Alteration of environment
  - Reduction of ammonia levels in the cage
- Bronchodilators
- Short-term use of corticosteroids

Bacterial Pneumonia

CLINICAL SIGNS

- Dyspnea
- Snuffling
- Abdominal breathing
- Sudden death
- ± Purulent respiratory exudate

DIAGNOSIS

- Clinical signs and history
- Gram staining or cytology (numerous diplococci on gram staining)
- Culture and sensitivity (usual cause is *S. pneumoniae*)

TREATMENT

- Aggressive use of antibiotics (β-lactamase resistant):
  - Cloxacillin
  - Oxacillin
  - Dicloxacillin

Hamsters

Respiratory disease is also common in hamsters. The causative agents may be either viral or bacterial in nature. Bacterial pneumonias caused by *Streptococcus* may be transmitted from children to hamsters during handling.

Bacterial Pneumonia

CLINICAL SIGNS

- Dyspnea
- Nasal discharge ± purulence
- ± Sticky eyelids

DIAGNOSIS

- Clinical signs and history
- Gram staining of nasal secretions: gram-positive for diplococci
- Culture and sensitivity
- Radiography

TREATMENT

- Antibiotics
  - Chloramphenicol palmitate or succinate every 8 hours until culture and sensitivity results are available

INFORMATION FOR CLIENTS

- Increased levels of ammonia in cages will damage the respiratory system of these rodents and predispose them to invasion by viral or bacterial agents, resulting in pneumonias.
- These diseases, especially the viral or chronic bacterial ones, may be impossible to cure. Treatment may only alleviate clinical symptoms.

• Children with streptoccal infections should avoid handling hamsters.

🔘 TECH ALERT

When handling animals with dyspnea, it often helps to place them into an oxygen-enriched environment before obtaining laboratory samples.

The Rabbit

The anatomy of the respiratory system of the rabbit is similar to that of the cat.

Pasteurellosis (Snuffles)

Snuffles is the most frequently diagnosed respiratory disease of rabbits, but it may, in fact, be overdiagnosed. Several serotypes of organism *Pasteurella multocida* are responsible for this disease, and these serotypes vary in virulence. Transmission of the disease is by aerosol from infected rabbits, by direct contact, or by fomites. A genital form that also exists can be transmitted to kits. Virulence may be increased when the immune system is compromised by stress, inadequate diet, or poor environment. It is believed that many pet rabbits are already infected with the organism at the time they are purchased, and that the disease becomes active at a later date. The clinical signs of this disease vary with the degree of immunosuppression of the rabbit. Pasteurellosis is a difficult disease to cure.

CLINICAL SIGNS

• Rhinitis (snuffles) (Fig. 23-2)
• Increased upper respiratory sounds
• Purulent nasal discharge
• Sneezing or snorting
• Anorexia
• Lack of grooming
• ± Otitis media
• ± Pneumonia

DIAGNOSIS

• Physical examination and history
• Culture and sensitivity of nasal passage (may require sedation to obtain a representative swab)
• Radiography

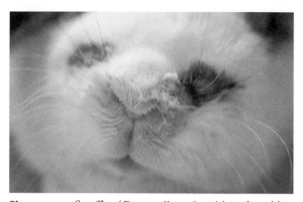

Figure 23-2 Snuffles (*Pasteurella multocida*) in the rabbit. (From Quesenberry KE, Carpenter JW: *Ferrets, rabbits, and rodents*, ed 2, St. Louis, MO, 2004, Saunders, by permission.)

TREATMENT

• Systemic antibiotic therapy:
  • Enrofloxacin
  • Tetracyclines
  • Trimethoprim sulfa
• Gentamicin nasal solutions
• Surgical trephination to drain excessive pus, if needed
• Maintenance of adequate hydration
• Nebulization
• Mucolytic agents (*N*-acetylcysteine)

INFORMATION FOR CLIENTS

• Avoid stress to rabbits by not overcrowding them, provide proper nutrition and water at all times, and avoid purchasing young rabbits with snotty noses.
• This disease is difficult to cure. Antibiotic therapy may result in remission of clinical signs, but they may reappear when the rabbit's immune system becomes stressed.
• Isolate all rabbits showing signs of upper airway disease.
• Currently, no vaccine against this disease is available.

Heatstroke

Depending on where your practice is located, you may see several cases of rabbit heatstroke per week.

Heatstroke may occur even in climates where the temperature reaches no greater than 80°F. Rabbits are unable to sweat and do not pant. They depend on the skin of their ears for heat exchange. If placed in conditions where they are unable to thermoregulate, heat stroke will develop (often, well-meaning owners take their bunnies to the park to play).

CLINICAL SIGNS

- Anorexia
- Increased respiratory rate
- Pulmonary edema
- Cyanotic mucous membranes
- Collapse
- Death

DIAGNOSIS

- Physical examination and history of heat exposure
- Increased rectal temperature (>104°F)

TREATMENT

- Reduce body temperature by:
  - Bathing the rabbit in tepid water
  - Wetting the ears
  - Using a fan
- Vasodilators; acetylpromazine
- Intravenous cooled fluids

INFORMATION FOR CLIENTS

- If you take your rabbit outside in the heat, make sure that the rabbit has a shady, cool place to rest frequently.

- Rabbits housed outside during the summer months must have a source of cooling water spray, fan, and shade.
- Heatstroke in the rabbit is an emergency. Take immediate measures to cool the rabbit and seek veterinary attention.

REVIEW QUESTIONS

1. Yearly flu vaccines for ferrets are recommended.
   a. True
   b. False
2. Treatment of *Mycoplasma* pneumonias will often cure the problem by removing the organism from the rodent's system.
   a. True
   b. False
3. Snuffles is a disease caused by:
   a. *Staphylococcus aureus*
   b. *Clostridium botulinum*
   c. *Pasteurella multocida*
   d. *Streptococcus pyogenes*
4. Children with strep infections should avoid handling ferrets and rodents.
   a. True
   b. False
5. Only feline distemper vaccines should be used when vaccinating ferrets.
   a. True
   b. False

Answers found on page 554.

Diseases of the Urinary System

Calculolytic
Debride
Diuresis

Hematuria
Hypercalciuria
Nephrosis

Oliguria
Urolithiasis

OUTLINE

Ferrets
    Acute Renal Failure
    Chronic Renal Failure
    Cystitis or Urolithiasis
Rodents
    Chronic Progressive Nephrosis
    Urethral Obstruction or Trauma in Mice

Rabbits
    Red Urine
    "Sludgy Urine"
    Urolithiasis

LEARNING OBJECTIVES

When you have completed this chapter, you will be able to:
1. Recognize signs of urinary disease in these species and be able to explain how a proper diet can prevent disease.
2. Explain the need for emergency evaluation of urinary obstruction in the affected pet.
3. Demonstrate knowledge of normal and abnormal urine in the rabbit.

Ferrets

Older ferrets may exhibit signs of renal failure, as do other animals. Urinary calculi, once common, are now rarely seen because of improved diets. Most urinary problems may be related to one or more of the endocrine abnormalities and may be treated as those of dogs or cats.

Urinary disease in aging ferrets is similar to the disease in cats and dogs. Renal failure may be classified as either acute (may be reversible) or chronic (usually not reversible).

Acute Renal Failure

Signs of acute renal failure in ferrets may develop secondary to lower urinary tract disease or obstruction.

CLINICAL SIGNS

- Polyuria or polydipsia
- Depression

- Lack of appetite
- Weight loss
- Hind-leg weakness
- Dehydration
- Pale mucous membranes
- Painful abdomen

DIAGNOSIS

- Physical examination
- Complete blood cell count (CBC)
- Serum chemistries: blood urea nitrogen (BUN) and creatinine level increases are seen but are not considered an accurate measure of renal failure; hyperphosphatemia, hyperkalemia, and hypocalcemia are considered signs of renal failure
- Urinalysis: active urine sediment
- Radiography: enlarged kidneys

TREATMENT

- Removal or correction of the underlying cause
- Correction of fluid balance: rehydration with lactated Ringer or normal saline if hyperkalemic; fluid rates of about 4 mL/kg/hr are suggested
- Diuretics if the ferret is oliguric: furosemide
- Adequate nutrition: Hill's Feline k/d or other high-quality meat protein diet
- Phosphorous binders when needed
- Antibiotics if indicated

INFORMATION FOR CLIENTS

- With rapid diagnosis and treatment, acute renal failure damage often can be reversed. Call your veterinarian immediately if you suspect urinary problems in your pet.
- A proper diet can reduce the incidence of lower urinary tract infection and acute renal failure.

Chronic Renal Failure

Chronic renal failure is a problem in aged ferrets. The result of the disease process is a slow, progressive loss of renal function, the cause of which is often unclear.

CLINICAL SIGNS

- Depression
- Lethargy
- Weight loss

- Pale mucous membranes
- Oral ulcers or halitosis
- Diarrhea or vomiting

DIAGNOSIS

- Physical examination; small kidneys
- CBC; anemia
- Serum chemistries: increased renal enzymes, hyperkalemia, hypocalcemia
- Urinalysis: increased protein, blood cells, low specific gravity
- Radiology: small kidneys

TREATMENT

- Rehydration
- Improved nutrition (diet should contain no less than 30% meat-based protein)
- Phosphorous-binding agents

INFORMATION FOR CLIENTS

- Chronic renal failure is a progressive disease. Treatment may improve the quality of life for the animal but will not reverse the lesions in the kidney resulting from the disease.

Cystitis or Urolithiasis

Cystitis, with or without the formation of bladder stones, may develop in the ferret. Signs may range from mild straining and pain during urination to complete obstruction.

CLINICAL SIGNS

Early clinical signs include the following:
- Straining to urinate
- Polyuria
- ± Hematuria

If stones form, affected animals will exhibit the following clinical signs:
- Straining to urinate
- Extreme pain due to obstruction
- Dribbling urine

DIAGNOSIS

- Physical examination; stones often can be palpated
- Radiography: most stones are struvite and visible on radiographs

- Urinalysis: increased crystals, blood, increased protein
- Urine culture and sensitivity

TREATMENT

- If obstruction is present, remove it either by catheterization or via cystotomy
- In the absence of obstruction, use a calculolytic diet such as s/d
- Antibiotics based on urine culture and sensitivity

INFORMATION FOR CLIENTS

- Urinary obstruction is an emergent, life-threatening condition. Have your pet seen by a veterinarian immediately if the animal is straining to urinate and not producing any urine.
- A proper diet may reduce the development of bladder stones.

Rodents

Staphylococcus aureus of the preputial glands in mice may cause urinary obstruction. Occasionally trauma to the penis is seen in mice that are aggressively fighting or as a result of aggressive breeding. In rats, chronic progressive nephrosis is the best-known age-related disease of the renal system. This disease may be more severe in male rats than in female rats. Little information is available on urinary problems in hamsters and gerbils.

Chronic Progressive Nephrosis

Chronic progressive nephrosis is primarily a disease of older rats.

CLINICAL SIGNS

- Enlarged, pitted kidneys
- Proteinuria >10 mg/day and progressively increasing with age

DIAGNOSIS

- Clinical signs and history
- Urinalysis (Table 24-1)
- Radiography or ultrasonography of the kidneys

TREATMENT

Supportive Care
- A low-protein diet which may slow progression of the disease
- Anabolic steroids

Urethral Obstruction or Trauma in Mice

CLINICAL SIGNS

- Failure to pass urine
- Traumatic injury to penis

DIAGNOSIS

- Physical examination and history
- Culture and sensitivity: to detect *S. aureus*

TABLE 24-1   Urinalysis Reference Values for Gerbils, Hamsters, Mice, and Rats

Value*	Gerbil	Hamster	Mouse	Rat
Urine volume (mL/24 hr)	A few drops (about 4)	5.1–8.4	0.5–2.5	13–23
Specific gravity	NA	1.060	1.034	1.022–1.050
Average pH	NA	8.5	5.01	5–7
Protein (mg/dL)	NA	NA	Males proteinuric	<30?

*Average reference values. Note that the ranges should be considered as guides; values are likely to vary among groups of animals according to such variables as strain, age, sex, fasting, and methodology.
NA, not available.
From Quesenberry KE, Carpenter JW: *Ferrets, rabbits, and rodents*, ed 2, St. Louis, MO, 2004, Saunders, by permission.

TREATMENT

- Cleaning and debriding wounds
- Antibiotics based on culture and sensitivity

INFORMATION FOR CLIENTS

- Proper diet and husbandry may prevent or slow the progression of the urinary problems in captive mice and rats.

Rabbits

Urinary disease and renal failure are common in the rabbit. Rabbits are extremely sensitive to disturbances of acid–base balance, pain, stress, dehydration, and anorexia. The rabbit kidney excretes large amounts of calcium that forms calcium carbonate in the urine, causing turbid, alkaline urine. In rabbits experiencing pain or stress, blood flow to the kidney, and hence glomerular filtration, is decreased. The rabbit kidney appears to be the main organ of regulation of calcium homeostasis, and as such, the secretion of calcium by the kidney matches that of calcium intake. Diets high in calcium may predispose the rabbit to hypercalciuria and the development of bladder stones.

Red Urine

Rabbits may excrete a porphyrin-related compound in their urine that will make the urine red. It is often mistaken by the owner for hematuria. This unusual urine color may be the result of pigments found in the normal diet of the rabbit and does not present a problem. Porphyrin products will fluoresce under a Wood lamp whereas hemoglobin will not.

CLINICAL SIGNS

- Dark brown, dark red, red-orange urine

DIAGNOSIS

- Physical examination and history
- Complete urinalysis will be normal
  - Check urine with a Wood light: porphyrin will fluoresce

TREATMENT

- No treatment is available.

INFORMATION FOR CLIENTS

- It is normal for rabbit urine to be colored red. Have your rabbit examined if any other signs of disease are present.

"Sludgy Urine"

It is normal for rabbit urine to be turbid; however, when the calcium carbonate deposits begin to build up in the bladder, urine may actually become sludgy (thick, pasty).

Urination may become difficult and painful, and the rabbit may strain to urinate. The sludge irritates the bladder, the urethra, and the perineum, and secondary infections may occur.

CLINICAL SIGNS

- Straining to urinate
- Depression
- Hunched stance
- Pain

DIAGNOSIS

- Physical examination and history
- Radiology or ultrasonography shows a distended bladder containing sludge
- Complete urinalysis

TREATMENT

- Empty the rabbit's bladder under anesthesia and flush until clean
- Decrease dietary calcium and increase diuresis (may include intravenous fluids)
- Improve any housing conditions that may result in retention of urine by the rabbit (such as dirty litter)
- Administer anti-inflammatory medications if urine retention is related to spinal pain
- Provide antibiotics for secondary infections

INFORMATION FOR CLIENTS

- Make sure your rabbit has a clean litter box for urination.
- Rabbits should have free access to clean water at all times.
- Increase moist, leafy greens in the diet if sludging has been a problem.

Urolithiasis

The formation of bladder stones may or may not be associated with sludgy urine in the rabbit. As with other animals, any condition that increases the urinary concentration of stone-producing minerals and promotes crystal formation may lead to the formation of uroliths. Normal rabbit urine contains many crystals. Almost 100% of the uric acid handled by the kidney is excreted in urine in the rabbit, as opposed to 40% in the dog; thus a supply of raw materials is available for the formation of stones. Restricted water intake, retention of urine, and infection may all cause urolithiasis.

CLINICAL SIGNS

- Straining to urinate or unable to pass urine
- Hematuria
- Depression
- Lethargy
- Hunched stance
- Grinding of teeth
- Anorexia and weight loss

DIAGNOSIS

- Physical examination and history
- Complete urinalysis—obtained by cystocentesis
  - Increased crystalluria
  - Proteinuria
  - Hematuria
  - ± Bacteria
- Complete CBC and serum chemistries:
  - Especially to evaluate renal function
- Culture and sensitivity of urine, if bacteria present
- Radiography (Fig. 24-1)

TREATMENT

- Cystotomy if stones are large
- Bladder flushing through a catheter to remove fine particulate matter
- Nephrectomy if stone is in renal pelvis
- Fluids to aid in flushing the bladder by increasing urination
- Urohydropropulsion of stones that are nonobstructive may be attempted under anesthesia
- Change in diet: decreased levels of calcium-containing foods
- Weight reduction or exercise increase
- Antibiotics, according to culture and sensitivity results

INFORMATION FOR CLIENTS

- A properly balanced diet of grass hay and vegetables may limit the formation of cystic calculi.
- Avoid letting your rabbit become overweight, and make sure it always has access to fresh water.
- If you notice your rabbit straining to pass urine or no urine is in the box, have your pet seen immediately by a veterinarian.

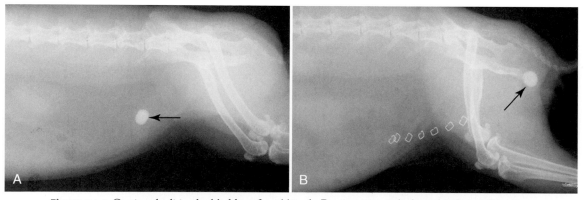

Figure 24-1 Cystic calculi in the bladder of a rabbit. **A,** Preoperative right lateral radiographic view. **B,** Cystotomy was unsuccessful because the calculus (*arrows*) moved into the distal urethra, probably at the time of anesthesia induction. (From Quesenberry KE, Carpenter JW: *Ferrets, rabbits, and rodents*, ed 2, St. Louis, MO, 2004, Saunders, by permission.)

REVIEW QUESTIONS

1. Recommended diets for ferrets should contain no less than ____ high-quality meat protein.
   a. 60%
   b. 30%
   c. 10%
   d. 50%
2. What is the most common type of bladder stone in the ferret?
   a. Urate stone
   b. Oxalate stone
   c. Struvite stone
   d. Mixed stone
3. Chronic progressive nephrosis is more severe in _____ rats.
   a. Male
   b. Female
4. Unlike in most other mammals, rabbit urine contains high amounts of _____, which makes urine turbid.
   a. Ammonium chloride
   b. Triple-phosphate crystals
   c. Calcium carbonate
   d. Sodium carbonate
5. As with other animals, chronic renal failure will result in a(n) _____ in packed cell volume (PCV).
   a. Increase
   b. Decrease
6. Rabbit urine that is red and fluoresces under UV light contains this pigment and is probably normal.
   a. melanin
   b. hemoglobin
   c. porphyrin
   d. myoglobin

Answers found on page 554.

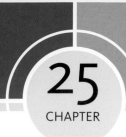

25

CHAPTER

Overview of the Bird as a Patient

LEARNING OBJECTIVES

When you have completed this chapter, you will be able to:
1. Discuss the suitability of certain species of birds as pets when asked by clients.
2. Advise clients on housing and diet for pet birds.
3. Become interested in these patients and begin to feel comfortable in handling them.
4. Appreciate how the unique anatomy of the avian patient contributes to the development of disease.

More than 9000 different species of birds exist, and many of them make excellent pets for people who live in urban environments. Of these species, the most common groups kept as pets include psittacines (hook-beaked parrots) and passerines (canaries and finches). As birds have become more popular, the number of birds treated in veterinary clinics has increased. For this reason, technicians must become familiar with the husbandry requirements, handling, and diseases of these pets.

It has been estimated that approximately 90% of all medical problems in birds are the result of poor husbandry. It is the responsibility of the veterinary staff to provide guidance to clients who wish to acquire a pet bird and to provide support to those clients who already own one.

Husbandry

Most pet bird owners know little about the housing and nutritional requirements of their new bird. Pet stores often do little in the way of counseling or educating new owners, and many birds are acquired as "impulse" purchases, with no thought of how that animal will be maintained during its adult life span (which can be quite long in some species). It is important that technicians who work in practices that treat avian patients have a working knowledge of these requirements.

Housing

Pet birds live in confined environments (usually a cage). The size of cage should be determined by the size of the bird, not by the cost of the cage. A bird should be able to spread its wings without touching the cage walls, and its tail should not drag the floor or hit the sides of the cage.

Because birds are social creatures, the cage should be placed in an area where interaction with the owner is possible; however, certain rooms should be avoided—especially the kitchen. The cage should be in an area away from air conditioning and heating vents and out of direct sunlight. Birds are quite hardy and will readily adapt to the usual temperatures in homes.

Cages may be constructed of metal, Plexiglas, or a suitable wire mesh. Cage materials include everything from bamboo to decorative wood and Plexiglas. The material used in the cage must be suitable for the size and strength of the bird, or else the cage will be destroyed by the natural tendency of the animal to chew. The construction and design must be simple and provide a safe environment for the bird, whether they are outside the cage or inside.

Perches should be of sufficient size and should not be covered with sandpaper because this can lead to foot trauma and infection. Newspaper is the best substrate for the bottom of the cage (unprinted newspaper can be purchased from many sources). Wood shavings, cat litter, or other particulate substrates may hide excreta and hold excess moisture, making it difficult for the owner to see changes that may be caused by disease or dietary changes.

Cages should be cleaned and bedding changed at least daily. Other items such as mite protectors and grit are unnecessary. Owners should bring the bird to the clinic in its own cage, whenever possible; the cage may provide important clues to the environment in which the pet lives.

Nutrition

Since the late 1980s, research in the area of avian nutrition has provided marked improvement in the diets of caged birds. Previously, seed mixtures were the only diets available to bird owners. Today, a varied diet of seeds, pellets, and table food is highly recommended by most avian veterinarians. This diversified diet should consist of vegetables, breads, cheese, cooked eggs, fruit, and even a small amount of meat together with seeds, peanuts, and or pellets. A well-balanced diet is just as important for a bird as it is for its owner! A diversified diet not only provides the necessary vitamin and energy requirements for the bird, but will also provide psychological stimulation through touch, feel, and color and keep the bird interested.

Birds produce little saliva and therefore require an adequate water intake to digest their foodstuff. Fresh water should always be available to the bird. Water containers must be cleaned several times daily because birds are prone to placing food and other things in their water.

Birds that receive a well-balanced diet probably need no other supplements such as vitamins and calcium. Laying hens or birds not eating well may need the addition of supplements during these periods of stress. Whenever supplements are used, they should be placed in the soft food and not in the water.

Exercise

All birds need exercise. However, because the home is an inherently dangerous place for birds, that exercise must be supervised at all times. Birds should never be left unattended when out of the cage. Large parrots can be quite destructive, and smaller birds may be injured by ceiling fans, by other pets, or by flying into windows or mirrors. Many owners set up play areas for their parrots, and some even have harnesses that allow them to take their birds outside without the danger of losing them. Owners may request a wing trim to keep their birds from flying, but this will not prevent flight; it serves only to provide less lift. Many birds are lost each year when owners take them outside, only to have them take off on wind currents and disappear.

Handling and Restraint

The goal of handling and restraint of the avian patient is to prevent trauma to the patient and to the veterinarian examining the patient. Therefore, it is important to control the head of the bird. Before trying to remove any bird from the cage, remove all perches, food and water bowls, and toys to prevent injury during the capture process. If possible, dim the lights in the examination room to slow down the bird's reactions. For small birds the technician may use a paper towel or wash cloth placed over the bird. Gently surround the head with the thumb and first finger while wrapping the cloth around the body of the bird with the opposite hand. Cradle the bird in the palm of your hand for support. For the larger parrots, use a bath towel or a beach towel. Large birds may require two persons for restraint; one to support and control the head and one to support and control the body and wings. Larger parrots can severely injure someone with their beak so head control is very important!

Several good texts on restraining and handling avian patients are available; we advise the technician to refer to these texts for more information. Remember, practice makes perfect (or at least improves your technique)!

Anatomy of the Avian Patient

Although humans have kept birds as pets for a long time, birds are not considered a "domesticated" animal as are dogs and cats. The unique structure and temperament of the bird makes it a challenging patient. Even if hand-raised, all birds retain their wild genes and will react to stress as their wild relatives have for thousands of years.

To understand the development of disease in the bird, the technician should become familiar with the unique anatomy of the bird (Fig. 25-1 and Fig. 25-2). A detailed description of the anatomic structures of the avian patient is beyond the scope of this text;

however, brief overviews are presented throughout Section III with the discussions of each body system.

Advice to Clients Wishing to Purchase a Bird

Veterinary technicians are often asked what species of bird will make the best pet. It is important, therefore, for the technician to be familiar with some of the most common species kept as pets (Box 25-1) and their personalities. In general, species with a reputation for being good talkers (parakeets, Amazon parrots, African gray, cockatoos, and macaws) also have a reputation for being noisy. The larger the bird, the larger and stronger is the beak and the more likely that their bite would be severe. Larger birds usually cost more to purchase and will be more costly to maintain. It may also be difficult to find boarding or someone to care for them when the owner is away. A client who wishes to purchase a bird as a pet should consider all of these issues before deciding on a species.

BOX 25-1 Psittacines and Passerines Commonly Kept as Pets

Psittacines (Birds with a Hooked Beak and Two Toes Pointing Forward and Two Pointing Backward)
Amazon parrots
Budgerigars and parakeets
Caiques
Cockatoos
Cockatiels
Conures
Eclectus parrots
Lorikeets
Lovebirds
African gray parrots
Monk parakeets
Pionus
Senegal parrots
Ring-necked parakeets

Passerines (Birds with Three Forward-Facing Toes)
Canaries
Finches
Mynas

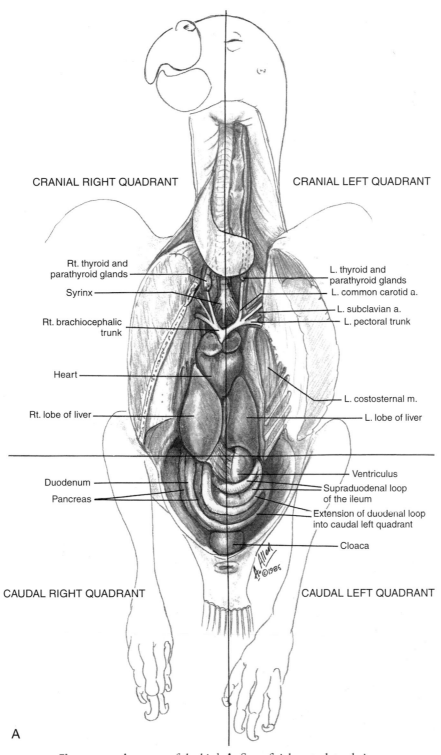

CRANIAL RIGHT QUADRANT

CRANIAL LEFT QUADRANT

Rt. thyroid and
parathyroid glands

Syrinx

Rt. brachiocephalic
trunk

Heart

Rt. lobe of liver

L. thyroid and
parathyroid glands

L. common carotid a.

L. subclavian a.

L. pectoral trunk

L. costosternal m.

L. lobe of liver

Duodenum

Pancreas

Ventriculus

Supraduodenal loop
of the ileum

Extension of duodenal loop
into caudal left quadrant

Cloaca

CAUDAL RIGHT QUADRANT

CAUDAL LEFT QUADRANT

A

Figure 25-1 Anatomy of the bird. **A,** Superficial ventrolateral view.

Continued

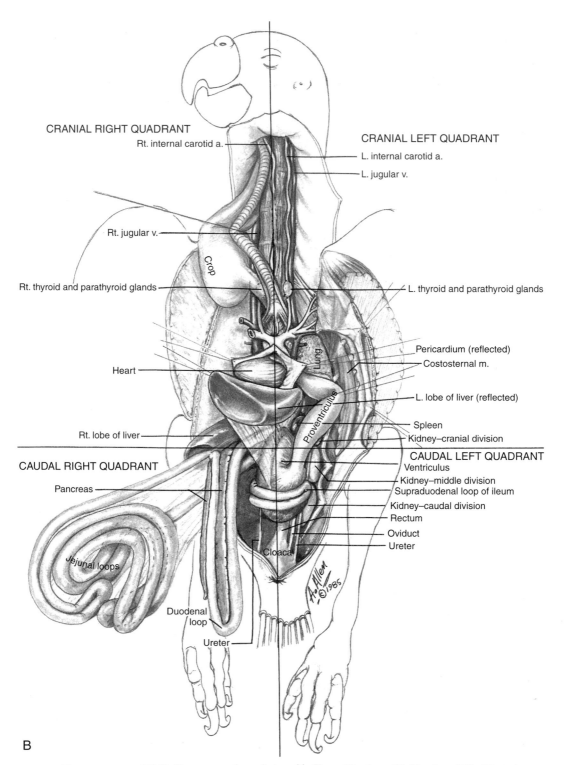

CRANIAL RIGHT QUADRANT

Rt. internal carotid a.

CRANIAL LEFT QUADRANT

L. internal carotid a.

L. jugular v.

Rt. jugular v.

Crop

Rt. thyroid and parathyroid glands

L. thyroid and parathyroid glands

Lung

Pericardium (reflected)

Costosternal m.

Heart

Proventriculus

L. lobe of liver (reflected)

Spleen

Kidney–cranial division

Rt. lobe of liver

CAUDAL RIGHT QUADRANT

CAUDAL LEFT QUADRANT

Ventriculus

Kidney–middle division

Supraduodenal loop of ileum

Kidney–caudal division

Rectum

Oviduct

Ureter

Pancreas

Jejunal loops

Cloaca

Duodenal
loop

Ureter

A. Allen
©1985

B

Figure 25-1, cont'd B, Deep ventrolateral view. (**A,** From Harrison GJ, Harrison LR: *Clinical avian medicine and surgery*, Philadelphia, 1986, Saunders, by permission.

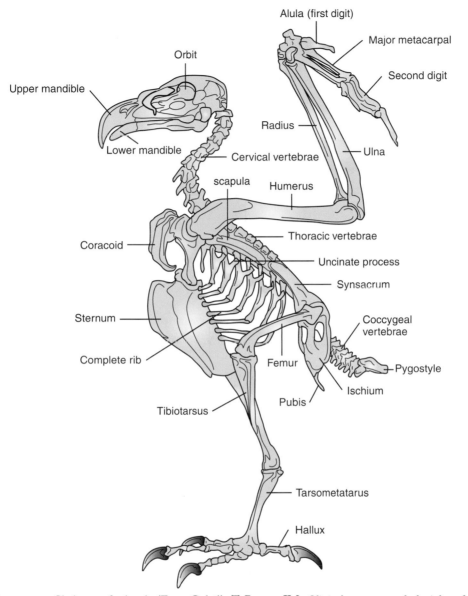

Figure 25-2 Skeleton of a hawk. (From Colville T, Bassert JM: *Clinical anatomy and physiology for veterinary technicians*, ed 2, St. Louis, MO, 2008, Mosby.)

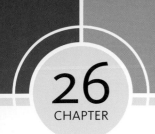

Diseases of the Cardiovascular System

LEARNING OBJECTIVES

When you have completed this chapter, you will be able to:

1. Auscultate the hearts of *all* avian patients even though it will be difficult to count the heart rate.
2. Practice listening to heart sounds in avian patients and recognize any abnormal sounds.
3. Relate clinical pathology changes to heart disease in the bird.

Anatomy of the Heart

The structures of the heart and vasculature of the bird are similar to those of the dog and the cat. The bird heart is larger than the mammalian heart compared with body mass, and the heart is designed for rapid depolarization, which is important with a rapid heart rate. The aortic arch is derived from the right arch, not from the left as in mammals, and the circulatory system contains two important portal systems: (1) the hepatoportal system and (2) the renal portal system. The avian heart is designed for high performance. However, heart disease in pet birds is rarely recognized. Abnormalities in chickens and turkeys have been linked to nutritional deficiencies, infectious diseases, hypertension, toxicities, and primary congestive heart failure, but cases of these diseases in pet birds have not been well documented for several reasons. The heart rate of the normal bird will vary by species (600–750 beats per minute (beats/min) in parakeets to 120–780 beats/min in parrots); thus it is often difficult to auscultate murmurs or other defects, and electrocardiography in the avian patient is cumbersome.

Heart Disease (General)

CLINICAL SIGNS

- Listlessness
- Ascites
- Exercise intolerance
- Cough
- Dyspnea
- Murmur or rhythm disturbance found on auscultation
- Syncope

DIAGNOSIS

- Complete history and physical examination
- Auscultation of the heart
- Radiography
- Electrocardiography
- Echocardiography
- Ruling out any bacterial or viral causes of systemic disease

TREATMENT

- Drugs used for other animals may be adapted for use in pet birds
- Digoxin (inotropic agents)
- Diuretics (to reduce fluid retention or to decrease preload and afterload on the heart)
- Bronchodilators
- Vasodilators (not commonly used in avian patients)
- Diet changes to prevent vitamin E, selenium, and amino acid deficiencies

INFORMATION FOR CLIENTS

- Primary cardiac disease is rare in pet birds.
- In large, expensive birds, a baseline electrocardiogram acquired at the time of purchase may be useful in diagnosing future problems.

Hemorrhage

In most cases, hemorrhage in birds is related to trauma. Head trauma may result in bleeding into the sinus cavities, and into the brain. Fractured bones, bites from other animals, and bruising of the skin may also cause significant blood loss, especially in small birds. Fractured beaks, broken nails, and injured blood feathers are the most common causes of bleeding in pet birds.

CLINICAL SIGNS

- Bleeding (external)
- Neurologic dysfunction (if brain is involved)
- Acute death

DIAGNOSIS

- History of trauma to site of bleeding
- History of head trauma
- Complete blood cell count (CBC), total protein (TP) may indicate chronic blood loss from disease processes

TREATMENT

External Hemorrhage
Pressure to site will often be enough to stop the hemorrhage. Owners can use a pressure bandage or digital pressure. If bleeding is severe, electrocautery, chemical cautery, or ligation may be used once the bird arrives at the clinic.

Blood Feather Injury
Blood feathers are immature feathers that contain a large blood vessel that will bleed if broken or cut. Once injured, blood feathers will continue to bleed unless pulled from the feather follicle. The feather must be grasped close to the skin and pulled out to stop the bleeding.

Internal Hemorrhage
Supportive measures including fluid therapy should be used to control internal hemorrhage. Most cases of this type of hemorrhage will be found on necropsy.

Pericarditis and Myocarditis

Pericarditis and myocarditis are seen infrequently in pet birds. The cause of both diseases is usually bacterial septicemia. Occasionally urate deposits will be found in the pericardial membrane in birds with visceral gout (see Chapter 36).

Arteritis

Arteritis has been reported in birds, usually as a result of thrombosis from a resulting infection such as bumble foot. It is, however, not a common disease.

Anemia

Most anemia cases in pet birds are the result of chronic disease or parasitism. Parasites are most commonly seen in birds imported from other countries (not common at this time) or birds living in contact with wild birds and feral animals. It is not a common finding in pet birds.

Acute Death Related to Stress

Acute death related to capture stress or fright is seen in birds, especially in budgies and smaller birds. This is related to excessive epinephrine release, and in some cases heart failure, aortic rupture, or both. The increased blood pressure seen in birds (300–400 mm Hg) may contribute to the morbidity.

● TECH ALERT

Avoid prolonged effort when trying to capture and restrain small birds. If it is difficult to catch the bird, darken the examination room, let the bird rest, and then try again.

REVIEW QUESTIONS

1. The release of the hormone _____ in the avian patient has been attributed to death resulting from handling a stressed bird.
   a. Epinephrine
   b. Insulin
   c. Parathyroid
   d. Oxytocin

2. Which of the following substances are important dietary components for good cardiac health in birds?
   a. Vitamins B and D
   b. Vitamin E and selenium
   c. Vitamin A and sodium
   d. Vitamins K and D

3. List the differences between the avian and mammalian cardiovascular systems.
   a. The aortic arch in avian anatomy is derived from the right arch, and not from the left as in mammals.
   b. Two portal systems affect blood flow through the liver and the kidney.
   c. The avian heart is larger with respect to body weight.
   d. The heart rates for most birds exceed those of mammals.

4. When a bird appears stressed with restraint, technicians should _____.
   a. Cover the head with a towel
   b. Release restraint of the head
   c. Put the bird back into the cage
   d. Continue restraint to finish the task

5. Birds have a _____ systemic blood pressure than mammals.
   a. Lower
   b. Higher

Answers found on page 554.

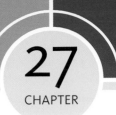
Diseases of the Digestive System

LEARNING OBJECTIVES

When you have completed this chapter, you will be able to:
1. Explain the basic anatomy of the avian digestive system to owners.
2. Recognize how similar gastrointestinal (GI) symptoms may be related to multiple, unrelated causes.
3. Explain why gram staining of the cloaca and choanal areas of the bird is an important screening test that should be part of our routine avian physical examinations.

Anatomy of the Digestive Tract

The digestive systems of birds are different from those of mammals. Birds have no teeth for cutting and grinding food. The esophagus, found on the right side of the neck in birds, contains a dilated portion called the *crop* used for food storage, allowing the bird to eat fast and travel at the same time. From the crop, the food passes into the proventriculus (the glandular stomach), to the ventriculus (the gizzard or grinding stomach), and then into the small intestine. After traveling through the small intestine, the large intestine, and the colon, feces pass into the cloaca. Because the renal and reproductive tracts also empty into the cloaca, feces are excreted mixed with urine and urates. Disturbances of the digestive system are among the most common problems in captive birds.

Regurgitation (Courtship Behavior)

CLINICAL SIGNS

- Bird seen regurgitating food onto shiny surfaces in the cage or onto the owner

- Usually a healthy-appearing male bird
- No other signs of disease, normal appetite, normal feces
- No vomiting or regurgitation seen at other times

DIAGNOSIS

- Gram staining of crop to rule out bacterial or fungal infection
- History of other breeding behavior

TREATMENT

- Removal of the surface from the cage
- Frequent changes in toys and cage furniture
- Avoidance of activities that stimulate behavior
- Extending the daily period of darkness to reduce mating behavior
- Hormone therapy, which however, has many adverse effects

INFORMATION FOR CLIENTS

- Unless the bird is losing weight, this is harmless behavior.
- The removal of shiny objects such as mirrors from the cage may cure most birds.
- Decrease the light period by covering the cage or placing it in a dark room.

Crop Stasis and Crop Burns

Crop stasis and crop burns are primarily problems in hand-fed baby birds. Failure of the crop to move the food into the lower digestive tract may result in malnutrition and death.

Crop Stasis

The primary causes of crop stasis are as follows:
- Foreign objects (such as bedding or large pieces of food)
- Infection
- Atony from overstretching
- Dehydrated food particles
- Low environmental temperatures
- Feeding food that separates in the crop
- Overfeeding in older birds

CLINICAL SIGNS

- Failure of the crop to empty in an appropriate time frame

- Regurgitation of food
- History of ingestion of foreign body

DIAGNOSIS

- Palpation of crop to rule out presence of foreign bodies
- Gram staining or culture and sensitivity for infectious agents
- ± Radiology to rule out foreign objects

TREATMENT

- Stop feeding the bird until crop motility returns to normal.
- Evacuate crop contents using a feeding tube and syringe.
- Lavage the crop by using warm saline and gentle massage to break down any impactions.
- Replace hand-feeding diet with warm fluids to prevent dehydration until crop motility returns.
- Administer antibiotics based on culture and sensitivity results.
- Foreign objects often may be removed using alligator forceps.
- As crop motility returns, slowly increase the consistency of the hand-feeding diet.
- Make sure the environment is temperature controlled (about 85°F to 90°F for most baby birds).
- For crops that are overstretched or pendulous, a "crop bra" may be fashioned to provide support.

INFORMATION FOR CLIENTS

- Seek instructions from the breeder or the pet store on how to hand-feed baby birds.
- Make sure the environmental temperatures of the food and cage are appropriate for the bird.
- Do not reheat used food. Throw away any unused food after each feeding.
- Do not feed new food over old food in the crop. Make sure that the crop is empty before feeding.

Crop Burns

Crop burns occur in birds when owners feed diets that are heated to extreme temperatures. This primarily is a result of using a microwave for heating the food. Microwaves produce high heat areas in the middle of the food, leaving cooler areas at the surface and sides of the container. If the food is not well mixed after heating, the very hot food may be placed into the crop, causing a severe burn. The damaged tissue will become necrotic and slough, often leaving a fistula in the crop (Fig. 27-1).

CLINICAL SIGNS

- Discolored areas in the skin over the crop
- Leakage of food or fluid from the crop onto skin
- Pain on palpation of the crop
- Reluctance to eat

DIAGNOSIS

- Good examination of crop and surrounding tissue
- Demonstration of a fistula opening in the crop

TREATMENT

Severe Burn

- Perform surgical debridement of the damaged area, with repair of fistulous opening.

Mild Burn

- Withhold food for several feedings.
- Replace food with a balanced electrolyte solution.
- Treat with antibiotics, if needed.

PREVENTION

- After heating hand-fed food, especially if using a microwave, make sure that the food is well mixed; and use a thermometer to ensure that the temperature is not greater than 105°F (normal temperatures should be between 98°F and 100°F).

INFORMATION FOR CLIENTS

- Before feeding, always check the temperature of the hand-feeding mixture by using a thermometer.
- Make sure that the food is well mixed to eliminate extremely hot areas.
- Young birds may reject food that is cooler than 98°F to 100°F.

Beak Deformities

Malformed beaks (Fig. 27-2) are the result of trauma, malnutrition, improper hand-feeding techniques, mite infestation, bacterial or viral disease, or liver dysfunction. Whatever the cause, a malformed beak may result in an inability to eat properly and digestive problems. Beak deformation in young hand-fed birds once thought to be related to hand-feeding from a single side of the beak is more likely related to poor nutritional balances in hand-feeding diets. In older birds, trauma to the germinal tissue of the beak will cause permanent beak deformities similar to those seen with damage to the cuticle of the fingernail or the coronary band of the hoof. Mite infestation with

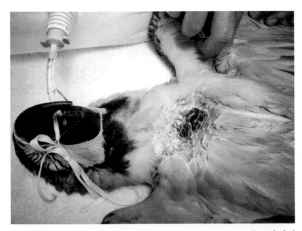

Figure 27-1 Crop burn with necrosis in a young hand-fed bird. From Donnelly, TM; Mayer J: Clinical Veterinary Advisor: Birds and Exotic Pets, St Louis, 2013, Saunders.

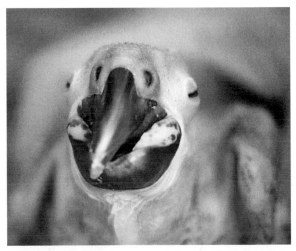

Figure 27-2 Lateral deviation of the maxilla in a macaw. (From Altman RB, Clubb SL, Dorrestein GM, Quesenberry KE: *Avian medicine and surgery*, Philadelphia, PA, 1997, Saunders, by permission.)

Knemidokoptes may also result in damage to the beak, resulting in deformities that are seen primarily in parakeets.

CLINICAL SIGNS

- Observation of uneven wearing of the beak
- Malocclusion of the beak
- Overgrowth of the beak (upper, lower, or both)
- History of trauma or signs of trauma: bite wounds, bruising of beak soft tissues, or disruption of the horny surface

DIAGNOSIS

- Complete physical examination
- Clinical chemistries, complete blood cell count (CBC) to rule out nutritional disorders
- Gram staining with culture and sensitivity—choanal slit

TREATMENT

- Treatment will depend on the cause of the malformation.
- Deformities that have become permanent may be partially corrected by corrective grinding using a Dremel (Dremel, Racine, WI)
- Early correction of malnutrition or calcium deficiencies may result in some improvement.
- Fractures or damage to the horny beak can be repaired with medical acrylics. Splinting has been successful in some cases.

INFORMATION FOR CLIENTS

- Malformation of the beak is usually manageable, but permanent return to normal shape and function is not possible.
- Birds with malformed beaks will need frequent corrective grinding.
- Birds adapt well to eating with malformed beaks.
- Diets may need to be adapted to maintain adequate nutrition.

Proventricular Dilatation Disease (Macaw Wasting Disease)

Proventricular dilatation disease (PDD) was first reported in the late 1970s in macaws. Initially, it was thought to affect only macaws, but we now know that it affects more than 50 species of parrots, Canadian geese, toucans, spoonbills, and weavers. Histologically, the disease is characterized by inflammation of both central and peripheral nervous tissues, with migration of lymphocytes and plasma cells into the nerve ganglia located in the proventriculus and other parts of the digestive system. The disease affects adult birds more than juvenile birds (3:1), and both sexes are equally affected. The cause of this disease has recently been identified as a polyomavirus, a double-stranded deoxyribonucleic acid (DNA) virus of the *Papoviridae* family. Transmission involves bird-to-bird contact, feces, feather dust, and contaminated environments. The virus appears to be somewhat unstable in the environment, and thus, bird-to-bird contact is probably the most successful means for the spread of the disease.

CLINICAL SIGNS

- Weight loss
- Regurgitation
- Depression
- Swollen abdomen, diarrhea
- Passage of undigested seeds in feces—most important sign
- Neurologic signs: ataxia, abnormal head movements, seizures, motor problems

DIAGNOSIS

- History and clinical signs
- Radiography: dilated proventriculus or dysfunction
- Increased creatine phosphokinase concentration may be suggestive
- Increase in barium transit time as seen on radiographs
- Proventricular or crop biopsy for typical histopathologic signs
- Polymerase chain reaction (PCR) test: best diagnostic test (uses whole blood and cloacal swab)

TREATMENT

- No cure exists for PDD.
- Cyclooxygenase-2 (COX-2) enzymatic antiinflammatory drugs may decrease the symptoms (watch out for adverse effects such as gastric bleeding, ulcers, etc.)
- Affected birds should be isolated from nonaffected ones.

INFORMATION FOR CLIENTS

- Proventricular dilatation disease currently has no cure. Any bird diagnosed with this disease should be placed in strict isolation to prevent contact with other birds.
- With proper diet and prevention of stress-related diseases, many birds can survive for long periods; however, many birds will die within months of diagnosis.
- Offspring and mates of infected birds should be considered at high risk for development of the disease.
- PCR and histology are currently the only means to obtain a positive diagnosis.
- A vaccine is available but is expensive.

Enteritis

Enteritis is common in pet birds (Fig. 27-3). It may be a primary disease condition or secondary to other generalized diseases.

As in other animals, a diet change may result in loose stool. The intake of increased fluids from either the diet (fruits, melons, or greens) or drinking water, as well as a change of seed, may result in loose stools. Fright or stress may cause diarrhea. One of the most common causes of diarrhea in the pet bird is a bacterial infection, which is usually caused by gram-negative organisms (such as *Esherichia*

coli, Pasturella, and Salmonella) commonly found in the environment.

Viral infections may also produce diarrhea in birds. Fatty liver disease, bacterial overgrowth from antibiotic treatment, pancreatitis, endocrine or metabolic disease, and mycotic infections may also result in alterations of the fecal material. It is important to isolate the cause because treatment should be specific for the disease producing the diarrhea.

CLINICAL SIGNS

- Anorexia
- Diarrhea
- Soiling of feathers around the vent
- Polyuria or polydipsia (Pu/Pd)
- Tenesmus (straining)
- Fluffing

DIAGNOSIS

- Gram staining (cloacal and choanal); culture and sensitivity, if required
- Ruling out other systemic diseases with serum chemistries, antibody–antigen titers, tests for toxins such as lead
- Ruling out mycotic infections
- History of diet change, excessive external temperatures, and so forth

TREATMENT

- Treatment will depend on the cause; if diet change is the only reason, decrease the amount of wet food (fruits, greens) being fed.
- Antibiotics administered should be based on gram staining, culture, and sensitivity tests.
- Yogurt or probiotics should be fed to normalize intestinal bacteria.
- Subcutaneous balanced electrolyte solutions should be given if needed.
- Intestinal protectants such as kaolin and pectin may be of some use.

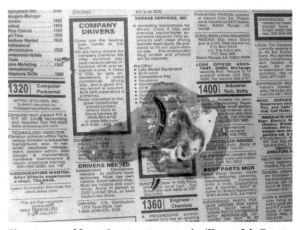

Figure 27-3 Normal psittacine stool. (From McCurnin DM, Bassert JM: *Clinical textbook for veterinary technicians,* ed 6, St. Louis, MO, 2010, Saunders, by permission.)

> ⊙ **TECH ALERT**
>
> Fecal swabs and samples should be obtained directly from the patient, not from the floor of the cage, to avoid inaccurate results.

INFORMATION FOR CLIENTS

- It is important to check the cage floor daily for droppings. Any change in number, color, or consistency may indicate a problem.
- All cases of diarrhea that do not self-correct within 24 hours should be seen by a veterinarian.
- Diet changes should be made slowly.
- Environmental temperatures should be increased to at least 85°F for fluffed birds.

Cloacal Prolapse

If diarrhea or tenesmus persists, it may lead to cloacal prolapse (Fig. 27-4). Efforts by female birds to pass retained eggs may also cause the cloaca to prolapse. Eversion of the cloaca to the outside of the bird prevents urine and feces from being passed; allows the tissue to become contaminated, dry, and necrotic; and may become a life-threatening condition for the bird. Cloacal prolapse should be handled as an emergency condition.

CLINICAL SIGNS

- Tenesmus and diarrhea
- Appearance of a pink to red blob of tissue from the cloaca

DIAGNOSIS

- Physical examination
- History

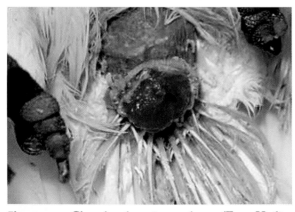

Figure 27-4 Cloacal prolapse in a cockatoo. (From Hnilica KA: *Small animal dermatology: A color atlas and therapeutic guide*, ed 4, St. Louis, MO, 2011, Saunders, by permission.)

TREATMENT

- Gently clean the exposed tissue.
- Reduce the swelling, and lubricate the exposed tissue (cortisone and antibiotic ointments, dimethyl sulfoxide, saturated sugar solution).
- Replace healthy tissue into the cloaca manually, and place a purse-string suture around the vent to prevent recurrence.
- Sutures are usually removed in 5 to 7 days.
- Treat the diarrhea or cause for straining.
- If tissue is necrotic when presented, surgical repair may be necessary.

INFORMATION FOR CLIENTS

- If you suspect a cloacal prolapse, have your bird treated immediately.
- Cloacal prolapse may recur if the bird strains for any reason (egg laying, diarrhea, or constipation, among other symptoms).

Cloacal Papillomas

Papillomas are neoplasms derived from nonglandular epithelium. Cloacal papillomas tend to occur most frequently in macaws, cockatoos, and some Amazon parrots. They can appear as protruding red masses from the vent (appear similar to a prolapse) or may be visualized only on internal examination of the cloaca. Birds with papillomas should not be used for breeding, and a breeding soundness examination should include ruling out the presence of papillomas.

CLINICAL SIGNS

- Tenesmus
- Soiled vent feathers
- Hemorrhage in the vent area
- Pasting of the vent area with feces, foul odor, and scalding of the area
- Some birds will not yet show signs when seen for treatment

DIAGNOSIS

- Visualization of masses in the cloaca (normal lining is smooth)
- Application of 5% acetic acid will turn abnormal tissue white
- Biopsy

TREATMENT

- Most birds respond to cryosurgery, but rapid regrowth may occur.
- Autogenous vaccines may be prepared from removed tissue.

INFORMATION FOR CLIENTS

- When buying a bird for breeding, always have a cloacal examination performed.
- Do not use infected birds for breeding because these papillomas may be transferred to the mate.
- Regrowth may occur rapidly after treatment.

Hepatitis

Most systemic avian diseases involve the hepatobiliary system. Clinical signs of liver disease may include inappetence and inactivity, weight loss, weakness, diarrhea, Pu/Pd, poor feathering, ascites, coagulopathy, green urates, and melena. Because of the large functional reserve of the liver, at least 80% of the liver tissue must be damaged for clinical signs to occur; therefore, liver disease is often a difficult diagnosis. Birds with liver disease do not experience development of jaundice; thus, this feature of mammalian liver disease is not helpful. Serum chemistries, radiography, and ultrasonography are the best means of determining liver dysfunction in the avian patient. Liver biopsy may be used to confirm the actual cause of the dysfunction. Some of the more frequent causes of hepatic disease are bacterial infections, chlamydial infection, viral infections, hepatic lipidosis, and toxins. Neoplasia may be seen in older birds, especially Amazon parrots.

CLINICAL SIGNS

- Weight loss
- Anorexia
- Weakness
- Pu/Pd
- Ascites
- Coagulopathy
- Melena or green urates

DIAGNOSIS

- CBC
- Bacterial cultures (usually from the liver biopsy sample)

- Serum chemistries:
  - Aspartate aminotransferase (AST) is found in high concentrations in hepatocytes but is also found in other tissues of the bird. Although not liver specific, most clinicians look at AST levels when assessing liver function. Alanine aminotransferase (ALT) is not useful in avian species.
  - Creatine kinase levels should be obtained to rule out muscle damage as the cause of increased AST levels.
- Bile acid level >120 micromolecules per liter (μmol/L); plasma levels of bile acids rely on the integrity of the enterohepatic circulation and the hepatobiliary system; disease of these pathways may interfere with the uptake of bile acids from the circulation
- Radiography: to identify hepatomegaly and ascites, if present; not all birds with liver disease will show signs of an enlarged liver
- Ultrasonography: may be useful in larger birds for localization of hepatic lesions such as granulomas or neoplasms
- Liver biopsy: not without potential risk but can confirm the diagnosis
- *Chlamydia* or viral serology

TREATMENT

- Lactulose is given orally to reduce ammonia levels.
- Colchicine may aid in limiting fibrosis of the liver.
- Eliminate the underlying cause of the disease, if possible.

Supportive Care
- Oxygen therapy
- Fluids
- Removal of ascetic fluids to aid in breathing
- Intravenous dextrose
- Colloid administration

⬤ **TECH ALERT**

Birds with hepatitis should be handled gently and should not be stressed!

Diet Therapy
- Hand-feeding with a protein-restricted diet
- Vitamin therapy, especially A, D, E, K, and B complex

INFORMATION FOR CLIENTS

- Birds with hepatitis are extremely ill, and many will die despite excellent treatment.
- Hospitalization and treatment may be a lengthy process.
- The prognosis will depend on the initial cause of the hepatic disease.

Internal Parasites

Internal parasites are not a major problem for captive birds raised and maintained in indoor environments. However, when birds are kept in enclosures with access to the ground or to wild birds, internal parasites may become a problem. Following is a partial list of internal parasites seen in captive birds (the technician is referred to a parasitology text for details of life cycles and transmission):
- *Ascarid* (Fig. 27-5)
- *Capillaria*
- *Cestodes* (Fig. 27-6)
- *Cryptosporidium*
- *Eimeria* (Fig. 27-7)
- *Giardia* (Fig. 27-8)
- *Isospora*

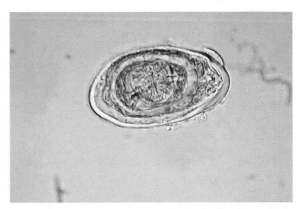

Figure 27-6 Cestode egg from a Lady Gouldian finch. (From Altman RB, Clubb SL, Dorrestein GM, Quesenberry KE: *Avian medicine and surgery*, Philadelphia, PA, 1997, Saunders, by permission.)

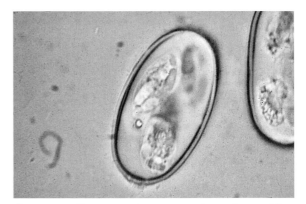

Figure 27-7 *Eimeria* species in a specimen from a blue-footed Amazon. (From Altman RB, Clubb SL, Dorrestein GM, Quesenberry KE: *Avian medicine and surgery*, Philadelphia, PA, 1997, Saunders, by permission.)

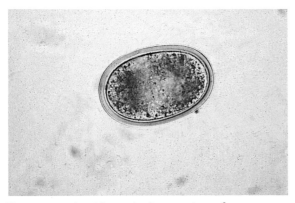

Figure 27-5 *Ascaridia* species in a specimen from a macaw. (From Altman RB, Clubb SL, Dorrestein GM, Quesenberry KE: *Avian medicine and surgery*, Philadelphia, PA, 1997, Saunders, by permission.)

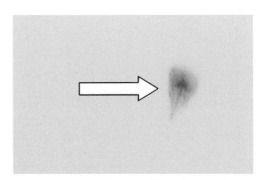

Figure 27-8 *Giardia* trophozoite. (From Bassert J, McCurnin DM: *McCurnin's clinical textbook for veterinary technicians*, ed 7, St. Louis, MO, 2010, Saunders.)

- *Sarcocystis falcatula*
- *Sternostoma tracheacolum* (air sac mite, tracheal mite)

CLINICAL SIGNS (WILL DEPEND ON PARASITE)

- Weight loss, depression
- Diarrhea, melena
- Bowel obstruction (ascarid)
- Debility
- Respiratory (*Cryptosporidium, Sternostoma, Sarcocystis*)
- Nervous system involvement (*Baylisascaris*)
- Feather picking (*Giardia*)

DIAGNOSIS

- Fecal flotation
- Direct smear, when it is necessary to identify the organism
- Clinical signs

TREATMENT

- Ivermectin
- Metronidazole (coccidia)
- Praziquantel (tapeworms and flukes)
- Cleaning up the environment
- Removal of the bird from the source of infection

INFORMATION FOR CLIENTS

- Prevention of exposure to wild birds will decrease the chance of exposure to internal parasites.
- If your birds will be housed outside, use elevated, covered cages to prevent fecal contamination.
- Periodic fecal examinations should be performed on all birds housed outside.

REVIEW QUESTIONS

1. Which of the following lists the proper order for treating crop stasis in a baby bird?
   a. Flush the crop using tap water, and refeed the bird using the normal feeding material.
   b. Flush the crop using warm saline, and re-feed the bird using the normal feeding material.
   c. Flush the crop using warm saline, and then refill the crop with a balanced electrolyte solution.
   d. Flush the crop using tap water, and then refill the crop with an antibiotic solution.

2. On finding papillomas in the cloaca of a blue and gold macaw, the veterinarian should tell the owners that:
   a. This disease is not treatable and they should sell the bird.
   b. This disease will eventually be fatal to the bird.
   c. This disease is contagious to humans.
   d. This disease is treatable, but the animal should not be used for breeding.

3. Describe how to determine the difference between "courtship regurgitation" and vomiting from a disease process.

4. Which of the following foods would most likely cause loose stools if added to a bird's diet?
   a. Watermelon
   b. Bread
   c. Meat
   d. Potato

5. Which of the following clinical chemistry tests is not useful for diagnosis of liver disease in the avian patient?
   a. ALT
   b. AST
   c. Bile acids
   d. γ-Glutamyl transferase (GGT)

6. The intestinal tract of birds contains predominately _____ bacteria.
   a. Gram +
   b. Gram −
   c. Acid-fast

7. Cloacal polyps should be treated before using the bird for breeding.
   a. True
   b. False

8. This organ is the glandular stomach of the bird.
   a. Crop
   b. Proventriculus
   c. Ventriculus

Answers found on page 554.

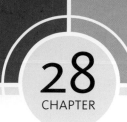

Diseases of the Endocrine System

LEARNING OBJECTIVES

When you have completed this chapter, you will be able to:
1. Discuss how iodine-poor diets affect some species of avian patients.
2. Relate symptoms of diabetes in the bird to pancreatic islet cell dysfunction seen in other species.

3. Recognize the presence of unique hormones and their function in the avian patient.

Anatomy of the Avian Endocrine System

The endocrine glands and hormones in birds are similar to those found in mammals (Box 28-1). The glands release hormones into the circulation. These hormones activate a target organ to produce changes within the body. As in mammals, a hypothalamohypophysial axis is composed of the hypothalamus and the pituitary gland. Releasing hormones are produced in the hypothalamus and are carried by the portal circulation to the anterior pituitary, where they stimulate the release of the appropriate stimulating hormone into the general circulation. Stimulating hormones released from the anterior pituitary (the adenohypophysis) include follicle-stimulating hormone (FSH) luteinizing hormone (LH), thyroid-stimulating hormone (TSH), prolactin, growth hormone (GH), and adrenocorticotropic hormone (ACTH). The posterior pituitary (the neurohypophysis) releases arginine vasotocin (AVT) and mesotocin (MT).

Both AVT and MT are produced in the hypothalamus and stored in the posterior pituitary. The effect of AVT is similar to antidiuretic hormone in mammals. It acts to control water resorption and oviductal contraction during oviposition. AVT

BOX 28-1   Endocrine Organs of the Avian Species

Thyroid
Parathyroid
Ultimobranchial gland
Thymus
Adrenal
Pituitary
Pineal
Pancreas
Testes or ovaries
   The following organs produce some hormones in addition to performing their other functions:
Liver
Small intestine
Kidneys
Uterus

also decreases glomerular filtration, which causes increased water retention. The role of MT currently is unknown.

Diseases of the Thyroid Gland

The thyroid glands are located just cranial to the thoracic inlet and lateral to the trachea. They are innervated by both the parasympathetic and sympathetic systems. As in mammals, the glands are composed of follicles that produce both triiodothyronine (T_3) and tetraiodothyronine (T_4). The thyroid glands of birds do not contain C-cells for the production of calcitonin. In birds, calcitonin is produced by C-cells found in the ultimobranchial bodies that are just caudal to the parathyroid glands. The function of calcitonin is unknown and does not appear to reduce the serum levels of calcium as it does in mammals. Iodine is concentrated in the gland, but thyroid hormones contain a greater percentage of iodine compared with those of mammals. The most common disease associated with the thyroid gland is related to iodine deficiency, resulting in formation of goiter. This disease is more commonly associated with parakeets, budgies, canaries, pigeons, and cockatiels than the larger parrots.

CLINICAL SIGNS

- Dyspnea
- Characteristic squeaking noise on inspiration
- Regurgitation or repeated swallowing attempts when eating

DIAGNOSIS

- History of a diet low in iodine (all-seed diet)
- The enlarged thyroid usually not palpable

TREATMENT

- Increase the level of iodine in the diet by oral administration of a dilute Lugol iodine solution via the water.
- Improvement in diet can be achieved by addition of vegetables that contain iodine or through formulated pelleted diets that contain iodine.

⬤ TECH ALERT

Dyspneic birds may need supplemental oxygen before they are handled. Be careful to avoid causing stress in these birds.

INFORMATION FOR CLIENTS

- All birds should be on a well-balanced diet that contains iodine. Avoid seeds as the primary diet because many are grown in iodine-deficient soil.
- Vegetables and fruits that contain iodine include dark leafy greens.
- It will not be easy to retrain your bird to eat properly. Start by adding a small amount of one food to a familiar food cup daily for up to a week. Leave this cup in the cage all day, but remove the normal diet 15 to 20 minutes after placing it in the cage. Do not offer seeds during this period. As the bird begins to eat this new item you can add others slowly using the same method. Do not give up; it may take a while to successfully implement a better diet.
- Most formulated pelleted diets contain iodine and other vitamins that are easy to use.
- A well-balanced diet will increase the life span of your pet bird.

Hypothyroidism

Primary hypothyroidism is not a common disease in pet birds.

Disease of the Pancreas: Diabetes Mellitus

The endocrine portion of the pancreas contains three types of Islet cells: (1) α-cells (secrete glucagon), β-cells (secrete insulin), and δ-cells (secrete somatostatin). As in mammals, insulin reduces blood glucose levels, glucagon increases blood glucose levels, and somatostatin regulates the release of both hormones. A fourth hormone, avian pancreatic polypeptide, is also produced by the pancreas, although its function is unknown.

Spontaneous occurring diabetes mellitus has been reported in several species of birds, including budgerigars, toucans, Amazon parrots, African grays, and cockatiels. Some controversy has existed about the roles of insulin and glucagon in the development of diabetes in birds. Because the avian pancreas contains more glucagon-secreting cells and the glucagon–insulin ratios in birds are 5 to 10 times greater than in mammals, it was thought that glucagon was the most important hormone in blood glucose regulation, but newer research has shown that insulin does play an important role in carbohydrate homeostasis. Lack of insulin results in impaired glucose tolerance, and lack of glucagon leads to hypoglycemia.

CLINICAL SIGNS

- Polyuria or polydipsia
- Weight loss in the presence of a voracious appetite
- Depression, lethargy

DIAGNOSIS

- Persistent glycosuria: it is often difficult to obtain a pure urine sample from a bird; successful urine samples can be obtained by using waxed paper on the bottom of the cage and carefully collecting only the liquid portion of the fecal sample using a syringe or eyedropper
- Serum glucose levels are persistently increased to >600 milligrams per deciliter (mg/dL)
- Serum glucagon levels should be obtained

TREATMENT

- Supportive care should be implemented: fluids, hand-feeding, correction of electrolyte disorders.
- A serial blood glucose curve should be performed.
- Insulin therapy should be instituted; twice daily injections usually are required.
- Addition of a high-fiber diet to decrease postprandial hyperglycemia should be considered.

INFORMATION FOR CLIENTS

- Treatment of the bird will be lifelong.
- Blood glucose levels will need to be reevaluated periodically to ensure adequate insulin levels.
- Signs of hypoglycemia due to insulin overdose include weakness, ataxia, disorientation, lethargy, and seizures. You should keep Karo syrup on hand to treat hypoglycemic crises. It can be rubbed onto the roof of the mouth (take care not to get bitten) or given directly by crop tube if the bird is not experiencing a seizure.

Diseases of the Adrenal Glands

No cases of naturally occurring hypoadrenocorticism or hyperadrenocorticism have been reported in pet birds.

REVIEW QUESTIONS

1. Blood glucose levels in the range of _____ should suggest diabetes mellitus in the bird.
   a. 250 mg/dL
   b. 600 mg/dL
   c. 300 mg/dL
   d. 150 mg/dL
2. Goiter is a common problem in parakeets because of:
   a. A seed diet low in iodine
   b. Lack of leafy green vegetables in the diet
   c. An excess of calcium and vitamin D in the diet
   d. An inherited trait
3. Compared with mammalian thyroid glands, which type of cell is missing from the avian thyroid gland?
   a. Follicular cells
   b. Parathyroid cells
   c. C-cells

4. The most common thyroid problem seen in pet birds is related to:
   a. Hygiene problems
   b. An iodine-deficient diet
   c. Exposure to ultraviolet light
   d. Oversupplementation of the diet

5. Lack of the hormone glucagon in the avian patient may result in:
   a. Hyperglycemia
   b. Hyperproteinemia
   c. Hypoglycemia
   d. Hypercalcemia

Answers found on page 555.

Diseases of the Eye and Ear

LEARNING OBJECTIVES

When you have completed this chapter, you will be able to:
1. Locate the ear canal in the avian patient.
2. Examine the structures of the avian eye.
3. Appreciate how eye color may be used to determine the age of a bird.
4. Treat hospitalized avian patients with eye problems.

The Eye

The structures of the eye in the bird are similar to those in mammals. Upper and lower eyelids and a nictitating membrane are present. Modified feathers called *filoplumes* are present at the margins of the lids and function like eyelashes, for protection and tactile stimulation. The leading edge of the nictitans is pigmented. The Harderian gland, the major source of tear production, is located at the base of the nictitating membrane.

The cornea resembles that of the mammalian animal. The iris of most birds is brown, although other colors may be seen. The iris of cockatoos is sexually dimorphic, with female birds having red irises and male birds having brown ones. Young African gray parrots have brown irises, whereas the irises of adults are more grayish. Young Amazons will have brown irises that become red-orange as they age, and macaws have brown irises that become gray between 1 and 3 years of age, and then turn yellow in older birds. Direct pupillary light reflexes are demonstrable, but consensual reflexes are absent in avian species. The vitreous body is large and transparent. The fundus is usually gray or red. The optic disk is elongated and barely visible because of the presence of the pecten. The pecten is a vascular structure believed to be involved in the nutritional support of the retina, in the acid–base balance of the inner eye, and it may agitate the vitreous during eye movement. No tapetum is present in the avian retina. Color vision is well developed in pet birds.

Abnormal Palpebral Fissures

Cryptophthalmos, the abnormal fusion of skin over the globe and orbit, is seen in cockatiels (Fig. 29-1). This fusion reduces the palpebral fissure in both length and width.

DIAGNOSIS

- Physical examination will show abnormal tissue covering the cornea.

TREATMENT

- Surgical removal of the excess tissue has not been successful in curing this condition.
- Topical application of cortisone-containing eye ointments may help after surgery.

INFORMATION FOR CLIENTS

- Avoid purchasing a bird with this condition.
- Although treatment may help temporarily, complete cure is unlikely. *Do not* use a bird with this problem for breeding.

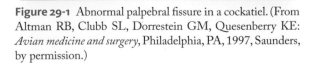

Figure 29-1 Abnormal palpebral fissure in a cockatiel. (From Altman RB, Clubb SL, Dorrestein GM, Quesenberry KE: *Avian medicine and surgery*, Philadelphia, PA, 1997, Saunders, by permission.)

Periocular Swelling

Periocular swelling occurs frequently in the bird. It may result from disorders of the eyelids, the infraorbital sinuses, or less commonly, the conjunctiva. Trauma to periocular tissue may also cause swelling. Bacterial, viral, and parasitic infections may cause periorbital swelling as well.

CLINICAL SIGNS

- Eyelids or periocular tissue will appear swollen and red or scaly.
- Palpebral fissure may be reduced, and the nictitans may be prolapsed.
- Feather loss around the eye may be present
- Facial swelling may be present with evidence of rubbing.
- ± Scabbing of tissues is seen

DIAGNOSIS

- Complete ocular examination
- Skin scraping to rule out *Knemidokoptes* infection
- Skin biopsy if necessary
- Good dietary history
- Gram staining or culture and sensitivity of the infraorbital sinuses to rule out bacterial infection

TREATMENT

- Therapy should be aimed at the causative agent
- Maintain adequate corneal lubrication with the use of ophthalmic ointments
- Repair eyelid lacerations if present
- Vitamin A therapy may help some birds
- Flush the sinuses; some may have to be trephined to remove debris.

INFORMATION FOR CLIENTS

- Therapy may involve multiple treatments daily. If it is difficult to handle the bird, it should be admitted to the hospital.
- The periorbital swelling is usually secondary to another disease process that may not respond well to treatment.

Conjunctivitis and Keratoconjunctivitis

Conjunctivitis caused by trauma, bacterial infections, viral infections, and vitamin A deficiencies are seen in birds. Cultures of the conjunctiva of normal psittacines indicated no bacteria in half the birds, and the remainder had mostly gram-positive isolates. Organisms capable of causing conjunctivitis include *Chlamydia*, *Mycoplasma*, *Escherichia coli*, *Pseudomonas*, *Bordetella*, *Mycobacterium*, and *Streptococcus* spp. Conjunctivitis in cockatiels believed to be caused by *Mycoplasma* and adenovirus infection has been reported. Conjunctivitis may accompany any respiratory infection as well. Keratoconjunctivitis is usually the result of trauma, infectious agents, or general anesthesia (lack of protection and lubrication during the process).

CLINICAL SIGNS

- Hyperemia
- Blepharospasms
- Photophobia
- Ocular discharge
- Swelling

DIAGNOSIS

- Thorough history and physical examination
- Culture and sensitivity of the conjunctiva and cornea
- Complete ocular examination under magnification
- Corneal staining
- Cytology of the conjunctiva
- Viral serology or cultures to rule out systemic causes

TREATMENT

- Broad-spectrum topical ophthalmic antibiotics
- Oral or systemic antibiotics if respiratory disease or systemic disease is involved
- Corticosteroids if conjunctivitis is nonsuppurative and if no corneal ulceration is present

INFORMATION FOR CLIENTS

- Birds with conjunctivitis should be isolated from other birds in the household to prevent the spread of disease.
- Birds will need four to six treatments daily with topical ophthalmic ointments. If it is difficult to treat the bird at home, it will have to be admitted to a hospital.
- You may need to prevent further trauma to the bird's eyes and to limit light until the photophobia decreases.

Cataracts

Cataracts are frequently noted in long-living psittacines. Cataracts may also be seen in response to trauma, nutritional deficiencies, and other ocular disorders. As in mammals, cataracts mature over time with the lens gradually becoming opaque.

CLINICAL SIGNS

- Lens opacity identified visually
- Owner may report vision loss
- ± History of ocular trauma or disease

DIAGNOSIS

- Physical examination with complete ocular examination

TREATMENT

- Surgical removal of the lens if other intraocular disease is absent
- Treatment of any related ocular disease if present

INFORMATION FOR CLIENTS

- Handle vision-impaired birds carefully because they may be more likely to get startled and bite.
- Consult an ophthalmic specialist to determine whether surgery is an option.
- Prevent trauma to the bird's eyes, and aggressively treat any inflammatory disease of the eyes to decrease the formation of cataracts.

The Ear

As in mammals, the ear of the bird consists of outer, middle, and inner parts. The pinna is absent, and the middle ear has only one ossicle. The cochlear duct of the inner ear is not coiled as in mammals. The external ear is hidden by feathers and a loose flap of skin. The external canal is examined using an otoscope.

Otitis Externa

Otitis externa has been diagnosed in pet birds. It is usually related to a bacterial infection.

CLINICAL SIGNS

- Pruritus
- Serous or purulent discharge with or without soft-tissue swelling

DIAGNOSIS

- Examination of the external ear canal
- Swab of discharge for cytology and culture and sensitivity testing

TREATMENT

- Topical antibiotics applied into the ear canal after cleaning (three to four times daily)

INFORMATION FOR CLIENTS

- If the bird cannot be treated at home, it should be admitted to a hospital.
- Untreated otitis externa may progress to otitis media or interna with signs of head tilt, loss of balance, and inability to fly. Report the development of these signs to your veterinarian immediately.

REVIEW QUESTIONS

1. "Eyelashes" in the bird are actually:
   a. Hairs
   b. Feathers
2. The color of a female cockatoo's eye is:
   a. Brown
   b. Black
   c. Red
   d. Yellow
3. The _____ is a vascular structure involved in nutritional support of the retina. It may be seen by using the ophthalmoscope.
   a. Optic disc
   b. Pecten
   c. Vitreous body

4. Bacterial isolates from most normal birds will contain mostly _____ bacteria.
   a. Gram-negative
   b. Gram-positive
   c. Both gram-positive and gram-negative
5. What structure is missing from the avian ear but is found in mammals?
   a. Pinna
   b. External ear canal
   c. Ossicles
   d. Cochlear duct
6. This vitamin is important for normal visual health in avian patients.
   a. Vitamin B
   b. Vitamin A
   c. Vitamin K
   d. Vitamin E
7. Surgical correction of abnormal palpebral fissures in the cockatiel is always successful.
   a. True
   b. False
8. Birds have excellent color vision.
   a. True
   b. False

Answers found on page 555.

30
CHAPTER

Hematologic and Immunologic Diseases

LEARNING OBJECTIVES

When you have completed this chapter, you will be able to:
1. Begin a study of avian blood cells.
2. Attempt to draw blood from avian patients.

3. Discuss diagnostic hematology with avian owners.

Review of Avian Hematology

Hematology is an important part of the diagnostic workup in the ill bird. With a little practice and a minimum amount of equipment, a technician can perform a complete blood cell count (CBC) as for the mammalian patient. Blood collection is practical even from small birds. Up to 1% of the bird's body weight can be collected safely unless the bird is anemic or hypovolemic (Box 30-1). The preferred collection site for samples is the jugular vein (accessed from the right side of the neck), but the basilic (wing vein) vein and the medial metatarsal veins also may be used. Hematoma formation from venipuncture of the basilic or metatarsal veins may become a serious problem in small birds if not addressed promptly. A toenail clip

is the least desirable method for blood collection because it is painful for the bird and the site is usually contaminated with feces and other debris.

Evaluating blood smears for the avian patient takes some practice because the cells are slightly different from those of the mammal. They are more fragile and tend to be easily damaged during preparation of the blood smear. The use of glass coverslips for the preparation of the smear will decrease the amount of cell damage. (The technician should refer to a hematology text for the exact description of each cell type found in the avian sample.)

Anemia

Causes of anemia in birds include blood loss caused by trauma, toxicosis resulting in coagulopathy,

BOX 30-1 Calculations of Blood That Can Be Collected for Hematology Testing

- Average total volume of blood in the avian patient = 6% to 13% body weight (can use 8% as a general value for calculation)
- Body weight (in kg) $\times$ 0.08 $\times$ 1000 mL/kg = total blood volume (in mL)
- Total blood volume (in mL) $\times$ 0.10 = total amount that can be obtained for testing
- Most testing will require less than the calculated amount.

parasites, and organic disease. Chronic diseases such as chlamydiosis, mycobacteriosis, nephritis, aspergillosis, and others may also result in a decrease in blood cell production and anemia. Most anemias in birds are nonregenerative.

CLINICAL SIGNS

- Weakness
- Lethargy
- Clinical signs of systemic disease related to the specific organ system involved

DIAGNOSIS

- Good history and complete physical examination
- Complete blood cell count (CBC) and serum chemistry panel
- Should include a reticulocyte count (normally <10% of total red blood cell count)
- Bone marrow aspirate if other tests are inconclusive

TREATMENT

- Involves treating the underlying cause of the anemia
- Blood transfusions may be performed in critical patients
- Iron dextran and B vitamins if needed

INFORMATION FOR CLIENTS

- Anemia is almost always caused by systemic disease in the avian patient.
- Diagnosis of the underlying disease may be time-consuming, expensive, and difficult.

- Make sure the anemic bird is being fed a well-balanced diet and vitamin supplement, and protect it from stress and injury.

Hemochromatosis (Iron Storage Disease)

Although not actually a disease of the heme system, hemochromatosis does involve blood. The disease results from an excessive amount of iron stored in various tissues of the body, especially the liver. It is an inherited metabolic defect common in toucans and mynahs but rarely is seen in psittacines.

CLINICAL SIGNS

- Weakness
- Lethargy
- Ascites
- Coughing
- Dyspnea
- $\pm$ Hepatomegaly
- Sudden death in toucans

DIAGNOSIS

- Physical examination
- Susceptible species
- Greatly increased packed cell volume (polycythemia)
- Abdominocentesis yields a yellow transudate or modified transudate
- Liver biopsy: definitive for diagnosis

Radiography

- Enlarged liver
- Ascites
- $\pm$ Cardiomegaly and splenomegaly

TREATMENT

- Aspiration of ascetic fluid to relieve dyspnea
- Phlebotomies to decrease circulating blood volume
- Recommended weekly withdrawal of 1% of circulating blood volume
- Low-iron pelleted diet or soft foods low in iron (egg whites, potatoes, corn, wheat, apples, bananas, pears, berries, melons, among others)

INFORMATION FOR CLIENTS

- Hemochromatosis is an inherited metabolic defect and is incurable.

- This disease carries a poor prognosis even with extensive therapy.
- Treatment will be required for the life of the bird.
- Do not use birds with hemochromatosis for breeding.

Splenomegaly

In the bird, the spleen functions in the phagocytosis of aged erythrocytes, lymphocytosis, and in antibody production. Primary disease of the spleen is uncommon; however, the spleen can become involved in many systemic disorders. Splenic enlargement is associated with various conditions such as viral infections (most commonly polyomavirus and herpesvirus), bacterial infections (chlamydiosis, gram-positive and gram-negative infections), and disseminated mycotic infections.

CLINICAL SIGNS

- With or without clinical signs; signs usually characteristic for specific disease state

DIAGNOSIS

- Physical examination for existing disease
- Radiography
- Necropsy finding

TREATMENT

- Treat the existing systemic disease.

INFORMATION FOR CLIENTS

- Splenic enlargement is common with many systemic diseases.

Immune-Mediated Conditions

Immune-mediated conditions are suspected in birds but have not been proven to exist. It is believed that some birds that feather-pick and are pruritic have an autoimmune dermatitis because they have lesions consistent with that form of disease. A severe pneumonitis reported in blue and gold macaws is also believed to be immune-mediated, the allergens being powder down or feather fragments from other birds, endotoxins, or fungal organisms. Immune mediation may play a role in the development of proventricular dilation syndrome in psittacines as well.

CLINICAL SIGNS

- Dermatitis: pruritus, feather picking
- Respiratory: acute onset of severe dyspnea (emergency situation)

DIAGNOSIS

- No adequate way to diagnose immune-mediated conditions exists
- Skin biopsy may be of value for dermatitis cases
- Frequent occurrence of symptoms

TREATMENT

- Steroids and nonsteroidal antiinflammatory drugs
- Oxygen therapy when needed

● TECH ALERT

Avoid topical products that are not water soluble for use on the skin of birds. Sprays that contain oral irritants or antiitch substances may irritate the skin and actually increase picking.

INFORMATION FOR CLIENTS

- Autoimmune or allergic diseases in birds are suspected but have not been proven.
- Treatment is aimed at decreasing the allergic reaction within the animal and making the animal more comfortable.
- Acute development of severe difficulty breathing is serious, and veterinary care should be obtained immediately.

REVIEW QUESTIONS

1. Assuming your bird patient weighs 378 g, how much blood can you safely remove for laboratory testing?
   a. 38 mL
   b. 3.8 mL
   c. 0.38 mL
2. What is the recommended site for blood collection from the avian patient?
   a. Medial metatarsal vein
   b. Jugular vein
   c. Basilic vein
   d. Heart

3. Which of the following methods is the least desirable for collection of blood in the avian patient?
   a. Jugular venipuncture
   b. Toenail clip
   c. Basilic vein puncture
   d. Medial metatarsal venipuncture

4. Most anemias in birds are:
   a. Regenerative
   b. Non-regenerative

Answers found on page 555.

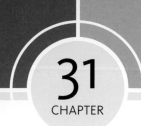

Diseases of the Integumentary System

LEARNING OBJECTIVES

When you have completed this chapter, you will be able to:
1. Distinguish normal feathering from abnormal feathering.

2. Discuss with owners proper husbandry to maintain good health of skin and feathers.

Anatomy and Physiology of Avian Skin

Avian skin is much thinner and more easily damaged than that of mammals. The layers of skin (epidermis, dermis, and subcuticular) are the same as in other animals. The horny beak is composed of hard keratinized epithelium and the underlying dermis that is continuous with the periosteum of the mandible and premaxilla. The beak contains sensory receptors that provide for food discrimination and tactile sensation. Claws are also extensions of the hard keratinized epithelium. Some species of birds have the uropygial gland located at the base of the tail. This gland produces an oily substance for waterproofing of the feathers (African gray

parrots and budgies have this gland whereas Amazon parrots do not). This gland may become obstructed and cause a swelling above the tail head in some birds.

The most obvious difference in avian skin is the presence of feathers. Several different types of feathers exist, and each has a specific purpose. The feathers are aligned in tracts with bare skin in between each tract. Feathers are molted by extrusion of the old feather from its base and replacement with new feather growth from the dermis. The newly developing feather is known as a *blood feather* because it contains large vessels that will retreat as the feather ages. Normally, except the face in some species, no area of the bird's body is not covered by feathers.

Feathers serve many functions: They give the body its shape; allow for flight; provide balance during landing and takeoff; offer thermal insulation; and in some species, provide for sexual recognition. Feathers also provide the beautiful colors that bird owners appreciate. Any topical medications that would interfere with the normal fluffing of the plumage for insulation may cause problems in birds. For this reason, oil-based topical medications should be avoided in the treatment of skin problems.

Diseases of Feathers

Feather Mutilation

Feather picking, plucking, and chewing are common problems seen in the veterinary clinic (Fig. 31-1). They are also some of the most frustrating and difficult problems to treat. It is believed that some of these behaviors may develop from boredom and excessive grooming behavior that gets out of hand (similar to cage walking and other captive behavior problems seen in mammals). In some species—the passerines—feather plucking may be related to aggression, with male birds plucking the feathers of female birds or other subservient male birds. In psittacines, feather mutilations appear to be more complex. Feather picking should be suspected in birds that have normal head feathers with varying degrees of body feather loss or damage. African gray parrots appear to be involved in feather mutilation more frequently compared with Amazon or Macaw parrots.

CLINICAL SIGNS

- Loss or damage to body feathers with normal head and neck
- Change in plumage
- History of recent wing clip, change in environment, change in diet
- Signs of systemic disease

DIAGNOSIS

- History of poor diet, low humidity, or poor environmental conditions
- Complete blood cell count (CBC) and biochemical profile
- Bacterial or fungal skin cultures and sensitivities
- Skin scrape to rule out mites
- Biopsy

TREATMENT

- Occupational therapy: find something to occupy the bird's attention
- Change the environment; increase humidity, improve diet, more companionship.
- Decrease emotional and physical stress
- Provide drug therapy with anxiolytics, tranquilizers, or opioids:
  - Clomipramine (Anafranil)
  - Haloperidol (Haldol)
  - Fluoxetine (Prozac)
  - Naltrexone (Trexan)
- Apply restraint collars to prevent further trauma (may increase stress to bird).
- Add chewable toys to the cage as substitutes for feathers

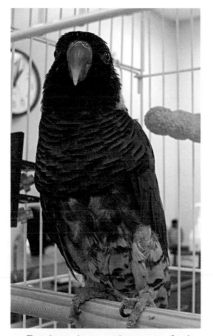

Figure 31-1 Rainbow lory with severe feather picking. (From Hnilica KA: *Small animal dermatology: A color atlas and therapeutic guide*, ed 3, St. Louis, MO, 2011, Saunders, with permission.)

- Feather mutilation is a problem that will not be easily solved; it will require creativity on the part of the owner.
- Do not expect a cure even with extensive therapy.
- Therapy for this condition will be lifelong.

Feather Cysts

Feather cysts are common in canaries and are thought to be a genetic problem. The cysts present as smooth masses on the body or wing. They may be quite large, be covered partially with skin, and have filamentous-appearing content.

CLINICAL SIGNS

- Smooth, dry, often crusted mass on the skin of the body or wing
- Multiple cysts

DIAGNOSIS

- Appearance and characteristic species
- Needle biopsy (use care because tumors may bleed excessively)

TREATMENT

- Surgical removal of the feather from the cyst or surgical removal of the entire feather follicle or tract
- Radiosurgical ablation of the cyst lining

INFORMATION FOR CLIENTS

- Removal of feather cysts may be a long-term management problem for the bird.
- Avoid using these birds for breeding.

Skin Abnormalities

Bumblefoot (Pododermatitis)

Bumblefoot (pododermatitis) is a common problem in captive, heavy-bodied birds, particularly cockatiels, budgies, and Amazon parrots (Fig. 31-2). Development of the infection is secondary to trauma to the plantar surfaces of the feet.

CLINICAL SIGNS

- Abnormal appearance of the plantar surface of the foot

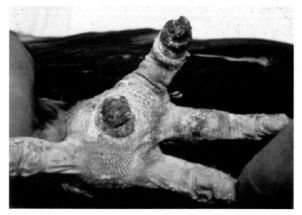

Figure 31-2 Bumblefoot lesion in an obese parakeet maintained on improper perches. (From Hnilica KA: *Small animal dermatology: A color atlas and therapeutic guide*, ed 3, St. Louis, MO, 2011, Saunders, with permission.)

- ± Swelling
- Central lesion of necrosis

DIAGNOSIS

- Physical examination
- Environmental history or heavy bird
- Culture and sensitivity of lesion

TREATMENT

- Correct inadequate husbandry
- Apply wet bandages to protect tissue after debridement of necrotic tissue.
- Apply antibiotic ointment as wound dressing
- Provide systemic antibiotic therapy

INFORMATION FOR CLIENTS

- Perches should be wrapped in a safe, padded material that can be changed or washed frequently.
- To prevent the disease, make sure that the perches in the cage are of varying diameters and materials to prevent constant trauma to the same area of the foot.
- *Do not cover perches with sandpaper*!

Viral Skin Conditions

Pox Virus Infection

Pox virus infections are common in many species of pet birds. Most lesions are found on the head around the eyes and beak. Lesions include crusts or plaques that may be white or honey colored. The infection is common in canaries, lovebirds, and blue-fronted Amazon parrots.

CLINICAL SIGNS

- Presence of large, crusty lesions around the eyes and beak in recently imported birds

DIAGNOSIS

- History and species
- Biopsy if possible

TREATMENT

Nonspecific
- Effective nursing care
- Improved nutrition
- Hand-feeding if necessary
- Gentle cleaning of lesions and application of broad-spectrum antibiotic ointment
- Systemic antibiotics to prevent secondary infections

INFORMATION FOR CLIENTS

- Avoid purchasing a bird with crusty lesions around the eye or beak.
- Buy domestically raised birds if possible.

Psittacine Beak and Feather Disease

Psittacine beak and feather disease (PBFD) is an infectious viral disease documented in more than 42 species of parrots. Initially believed to be a disease affecting only cockatoos, eclectus parrots, and African gray birds, it is now known that many bird species are susceptible to this disease. Most birds that acquire the chronic form of PBFD experience development of signs of the disease between 6 months and 3 years of age. Initial signs are subtle but progress with time. Lack of powder down, progressive loss of feathers on the entire body, delayed molts, and dysplastic feather formation may be early signs. Beak and nail lesions are also seen. Beak lesions often make it painful for the bird to eat. Secondary infections are common in the beak and nails. The cause of this disease is a non-enveloped single-stranded deoxyribonucleic (DNA) virus that is naturally occurring in wild Australian parrots. The exact route of transmission is unknown; however, the virus remains infective in the environment for long periods. The virus is shed in the feces and feather-down dust. The incubation period may be as short as 3 weeks in young nestlings to years in older birds. Most infections will eventually be fatal, but birds may live for extended periods after the onset of symptoms.

CLINICAL SIGNS

- Feather loss, dysplastic feathers, prolonged molt
- Beak lesions
- Absence of feather dust on the beak

DIAGNOSIS

- Clinical signs
- Polymerase chain reaction (PCR) based diagnostic test using whole blood

TREATMENT

- No cure currently exists for PBFD. These birds may live for years with good supportive care.

INFORMATION FOR CLIENTS

- Birds with this condition are infectious to other birds in the household.
- All new birds susceptible to PBFD should be tested before purchase.
- Birds may be infected at bird shows, in breeding facilities, and when boarding. Avoid exposing your bird to other birds.
- Proper cleaning of surfaces, air ducts, and the facility is necessary to decrease viral numbers.
- Vaccination is not currently available.

External Parasites

The most commonly seen external parasite in captive birds, especially budgies, is *Knemidokoptes pilae* (the scaly face mite) (Fig. 31-3). The mites burrow under the skin in featherless areas of the legs and the cere. Lesions have a sandy, honeycomb appearance and may progress to cover the entire beak and eye area. The mites may damage the beak if the disease is left untreated.

CLINICAL SIGNS

- Sandy, scaly lesions on cere or feet, or both; may be seen on cloaca
- Abnormal beak growth

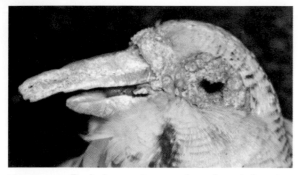

Figure 31-3 Beak damage in a parakeet from infestation with *Knemidokoptes* mites. (From Hnilica KA: *Small animal dermatology: A color atlas and therapeutic guide*, ed 3, St. Louis, MO, 2011, Saunders, with permission.)

DIAGNOSIS

- General appearance of lesions
- Scraping positive for mite or eggs

TREATMENT

- Ivermectin given orally or transdermally until lesions are gone or scrapings are negative

INFORMATION FOR CLIENTS

- Mites may be transmitted by direct contact or by fomites in the cage.
- Remove all wood perches and toys from the cage and dispose of them.
- Clean all cage surfaces using an effective disinfectant and allow cage to dry in the sun if possible.
- Treat all birds that have contact with the infected bird.
- This disease is easily cured with proper care.

Fungal Infections

Dermatophyte infections are uncommon in pet birds but they have been reported, *Trichophyton* being the most common organism found.

CLINICAL SIGNS

- Feather loss
- Dry, thickened, scaly skin lesions
- Lesions may be weeping

DIAGNOSIS

- Cytology (wet mounts or Gram staining)
- Culture
- Biopsy

TREATMENT

- Antifungal creams or sprays

INFORMATION FOR CLIENTS

- *Trichophyton gallinae* infection is a zoonotic disease; it can be transmitted to humans.
- Improve the general health and hygiene of the infected bird.

Tumors of Skin

Although not common, tumors of skin do occur in pet birds. The specific cause for most of the tumors is not known, and most may occur anywhere in the skin. Types of tumors reported include papillomas, carcinomas, lipomas, adenomas, basal and squamous cell carcinomas, and lymphosarcomas. (The technician should refer to the literature for detailed descriptions of each tumor.)

CLINICAL SIGNS

- Physical examination to find a mass in the skin

DIAGNOSIS

- Cytology
- Biopsy

TREATMENT

- Surgical removal
- Cryosurgery
- Radiation therapy
- Chemotherapy; doxorubicin, cisplatin, chlorambucil, and combination therapy have been used in pet birds

INFORMATION FOR CLIENTS

- Prognosis will depend on the type of tumor.
- Chemotherapy and radiation therapy are new in avian medicine and techniques are extrapolated from treatments for other species.
- Surgical removal is the treatment of choice whenever possible.
- Treatment may be prolonged and expensive.

REVIEW QUESTIONS

1. Some species of birds have a gland that produces oil to waterproof the feathers. It can become blocked, producing a swelling just above the tail. What is the name of this gland?
   a. The anal gland
   b. The uropygial gland
   c. The meibomian gland

2. Which of the following products should be avoided in treating skin lesions in birds?
   a. Otomax ointment
   b. Gentocin spray
   c. Silvadene cream

3. Which of the following findings from physical exam should cause technicians to suspect feather picking?
   a. Feathers are occasionally missing from random feather tracts.
   b. Feathers are missing from multiple tracts from all parts of the body.
   c. Feathers are missing from tracts on the body only.
   d. Feathers are missing from tracts on the head only.

4. What class of drug is being used more frequently today to treat feather-picking in birds?
   a. Antibiotics
   b. Antihistamines
   c. Anxiolytics
   d. Antiparasitics

5. In what species of bird are feather cysts common?
   a. Parakeet
   b. Canary
   c. Cockatiel
   d. Amazon parrot

6. What is the most common external parasite seen in captive birds?
   a. *Ctenocephalides canis*
   b. *Sarcoptes scabiei*
   c. *Knemidokoptes pilae*
   d. *Psoroptes communis*

7. Bumblefoot in birds is often related to trauma from _____ . (Choose all that apply):
   a. Improper perch materials
   b. Improper diet
   c. Improper perch size
   d. Improper cage size
   e. Improper exercise

Answers found on page 555.

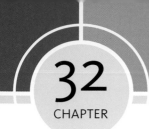

Diseases of the Musculoskeletal System

LEARNING OBJECTIVES

When you have completed this chapter, you will be able to:
1. Recognize causes of common skeletal problems seen in the avian patient.

2. Discuss with clients how diet and husbandry affect the bird's musculoskeletal system.

Anatomy and Physiology of the Avian Musculoskeletal System

Disorders of the musculoskeletal system are common in pet birds. Trauma is a frequent cause of these disorders, although many systemic diseases also involve this system. Malnutrition, metabolic diseases, parasites, and neoplasia may all affect the musculoskeletal system.

The skeletal anatomy of avian species is well developed for flight (Fig 32-1). Bones are lightweight, air-filled structures (pneumatic bones), and other structures are fused for increased rigidity. The keel bone is adapted for support of the large pectoral muscles, and flight muscles have an increased anaerobic metabolic ability. However, the same structures that are useful in flight also predispose the avian animal to traumatic injuries.

Trauma

Traumatic injuries include damage of both soft tissue (Fig 32-2) and bony tissue. Soft-tissue injuries frequently involve bite wounds, caused by other birds or by mammalian pets in the household. Cat bites can be extremely problematic because they are commonly associated with *Pasteurella multocida* infections and a guarded prognosis. Injuries from falls during flight are also common. Heavy-bodied birds with extensive wing trims often land hard on the sternum, splitting the skin and damaging the underlying muscles. Traumatic wing or leg injuries may occur while flying, landing, or playing in the cage. Ceiling fans are particularly dangerous for flying birds. Self-mutilation occurs in several species of birds, most commonly cockatoos (sternum), lovebirds, conures, Quaker parakeets (flank and axilla),

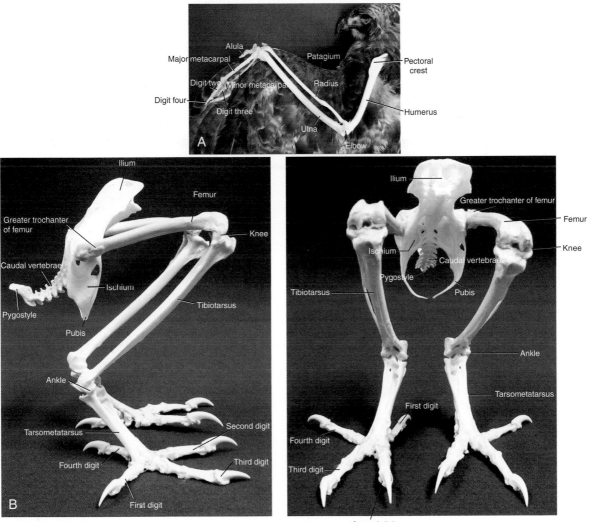

Figure 32-1 Avian Structures. **A,** Wing bones identified in a red-tailed hawk. **B,** Anatomy of the leg bones and pelvic girdle of a great horned owl, lateral and ventral views. (From Colville T, Bassert JM: *Clinical anatomy and physiology for veterinary technicians*, ed 2, St. Louis, MO, 2008, Mosby, with permission.)

and Amazon parrots (feet). The cause of this problem is not well understood.

Hens that are excessively laying eggs may deplete calcium levels within their blood and begin to break down bone to supply the eggs. Lameness caused by stress fractures in the legs may be seen in these birds.

CLINICAL SIGNS

- Bleeding, bruising at site of injury
- Swelling
- Feather loss or feathers pasted with blood
- Lameness or wing droop
- History of interaction with other pets, usually dog or cat

DIAGNOSIS

- Physical examination (may need to wet feathers to find lesion)
- Radiography
- History

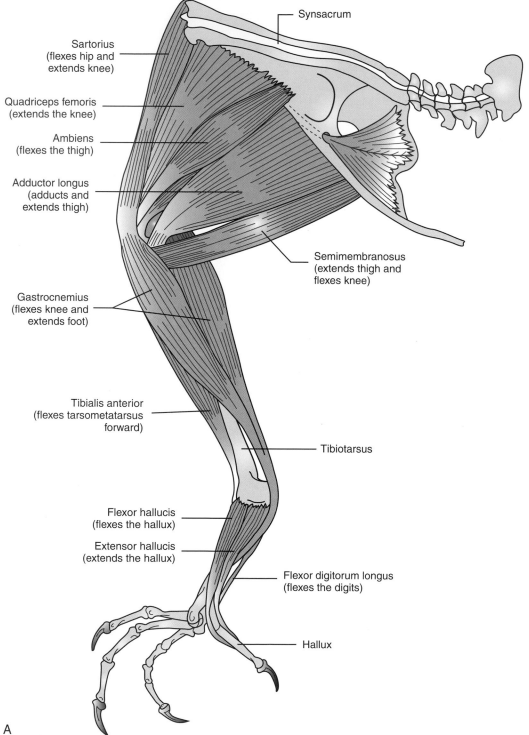

Figure 32-2 A and B, Leg muscles and their function, lateral and medial views.

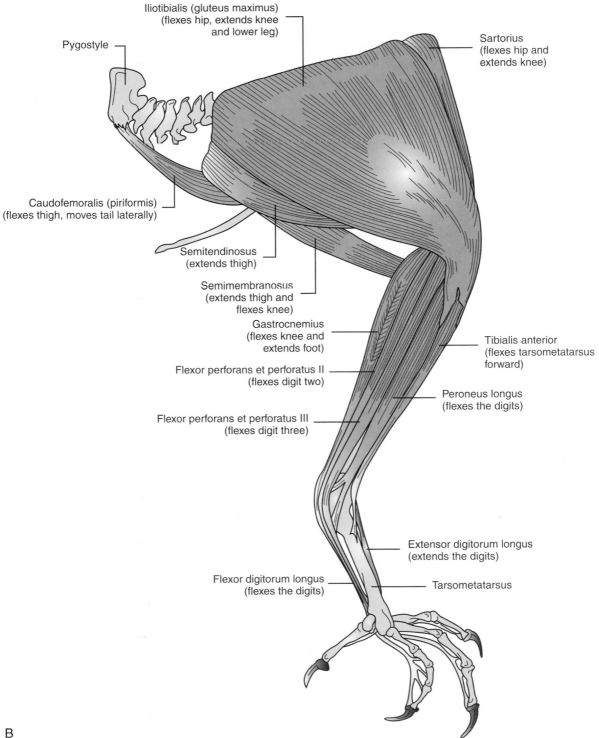

Iliotibialis (gluteus maximus)
(flexes hip, extends knee
and lower leg)

Sartorius
(flexes hip and
extends knee)

Pygostyle

Caudofemoralis (piriformis)
(flexes thigh, moves tail laterally)

Semitendinosus
(extends thigh)

Semimembranosus
(extends thigh and
flexes knee)

Gastrocnemius
(flexes knee and
extends foot)

Tibialis anterior
(flexes tarsometatarsus
forward)

Flexor perforans et perforatus II
(flexes digit two)

Peroneus longus
(flexes the digits)

Flexor perforans et perforatus III
(flexes digit three)

Extensor digitorum longus
(extends the digits)

Flexor digitorum longus
(flexes the digits)

Tarsometatarsus

B

Figure 32-2, cont'd

Continued

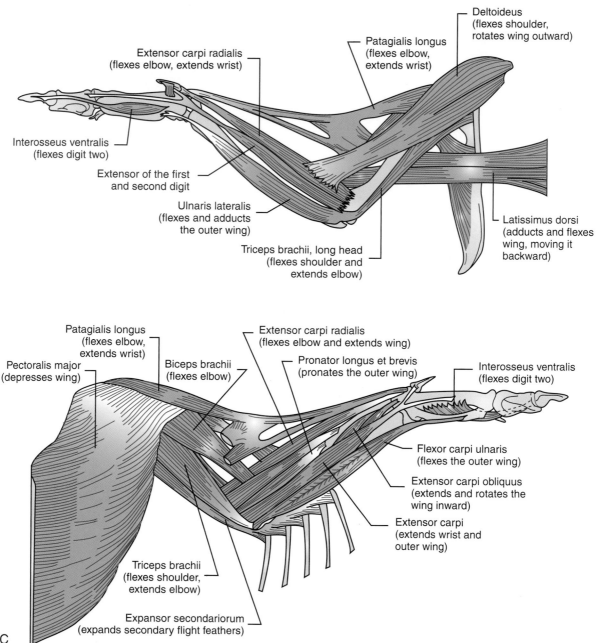

Figure 32-2, cont'd C, Wing muscles and their function, dorsal and ventral views. (From Colville T, Bassert JM: *Clinical anatomy and physiology for veterinary technicians*, ed 2, St. Louis, MO, 2008, Mosby, with permission.)

TREATMENT

- Supportive care (fluids, warmth, oxygen)
- Clean wounds with lavage
- Antibiotic therapy (culture of wound may be necessary)
- Protective dressings
- Use of collar, if necessary, to prevent further damage
- Calcium supplements

INFORMATION FOR CLIENTS

- Birds should be protected from their environment at all times. Mirrors, ceiling fans, windows, doors, and other pets all present a danger to free birds.
- Small external wounds may hide larger, more serious internal problems. Have all injured birds examined by a veterinarian as soon as possible.

Lameness

Lameness in pet birds may have many causes. Fractures or luxations, joint infections, metabolic diseases, trauma, neoplasia, and nutritional problems may all cause lameness. Fractures or luxations are frequently the result of trauma. The onset of the lameness is usually acute. Septic joints will appear swollen and painful with or without bone involvement. Lameness as a result of metabolic disease or neoplasia may have a slower onset or appear to be acute.

CLINICAL SIGNS

- Lameness
- Swollen joint(s)
- Pain on palpation
- Other signs of systemic disease
- Reluctance to perch or shifting leg perching

DIAGNOSIS

- Physical examination
- Radiography
- Complete blood cell count (CBC) serum chemistries
- Culture and sensitivity of joint aspirate
- Cytology of aspirate (mass)

TREATMENT

Fractures or Luxations

- Replace luxations and apply a splint.
- Fractures can be repaired using a splint or internal or external fixation technique.

Infected Joints

- Perform joint lavage after culture and sensitivity.
- Surgical removal of necrotic tissues is a treatment option.
- Intraarticular injection of antibiotics may provide benefit.
- If the lesions are related to gout, treat with allopurinol, colchicines, and special diet.

Metabolic

- Correct any imbalances found on serum chemistries (usually involving calcium, phosphorus, and vitamin D levels).
- Support and protect bones until the disease is corrected.

Neoplasia

- Treatment may not be possible, especially in the case of renal neoplasia in budgerigars.
- Surgical removal, where possible, may be effective in some cases.

INFORMATION FOR CLIENTS

- Trauma is a frequent cause of fractures and luxations in pet birds. As much as is possible, traumaproof the bird's environment and supervise all play time.
- Have your veterinarian examine the bird for all lameness, swellings, or acute signs of pain.

Constrictive Injuries

Constrictive injuries are frequently seen in finches, canaries, and budgies, but they may also occur in larger species. Leg bands, nesting materials, and toys are usually involved. Plastic or metal leg bands, often applied when the bird is very young, may become too tight as the animal matures, or swelling of the leg from another cause may result in tightening of the band. As the band tightens on the leg, poor circulation causes increased swelling of the leg and further tightening of the band. If the pressure is not released, necrosis of the leg and foot may occur, resulting in loss of the foot. These bands should be removed by the veterinarian at the time of purchase to prevent these injuries. Fibrous nesting materials commonly sold for finches and canaries may become wrapped around the foot, causing excessive swelling and eventually necrosis. These fibers are often difficult to see because of the swelling—so use a magnifying head loop and a bright light to examine the bird. The material should be removed gently from the leg by teasing using a blunt probe or a 22-gauge needle. Toys composed of fibers (ropes, material) or small chains also may become wrapped around the foot, causing constrictive lesions. Most of these lesions will heal with proper treatment if the constrictions are removed before necrosis of the tissue occurs.

CLINICAL SIGNS

- Presence of band, and fiber on physical examination
- Lameness
- Swelling and discoloration of the tissue on the leg or foot
- No other signs of systemic disease

DIAGNOSIS

- Examination of injured leg under magnification

TREATMENT

- Carefully remove the band or fibrous material (tissue may be friable).
- Gently clean the wound.
- Apply bandage loosely with an antibiotic wound dressing.
- Administer systemic antibiotics for severe wounds.
- If necrotic tissue does not bleed, amputation may be required. Wait a few days to a week before deciding to amputate because some return of circulation may occur during healing.

INFORMATION FOR CLIENTS

- Have all bands removed at the time of purchase. This should be done by a veterinarian to avoid fracture of the limb.
- Avoid fibrous nesting materials and examine nesting birds frequently for constrictive lesions.

- Open bands found on many larger psittacines can become caught on toys or cage bars. They should be removed and kept with the bird's record for identification as a captive-bred bird.

REVIEW QUESTIONS

1. In which species of pet birds are constrictive injuries from leg bands or nesting materials frequently seen?
   a. Finches and canaries
   b. Macaws and cockatoos
   c. Amazon and African gray parrots
2. Which of the following conditions will develop if constrictive bands are not removed from the bird's leg?
   a. Infection of the area proximal to the band
   b. Necrosis of the area distal to the band
   c. Hypertrophy of the area under the band
   d. Nothing will happen
3. What type of bone results in a lighter skeleton designed for flight?
   a. Cortical bone
   b. Pneumatic bone
   c. Spongy bone
4. This bone is the "breast bone" in the bird.
   a. The sternum
   b. The manubrium
   c. The keel
5. Excessive egg laying may result in wing droop or lameness caused by _____.
   a. Depletion of calcium
   b. Depletion of albumen
   c. Depletion of sodium

Answers found on page 555.

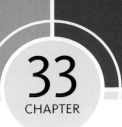

Diseases of the Nervous System

LEARNING OBJECTIVES

When you have completed this chapter, you will be able to:
1. Recognize a neurologic disturbance in an avian patient.
2. Assist the veterinarian in diagnosis and discuss the given prognosis with the client.

Anatomy of the Avian Nervous System

The nervous system of the bird is arranged in a similar manner to that of mammals, but with some major differences. The neocortex, developed on the surface of the cerebral cortex of mammals, is not superficial in birds; cortical cells are found deep within the cortex. Also, birds have the ability to repopulate neurons and reestablish tracts within the central nervous system. The cranial nerves are similar to those in mammals. Birds are intelligent and can outperform mammals in many problem-solving experiments. Alex, an African Gray parrot which belonged to Dr. Irene Pepperberg (Department of Psychology, Brandeis University, Waltham MA), was used to study the cognitive and learning abilities of birds as related to great apes and other animals. Alex showed avian intelligence levels close to that of a 4-year-old human child. Birds have highly developed color vision, good hearing, and the ability to vocalize. Vocalization may be inherited, learned, or invented. Anyone who has owned one of the talented breeds of talkers can vouch for their vocal ability! Vocalization is used by the bird to attract other birds, to gain the attention of the owner, for song, and for amusement.

Neurologic disease is common in pet birds; however, diagnosis is more difficult than in mammals because most of the tests used in mammals are not applicable to avian species. As in other animals, the age of the animal may provide a list of ruled-out diseases (e.g., epilepsy in younger birds, neoplasia in older ones).

Seizures

Seizures are defined as paroxysmal, uncontrolled, electrical discharges from the brain. They may be mild to severe, generalized or partial, frequent or infrequent. Seizures may progress, as in mammalian patients, with a variable postictal period. During the seizure, birds may fall off their perch, lose consciousness, become rigid, or have excessive motor activity.

CLINICAL SIGNS

- Abnormal motor activity
- Loss of consciousness and disorientation
- Falling off perch
- Tremors of wings or legs

DIAGNOSIS

- Aimed at determining whether a seizure has occurred and the reason for the seizure
- Complete physical examination
- Complete blood cell count (CBC) and serum chemistries, including heavy metals levels in blood
- Calcium levels, especially in African gray parrots
- Gram staining culture and sensitivity (cloacal and choanal)
- Fecal examination
- Environmental history (to rule out toxins)
- Computed tomography (CT) or magnetic resonance imaging (MRI) to rule out brain lesions

TREATMENT

- Treatment is designed to treat abnormalities found on diagnostic testing.

Hypocalcemia and Hypoglycemia
- Replacement involves using oral or injectable calcium and oral or injectable dextrose solutions.

Heavy Metal Toxicity
- Use chelating agents to remove the heavy metals (calcium disodium ethylene-diaminetetraacetate [CaEDTA]).

Systemic Bacterial or Viral Disease
- Treat specifically on the basis of laboratory results.

Brain Tumor
- No treatment currently is available.

INFORMATION FOR CLIENTS

- Lack of any laboratory finding for the cause of seizures indicates "idiopathic" epilepsy, that is, the cause of the seizures is unknown.
- Exposure to heavy metals may occur from chewing paint, toys, and cage materials that contain zinc or lead. Jewelry may also contain heavy metals that may leach out after being swallowed.
- Treatment will involve medications related to the specific cause of the seizure. If no specific cause is found, phenobarbital or diazepam (Valium) may be used to control the seizures. Phenobarbital may need to be given twice daily.

Paresis of One Limb

Paresis of a leg or wing is common in pet birds. Paresis of one limb usually involves an injury to the brachial or sacral plexus or neoplasia.

CLINICAL SIGNS

- Weakness or paralysis of the wing or leg in the absence of fractures
- Muscle atrophy; inability to grasp
- Acute onset
- ± Signs of systemic disease

DIAGNOSIS

- Complete physical examination
- CBC, serum chemistries
- Heavy metal screening
- Radiography to rule out fracture, tumor (budgies with renal tumor)
- Nutritional history
- Gram staining; culture and sensitivity (cloacal and choanal)

TREATMENT

- Treatment is based on the laboratory test results.

INFORMATION FOR CLIENTS

- Birds demonstrating paresis of one or more limbs should be examined by the veterinarian.
- Remove any toys or perches from the cage if the bird might be injured interacting with them.

Ataxia and Head Tilt

Head ataxia and head tremors are the result of cerebellar disease, whereas head tilt is usually related to the vestibular system. Most diseases that involve the cerebellum are diagnosed at necropsy. It is important to differentiate between cerebellar signs and those of vestibular disease when examining the animal.

CLINICAL SIGNS

- Head tilt, circling, ataxia, nystagmus
- Inability to perch
- Signs of other systemic disease or abnormalities

DIAGNOSIS

- Complete physical examination
- CBC, serum chemistries
- Heavy metal screen
- Gram staining; culture and sensitivity (choanal and cloacal)
- Nutritional history
- Radiology
- CT or MRI, if needed

TREATMENT

- Supportive care
- Shallow feed pans and water pans or tube feed
- Antibiotic treatment (systemic)
- Chelation, if heavy metal toxicity exists
- Corticosteroids to reduce swelling
- Treatment of specific systemic disease

INFORMATION FOR CLIENTS

- Diagnosis and treatment of neurologic disease in the avian patient may be extremely difficult.
- A cure may not be possible.
- Birds with neurologic symptoms may be unable to perch or to obtain food without assistance. These birds may require 24-hour care.
- Use care in handling a bird having a seizure; you may be injured.

REVIEW QUESTIONS

1. Unlike mammals, avian species are able to repopulate the neurons within the central nervous system.
   a. True
   b. False
2. Avian species have the ability to see color.
   a. True
   b. False
3. Head tilt seen in avian patients is usually related to disease in the:
   a. Cerebral cortex
   b. Vestibular apparatus
   c. Cerebellum
   d. Peripheral nervous system
4. Seizures in African gray parrots may be related to:
   a. Hypophosphatemia
   b. Hypocalcemia
   c. Hyponatremia
   d. Hypokalemia
5. Paint, jewelry, cage materials, and building materials often contain heavy metals which when ingested may cause seizures in pet birds.
   a. True
   b. False
6. Changes in voice of a bird might be due to: (Choose all possible answers.)
   a. *Aspergillus* granulomas
   b. *Mycobacterium* granulomas
   c. *Candida* lesions
   d. Parrot fever
7. Splenomegally seen on necropsy may be a sign of bacterial infection
   a. Megabacteria
   b. *Chlamydia*
   c. *Aspergillus*

Answers found on page 555.

34 CHAPTER

Pansystemic Diseases

KEY TERMS

Basophilic
Cachexia

Emaciation
Leukocytosis

Saprophyte
Subclinical

OUTLINE

Viral Diseases
    Psitticine Beak and Feather Disease
    Avian Polyomavirus
    Pacheco Disease (Herpes Virus)
    Exotic Newcastle Disease
Fungal Diseases
    Aspergillosis
    Candidiasis

Bacterial Diseases
    Mycobacteriosis
    Megabacteriosis
    Chlamydiosis (Psittacosis, Parrot Fever)

LEARNING OBJECTIVES

When you have completed this chapter, you will be able to:
1. Differentiate among viral, bacterial, and fungal diseases of birds.
2. Know when protective measures should be taken if handling infected materials or during necropsy.

3. Know which diseases are considered "reportable" to health officials.
4. Explain zoonotic diseases to owners of affected pet birds.

Pansystemic diseases are usually viral, bacterial, or fungal diseases that involve multiple body systems. These diseases are devastating to the bird and to the owner, resulting in losses of pet birds and valuable breeding stock. Unlike with mammalian pets, few vaccines are available to protect avian species from these diseases.

Viral Diseases

Viral diseases of pet birds are common. Many of these viruses have a complex biology and are difficult to prevent and treat. Prevention of viral diseases involves quarantine and testing of all new additions to the household, limiting the number of species housed together, prepurchase examinations of all new birds, obtaining new birds from reputable breeders (avoid imported birds and previously owned birds), and common sense. Viral diseases may be subclinical in some birds but may cause disease in other species. Some birds may be carriers and yet show no clinical signs of disease. Because disease may be unapparent, all new birds should be quarantined for a minimum of 60 to 90 days (this means in a separate room or facility, worked on last for cleaning and feeding, etc.). A prepurchase examination including a complete blood cell count (CBC), serum chemistries, fecal tests, and Gram staining may identify birds with early signs of disease. Viral testing is available for some diseases that are species specific.

Psittacine Beak and Feather Disease

See Chapter 31 for a detailed discussion of psittacine beak and feather disease.

Avian Polyomavirus

Avian polyomavirus disease (APVD) is a recognized cause of high nestling mortality in budgerigar aviaries. Affected birds are stunted and have dysplastic feathers, abdominal distension, hepatomegaly, and discolored skin. The disease may persist within the aviary from breeding season to breeding season. The disease also occurs in nonbudgerigar parrots. Macaws, conures, electus parrots, and ring-necked parakeets are most susceptible, but Amazons, cockatoos, and lories may also be infected (proventricular dilatation disease). Most small birds die suddenly as nestlings or young fledglings (2–14 weeks of age). APVD is endemic in many lovebird collections.

APVD is caused by a nonenveloped, double-stranded deoxyribonucleic acid (DNA) virus capable of infecting numerous species of birds. The virus is shed in droppings and in feather and skin dander. The virus is capable of replicating in many tissues.

CLINICAL SIGNS

Budgerigars
- Stunted growth
- Dysplastic feathers
- High nestling mortality in aviary
- Abdominal distension, hepatomegaly
- "French molt"

Nonbudgerigars
- Sudden death with no signs of disease
- Weakness, pallor, subcutaneous hemorrhages
- Anorexia
- Dehydration
- Crop stasis

DIAGNOSIS
- History
- Necropsy findings (necropsy must be performed on all dead birds)

- Histology of infected tissues (pathognomonic)
- Serology testing

TREATMENT
- Serology testing of all birds in the aviary or collection
- Removal of all seropositive birds
- Complete disinfection of the aviary; leaving aviary unused for 3 to 6 months
- Vaccination: two doses given 2 to 3 weeks apart for protective antibody levels; vaccinations to begin at 6 weeks of age or older in high-risk situations

INFORMATION FOR CLIENTS
- Quarantine all new birds for a minimum of 60 days.
- Avoid species that are especially susceptible to APVD.
- Buy new birds from reputable dealers and have them tested before introducing them into your aviary or home.
- Consider vaccination for breeding stock or birds in high-risk situations.
- Viral diseases do not respond to antibiotic therapy.

Pacheco Disease (Herpes Virus)

In the past, Pacheco disease was seen predominately in aviaries or in quarantine stations that housed imported psittacines. Infection of birds in pet shops and of individual pet birds have also been reported, especially in birds that have been exposed to newly added conures (Patagonian, nanday, and mitred). The cause of the infection is an enveloped, double-stranded DNA herpes virus. The virus is shed in the feces and respiratory secretions of the infected bird. The incubation period is between 5 and 14 days. Affected birds may exhibit latent infections and shed virus when stressed. A vaccine is available but it has not been well accepted in the United States because of the severity of its adverse effects (sudden death, vaccine granulomas). Other control measures that help prevent infection include effective management practices, testing of all new birds, and keeping a closed aviary.

CLINICAL SIGNS
- Sudden death with no previous signs of illness
- Lethargy

- Depression
- Sulfur-colored urates
- Bloody diarrhea
- Regurgitation
- Central nervous system disorders

DIAGNOSIS

- History of addition of a new bird, stress, or exposure to conures
- Clinical appearance
- Necropsy of dead birds in the collection
- Isolation of the virus from feces

TREATMENT

- Acyclovir may limit the spread and the mortality rate of the disease

INFORMATION FOR CLIENTS

- Purchase only captive-raised birds. Avoid mixing conures with other psittacine parrots in your collection.
- Pacheco disease is usually diagnosed at necropsy, thus it is important to have dead birds examined by your veterinarian.
- Limit access to your aviary, keep sufficient distance between cages, and use effictive sanitation procedures to prevent the spread of infections.
- Consider vaccination of birds in breeding facilities or where other birds have died of Pacheco disease.

Exotic Newcastle Disease

Because of good quarantine procedures and the limiting of importation of all bird species, current outbreaks of exotic Newcastle disease are usually related to smuggled birds. The disease can be spread to poultry; previous outbreaks have been devastating for the poultry industry. Mexican and Central American parrots and fighting cocks are commonly implicated in outbreaks.

The disease is caused by an enveloped, single-stranded ribonucleic acid (RNA) virus (five strains of varying virulence and species specificity). Infected birds shed large amounts of virus in feces and respiratory secretions. Recovered birds may continue to shed viral particles for up to 1 year. The disease has been eradicated in the United States because of quarantine

procedures; however, in states where smuggling of birds is common (e.g., southwestern states), the possibility of an outbreak of infection is always a concern. This is a reportable disease.

CLINICAL SIGNS

- Depression
- Anorexia
- Diarrhea
- Weight loss
- Respiratory signs: may be intermittent
- $\pm$ Neurologic signs
- Death may occur in as little as 1 to 2 days

DIAGNOSIS

- Clinical signs, history of exposure to imported birds
- Viral isolation (cloacal swabs)
- CBC (may be normal)
- Serum chemistries
- Necropsy of dead birds

TREATMENT

- No treatment is available. Because this is a reportable disease, all infected birds are destroyed. All birds in contact with the infected bird are destroyed.

INFORMATION FOR CLIENTS

- Avoid "low-cost" birds and birds offered in large numbers for less than market value. Infected birds are typically found at swap meets or flea market sales.
- Quarantine all newly acquired birds for a minimum of 60 days. Have necropsy performed on all birds that die during quarantine.
- Exotic Newcastle disease is a reportable disease. The U.S. Department of Agriculture must be informed if this disease is found.

Fungal Diseases

The two most frequently seen fungal diseases are aspergillosis and candidiasis. Fungal infection is almost always an opportunistic disease, developing in cases of immunosuppressed birds or overwhelming exposure.

Aspergillosis

Aspergillus spp. are ubiquitous soil saprophytes that enter the bird through the respiratory system. After inhalation of spores, phagocytotic cells transfer the organisms to other tissues of the body or clear the infection completely. Environmental factors play an important role in infection. Damp litter, dirty nesting boxes, improper storage of seeds, poor ventilation, and dusty environments all contribute to the risk of disease. Aspergillosis can be acute or chronic, with the chronic form being most frequent in pet birds. Fungal colonization of the respiratory tract or other tissues in the body results in the formation of granulomas. Treatment is often difficult, and the disease has a poor prognosis, depending on the location of the lesion.

CLINICAL SIGNS

- Anorexia
- Polyuria or polydipsia (in acute form)
- Dyspnea
- Cyanosis
- Change of voice, reluctance to talk
- Weight loss
- ± Diarrhea
- ± Biliverdinuria
- ± Central nervous system signs

DIAGNOSIS

- Environmental history
- Clinical signs
- CBC (usually a severe leukocytosis: white blood cell count [WBC] of 20,000–100,000/μL)
- Serum chemistries
- Endoscopy (tracheal, air sacs)
- Radiography (later in the disease)
- Identification of organisms from lesions (cytology and culture)

TREATMENT

- Surgical removal of isolated lesions when possible
- Antifungal medications (amphotericin B, flucytosine, ketoconazole, and itraconazole have been used); requires long-term (months) treatment
- Supportive care; birds are usually immunosuppressed; treatment includes:
  - Fluids
  - Antibiotics
  - Tube feeding
  - Supplemental heat

INFORMATION FOR CLIENTS

- Development of this disease is strongly related to poor hygiene.
- Check the living environment before purchasing a bird.
- Have all newly purchased birds examined by your veterinarian.
- Change of voice in your bird should be reported immediately to your veterinarian.
- Aspergillosis often has a poor prognosis, and treatment may be expensive and prolonged.
- To prevent infection, reduce stress, maintain good nutrition, house birds in a well-ventilated area, store seeds and peanuts properly, and change bedding daily.

Candidiasis

Candidiasis is a frequently seen fungal problem involving the gastrointestinal tract of pet birds. Like *Aspergillus* spp., *Candida* spp. are opportunistic organisms. *Candida albicans* is a normal inhabitant of the avian digestive tract, but in immunosuppressed birds, it may colonize deeper tissues as well. Antibiotic therapy, corticosteroids, and stress of another disease may all predispose the bird to fungal infection. Infection usually involves the gastrointestinal tract. Lesions have been reported in the small intestine, crop (especially in young, hand-fed baby birds), mouth, esophagus, proventriculus, and the ventriculus, as well as the skin, respiratory tract, cloaca, and beak.

CLINICAL SIGNS

- Anorexia
- Regurgitation
- Delayed crop emptying
- Vomiting, weight loss
- Diarrhea
- Oral plaques (white and cottonlike)
- Sinusitis or dyspnea

DIAGNOSIS

- History of immunosuppressive state
- Visualization of Turkish towel–like lesions orally
- Identification of large numbers of yeast on Gram staining of feces

- Demonstration of pseudohyphae in lesions (with staining)

TREATMENT

- Oral nystatin
- Oral flucytosine
- Ketoconazole or fluconazole orally in acidic juice
- Topical treatment after debridement of cutaneous or oral lesions

INFORMATION FOR CLIENTS

- Reducing stress on birds, good nutrition, and good hygiene will reduce the chance of infection.
- Clean feeding equipment and disinfect after every use when hand-feeding baby birds.
- If prolonged antibiotic therapy has been prescribed for your pet, be on the lookout for fungal lesions.
- Treatment and supportive care are effective in curing the infection.

Bacterial Diseases

Birds are primarily "gram-positive" animals, unlike mammals, which are "gram- negative." It is important for the technician (and the veterinarian) to be familiar with the normal flora of the avian species when determining treatment for bacterial infections. It is also important for the commercial laboratory performing the culture and sensitivity to know what is normal and abnormal for that species. Although a complete description of bacterial infections is beyond the scope of this text, several organisms that frequently cause pansystemic symptoms are discussed.

Mycobacteriosis

Mycobacterium spp. are found in many species; *Mycobacterium bovis* in cattle, and *M. tuberculosis* and *M. leprae* in humans. The organism is a rod-shaped gram-positive, acid-fast staining bacterium that tends to form branching structures resembling filaments. Although *M. avium* has not frequently been reported to infect humans, the other members of this family are zoonotic, so care should be taken when handling these patients.

M. avium infections have been reported in Amazon parrots, gray-cheeked parakeets, and other species. The organism is very stable in the environment and difficult to eradicate once an area is infected. Transmission is via aerosol exposure of dried feces and urine. Infection in birds results in a chronic wasting disease.

> ### ⬤ TECH ALERT
>
> This is a potentially zoonotic disease! Human infections have been reported in patients with acquired immunodeficiency syndrome (AIDS) or other immunosuppressive disease.

CLINICAL SIGNS

- Weight loss
- Depression
- Diarrhea
- Polyuria
- Cachexia
- ± Abdominal distension
- ± Dyspnea
- Signs of specific organ involvement

DIAGNOSIS

- Finding acid-fast organisms in feces or cytology smears
- Radiography; granulomas seen in organs, air sacs
- CBC and serum chemistries (very high WBC)
- DNA–RNA probe testing

TREATMENT

- Treatment is not recommended because this disease may be contagious to humans, especially to children and immunosuppressed patients.
- Drugs used to treat human patients are often successful in birds as well:
  - Rifabutin
  - Azithromycin
  - Ethambutol
- Treatment is long term, often up to a year or more.
- Euthanasia should be considered.

> ### ⬤ TECH ALERT
>
> This is potentially a zoonotic disease. When assisting in a necropsy of a bird, always wear a mask, gloves, and protective eyewear. You never know when you may find a tubercular lesion!

INFORMATION FOR CLIENTS

- *M. avium* infection is a zoonotic disease. Children and immunosuppressed individuals may become infected.
- Euthanasia should be considered after a positive diagnosis is made.
- Birds in contact with infected birds should be removed from the contaminated area, quarantined for up to 2 years, and tested at regular intervals for acid-fast bacteria.
- This organism may remain viable in the environment for years.
- Treatment, if desired, involves long-term administration of medication. Birds undergoing treatment must be isolated from others, and care should be used when handling them.

Megabacteriosis

Megabacteria are large, gram-positive, rod-shaped organisms found in the proventriculus or feces of several avian species. These bacteria have been associated with proventricular disease, poor digestion, and chronic emaciation. The organisms appear to be resistant to most common antibiotics.

CLINICAL SIGNS

- Chronic emaciation over a 12- to 18-month period
- Diarrhea; passing undigested seeds

DIAGNOSIS

- Finding organisms in feces
- Culture (facultative anaerobes)
- Radiology (proventricular dilation)
- History of chronic emaciation

TREATMENT

- Acidification of the drinking water
- Nutritional support
- Oral nystatin; some species may be sensitive to antibiotics
- Oral *Lactobacillus* may help

INFORMATION FOR CLIENTS

- Megabacteriosis may be found in both normal and abnormal birds. Treatment may be unnecessary unless clinical signs are seen.

Chlamydiosis (Psittacosis, Parrot Fever)

Chlamydia psittaci organisms are intracellular bacteria that cause psittacosis or parrot fever. Many strains of the bacteria exist, and clinical signs depend on the virulence of the strain involved. The disease affects all avian species, but Amazons and macaws appear to be more susceptible than other species. A carrier state exists, and cockatiels are frequently implicated. Stress may increase shedding of the organism in feces. The organism is stable in the environment in dried feces and oral secretions. Treatment of infected birds may result in remission of clinical symptoms and shedding of organisms, but it may not cure the infection.

⬤ TECH ALERT

Psittacosis is a zoonotic disease that produces serious flulike symptoms in infected humans. Some infected individuals may require hospitalization. Death has been reported in infected individuals.

CLINICAL SIGNS

- May depend on the strain of bacteria
- Diarrhea
- Anorexia
- Depression
- Biliverdinuria (lime-green feces)
- Dyspnea
- Conjunctivitis, sinusitis, sneezing

DIAGNOSIS

- Clinical signs
- Positive test result (little agreement currently exists on testing modalities)
  - Cytology of infected tissues—intracytoplasmic, basophilic inclusions
  - Serology (enzyme-linked immunosorbent assay (ELISA) complement fixation (CF), latex agglutination, titers)
  - Culture (egg inoculation)
  - Kodak SureCell Chlamydia test may be done in-house for screening patients
- CBC (severe leukocytosis seen in active infections)

- Serum chemistries (aspartate aminotransferase [AST], lactate dehydrogenase, creatine kinase levels may be increased)
- Radiology may show splenomegaly

TREATMENT

- Tetracycline, doxycycline (orally or intramuscularly) given long term
- Enrofloxacin (may not eliminate the organism)
- Supportive care

INFORMATION FOR CLIENTS

- Psittacosis is a zoonotic disease. It can produce serious atypical pneumonia in humans.
- All newly acquired birds should be quarantined and tested for *Chlamydia*, especially cockatiels and Amazon parrots.
- Treatment may eliminate shedding of the organism but not result in a complete cure. The bird may remain a carrier for life.
- Because of stress, newly acquired birds may exhibit shedding of the organism and clinical signs of disease. Have all sick and new birds checked immediately by your veterinarian.
- Treatment is recommended for all suspected cases.
- Good hygiene and well-ventilated areas may help to prevent the spread of the disease. Wear a mask when cleaning cages.

● **TECH ALERT**

In most states, this is a reportable disease.

REVIEW QUESTIONS

1. Candida infection might be seen in birds given:
   a. High levels of dietary carbohydrates
   b. High levels of dietary seeds
   c. High levels of antibiotics
   d. High levels of vitamin D
2. Birds have predominantly _____ intestinal flora.
   a. Gram-positive
   b. Gram-negative
3. Which of the following diseases has zoonotic potential?
   a. Psittacine beak and feather disease
   b. Proventricular dilatation disease
   c. Newcastle disease
   d. Psittacosis
4. All new birds should be quarantined for a minimum of _____ before being placed into the collection.
   a. 14 days
   b. 190 days
   c. 60 days
   d. 90 days
5. Prevention of what viral disease is important for the poultry industry and is the main reason for quarantine of all imported birds?
   a. Pacheco disease
   b. Chlamydia
   c. Exotic Newcastle disease
   d. APVD

Answers found on page 555.

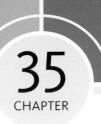

Diseases of the Respiratory System

Concretions   Infraorbital   Syrinx
Emphysema   Nebulization

**Anatomy and Physiology of the Avian
    Respiratory System**
    Rhinitis

Periorbital Swelling
Air Sacculitis and Pneumonia

When you have completed this chapter, you will be able to:
1. Understand how the uniquely designed respiratory
system of the avian patient predisposes it to disease.

2. Recognize that a dyspneic avian patient requires
oxygen therapy and special handling.

Anatomy and Physiology of the Avian Respiratory System

The respiratory system of birds is uniquely designed for
flight. The nostrils are found in the cere, the area around
the most dorsal surface of the upper beak. The cere of
male budgies is usually blue, whereas in females it is
pink. Discoloration of the cere may indicate gonadal
tumors in budgerigars. The nasal cavity is divided by a
septum. An infraorbital sinus is located ventromedial to
the orbit of the eye—this is the site of swellings involved
in sinusitis. The glottis (the opening to the trachea) is
located on the dorsum of the tongue and is not covered
by an epiglottis. The trachea bifurcates immediately after
the thoracic inlet, and the bifurcation is the location of
the syrinx, the voice box of birds. The lungs are paired
and are firmly attached to the dorsal body wall.

Birds do not have a diaphragm, so they must
be able to expand their chest wall to breathe (be
careful not to impede chest movements during
restraint procedures). Birds have a series of air sacs
that are connected to the lungs. The air sacs are
thin-walled structures that extend throughout
body cavities and into the pneumatic wing and leg
bones. Most birds have two cervical, two anterior
thoracic, two posterior thoracic, two abdominal,
and one interclavicular air sacs. The air sacs make
possible the continuous flow of oxygen to the
lungs. With each breath, the bird replaces 50% of
the air in the lungs with fresh air—fresh air enters
the lungs on both expiration and inspiration. This
highly efficient system allows for oxygen transport
throughout the body even at high altitudes during
flight.

Respiratory problems are frequently seen in pet birds. The design of the respiratory system predisposes birds to these problems. Bacterial, viral, and mycotic causes of respiratory symptoms are addressed in Chapter 34. This chapter deals with diseases that are specific to structures in the respiratory system: the nasal cavity, sinuses, trachea, syrinx, lungs, and air sacs.

Rhinitis

Nasal discharge seen in birds may vary from clear to opaque, yellow mucus. It is usually the result of infection or irritation to the nasal cavity. Birds on a poor diet or those housed in dry environments may experience development of nasal plugs, that is, concretions of dust and debris that block the openings to the nares.

CLINICAL SIGNS

- Nasal discharge
- ± Sneezing or cough
- ± Signs of systemic disease
- ± Nasal plugs

DIAGNOSIS

- Clinical signs
- Complete physical examination
- Gram staining of nasal area and choanal slit
- ± Culture and sensitivity
- Cytology of nasal flush or exudates
- Complete blood cell count (CBC) and serum chemistries
- Viral serology or *Chlamydia* testing if indicated

TREATMENT

- Based on diagnostic test results
- Gently clean nares; remove nasal plugs by moistening first with wet cotton swabs; then gently tease them loose using a small curet or blunt probe
- Topical antibiotic therapy (ophthalmic solutions may be used in the nostrils; avoid those that contain steroids)
- Exposure to steam in the shower will help to loosen secretions
- Systemic antibiotics if indicated
- Improved environment and diet

INFORMATION FOR CLIENTS

- Avoid keeping birds in dusty, smoke-filled environments.
- Good nutrition (especially vitamin A) is important for normal nasal epithelium. Lack of vitamin A may thicken the nasal lining and predispose the bird to disease.
- An air filter system or a humidifier, or both, will provide a cleaner environment for your bird.
- Regular bathing will help maintain hydration of nasal tissues.

Periorbital Swelling

Periorbital swellings are commonly caused by disease of the infraorbital sinuses. Bacterial, fungal, or viral infections and trauma are frequently implicated in these swellings.

CLINICAL SIGNS

- Unilateral or bilateral swelling ventral to the eye
- ± Signs of respiratory disease
- ± Bruising of the soft tissue of the eye

DIAGNOSIS

- Clinical signs
- Complete physical examination and history of problem
- Radiography
- Fine-needle aspiration of contents of swelling, if possible
- ± Biopsy of sinus epithelium
- *Chlamydia* or viral testing

TREATMENT

- Treat swelling as an abscess: lance and drain, flush the pocket
- Antibiotic therapy (topical, systemic, or both)
- Improve diet: supplement vitamin A
- Sinus trephination may be required in severe cases: daily flushing

INFORMATION FOR CLIENTS

- Any periorbital swelling should be examined by a veterinarian.
- Bacterial cultures may be required to isolate the specific cause of the infection.

- Owners may have to handle the bird several times daily for treatment. If this cannot be done, the bird should be placed in a hospital

Air Sacculitis and Pneumonia

Birds with air sacculitis or pneumonia will present with dyspnea. Care should be taken when handling dyspneic birds because any added stress may result in death. Dyspneic patients should be placed in an oxygen-enriched environment for several hours before physical examination or diagnostic testing. Birds may be anesthetized and an air sac tube placed if upper respiratory disease is present. Nebulization is the best method for delivery of antibiotics to the lower respiratory tract of the avian patient. Air sacculitis may also develop with exposure to environmental toxins, especially from burning nonstick Teflon pans. A high mortality rate is associated with this toxicity. Other fumes from paint, perfumes, smoke, and other household chemicals are concentrated in the air sacs and may also result in serious air sacculitis and pneumonia.

CLINICAL SIGNS

- Dyspnea
- ± Nasal discharge, cough, sneezing
- ± Subcutaneous emphysema
- Tail bobbing, open-mouth breathing
- Abnormal voice or breathing noise

DIAGNOSIS

- Clinical signs
- Physical examination and history
- Radiography
- Gram staining (choanal and cloacal)
- ± Culture and sensitivity
- CBC and serum chemistries
- Chlamydial and viral serology, if indicated

TREATMENT

- Nebulization
- Systemic antibiotic therapy if indicated
- Removal from toxic environment (no treatment for Teflon toxicity)
- Placement of air sac breathing tube until inflammatory process can be corrected

- Surgical removal of granulomas seen on the radiographs

INFORMATION FOR CLIENTS

- The design of the bird's respiratory tract predisposes it to irritation by *all* airborne irritants. Avoid using aerosols in the area where the bird lives.
- Never leave a Teflon pan on the stove unattended.
- If your bird is having trouble breathing (dyspnea), veterinary care should be sought immediately.

REVIEW QUESTIONS

1. What is the usual color of the cere of the female parakeet?
   a. Blue
   b. Pink
   c. Brown
2. Discoloration of the cere of the budgerigar may indicate disease of the _____ system.
   a. Respiratory
   b. Integumentary
   c. Reproductive
   d. Cardiovascular
3. Periorbital swelling is usually seen when the _____ is infected.
   a. Syrinx
   b. Air sac
   c. Infraorbital sinus
   d. Nostril
4. Which of the following vitamins is important for healthy nasal epithelium?
   a. Vitamin B
   b. Vitamin D
   c. Vitamin A
   d. Vitamin E
5. Owners of pet birds should avoid overheating _____ cooking utensils in the area where the bird is caged.
   a. Plastic coated
   b. Stainless steel
   c. Copper bottomed
   d. Teflon-coated

6. If presented with a dyspneic patient, the technician should:
   a. Place the bird in an oxygenated environment before evaluation
   b. Obtain radiographs immediately to discover the cause of dyspnea
   c. Obtain a CBC and clinical chemistry sample
   d. Not handle the patient; wait for the veterinarian

7. Nebulization is the best way to treat _____ respiratory disease.
   a. Upper airway
   b. Lower airway

Answers found on page 555.

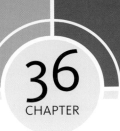

Diseases of the Urogenital System

LEARNING OBJECTIVES

When you have completed this chapter, you will be able to:
1. Diagram the reproductive system of female and male birds.

2. Explain to owners the methods used for sexing avian patients.

Anatomy and Physiology of the Avian Urogenital System

The urinary system of the bird is composed of two kidneys located along the dorsal body wall, two ureters, and the cloaca. There are two types of nephrons in birds: (1) the cortical, which is reptilian in form, and (2) the medullary, which is mammalian in form. The cortical form produces urates, and the medullary form produces urine. The renal portal system allows blood to be shunted from the caudal abdominal structures directly to the kidney, bypassing the rest of the body. As a result of the renal portal system, any medications injected in the caudal portion of the bird will be eliminated by the kidney before distribution to the body. The ureters empty into the cloaca.

The reproductive system of the bird is quite different from that of mammals. The female system is composed of two ovaries (although the right one is usually inactive in adult birds), the oviduct, and the cloaca. The oviduct is divided into segments: the infundibulum, the magnum, the isthmus, and the shell gland. The male reproductive system consists of two testicles located internally, the ductus deferens, the seminal glomus, and the ejaculatory duct that opens into the cloaca. A phallus may be present in some species but is absent in psittacines. In both female and male birds, the cloaca is divided into the coprodeum,

351

the urodeum, and the proctodeum. The coprodeum, the most cranial portion, is a continuation of the rectum or large intestine. The urodeum contains the openings from the ureters and genital ducts. The proctodeum contains the bursa of Fabricius, or the cloacal bursa, the site of B-lymphocyte production. The vent is the opening of the cloaca to the external surface of the bird. It is located under the tail.

Seasonal changes in the photoperiod affect the reproductive system of the bird. Breeding and laying of eggs increase during periods of increased light in the spring. After breeding, shortening periods of light seen in the autumn stimulate molting. By housing birds under artificial light, some owners influence the breeding periods, sometimes to the detriment of the pet bird.

Renal Disease

Renal disease, usually as a consequence of another systemic disease, is seen in pet birds. Signs of renal disease are similar to those in mammals, but lameness may be the only sign of renal enlargement seen in some birds. It is important to recognize the early signs of renal disease, but this is often difficult because the symptoms are nonspecific and obtaining a urine sample is not easy.

CLINICAL SIGNS

- Lethargy, anorexia
- Weakness
- Regurgitation or vomiting
- Dehydration
- Abdominal distension or swelling
- Lameness
- Inability to fly
- Constipation

DIAGNOSIS

- Complete physical examination and history
- Complete blood cell count (CBC), serum chemistry (plasma uric acid concentration increased; blood urea nitrogen and creatinine have little value in evaluating avian kidney function)
- Urinalysis: must be sure to collect just urine when obtaining sample (replace cage lining with waxed paper or tile, and collect only the clear liquid portion of the sample)
- Cytology and dipstick evaluation

- Radiology may indicate enlarged kidneys, mineralization, or other abnormalities
- Ultrasonography ± dye studies
- Endoscopy and renal biopsy

TREATMENT

- Supportive care: fluids
- Antibiotics if indicated
- Control of hyperuricemia with allopurinol
- Introduction of a low-protein diet

INFORMATION FOR CLIENTS

- Renal disease is often difficult to diagnose until late in the disease, making treatment difficult.
- In most cases, renal disease is the result of other bacterial, viral, or neoplastic disease in the bird.
- Good nutrition and disease-preventative measures may help to avoid renal disease.

Visceral and Articular Gout

This syndrome is common in psittacines. Uric acid deposits may be deposited around joints, the pericardial sac, and in other viscera. Treatment is usually unsuccessful.

Diseases of the Reproductive System

Diseases of the reproductive system are common in pet birds. Egg binding and dystocia, prolapse of the oviduct, excessive egg laying, ectopic eggs, and egg yolk peritonitis are diseases that affect the female bird, whereas neoplasia, papillomas, and infertility are seen in male birds.

Egg Binding and Dystocia

The failure of an egg to pass through the oviduct at a normal rate is termed *egg binding*, whereas dystocia is related to mechanical obstruction of the cloaca related to the presence of the egg (egg is stuck in cloaca). Many factors predispose birds to egg binding and dystocia: obesity, excessive egg laying (oviduct fatigue), inadequate nutrition, inadequate exercise, genetic predisposition, and other stressors.

CLINICAL SIGNS

- Depression
- Abdominal straining

- Spending excessive time on the floor of the cage
- History of excessive egg laying
- ± Lameness

DIAGNOSIS

- Clinical signs and history of egg laying
- Physical examination (use care; birds are usually unstable)
- Radiography or ultrasonography (Fig. 36-1 and Fig. 36-2)
- CBC and serum chemistries

TREATMENT

- Stabilization of the patient (heated environment, oxygen, quiet)
- Supportive care (fluids)

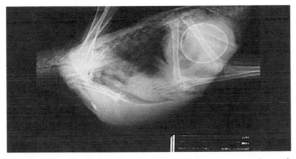

Figure 36-1 Radiograph of a macaw that was egg bound. (From Altman RB, Clubb SL, Dorrestein GM, Quesenberry KE: *Avian medicine and surgery*, Philadelphia, PA, 1997, Saunders, by permission.)

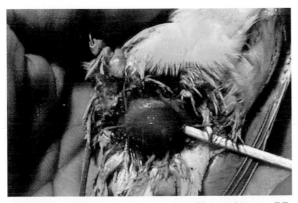

Figure 36-2 Egg-bound budgerigar. (From Altman RB, et al: *Avian medicine and surgery*, Philadelphia, PA, 1997, Saunders, by permission.)

- Parenteral calcium supplementation
- Manual delivery of the egg with careful digital pressure
- Ovocentesis and collapse of the egg internally with digital removal
- Drug therapy
- Oxytocin if no physical obstruction to egg passage
- Prostaglandins
- Surgical removal of eggs in larger birds

INFORMATION FOR CLIENTS

- To decrease the incidence of egg binding, keep your bird on a good plain of nutrition, give her plenty of exercise, and limit the photoperiod to about 8 hours daily.
- Discuss with your veterinarian what is excessive laying for your species of bird, and have the bird examined if the number of eggs exceeds that level.
- Never hold your egg-bound bird over boiling water to try to steam the egg loose. It will only increase the stress and may, in fact, harm the bird. Do not use grease or oil on the bird to facilitate egg removal.
- Consider spaying a female bird that continually has egg binding.

Prolapse of the Oviduct

Prolapse of the oviduct is usually seen in conjunction with egg binding and dystocia.

CLINICAL SIGNS

- Presence of red, moist tissue protruding from the vent
- ± Egg present in the vent
- Straining

DIAGNOSIS

- Physical examination and history

TREATMENT

- Gently clean the prolapsed tissue; remove any egg remnants.
- Lubricate the tissue using a water-soluble product containing an antiinflammatory (ophthalmic ointments work well).
- Repair any lesions or tears.
- Replace tissues with or without purse-string suture if needed.

INFORMATION FOR CLIENTS

- Most birds will return to breeding function after treatment of a prolapse.
- Have your bird seen immediately by your veterinarian if a prolapse is suspected.

Excessive Egg Laying

Excessive egg laying is frequently seen in cockatiels, budgerigars, and lovebirds. The hen will lay a larger-than-normal clutch or will have closely repeated laying periods. Excessive laying depletes the body of calcium and other nutritional elements that eventually may predispose the hen to egg binding, osteoporosis, malnutrition, or all of these.

CLINICAL SIGNS

- Hen that has laid excessive amounts of eggs during that specific laying period
- Lameness with or without fractures of long bones
- Development of other nutrition-related problems

DIAGNOSIS

- History and physical examination
- Radiology may indicate stress fractures or cortical thinning of long bones

TREATMENT

- Perform environmental manipulation (decrease photoperiods, improve diet, change cage).
- *Do not* remove the eggs from the nest; remove the entire nest or any toys that sexually stimulate the bird.
- Provide drug therapy:
  - Medroxyprogesterone injections (have adverse effects of polyuria or polydipsia, diabetes, obesity)
  - Oral testosterone
  - Leuprolide acetate to prevent egg laying in cockatiels
  - Human chorionic gonadotropin
  - Oral calcium supplementation if needed

INFORMATION FOR CLIENTS

- Prevention of excessive egg laying is important in susceptible species.
- Limit daylight hours to 8 to 10 hours daily; cover the bird or move to a dark room to shorten exposure to light.

- *Do not* remove eggs from the nest; it may result in "double-clutching," or the laying of more eggs. (Birds have a genetic knowledge of the number of eggs in the normal clutch. If eggs are removed, they never reach that magic number and will continue to lay more eggs.)
- Changing the cage, toys, and location may help some birds.
- The addition of egg shells or oral calcium supplement to the diet will help to maintain calcium levels in bones.
- Birds that do not respond to medical therapy may need to be spayed.

Egg Yolk Peritonitis

Egg yolk peritonitis occurs when egg yolk material is found free in the abdominal cavity. It results from internal laying (ectopic egg does not reach the oviduct), oviduct disease, or both.

CLINICAL SIGNS

- Gradual weight loss
- Depression
- Abdominal distension or ascites
- History of egg laying

DIAGNOSIS

- Clinical signs and physical examination
- CBC and serum chemistries
- Leukocytosis
- Cytology of abdominal tap reveals yolk material

TREATMENT

- Supportive care
- Abdominocentesis
- Broad-spectrum antibiotics
- Surgical exploration and removal of yolk material
- Salpingohysterectomy

INFORMATION FOR CLIENTS

- Have your bird seen immediately by your veterinarian if you notice any of the above symptoms in your laying hen.

Ovarian Neoplasia

Ovarian neoplasia, most commonly seen in the budgerigar, carries a poor prognosis.

CLINICAL SIGNS

- Abdominal enlargement
- Discoloration of the cere

DIAGNOSIS

- Physical examination
- Radiography or ultrasonography
- Exploratory laparotomy

TREATMENT

- Provide supportive care
- Therapy is usually unsuccessful

Testicular Neoplasia

Clinical signs of testicular neoplasia may be similar to ovarian neoplasia in the female, although most testicular neoplasms are unilateral. Treatment, if the disease is detected early, involves orchiectomy.

Sexing

Psittacines are not dimorphic—it is difficult to determine the sex simply by looking at the bird. Electus parrots are exceptions; the male is green and the female is red but it is not so easy with other species. It is therefore necessary to determine the sex either by surgical sexing or with deoxyribonucleic acid (DNA) testing. Surgical sexing involves anesthesia and the use of an endoscope to observe the ovaries or testicles within the body cavity. This entails some risk for the patient.

DNA sexing using blood or feather epithelium is much easier and safer. Several companies offer this service. (The technician is referred to the Internet for information on these companies.)

REVIEW QUESTIONS

1. One should never inject medications in the rear portion of the bird because of the existence of the:
   a. Hepatoportal system
   b. Caudal air sac system
   c. Renal portal system
   d. Medullary reflux system
2. The cortical portion of the kidney in birds is responsible for the production of:
   a. Liquid urine
   b. Solid urates
   c. Both urates and urine

3. What three organ systems empty into the cloaca of the bird? (You may have to look back to discussions of other systems to determine this answer.)
   a. Renal, digestive, reproductive
   b. Digestive, reproductive, cardiovascular
   c. Renal, respiratory, digestive
   d. Reproductive, respiratory, renal
4. Which of the following serum chemistries is the most accurate measurement of renal function?
   a. Creatine
   b. Blood urea nitrogen
   c. Uric acid
5. Mechanical obstruction of the cloaca secondary to the presence of an egg is known as:
   a. Dystocia
   b. Egg binding
   c. Constipation
6. Prolapse of the oviduct should not be considered an emergency and can wait up to 3 days for repair.
   a. True
   b. False
7. Excessive egg laying will deplete the body of _____ and predispose the bird to muscle weakness and stress fractures.
   a. Potassium
   b. Protein
   c. Sodium
   d. Calcium
8. An "off-color" brown cere in a parakeet may indicate:
   a. Gonadal tumor
   b. Kidney disfunction
   c. Vitamin A deficiency
9. White, granular accumulations within body tissues and joints would be termed _____.
   a. Granulomatous neoplasia
   b. Visceral gout
   c. Calicum granuloma

Answers found on page 555.

37

CHAPTER

Overview of Reptiles as Pets

LEARNING OBJECTIVES

When you have completed this chapter, you will be able to:

1. Describe how differences in anatomy and physiology of reptiles make them interesting pets but challenging patients.
2. Discuss with owners the possibility of zoonotic diseases when handling reptiles.
3. Explain the importance of the POTZ to owners of reptiles.

Like birds, reptiles hold a special place in the hearts of many pet owners. They are different from dogs and cats, they require little space, and they are quiet. Many reptiles make very good pets if properly maintained; however, as with birds, many owners purchase reptiles without knowledge of their needs. This results in the needless death of many of these pets. Many different species of reptiles exist, and a discussion of all of them is beyond the scope of this book. The technician is referred to several good texts on reptile medicine for detailed information. In this section, we will cover the general husbandry requirements and specific diseases for the most common reptiles kept as pets.

For many years, pet stores have been the prime source of information concerning captive reptiles. Veterinarians have played a smaller role in this area (either from lack of a desire to have these animals as patients or lack of knowledge). Today, the availability of massive amounts of information on the Internet has created the owner who requires better medical care for their valuable pets than generally provided by the pet store. It is time for veterinarians who are interested in these species to step forward and provide improved care.

Obtaining a New Reptile

Potential owners should consider many factors when deciding to purchase a reptile as a pet, including the following:
- The type of reptile to purchase
- Housing considerations
- Eventual size of the animal
- Temperament of the animal
- What the animal will be used for
- Family constraints (children, other pets)

Most reptiles are purchased from pet stores or private breeders. All new reptiles should be quarantined for a minimum of 60 to 90 days to prevent introduction of disease into the collection. During this period, the animals should be given a complete physical examination, including diagnostic laboratory testing to rule out disease, parasites, or nutritional problems. The quarantined animal should be housed in a separate area of the house; be fed, cleaned, and handled last; and have no exposure to animals already

in the collection until it is proven free of disease. New animals should be housed separately because many reptiles are carnivores and may eat cage mates when stressed.

General Environmental Requirements

Each species of reptile has what is known as the "preferred optimal temperature range" in which they thrive. It is important, therefore, for the owner to know what species is being kept and what that temperature range is. The preferred optimal temperature ranges for some frequently kept reptiles are as follows:
- Snakes: 80–85°F (day); 65–80°F (night)
- Lizards: 80–90°F (day); 65–80°F (night)
- Turtles: 80–85°F (day); 65–80°F (night)

This generally means that the entire environment must be at this temperature, not just the floor of the cage or the house. Heat lamps, heat tape, and hot rocks have all been used to maintain these temperatures.

Reptiles come from a variety of climates. Some require increased humidity, and some desert conditions; some reptiles are carnivores, whereas others may be herbivores. Most will require exposure to full-spectrum light or sunlight.

Most reptiles are kept indoors in cages. The cages are generally made of wood, wire, glass, or Plexiglas. Whatever the cage is constructed from, it should be easy to clean and disinfect, and it should be strong enough to contain the animal. A locking mechanism will prevent the accidental escape of the animal. The cage should have adequate "cage furniture" to allow for basking or hiding. It should have a source for clean water for drinking or bathing. That is, the cage should replicate the natural environment of the animal. Owners should avoid sand, wood shavings, or kitty litter as a substrate for the cage because they may be swallowed by the pet and are difficult to clean. Newspaper or indoor–outdoor carpet provides for easy cleaning in most cages. Some reptiles require nonporous materials that will allow for burrowing. The cage should be designed to provide temperature gradients that will provide both cooler and warmer areas for the pet. It should also have an artificial full-spectrum light source. Many reptiles kept as pets will eventually grow to large sizes and will need even larger habitats, so the eventual size of the animal should be kept in mind when choosing a cage.

Diet

Many beginning owners will not be familiar with the dietary requirements or feeding habits of their pets. It is important that they receive correct information concerning diet, methods of feeding, and number of feedings. The following comments are general; however, exact dietary requirements will be discussed with each species.

In general, all snakes are carnivores. They will eat pinky mice, adult rodents, chickens, ducks, and rabbits (depending on the size of the snake). Some lizards are also carnivores and require insects or small rodents for food, whereas others are herbivores and have little requirement for protein (meat). Many reptiles will not feed unless the prey is presented alive; others prefer killed prey. Adult snakes generally eat one to three times per month, whereas iguanas and other lizards eat daily. It is important for the owner to know the requirements for the species being kept as a pet. Handling snakes after feeding can result in regurgitation of the entire meal and, eventually, loss of condition. All food sources should be fresh and clean. If frozen, they should be allowed to thaw in the refrigerator rather than in the microwave. Powdered vitamins may be hidden in or dusted on the food if desired.

Water

Reptiles require water for drinking and bathing (soaking). The water bowl should be large enough to allow the animal to submerge its entire body. The sides of the container should be low enough to provide easy entry. Water containers must be cleaned daily because many reptiles will defecate when soaking. The bowls should be disinfected weekly.* Misting systems may help increase the humidity in the habitat for those species from rainforest environments.

---

*Dilute chlorox solutions or chlorhexadine solution can be used to disinfect bowls.

Reptile Zoonoses

Zoonoses are diseases that may be transferred from pets to humans, and vice versa. Owners and veterinary staff should be aware of some pathogens when handling reptiles. Adults who are immunosuppressed (because of chemotherapy for cancer or AIDS) or young children are at greatest risk for infection. Humans come into contact with the infectious organisms when handling the pet, while cleaning the cage, or from airborne dust from feces and cage bedding. Caught wild animals frequently have parasites that are infectious to humans as well. For these reasons, certain precautions should be taken when keeping reptiles as pets. Avoid housing the animals in the kitchen or other areas where food is handled. Always wash your hands after handling the pet, and never let children kiss the pet. Wear protective clothing when cleaning the cage, and properly dispose of all cage bedding and uneaten prey. Do not allow reptiles to soak in bathtubs or sinks used by humans, do not ignore bite wounds from your pet, and have your pet examined frequently to screen for potentially harmful organisms.

The most recognized zoonosis of reptiles is salmonellosis. The gram-negative bacterium causes severe intestinal diseases in people and can be fatal. Many cases of salmonellosis can be traced to turtles and other reptiles. *Every reptile should be considered positive for* Salmonella *until proved otherwise by laboratory testing.* Other enteric bacteria isolated from reptiles include *Clostridium, Klebsiella, Enterobacter, Escherichia coli, Pasteurella, Pseudomonas,* and others. *Protozoa, Cryptosporidia,* and pentastomes are also passed from reptiles to humans.

Although not truly a zoonotic problem, venomous reptiles represent a threat to humans. The majority of owners should NEVER keep venomous reptiles as pets. Venomous reptiles present a danger to both the owner and those living in the surrounding environment. Even highly trained persons have been seriously injured handling venomous reptiles.

Snakes

Snake species kept as pets include boas, pythons, corn snakes, rat snakes, king snakes, and garter snakes.

Anatomy

The anatomy of the snake is unique because everything is linear in design (Fig. 37-1). Snakes have a three-chambered heart whose position is somewhat variable in that it is movable within the rib cage to allow for passage of large food items. One would think that three chambers would mean that oxygenated and unoxygenated blood would mix together; however, there is, in fact, separation within the heart that effectively does what the atrioventricular septum does in mammals. Heart rate varies with respect to the body temperature of the snake—slowing when cold and increasing when warm. The technician can locate the heart by palpation on the ventral side of the snake about one-third of the distance from head to tail. Snakes have both renal and hepatic portal circulatory systems. They have an abdominal vein that runs along the ventral midline. Snakes have two lungs, but the left one is usually smaller than the right one. The trachea opens on the midline of the tongue as in

the bird. The digestive system is linear from the oral cavity to the cloaca. Six rows of teeth are generally present and are replaced throughout the life of the reptile. Paired kidneys are located in the dorsal caudal abdomen. They are lobulated and elongated, and the ureters empty into the cloaca. Like birds, snakes pass urates with their feces. All male snakes have two intromittent organs (hemipenes), which lie in invaginated pouches on the ventral surface at the base of the tail. The depth of these pouches is used in sexing snakes; the deeper pouches are found in male snakes, the more shallow ones in female snakes. Female snakes are either *oviparous* (egg-laying) *or viviparous* (live birth), depending on the species. Ovaries are located internally and both are active.

Housing

Snakes are ectotherms; they assume the temperature of the environment. Snakes must be housed in temperatures that are within their preferred optimal temperature zone (POTZ), or eating, digestion, basking, breeding, and many other physiologic activities will be adversely affected.

Iguanas

One of the most popular species of lizard kept as a pet is the green iguana (*Iguana iguana*). Many other species of lizards are seen in the pet trade, but this section concentrates on the green iguana as an example of the "typical" lizard. When necessary, the gecko is also discussed in this text.

The green iguana, an arboreal herbivore, has been a popular pet for many years. Its size, color, and general "prehistoric" appearance appeal to reptile lovers throughout the world (Fig. 37-2). Green iguanas have been known to live up to 12 to 13 years in captivity, whereas other species may live well into their thirties. If an owner wants to maximize the life span of his or her pet, it is imperative that he or she maintain the pet in optimum condition at all times.

Excessive handling of lizards should be avoided. Male iguanas may become aggressive during breeding season, and all iguanas may exhibit defensive aggression when threatened. (Beware of the tail lash!) Iguanas are best restrained by light-touch methods. Smaller iguanas may be wrapped in a towel

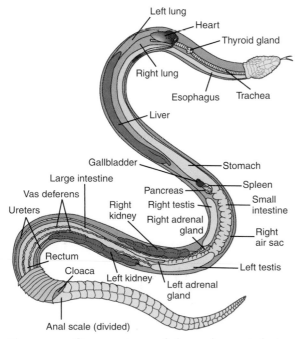

Figure 37-1 Gross anatomy of the snake, ventral view. (From Colville T, Bassert JM: *Clinical anatomy and physiology for veterinary technicians*, ed 2, St. Louis, MO, 2008, Mosby, by permission.)

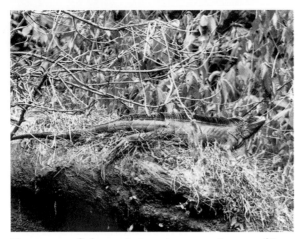

Figure 37-2 Color variations in green iguanas. (From Mader DR: *Reptile medicine and surgery*, ed 2, St. Louis, MO, 2006, Saunders, by permission.)

(burrito fashion) before examination. Larger species may require two people for restraint—one to restrain the body and one to restrain the tail. *Do not grasp the tail for restraint.*

Anatomy

The anatomy of the lizard is similar to that of the snake in many ways (Fig. 37-3). The cardiovascular system is similar; a three-chambered heart and a renal portal system are the same, but lizards have a large ventral abdominal vein that lies along the inner surface of the abdominal wall on the midline. This difference is important when considering surgical approaches to the abdomen in the lizard. The teeth of the lizard are pleurodont (they attach to the sides of the mandible without sockets). They are regularly shed and replaced. The tongue is mobile and aids in bringing scent into the olfactory organ. In iguanas, the tip of the tongue is darker than the rest of the tongue. The colon in herbivorous species may be sacculated to facilitate hindgut fermentation. Lizards have a cloaca divided into three areas: (1) the coprodeum (for feces), (2) the urodeum (for urine), and (3) the proctodeum (final chamber before elimination). Lizards excrete nitrogenous wastes as uric acid, urea, or ammonia. Their kidneys lack the ability to concentrate urine (no loop of Henle). Most species have a small, thin-walled bladder. Male lizards have

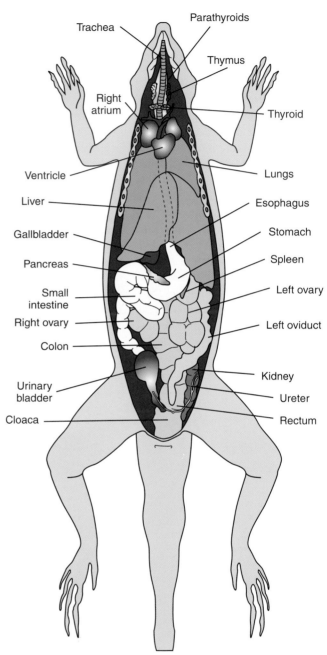

Figure 37-3 Anatomy of the green iguana (*Iguana iguana*), ventral view. (From Mader DR: *Reptile medicine and surgery*, ed 2, St. Louis, MO, 2006, Saunders, by permission.)

paired hemipenes as in snakes. Female lizards have paired ovaries and oviducts. Sexing can be performed by observing the hemipenes bulging at the base of the tail, or by observing enlarged femoral pores in the male lizard (Fig. 37-4). Male iguanas tend to have larger dorsal spines and larger dewlaps as well.

The lizard ear is both auditory and vestibular in function, and the tympanic membrane can be visualized in the shallow depression on each side of the head. The eyes usually have eyelids, except in some geckos and skinks. Iguanas have a well-developed parietal eye found on the dorsal midline of the head. This degenerate eye contains a lens and retina, and connects to the pineal gland, which plays a role in reproduction, thermoregulation, and basking (light sensitive) but is not visual.

Iguanas have nasal salt glands that excrete sodium when the plasma osmotic pressure is increased. The fine white powder (sodium chloride) may be seen on the head and around the nares. Some species have vocal cords and can produce loud vocalizations (geckos). Lizards will typically inflate their lungs to appear larger and more frightening when threatened. Iguanas and many other lizards are capable of tail autotomy (loss of the tail). This is an escape mechanism but is an important consideration when handling them because the tail may also fracture off when accidentally grabbed or twisted during physical examination. The lost tail may be replaced eventually, but the new tail will usually be smaller and of a different color. (This usually makes owners unhappy as you might well imagine.)

Lizards undergo regular shedding periods with the skin coming off in pieces instead of one piece as in the snake. Iguanas have large claws that require frequent trimming to prevent human injury.

Housing

Iguanas are arboreal lizards which typically retreat high into the trees to bask in the sun as daylight increases. Cages should mimic the natural habitat and should contain a tree or place for them to bask that is close to the heat source. It is also important to have cooler areas in the cage for the iguana. These jungle species also require increased humidity in the environment, and cages may need misting frequently to provide 50% to 70% humidity levels.

Green iguanas grow to extremely large sizes. This should be kept in mind when deciding to purchase the cute little baby animal in the pet store. Adults are strong and active and will require strong, secure caging that is easy to clean. The cage should contain climbing branches, an ultraviolet light source, a heat and humidity source, and an adequate substrate on the floor. An ideal substrate would be one that is easy to clean, inexpensive, and pleasing to look at. It should also be digestible in the event that the lizard decides to eat it. Indoor–outdoor carpet, flat newspaper, or alfalfa pellets make good choices for floors of iguana cages.

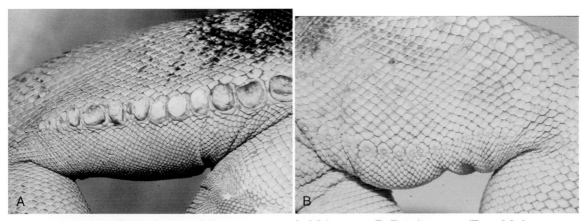

Figure 37-4 Femoral pores of the green iguana. **A**, Male iguana. **B**, Female iguana. (From Mader DR: *Reptile medicine and surgery*, Philadelphia, PA, 1996, Saunders, by permission.)

Hide boxes should be provided. Many lizards are territorial and are stressed when housed with another lizard. Most lizards do best if housed alone.

Nutrition

Green iguanas are herbivores and feed mostly on leaves and vines in the wild. In captivity they should be fed a variety of chopped, mixed vegetables and fruits. If proteins are fed in the diet, they should be plant-based proteins, not animal-based proteins (and they are not recommended as part of the diet by many experts). Geckos are carnivores and must be fed animal-based proteins (e.g. pinky mice)

Turtles

Is it a turtle, a tortoise, or a terrapin? That depends on which area of the world you are located. Each of these animals has a slightly different name, depending on the country of origin. However, for the purpose of this section, the term *turtle* refers to both aquatic and terrestrial chelonians, and *terrapin* refers to fresh-water or marine chelonians.

Turtles are commonly seen in exotic veterinary practice, but many veterinarians know little about the husbandry of these animals. (References given in the Bibliography will provide the technician with a more comprehensive view of chelonians.)

Anatomy

Chelonians are vertebrates, but because they "carry their houses on their backs" they are significantly different from other vertebrates (Fig. 37-5). The shell of the turtle consists of two separate pieces: the upper *carapace* and the lower *plastron* (Fig. 37-6). These structures are composed of bones derived from the ribs, vertebrae, sternum, clavicles, and dermal tissue of the skin. The bony shell is covered by *scutes*, composed of layers of keratin. These scutes are capable of regeneration. During growth periods, new scutes are produced, and many old ones are shed. The scutes are named for the underlying body parts.

The weight of the shell adds significantly to the body weight of the turtle and should be taken into account when calculating drug doses. It is suggested that because bone is metabolically active, the dose should be calculated on the *total* body weight, not compensating for the weight of the shell.

Turtles have a typical reptilian, three-chambered heart and a renal portal system. The rest of the cardiovascular system is similar to those of other vertebrates.

Chelonians lack teeth, and instead have a sharp, scissors-like beak for biting off pieces of food, which are then swallowed whole. The gastrointestinal system is arranged as in other animals.

In herbivorous species, the large intestine is the site of fermentation. The digestive tract terminates at the cloaca. Transit time in the gastrointestinal tract is affected by fiber content of the food, temperature, and frequency of feeding, and may reach up to a month on high-fiber diets. These animals have a pancreas and a gall bladder that aid in producing digestive enzymes.

The respiratory system of turtles is similar in arrangement to those of mammals. Turtles breathe in and out through the nostrils. The trachea is short and bifurcates high on the neck into two main stem bronchi. This allows the turtle to breathe when the neck is withdrawn into the shell. Turtles have no diaphragm, and respiration involves many structures. Turtles do not rely on negative pressures in the thorax for lung expansion. Because of the structure of the respiratory system, it is difficult to remove substances from the lungs and pneumonias are often life-threatening for these animals. Aquatic turtles are able to breathe underwater during periods of low activity via a cloacal bursal vascular complex that allows for oxygen absorption. When active, these turtles must return to the surface to obtain adequate oxygen. Turtles are able to sustain long periods of apnea, which makes gas induction of anesthesia often difficult (Fig. 37-7).

The urinary system of the turtle is composed of two kidneys (which are metanephric) and a bi-lobed bladder that empties into the cloaca. The kidneys are not capable of concentrating urine because they have no loop of Henle. Waste materials are converted to insoluble products such as uric acid and urate salts and are passed from the body in a semisolid state. The cloaca, bladder, and distal colon can all resorb urinary water when necessary.

Male turtles have two testicles located anterior to the kidneys. They have a single, large, dark-colored penis that lies on the floor of the proctodeum and may often be seen extended when engorged. The penis is not used for urine excretion.

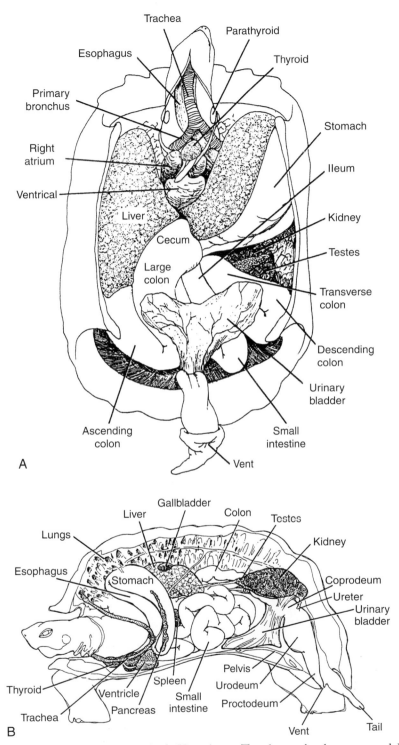

Figure 37-5 Gross anatomy of the turtle. **A,** Ventral view. The plastron has been removed. **B,** Mid-sagittal view. (From Mader DR: *Reptile medicine and surgery*, ed 2, St. Louis, MO, 2006, Saunders, by permission.)

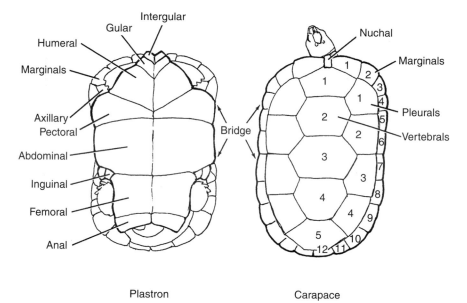

Plastron   Carapace

Figure 37-6 Nomenclature of plastron and carapace scutes. (From Mader DR: *Reptile medicine and surgery*, ed 2, St. Louis, MO, 2006, Saunders, by permission.)

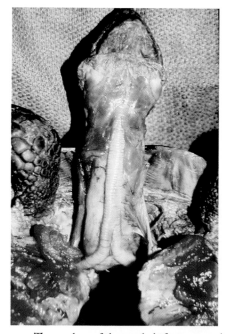

Figure 37-7 The trachea of the turtle bifurcates at the thoracic inlet and has complete cartilagenous rings. (From Mader DR: *Reptile medicine and surgery*, ed 2, St. Louis, MO, 2006, Saunders, by permission.)

The female gonads are also located internally. Turtles lay eggs, and the reproductive tract is similar to those of birds. Fertilization occurs internally before the shell is laid down in the oviduct. Unlike most avian species, sexual dimorphism exists in turtles. Male turtles typically have a longer and thicker tail compared with female turtles. Differences in eye color may exist, and male turtles have a concave plastron whereas female turtles have a flat one.

Husbandry

Turtles are heliotherms, which means they bask in sunlight to control body temperature. The POTZ for most of these species is between 75°F and 100°F. Turtles should be provided basking areas and full-spectrum ultraviolet light in captivity. They should have constant access to water for soaking.

Turtles are susceptible to many predators, especially dogs, coyotes, raccoons, and opossum. They are good diggers and climbers, and outdoor enclosures must be properly constructed to prevent escape.

Most turtles hibernate during the winter months; this is called *brumation*. Captive turtles in subtropical climates may skip brumation, but those in colder climates need to hibernate. (The technician is referred once again to the Bibliography for details of this process.)

Box Turtles

Box turtles are one of the most popular reptilian pets. They have long natural life spans (up to 40 years), but many die because of improper care.

Box turtles may be housed outdoors in warmer months but require a perimeter that is sealed against digging and a fence that is higher than 12 inches to prevent climbing. The area should have grass, shrubs, or a wooden shelter for escape from the sun, when needed. Indoors, turtles may be kept in large aquariums, plywood containers, or other large animal water troughs. These should be filled with humid substrate such as wood chips, peat moss, and sand and soil mixtures. A shallow water pan big enough to fit the turtle should be placed in the container.

Box turtles are omnivorous and will eat beetles, grasshoppers, worms, snails, spiders, pillbugs, small mammals, birds, fish, lizards, snakes, and many other sources of protein. They also enjoy fruits and vegetables such as mushrooms, tomatoes, and greens. Turtles, in general, have a need for vitamin A, so the diet should contain rich yellow or orange vegetables and dark, leafy greens.

Tortoises

Tortoises are land dwellers and should be kept outdoors, when possible. They need sunlight for synthesis of vitamin D, and they love to graze and bask in the sunlight. They will consume all vegetation enclosed in their pen, so avoid spraying chemicals on it. They are also prone to eat nonfood items such as plastic, wire, nails, and other trash, so the pen must be kept clean. Water should be available at all times.

Aquatic Turtles

Turtles kept in aquatic environments often are the most difficult to maintain. Water quality is important to the turtle's health. Proper depth and temperature must be maintained, and an adequate filtration system should be available for cleaning. Each area

should have a dry haul-out area that can be used for basking. Most of these turtles require a diet with adequate calcium. Chopped whole fish, skinned pinky mice, and guppies are a few favorite foods of turtles. Avoid goldfish because they have a high incidence of mycobacteriosis and hamburger because it is deficient in calcium.

REVIEW QUESTIONS

1. What does the abbreviation POTZ stand for?
2. With respect to dietary requirements, all snakes are:
   a. Herbivorous
   b. Carnivorous
   c. Omnivorous
3. All reptiles should be considered positive for _____ until proven otherwise.
   a. *Pseudomonas*
   b. *Shigella*
   c. *Mycobacterium*
   d. *Salmonella*
4. What is the optimal temperature range for most turtles?
   a. 75–100°F
   b. 60–80°F
   c. 50–75°F
   d. 45–75°F
5. Most chelonians kept as pets will become less active during:
   a. October to April
   b. June to September
   c. December to June
   d. January to July
6. The diet of aquatic turtles should contain:
   a. Chopped whole animals such as mice, worms, or guppies and vegetables
   b. Only leafy green vegetables such as spinach and lettuce
   c. Hamburger and leafy green vegetables with worms or insects
   d. Feeder goldfish and leafy, green vegetables
7. The upper shell of the turtle is called the _____.
   a. Plastron
   b. Osteoplast
   c. Carapace
   d. Carastron

8. Adult snakes should eat _____ times per month.
   a. 4–6
   b. 1–3
   c. 3–4
   d. 8–10

9. The fine white powder seen around the nares in iguanas is _____.
   a. Calcium
   b. Potassium
   c. Sodium

Answers found on page 556.

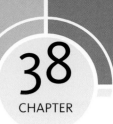

Diseases of the Cardiovascular System

LEARNING OBJECTIVES

When you have completed this chapter, you will be able to:
1. Recognize and explain the need for a complete cardiovascular assessment as a component of the examination of any sick reptile.

Snakes

Clinical cardiac disease in reptiles may be primary or secondary to metabolic or nutritional problems. This type of disease has been poorly reported in the past, possibly because no one has looked for it.

Although the anatomy of the heart (two atria and one ventricle) suggests a singular circulatory system, the function of the heart actually provides a dual system similar to those in other animals. Heart rate depends on a number of variables: body temperature, body size, metabolic rate, respiratory rate, and sensory stimulation. The heart functions most effectively within the preferred optimal temperature zone (POTZ). Heart rate tends to increase during active respiration and decrease during apnea.

Monitoring of the cardiac activity is possible in snakes using electrocardiographic equipment already in the hospital.

Another difference in the cardiovascular system is the presence of nucleated red blood cells. The hemoglobin in these cells is similar to that in mammalian cells; however, the oxygen affinity of hemoglobin tends to decrease with the age of the animal. It is important for the veterinarian and the technician to understand the anatomy and physiology of the cardiovascular system and how it relates to the development of disease to diagnose cardiovascular diseases in the snake.

Nutritional Diseases That Affect the Heart

Dietary deficiencies may affect the function of the cardiovascular system. Hypocalcemia, vitamin E deficiency, and excessive amounts of vitamin D_3 and calcium may all affect the cardiovascular system.

CLINICAL SIGNS

- May be nonspecific for cardiac disease
- Muscle tremors (hypocalcemia)
- Peripheral edema
- Ascites
- Cyanosis
- Petechial hemorrhages
- Weight loss
- Peracute death

DIAGNOSIS

- Dietary history
- Physical examination
- Biopsy of skeletal muscle
- Radiography may show calcification of vessels (excess vitamin D and calcium)
- Necropsy

TREATMENT

- Vitamin E and selenium products to correct imbalance
- Correct dietary imbalances

INFORMATION FOR CLIENTS

- A proper diet and correct environmental temperatures are important for maintaining good cardiovascular health.

Infectious Diseases of the Cardiovascular System

Septic endocarditis has been reported in animals with gram-negative systemic disease. *Salmonella*, *Corynebacterium*, *Chlamydia*, and *Mycobacterium* have all been reported to cause either endocarditis or myocarditis in the snake.

CLINICAL SIGNS

- Peripheral edema
- Ascites
- Weight loss
- Signs of the specific systemic infection

DIAGNOSIS

- Blood culture collected from cardiocentesis
- Complete blood cell count
- Ultrasonography or angiography

TREATMENT

- Systemic antibiotics specific to cultured organism
- Supportive care

INFORMATION FOR CLIENTS

- Have your pet examined immediately if you suspect illness.
- Laboratory workups may be expensive but are necessary to diagnose these conditions.

Congenital Cardiovascular Disease

Several congenital cardiac anomalies have been reported in snakes. Congestive heart failure and cardiomyopathy, although uncommon, do occur. The use of cardiac drugs in reptiles has not been well studied, and veterinarians should be careful in extrapolating doses from those for mammalian species.

Turtles

Whereas cardiac disease has been documented in most reptiles, it is not seen as a common problem in pet turtles except as a result of other diseases such as renal gout. The technician should refer to more detailed descriptions of cardiac function in reptile texts.

REVIEW QUESTIONS

1. In reptiles housed below the POTZ, one would expect the heart rate to be:
   a. Increased from normal
   b. Decreased from normal
   c. Normal
2. The reptile heart has ____ atria and ____ ventricle(s).
   a. Two; two
   b. One; two
   c. Two; one

3. Red blood cells of older reptiles are less functional than those of younger animals because:
   a. Their red cells are not able to carry as much oxygen
   b. The lungs are not able to oxygenate the cells properly
   c. The red cells do not give up their oxygen at the tissues easily

Answers found on page 556.

Diseases of the Digestive System

LEARNING OBJECTIVES

When you have completed this chapter, you will be able to:

1. Demonstrate knowledge of diseases related to the digestive system in reptiles.
2. Implement treatment plans to correct deficits related to gastrointestinal diseases.
3. Relate to clients how inadequate husbandry can result in gastrointestinal disease in reptile patients.

4. Understand that reptiles will require extended periods of antibiotic treatment before positive results will be seen.

Snakes

Snakes are frequently seen in the clinic for digestive problems.

Infectious Stomatitis (Mouth Rot)

Infectious stomatitis, commonly called "mouth rot," is a frequently seen problem in captive snakes (Fig. 39-1).

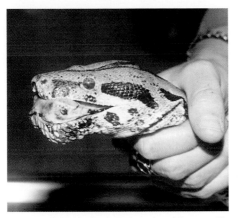

Figure 39-1 Infectious stomatitis is a problem in all reptiles but is most commonly seen in snakes. (From Mader DR: *Reptile medicine and surgery*, ed 2, St. Louis, MO, 2006, Saunders, by permission.)

This is not a primary disease but, rather, is usually secondary to stress, trauma, or husbandry problems such as overcrowding, low environmental temperatures, and poor nutrition. Suppression of the immune system in snakes kept in inappropriate conditions allows for opportunistic pathogens to infect the oral tissues.

CLINICAL SIGNS

- Swollen, red oral tissue
- Petechia may be present
- Changes in color of gum tissue
- Mucus, thick ropy exudates; excessive salivation
- Anorexia
- Dysphagia
- Respiratory signs if glottis is involved

DIAGNOSIS

- Physical examination and history
- Culture and sensitivity of oral mucosa
- Complete blood cell count (CBC) and serum chemistries
- Radiology of the oral cavity
- Biopsy of gingiva

TREATMENT

- Correction of environmental and nutritional problems
- Gentle cleansing of the oral mucosa

- Systemic antibiotics (injectable aminoglycosides are recommended)
- Surgical debridement of severe cases or those with bony involvement

Topical

- Antibiotic cream: silver sulfadiazine (Silvadene) 1%, gentamicin ophthalmic
- Dilute povidone-iodine (Betadine) or chlorhexidine flushes

Supportive Care

- May include tube feeding if animal is unable to eat

INFORMATION FOR CLIENTS

- Prevention of infectious stomatitis is easier than treating it.
- Treatment of infectious stomatitis may require long-term therapy.
- Viral or fungal stomatitis will not respond to antibiotic therapy. It is important that an accurate diagnosis be made before treatment is started.
- Infections in the oral cavity may quickly spread to the lungs if left untreated.

Vomiting and Regurgitation

Vomiting is defined as the forceful expulsion of food from the stomach or anterior intestine, whereas *regurgitation* involves bringing up food immediately after eating. It is often difficult to distinguish these conditions in the reptile patient. Regurgitation is frequently the result of handling just after eating and represents no threat to the animal unless it is frequent or aspiration pneumonia develops. Vomiting, in contrast, is frequently related to gastrointestinal (GI) disease and should be investigated.

CLINICAL SIGNS

- Vomited or regurgitated food found in the cage
- Weight loss
- ± Diarrhea
- Signs of systemic disease

DIAGNOSIS

- Physical examination and environmental history
- CBC and serum chemistries
- Radiography ± contrast

- Culture and sensitivity
- Fecal flotation

TREATMENT

- Depends on the problems identified
- Correction of husbandry and diet deficiencies
- Avoidance of handling snakes that have been fed recently
- Systemic antibiotics for bacterial infections
- Antiparasitics for GI parasites
- Surgical removal of any foreign objects or neoplasia
- Correction of fluid and electrolyte imbalances
- Metoclopramide for vomiting

INFORMATION FOR CLIENTS

- Avoid handling snakes after feeding.
- Make sure that all snakes are kept in ideal environmental conditions.
- If vomiting or regurgitation occurs, have your snake examined immediately by your veterinarian.
- Never feed spoiled or contaminated food. Make sure all food has been warmed to body temperature before feeding.

Diarrhea

Diarrhea may be a result of many disease states and is usually not a primary disease entity. As in the avian patient, it must first be determined whether diarrhea actually exists. Vomitus, urine, or respiratory secretions often appear similar to loose feces and are often not observed by the owner until cage cleaning. Loose stools must also be evaluated by what is normal for that species because some snakes (boas and pythons) have firm stools, whereas indigo snakes and cobras have soft stools. Normal stool of the snake will contain feces, whitish urates, and some urine as in birds.

CLINICAL SIGNS

- Loose stools found in the cage
- Weight loss
- Acute or chronic loose stools
- ± Vomiting
- ± Blood, fat in feces

DIAGNOSIS

- Physical examination and history

- Fecal examinations (floats and direct smears)
- Fecal culture and sensitivity (cloacal flush or swab)
- Radiology
- CBC and serum chemistries
- Endoscopy
- Exploratory surgery with biopsies

TREATMENT

- Depends on severity and cause
- Antiparasitics
- Antibiotics, if needed
- Narcotic agents to slow the bowel

Supportive Therapy

- Fluid and electrolyte replacement
- Warmth

INFORMATION FOR CLIENTS

- Any change in diet may cause diarrhea. Avoid foods with high water content or abrupt dietary changes.
- Keep your snake at preferred optimal temperature zone (POTZ) and the cage environment clean to prevent bacterial contamination.
- Have frequent stool tests performed to remove parasites.
- Wear protective gloves when cleaning the cage of an animal with diarrhea. Wash hands thoroughly after handling.

Intestinal Parasites

Almost every snake will harbor some type of internal parasite at the time of purchase. These parasites typically have complex life cycles, which the technician should review. Captive snakes are, by nature of their habitats, exposed to a greater parasite load compared with snakes in the wild, and this creates a greater problem. These animals have higher stress levels that result in immunosuppression, again predisposing them to parasitic infestation. Some of the most frequently found intestinal parasites of snakes are listed in Box 39-1. As shown in Box 39-1, parasitic infestation in snakes may involve multiple organisms. Parasitized animals are *unthrifty* (failing to grow or develop normally), have shorter life spans, and may act as a reservoir for human infestation.

BOX 39-1   Frequent Intestinal Parasites of Snakes

Protozoa
- *Entamoeba invadens*
- *Coccidia* spp.
- *Cryptosporidium* spp.
- *Giardia* spp.
- *Hexamita* spp.
- *Trichomonas* spp.

Trematodes
- *Renifer* spp.
- *Dasymetra* spp.
- *Ochetosoma* spp.
- *Stomatrema* spp.
- *Pneumatophilus*
- Renal flukes

Cestodes
- Crepidobothrium
- *Ophiotaenia*
- *Bothridium*
- *Spirometra*
- *Dilepididae*
- *Mesocestoididae*

Nematodes
- Ascarids
- *Strongyloides* spp.
- *Rhabdias* spp.
- *Diaphanocephalus* spp.
- *Kalicephalus* spp.
- *Macdonaldius* spp.
- Oxyurids
- *Capillaria* spp.
- Pentastomids

CLINICAL SIGNS

- Weight loss
- Failure to thrive
- Anorexia
- Dehydration
- ± Diarrhea
- Blood in feces
- ± Vomiting or regurgitation
- ± Anemia

DIAGNOSIS

- Fecal flotation, cloacal flush, and direct smear
- Finding adult parasites in feces

TREATMENT

- Depends on the parasite's life cycle:
  - Antiparasitic drug therapy (to eliminate parasites with a direct life cycle)
  - Eliminate any indirect host
- Cleaning the cage on a regular basis
- Ivermectin (effective in snakes; *do not use in turtles*)
- Feeding only parasite-free prey to prevent infection

INFORMATION FOR CLIENTS

- Have all snakes examined for parasites at least yearly.
- Keep cages clean. Do not allow fecal matter to accumulate.
- Feed parasite-free prey, when possible.
- If using an oral wormer, you can administer it to the prey before feeding the snake (stuff the prey with oral paste or liquid wormer).
- Several of these parasites are infectious to humans. Wash your hands, and wear protective gloves when cleaning the cages.

Failure to Feed

One of the most common problems reported to the veterinarian is failure to feed. Most of the time, this is a problem created not by the snake but, rather, by the owner. The new reptile owner may not know the proper diet for the snake, the proper feeding interval, the proper feeding technique, or the correct amount to feed the snake. The environmental temperature or the temperature of the food, or both, may be too low to initiate the feeding response. Snakes, like other animals, are not all alike; some prefer live prey and others dead prey. Some like to be hand-fed, and others like to be fed using tongs. Owners must get to know their snakes' preferences before determining whether a problem exists.

Feeding live prey is not recommended because often the prey may injure the snake. Live prey should be stunned before being fed; prekilled prey is available frozen or fresh from specialty pet stores.

Snakes should not be handled for several days after feeding. Meal size varies with the species; smaller snakes require smaller prey. The timing of feedings also varies with individual snakes; certain species will eat at any time, whereas others eat only in daylight or darkness. Some eat often (usually small snakes), whereas larger animals may eat once every 2 to 3 weeks. Several species may fast for months without harm.

CLINICAL SIGNS

- Lack of feeding response when prey is provided
- Weight loss
- Signs of shedding (either before or after shedding)

DIAGNOSIS

- Physical examination and history
- CBC and serum chemistries to rule out disease
- Fecal examination to rule out parasites

TREATMENT

- Adjust environmental temperature and photo-period.
- Try alternative prey (live or dead, rodents, birds, etc.).
- Consult a herpetologist for information concerning feeding a specific type of snake.
- Provide vitamin supplementation.
- Try force-feeding

INFORMATION FOR CLIENTS

- Snakes can undergo prolonged periods without feeding. In the absence of any signs of disease, it may be normal for them not to feed.
- Consult experts if you do not know what is normal for a particular species.
- Make sure your snake is kept at the POTZ.
- Have your snake examined by your veterinarian if you suspect a medical problem.

Iguanas

Like snakes, iguanas are also prone to diseases of the digestive system. Most diseases of the oral cavity and upper GI tract are due to stress and improper husbandry, low environmental temperatures, dehydration, and poor diets.

Infectious Stomatitis (Mouth Rot)

Iguanas, like snakes, are susceptible to mouth rot (Fig. 39-2). The condition is usually the result of stress depressing the immune system, trauma, and opportunistic bacteria. Bacteria such as *Pseudomonas*, *Aeromonas*, and *Klebsiella* are commonly identified from patients with infectious stomatitis. Lack of necessary vitamins and minerals may also predispose the iguana to infectious stomatitis.

CLINICAL SIGNS

- Swollen, sore gingival membranes
- Bleeding of oral tissues
- Excessive mucus production (excessive salivation)
- Reluctance to eat
- ± Regurgitation
- ± Pneumonia

DIAGNOSIS

- Physical examination and thorough history
- CBC and serum chemistries
- Radiography to rule out bony involvement
- Bacterial cultures and sensitivity: oral cavity

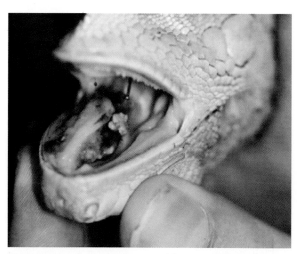

Figure 39-2 A green iguana with stomatitis and pneumonia. The oral cavity is congested, and the pharynx is full of excessive white foam. (From Mader DR: *Reptile medicine and surgery*, ed 2, St. Louis, MO, 2006, Saunders, by permission.)

TREATMENT

- Will depend on the cause
- Correction of husbandry and dietary causes
- Systemic antibiotics based on culture and sensitivity testing (gram-negative spectrum usually best)
- Flushing the mucous membranes twice daily with chlorhexidine or dilute iodine solution (1:10 dilution)
- Surgical debridement of infected or necrotic tissue

⬤ TECH ALERT

Reptiles do everything slowly—they get ill slowly, and they recover slowly. Make sure that owners maintain treatments for the necessary periods required to cure the problem.

Vomiting and Regurgitation

Lizards have a better developed cardiac sphincter compared with that of snakes, so vomiting or regurgitation is rare in lizards. If vomiting or regurgitation occurs, the animal is usually in poor condition and may be near death. GI foreign bodies, systemic infections, and enlarged kidneys that are pressing on the colon are among the few causes of vomiting in lizards.

Diarrhea

Low environmental temperatures, systemic infections, parasites, and an acute diet change may all cause diarrhea in the lizard (Fig. 39-3).

CLINICAL SIGNS

- Loose stools
- ± Foul-smelling feces
- Weight loss
- ± Dehydration

DIAGNOSIS

- Good dietary history
- Fecal flotation
- Direct smear to rule out amoebas, protozoa
- Culture and sensitivity, especially for *Salmonella* spp.

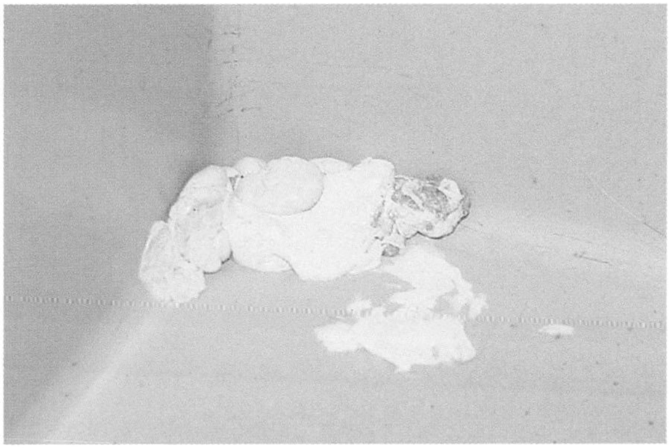

Figure 39-3 Feces from reptiles contain uric acid salts, which are white. (From Mader DR: *Reptile medicine and surgery*, ed 2, St. Louis, MO, 2006, Saunders.)

TREATMENT

- Improved husbandry and dietary conditions
- Antibiotics based on culture and sensitivity results
- Rehydration of the patient, if needed (intravenous [IV] or oral balanced electrolyte solutions)
- Antiparasitic drugs, if needed
- Feeding small amounts of a probiotic or plain, nonfat yogurt containing live bacterial cultures

Constipation

The problem in iguanas often is the opposite of diarrhea—constipation or lack of stool production. This also may be the result of improper husbandry, parasites, GI foreign bodies, or dehydration. Iguanas that eat every day should defecate every day.

CLINICAL SIGNS

- Lack of feces in the cage
- Distended abdomen
- Decreased appetite
- ± Straining to defecate
- ± Hard, small feces

DIAGNOSIS

- Physical examination and history
- Radiology to rule out foreign bodies
- Fecal flotation

TREATMENT

- Increase the ambient temperature.
- Feed foods with increased water content: fruits, wet greens, and so forth.
- Bathe or soak frequently to rehydrate; give oral or IV fluids.
- Administer small amounts of feline laxative or mineral oil.
- Treat any parasitic problems with ivermectin.

INFORMATION FOR CLIENTS

- Both diarrhea and constipation can be prevented by proper housing and feeding of your pet iguana.
- Iguanas frequently chew up flooring materials (bedding) in the cage. Make sure the substrate in your cage is digestible.
- If "home remedies" do not produce a normal stool within 1 to 2 days, have your pet seen by your veterinarian.

Cloacal Prolapse

The colon, urinary bladder (if present), penis, uterus, and oviducts may all prolapse through the cloaca (Fig. 39-4). Prolapse is usually the result of excessive straining from some secondary cause. Proper treatment depends on accurately determining which organ is prolapsed. The bladder may be identified as thin walled and translucent and can be aspirated. The penis or hemipenis will be a solid mass with no

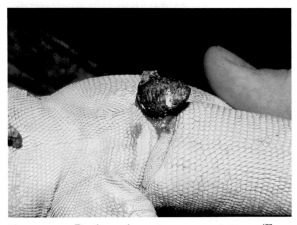

Figure 39-4 Penile prolapse in a green iguana. (From Mader DR: *Reptile medicine and surgery*, ed 2, St. Louis, MO, 2006, Saunders, by permission.)

lumen, whereas the colon will have an identifiable lumen. The shell gland will have a lumen but no feces inside the lumen.

CLINICAL SIGNS

- Presence of tissue protruding from the vent
- History of egg laying or straining
- Other signs of systemic disease

DIAGNOSIS

- Physical examination and history
- CBC and serum chemistries to rule out systemic disease
- Fecal examination to rule out parasites
- Radiography

TREATMENT

- Will depend on the diagnostic results
- Gentle cleaning of the prolapsed tissue with normal saline
- Manual replacement of the tissue
- Debridement of any necrotic tissue, if possible
- Purse-string suture, if possible, to retain the tissue until swelling decreases
- Systemic antibiotics
- Correction of the cause of straining
- Rehydration of the patient
- Raising the ambient temperature
- Treatment for intestinal parasites, if present
  - Some cases will require surgical correction through a celiotomy incision

INFORMATION FOR CLIENTS

- Prompt replacement of the prolapsed tissue has a good prognosis, whereas allowing the tissue to become dirty and necrotic has a poor prognosis.
- Veterinary assistance should be sought immediately if a prolapse is observed.

Intestinal Parasites

Several types of internal parasites live in the intestinal tract of iguanas. Protozoa, nematodes, and cestodes are typically identified in iguanas in captivity.

CLINICAL SIGNS

- Anorexia
- Lethargy

- Mucus in the feces
- Weight loss or failure to gain with a good appetite
- Worms visible in feces
- Frequent loose, smelly stools
- ± Regurgitation
- ± Bloating

DIAGNOSIS

- Fecal flotation
- Direct smear
- Rule out other systemic diseases

TREATMENT

- Ivermectin
- Deworming medication (pyrantel pamoate [Strongid], fenbendazole [Panacur])
- Metronidazole for protozoans
- Cleaning and disinfecting the iguana's enclosure and removing stools on a regular basis to prevent reinfection

Turtles

Diarrhea (Symptom, Not Disease)

It is important for the clinician to determine whether diarrhea is actually present. Each species has a characteristic form for feces, some softer than others, and the veterinarian or technician must have an idea of what is "normal." Most diarrheas should be classified as either acute or chronic. Chronic diarrheas are more severe and may lead to dehydration and electrolyte imbalances.

CLINICAL SIGNS

- Feces of a different consistency than normal
- ± Fat (steatorrhea)
- ± Flatulence
- ± Blood in feces
- Dehydration

DIAGNOSIS

- Complete physical examination and environmental and dietary histories
- CBC may show sepsis, anemia, heterophilia; serum chemistries
- Fecal flotation and smear
- Fecal culture and sensitivity

- Gastric and cloacal wash
- Radiography

TREATMENT

- Correct specific underlying problems.
- Improve husbandry.
- Parasiticides may be effective. (DO *not use ivermectin in turtles.*)
- Rehydrate the patient either orally or parentally.
- Oral pectin, aluminum hydroxide, or bismuth subsulfate solutions to coat the bowel may be used.

◉ TECH ALERT

Diarrhea is a symptom of more severe diseases. Avoid treating empirically without obtaining a diagnosis.

INFORMATION FOR CLIENTS

- Diarrhea is a symptom of a more severe disease. Have your animal examined by a veterinarian before beginning empirical treatment at home.
- Proper diet and husbandry practices should be maintained to prevent diarrhea.
- Have all new additions checked for intestinal parasites and cultured for *Salmonella* infection before adding them to the collection.

Anorexia (Symptom)

Lack of appetite is a symptom of many disease processes, poor husbandry conditions, or behavioral problems. Most frequently, anorexia is related to poor husbandry conditions and not to disease. In winter, turtles that hibernate will stop eating, and turtles kept at temperatures that are too low may do the same. Incorrect or improper presentation of food or improper food types may result in anorexia. It is important to rule out disease in an anorexic patient.

CLINICAL SIGNS

- Animal stops eating
- ± Other signs of systemic disease

DIAGNOSIS

- Complete history and physical examination
- CBC, serum chemistry analysis

- Radiography to rule out foreign bodies or tumors
- Endoscopy or ultrasonography

TREATMENT

- Correct the underlying disease process.
- Correct husbandry and dietary problems.
- Force-feed a high-calorie diet.

INFORMATION FOR CLIENTS

- Proper husbandry and diet are necessary for all reptiles.
- Owners must be willing to make changes for the health of the animal.

Internal Parasites

Turtles may be infested with a variety of internal parasites. Listed below are some of the species that may affect turtles:

- Protozoa (*Entamoeba* spp., *Coccidia*)
- Trematodes (flukes in freshwater turtles)
- Tapeworms (*Oochoristica* spp.)
- Nematodes (*Oxyuridae* spp., *Serpinema* spp., *Chapiniella* spp., *Spiroxis* spp., *Sulcascaris* spp.)

CLINICAL SIGNS

- Poor growth rate, weight loss
- ± Diarrhea
- Problems of the reproductive system
- Being unthrifty
- Increased susceptibility to disease

DIAGNOSIS

- Complete physical examination and history
- Cloacal wash with fecal flotation or direct smear (let stand 10 minutes before reading)
- Fixed samples of feces

TREATMENT

- Treatment should be based on the life cycle of the parasite. Eliminate intermediate hosts, if present; interrupt the life cycle and eliminate the adults.
- Parasiticides may be effective (DO *not use ivermectin in turtles!*):
  - Fenbendazole (may be given per cloaca or orally)
  - Albendazole
  - Mebendazole
  - Metronidazole (calculate dose carefully)
  - Piperazine
  - Pyrantel pamoate
  - Injectable wormers
- Freeze all prey animals for at least 30 days before thawing and feeding.
- Prevention is easier than correcting a problem.

INFORMATION FOR CLIENTS

- Most caught wild chelonians will have intestinal parasites. These parasites may also be found in other tissues where they may be difficult to remove with medication.
- Complete avoidance of parasitic infestation is impossible, but with proper husbandry, laboratory testing, and treatment, the parasitic load can be decreased significantly.
- All new additions to the collection should be quarantined for a minimum of 30 days to allow time for the diagnosis and treatment of parasitic infestation.

Hepatic Lipidosis

Hepatic lipidosis is a recognized disease in many reptiles. Chelonians store fat in fat bodies located in the caudoventral coelom. Fat is transported from the intestines to the fat bodies for storage and then moved to the liver when it is needed, especially during hibernation. Many factors may contribute to a buildup of fat within the liver: high-fat diet, decrease in activity, egg laying, prehibernation, and improper environmental temperatures. As fat stores build up in the liver, clinical signs become evident.

CLINICAL SIGNS

- Gradual reduction in appetite
- Gradual weight loss
- Hibernation problems
- Change in fecal character and color
- Decreased activity
- Decreased fertility
- Green urine or urates

DIAGNOSIS

- Complete physical examination and history
- CBC: increase in hematocrit usually indicates dehydration

- Serum chemistries: most liver function tests used in mammals are not definitive in turtles
- Radiography or ultrasonography: may or may not be of value because of the shell
- Endoscopy: visualize the liver, biopsy
- Magnetic resonance imaging (expensive)

TREATMENT

- Fluid and nutritional support are mandatory; avoid fluids that contain lactate in severe cases.
- Placement of an esophagostomy tube for long-term feeding may be necessary (Fig. 39-5).
- Addition of carnitine, choline, methionine, and thyroxine may be added to feeding solutions.
- Intramuscular nandrolone may be used to promote appetite and reduce catabolism.

INFORMATION FOR CLIENTS

- Proper feeding of turtles will prevent fat buildup in the liver, as will maintenance of normal environmental conditions.
- Stress and prolonged periods of anorexia may predispose to clinical signs of hepatic lipidosis.
- Treatment of hepatic lipidosis may be prolonged and require a lot of work.

Oral or Rostral Trauma

Rostral trauma with secondary bacterial infection is one of the most common presenting complaints in all

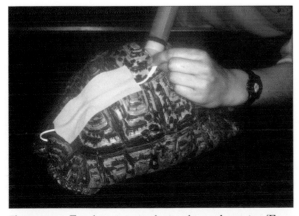

Figure 39-5 Esophagostomy tube in a leopard tortoise. (From Mader DR: *Reptile medicine and surgery*, ed 2, St. Louis, MO, 2006, Saunders. Courtesy of S. J. Hernandez-Divers.)

captive reptiles, and turtles are no exception. Constant rubbing of the face against the sides of the container is the most common cause. Thermal trauma from biting into electric cords or from ingestion of overheated food may also occur. Damage to the beak or overgrowth may result in anorexia. Tongue trauma may result from foreign material such as hair or string wrapping around the tongue causing swelling and necrosis.

CLINICAL SIGNS

- ± Swelling and inflammation at the tip of the beak or in the oral cavity
- ± Foreign objects wrapped around the beak
- Anorexia
- ± Abnormal growth of the beak

DIAGNOSIS

- Complete physical examination and environmental history
- Culture and sensitivity of any lesions
- Radiology if fracture is suspected

TREATMENT

- Cleaning and debridement of damaged tissues, as needed
- Antibiotics if infection is present (based on culture results)
- Correction of any dietary defects
- Force-feeding, if necessary
- Careful removal of any foreign materials

INFORMATION FOR CLIENTS

- It is important to examine your animals daily for signs of trauma. Catching a problem early prevents it from becoming critical.
- Viral diseases such as herpes virus, bacterial infections, and fungal infections may damage oral tissues and result in secondary infections. These should be ruled out before treatment for trauma.
- Make sure that the turtle enclosure is constructed in such a way to decrease the possibility of trauma because all animals tend to rub on cage walls.

Hypovitaminosis A

Turtles, especially aquatic chelonians, are susceptible to hypovitaminosis A. Lack of vitamin A in the diet may cause damage to mucosal surfaces. Lesions are commonly seen in the oral cavity or in the respiratory system (the nostrils).

CLINICAL SIGNS

- Lethargy
- Anorexia
- Blepharedema of the nasolacrimal ducts
- ± Oral infections
- ± Overgrowth of the beak

DIAGNOSIS

- Complete physical examination
- Dietary history
- Clinical signs

TREATMENT

- Correction of improper diet
- Vitamin A supplementation by injection
- ± Corrective beak trimming to improve food prehension

INFORMATION FOR CLIENTS

- Make sure that the diet being fed has adequate vitamin A levels for the particular species being housed.
- Vitamin supplements can be dusted onto or placed into foods before feeding. Avoid over-supplementation because toxicities may develop.

Gastrointestinal Tract Obstruction

Obstruction of the GI tract may develop in turtles housed on sand substrates. Sand impaction has been reported in tortoises. Many chelonians are prone to swallow woody substances and rocks.

CLINICAL SIGNS

- Anorexia
- Lethargy
- Dehydration
- Weight loss
- Absence of feces in the cage

DIAGNOSIS

- Complete physical and environmental history
- Radiography

- CBC: anemia, leukocytosis; increased hepatic and muscular enzymes on serum chemistries may be seen

TREATMENT

- Enema to remove sand
- Replacing sand substrate in cage with gravel or digestible material
- Surgical removal of nondigestible foreign bodies

INFORMATION FOR CLIENTS

- Proper housing of tortoises prevents the development of GI tract obstruction.

Gastritis and Enteritis

Bacterial, viral, and fungal gastritis or enteritis may be seen in turtles. Gram-negative organisms such as *Salmonella* are often found in these animals. Herpes-virus infection has been on the increase in chelonians in recent years. *Mycobacterium* spp. have also been implicated in cases of enteritis nonresponsive to antibiotics.

CLINICAL SIGNS

- Depend on the agent responsible
- In general:
  - Anorexia
  - Lethargy
  - Dehydration
- ± Oral lesions
- ± Signs of disease in the respiratory system or nervous system (herpes viral infection)

DIAGNOSIS

- Complete physical examination; dietary and environmental histories
- CBC
- Culture and sensitivity, viral isolation, or enzyme-linked immunosorbent assay (ELISA)
- Radiology
- Fecal flotation or smear

TREATMENT

Supportive Care
- Correction of dehydration
- Intestinal protectants

- Antibiotics based on culture results
- Force-feeding of easily absorbed nutrients and adequate fiber

INFORMATION FOR CLIENTS

- Proper quarantine, parasite evaluation, diet, and environment prevent many of the problems in captive turtles and tortoises.

REVIEW QUESTIONS

1. Ivermectin can be used to treat parasites in all species except the:
   a. Boa
   b. Green iguana
   c. Turtle
   d. Gecko
2. Infectious stomatitis in reptiles is usually a result of:
   a. Trauma
   b. Suppression of the immune system
   c. Viral infection
   d. Fungal infection
3. Many diseases of reptiles are the result of:
   a. Trauma
   b. Bacterial infection
   c. Poor husbandry
   d. Viral infection
4. Which of the following bacteria should be tested for in all reptiles prior to handling them as pets?
   a. *Chlamydia*
   b. *Salmonella*
   c. *Streptococcus*
   d. *Escherichia coli*
5. Lack of _____ in the diet of turtles may affect the mucosal membranes.
   a. Vitamin B
   b. Vitamin C
   c. Vitamin K
   d. Vitamin A
6. Hepatic lipidosis may occur in turtles that are _____.
   a. Too thin
   b. Anorexic
   c. Polyphagic
7. Chelonians store fat in _____.
   a. The liver
   b. Fat bodies
   c. The thorax
   d. The abdomen
8. Snakes should not be handled for _____ after feeding.
   a. 2 days
   b. 1 week
   c. 2 weeks
   d. 5 days
9. Young snakes will eat _____ frequently than older animals.
   a. More
   b. Less
10. Technicians should always wear gloves when cleaning any reptile cage.
   a. True
   b. False

Answers found on page 556.

Diseases of the Endocrine System

OUTLINE

Snakes   **Turtles**
Iguanas   Hyperglycemia
    Hypothyroidism

LEARNING OBJECTIVES

When you have completed this chapter, you will be able to:
1. Briefly discuss endocrine diseases seen in these species with clients.

Snakes

Snakes have a single thyroid gland or a pair that lies just anterior to the heart. Thyroid function is involved in shedding and growth. Unlike in most mammals, the thymus does not involute in the adult animal. Parathyroid tissue is embedded in the thymus and thyroid tissue and plays a role in calcium metabolism. The adrenal glands are associated with the gonads. The function of the endocrine system in snakes is poorly understood. Diseases of the endocrine system that affect other systems are discussed in Chapters 42 and 43.

Iguanas

Hypothyroidism

The thyroid gland is the only gland in the body that uses iodine. Some authors believe that iodine-deficient diets may result in hypertrophy of the thyroid gland and lead to disease. Foods commonly included in the diet of the green iguana are thought to contain substances that bind iodine, preventing the body from using it. Vegetables such as broccoli, cabbage, cauliflower, Brussels sprouts, and kale are a few of the more common species thought to bind iodine. Lack of iodine may result in hypothyroidism.*

CLINICAL SIGNS

- Sluggishness, lethargy
- Being overweight
- Slow growth

---

*Many references claim that endocrine disease in reptiles is poorly documented and do not mention hypothyroidism as being a problem.

DIAGNOSIS

- Complete blood cell count (CBC) and serum chemistries
- Thyroid hormone assay

TREATMENT

- Removal or reduction of fed amounts of the vegetables listed earlier
- Vitamin supplements that contain iodine

Turtles

Primary endocrine disease is uncommon in turtles; however, endocrine changes may be seen as part of a disease complex such as nutritional hyperparathyroidism. Hyperglycemia is a common finding in chelonians.

Hyperglycemia

Diabetes mellitus is an uncommon condition in reptiles. The presence of hyperglycemia may often be related to environmental conditions, stress, or other factors. Seasonal changes may also affect blood glucose levels. Animals with signs of hyperglycemia should be examined carefully to rule out these factors before making the diagnosis of diabetes. This condition will require more research before a complete diagnosis and treatment regimen can be suggested.

CLINICAL SIGNS

- Anorexia
- Weight loss
- Lethargy
- Depression (often severe)
- Muscle weakness
- ± Polyuria or polydipsia

DIAGNOSIS

- Complete physical examination and environmental history
- CBC
- Serum chemistries: increased blood glucose levels (reference range: 60–100 mg/dL)
- Radiology or ultrasonography
- Urinalysis (glycosuria may be present)
- ± Ketosis
- Pancreatic biopsy (not often performed)
- Necropsy

TREATMENT

- The cause of the hyperglycemia should be determined before treatment:
  - Eliminate stress, improve environmental conditions.
  - Treat any underlying metabolic disease process.
- If the case is determined to be true diabetes mellitus:
  - Insulin therapy should be provided

Supportive Care

- Maintain hydration
- Liver-supporting drugs
- Force-feeding

● TECH ALERT

Do not assume that all reptilian patients with hyperglycemia have diabetes. Rule out all other causes before treating with insulin.

INFORMATION FOR CLIENTS

- Many environmental factors may contribute to signs of hyperglycemia in reptiles.
- Because chronically affected animals are often in serious condition when diagnosed, necropsy may be needed to determine the cause of the problem.

REVIEW QUESTIONS

1. The upper portion of the shell is called the _____, and the lower portion is known as the _____.
2. Reptiles with hyperglycemia will always have diabetes and require treatment.
   a. True
   b. False
3. Which of the following vegetables should be fed in limited amounts to iguanas?
   a. Carrots
   b. Broccoli
   c. Leafy green lettuce
   d. Tomatoes

4. Which of the following hormones is necessary for normal shedding and growth?
   a. Thyroid hormone
   b. Insulin
   c. Cortisol
   d. Parathyroid hormone

5. One of the most frequent causes of endocrine disturbance in the reptile is:
   a. Poor husbandry
   b. Tumors
   c. Congenital defects
   d. Lack of vitamin D

Answers found on page 556.

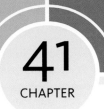

Diseases of the Special Senses

Cataract   Palpebral

Snakes
    Retained Spectacles
    Corneal Lesions Cataracts

Iguanas
    Ocular and Periocular Trauma

When you have completed this chapter, you will be able to:
1. Describe the special senses of reptiles and how diseases of these senses affect the animal patient.

Snakes

The ear has both auditory and vestibular functions in the snake. In many reptiles, the ear is located in a shallow depression on the side of the head and is covered by a thin piece of tissue that is shed during ecdysis. Snakes lack external ears and have no tympanic membrane or middle ear cavity. Although it has been the general belief that snakes have little hearing capability, they are able to hear sounds in the low-frequency range of 150 to 600 hertz (Hz).

The eye of the snake is different from that of mammals. The iris contains striated muscle and does not respond to common mydriatics. The pupil is round and relatively immobile in diurnal species and slitlike in nocturnal species. No consensual pupillary light reflex exists in the snake. Descemet's membrane is absent from the cornea. Fusion of the lids to form a protective

spectacle over the surface of the cornea allows tears to flow between the spectacle and the cornea to maintain moisture. The secretions drain into the lacrimal duct, which drains into the oral cavity. The retina is relatively avascular but contains the conus papillaris, a large vascular body that protrudes into the vitreus. Examination of the eye in reptiles is challenging.

Specialized infrared sensors called *heat pits* are found in Booidea and pit vipers. The location of these sensors depends on the species. These sensors allow the snake to navigate and find food in darkness and to sense small temperature variations.

Retained Spectacles

Spectacles cover the entire surface of the cornea in the snake. These spectacles undergo changes during the shedding cycle, becoming cloudy before the shedding and clearing after shedding is complete. Retention of the spectacles is a common condition seen in pet snakes and, in many cases, is a result of low humidity in the environment (Fig. 41-1).

CLINICAL SIGNS

- History of recent shedding
- Blue-white cap over cornea of one or both eyes
- Behavioral problems related to impaired vision; nervousness, striking when handled

DIAGNOSIS

- Physical examination

TREATMENT

- Removal of the retained spectacle without injuring the cornea may be done as follows:
  - Place snake in a warm container lined with damp paper, or soak the animal in warm water to loosen the spectacle; in some cases, wet cotton balls have been used over the spectacles to soak them.
  - Apply ointment to soften and loosen the spectacle.
  - When the spectacle is loose, gently lift it from the cornea; if it cannot be lifted easily, continue to soak it until it comes loose, or you may damage the cornea.
- Prevent the problem by educating the owner about maintaining proper humidity required by the species.

INFORMATION FOR CLIENTS

- Avoid retained spectacles by keeping the snake at its preferred optimal temperature zone (POTZ) and proper humidity.
- Do not attempt to remove the spectacles. Have the veterinarian remove them after they have been softened.
- Avoid handling snakes with retained spectacles because they may be more likely to strike because of poor visual capability.

Corneal Lesions

Corneal lesions are usually the result of attempts to remove retained spectacles or of ocular trauma.

CLINICAL SIGNS

- Cloudy cornea

DIAGNOSIS

- Positive staining results (as in mammals)

TREATMENT

- Antibiotic ointments (without steroids)
- Third eyelid flap or cyanoacrylate adhesive for deep ulcers

Cataracts

Both juvenile and senile cataracts have been reported in reptiles (Fig. 41-2).

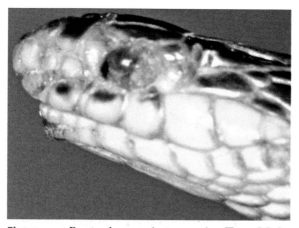

Figure 41-1 Retained spectacle in a snake. (From Mader DR: *Reptile medicine and surgery*, ed 2, St. Louis, MO, 2006, Saunders, by permission. Courtesy of S. Barten.)

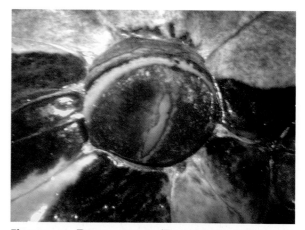

Figure 41-2 Dense cataract. (From Mader DR: *Reptile medicine and surgery*, ed 2, St. Louis, MO, 2006, Saunders, by permission.)

CLINICAL SIGNS

- White color, opaqueness of lens in papillary opening
- Behavior indicative of blindness; striking, failure to feed, nervousness

DIAGNOSIS

- Physical and ophthalmology examination

TREATMENT

- No treatment for cataracts is available.
- These animals must be hand-fed and handled carefully.

INFORMATION FOR CLIENTS

- Snakes with visual impairment may be more prone to strike when handled.
- These animals must be hand-fed.

Iguanas

Most problems that involve the eye in the green iguana are the result of infection or trauma. Restraining a struggling iguana by holding the back of its head can result in bilateral periorbital swelling from engorgement of the venous sinuses in the area (Fig. 41-3).

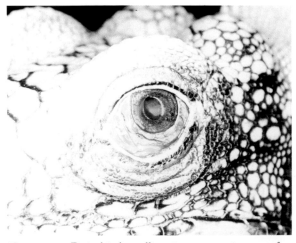

Figure 41-3 Periorbital swelling in a green iguana after struggling violently against vigorous restraint. (From Mader DR: *Reptile medicine and surgery*, ed 2, St. Louis, MO, 2006, Saunders, by permission.)

This swelling should disappear with time. Eyelids may be torn in fights with cage mates or by sharp projections in the cage. Blepharospasm may be caused by foreign material such as sand and bedding materials in the eyes. External parasites may be found around the eyes in some lizards. Keratitis is usually caused by a bacterial infection, and ulceration of the cornea may occur because of trauma.

Ocular and Periocular Trauma

CLINICAL SIGNS

- Periorbital swelling after handling
- Tissue damage to palpebrae after trauma
- Blepharospasm

DIAGNOSIS

- Physical examination and history
- Complete ophthalmic examination
- Complete blood cell count (CBC) and serum chemistries to rule out systemic disease
- Culture and sensitivity if bacterial cause suspected

TREATMENT

- Depends on outcome of diagnostic procedures
- If foreign body is suspected:
  - Flushing of the conjunctival tissue with eye wash solution
  - Antibiotic ophthalmic ointment
- If ulceration of the cornea is present:
  - Flushing to remove any foreign material
  - Antibiotic ophthalmic ointment
- If trauma to palpebrae has occurred:
  - Cleaning of the palpebrae with eye wash solution
  - Surgical repair of lacerations, if possible
  - Antibiotic ophthalmic ointment

REVIEW QUESTIONS

1. The most common cause of retained spectacles in the snake is:
   a. Inadequate diet
   b. Low environmental humidity
   c. Improper cage materials
   d. Lack of vitamin B

2. Care should be taken when handling snakes with visual impairment as they may be more prone to strike.
   a. True
   b. False
3. The large, vascular bundle that protrudes into the vitreus from the reptilian retina is known as the:
   a. Macula densa
   b. Conus papillaris
   c. Vitreous bundle
   d. Pectin vascularis

4. Retained spectacles should be removed by _____.
   a. Soaking until softened
   b. Use of a hemostat
   c. Pulled loose using thumb forceps
5. Improper restraint of the green iguana may result in _____.
   a. Bruising of the skin
   b. Periorbital swelling
   c. Hemorrhage in the mouth

Answers found on page 556.

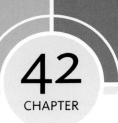

Diseases of the Integumentary System

LEARNING OBJECTIVES

When you have completed this chapter, you will be able to:

1. Recognize common causes for skin disease in reptiles.

2. Explain to clients how improper environment affects the skin of the pet.

Snakes

As in other animals, the skin of the reptile is the largest organ of the body and is important for the protection of internal structures, to prevent drying, and to prevent invasion by bacterial, fungal, and viral organisms. Normal reptilian skin consists of two layers, the epidermis and dermis. The epidermis is covered completely by keratin, forming scales and joints. The dorsal skin of some reptiles may be ornamental or defensive in structure (as in horned lizards).

The ventral surface skin is thin in some species and thick in others. The dermis consists of connective tissue and may contain small bones called *osteoderms*. Normal reptilian skin heals more slowly compared with mammalian skin, with lesions often taking up to 6 weeks to heal, and the speed of healing may be related to environmental temperatures. (Healing is faster at higher temperatures.)

Reptiles shed their skin periodically in a process known as *ecdysis*. The frequency of shedding is related to the species, age, state of nutrition, reproductive status, parasitic load, ambient temperature, and humidity. In snakes, the process normally replicates existing skin and replaces the entire epidermis, with the old skin usually shed in one piece. The process takes about 2 weeks. The animal may not feed and be cranky, so owners should limit handling them during this time. During ecdysis, the skin is much more permeable, and topical medications may be more readily absorbed.

Dysecdysis (Difficult or Incomplete Shedding)

Difficulty shedding or failure to completely shed is a common problem in snakes kept in excessively dry environments (Fig. 42-1). Areas of old scar tissue, suture lines, or areas heavily parasitized may also fail to shed completely.

CLINICAL SIGNS

- Dry, flaky skin
- Skin firmly attached at some points, loose at others
- Retained spectacles

DIAGNOSIS

- Physical examination
- History of recent shedding

TREATMENT

- Soak the snake in a warm-water bath until skin loosens.
- Gently remove the loosened skin.
- Improve environmental humidity to prevent recurrence.

INFORMATION FOR CLIENTS

- Snakes preparing to shed will often appear dull in color and be irritable.
- Keep environmental humidity within the proper limits for the species.
- Placing a rough object in the cage (carpet, brick, rough wood) will help the snake when shedding.
- Avoid using any topical medications during the shedding period.

Abscesses

Abscesses are one of the more common dermatologic problems seen in captive reptiles (Fig. 42-2). Bite wounds, cage trauma, prey bites, and attacks from cage mates may all result in infection with gram-negative bacteria. Reptiles, like birds, form caseous abscesses; they contain inspissated or dry pus that must be removed surgically. Culture and sensitivity are necessary for proper treatment.

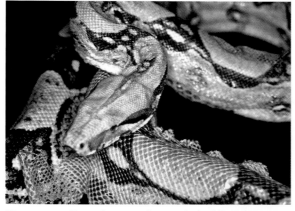

Figure 42-1 Dysecdysis, or abnormal shedding, has many causes. (From Mader DR: *Reptile medicine and surgery*, ed 2, St. Louis, MO, 2006, Saunders, by permission.)

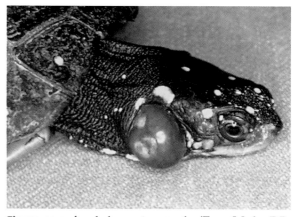

Figure 42-2 Aural abscess in a turtle. (From Mader DR: *Reptile medicine and surgery*, ed 2, St. Louis, MO, 2006, Saunders, by permission.)

CLINICAL SIGNS

- Firm, swollen mass on the surface of the animal; commonly on the head or trunk

DIAGNOSIS

- Physical examination and history of trauma or fighting
- Complete blood cell count (CBC)
  - Needle aspirate
  - Culture and sensitivity
- Radiology or ultrasonography

TREATMENT

- Surgical curettage of the abscess
- Flushing of the capsule until healing is well under way
- Topical antibiotics: silver sulfadiazine (Silvadene) ointment or other antibiotic ointment

INFORMATION FOR CLIENTS

- Avoid housing different species together.
- Feed only killed or recently killed prey; avoid feeding live prey.
- Some animals will ram their nose against glass or wire in an attempt to escape. This may cause a rostral abscess.

Discolorations

Discolorations frequently occur in animals with infections, trauma, or metabolic disease. The most common discolorations are brownish, greenish, reddish, or yellowish discolorations of the scales.

CLINICAL SIGNS

- Discoloration of scales in a previous healthy-appearing animal
- Clinical signs of other diseases

DIAGNOSIS

- Physical examination and history
- CBC, serum chemistry
- Culture and sensitivity of discolored areas

TREATMENT

- Depends on diagnostic workup results

INFORMATION FOR CLIENTS

- If you treat the problem, the discoloration may disappear with the next shedding.

Parasites

The most common dermal parasites seen in snakes are ticks (*Ixodes*, *Argasidae*, *Amblyomma*) (Fig. 42-3) and mites (*Ophionyssus natricis*; the snake mite). Numerous species inhabit reptiles, but the treatment is the same for all infestations.

CLINICAL SIGNS

- Scales that are lifted from the surface (ticks)
- Small red or brown dots moving under scales or between scales, especially around the eyes and cloaca (mites)

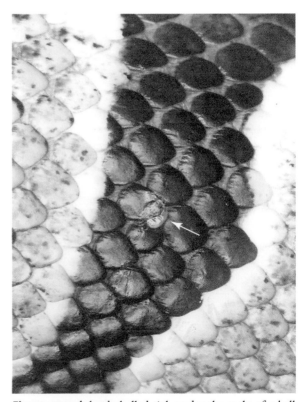

Figure 42-3 A hard-shelled tick under the scale of a ball python. (From Mader DR: *Reptile medicine and surgery*, ed 2, St. Louis, MO, 2006, Saunders, by permission.)

- Rubbing or twisting of bodies or remaining in water for extended periods
- Anemia (both ticks and mites)

DIAGNOSIS

- Observation of the parasite on the surface of the skin

TREATMENT

- Ticks: Manually remove all ticks.
  - Treat the area topically with antibacterial ointment
  - ± Systemic antibiotics
- Mites: Place the animal in 5% Sevin dust for 4 to 5 hours; then rinse the animal with a 1% ivermectin spray (prepared by mixing 5 mg ivermectin with 1 quart water).
- Thoroughly clean and disinfect the cage and cage furniture; remove any wood where mites might hide.

INFORMATION FOR CLIENTS

- Prevent infestation with parasites by housing the reptile in a clean environment.
- Treat all new additions to the collection before adding them to the cage.
- Examine your reptile frequently for external parasites.
- Never add caught wild snakes to your collection.

Trauma

Types of trauma commonly seen in reptile patients include cage trauma (usually to the nose and facial area), prey trauma (from the prey attacking the snake), and thermal trauma (caused by burns from hot rocks or heating lamps). As a result of the snake's environment, almost all wounds become infected and will require treatment. Bacteria such as *Aeromonas*, *Corynebacteria*, *Mycobacterium*, *Pseudomonas*, and *Salmonella* have been associated with both abscesses and superficial lesions in snakes.

Prey Trauma

Trauma from prey occurs when a live animal is fed to the snake and ends up attacking the snake instead (Fig. 42-4). Wounds may be superficial, but snakes may be critically injured or even killed by larger prey with a desire to survive. This type of trauma can be

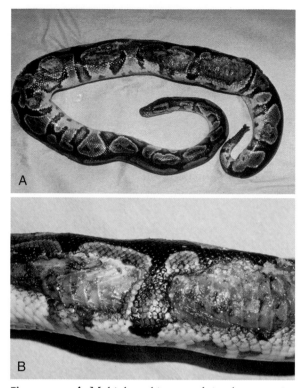

Figure 42-4 A, Multiple rat bite wounds in a boa constrictor. **B,** Close-up of some of the wounds on the same snake. (From Mader DR: *Reptile medicine and surgery*, ed 2, St. Louis, MO, 2006, Saunders, by permission.)

prevented by feeding killed or stunned prey and carefully monitoring the feeding process until the end.

CLINICAL SIGNS

- Fresh wounds anywhere on the body immediately after feeding

DIAGNOSIS

- History and physical examination
- Culture and sensitivity if infected

TREATMENT

- Wet-to-dry bandages of all wounds
- Surgical repair, if necessary, to close the wounds
- New-Skin (Prestigebrands, Irving, NY) to protect healing tissue
- Antibiotics (systemic), if needed

INFORMATION FOR CLIENTS

- Never leave live rodents in a reptile cage overnight, or preferably feed only killed or stunned prey.
- Serious wounds are an emergency and should be seen by your veterinarian immediately.
- Most of these lesions will heal well in time and with proper treatment.

Cage Trauma

Cage trauma is usually the result of the active snake attempting to escape confinement by butting against or hitting the cage with its nose, which results in abrasions that may become infected. These infections often spread to the oral cavity if left untreated.

CLINICAL SIGNS

- Abrasions or abscesses in the rostral area
- Swelling and inflammation of oral, nasal tissues

DIAGNOSIS

- Observation of traumatic behavior
- Physical examination
- Culture and sensitivity if infected

TREATMENT

- Clean the wounds.
- Apply Silvadene cream or other antibiotic agents.
- Prevent further trauma by:
  - Keeping the pet in a larger enclosure with smooth, high sides.
  - Avoiding the use of wire cages. (*Do not tap on the glass.*)

INFORMATION FOR CLIENTS

- Keep your pet in the largest enclosure possible.
- Discourage others from tapping on the glass.
- The sides of the enclosure should be smooth.
- Give the snake lots of places to hide.

Thermal Trauma

Thermal trauma is usually the result of improper use of hot rocks or heat lamps and is frequently seen in captive snakes and lizards (Fig. 42-5). Large areas of necrotizing dermatitis are found on the ventral surface where the animal has contacted the heat source. These wounds typically become infected with multiple gram-negative bacteria.

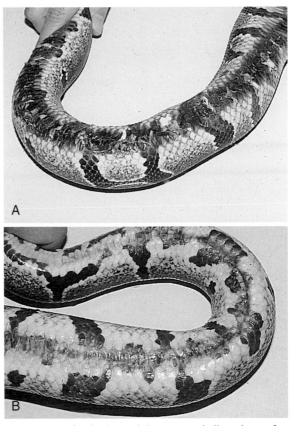

Figure 42-5 A, A thermal burn in a ball python after 4 weeks of healing and just before shedding. **B,** The same ball python 15 minutes later after shedding was completed. (From Mader DR: *Reptile medicine and surgery*, ed 2, St. Louis, MO, 2006, Saunders, by permission.)

CLINICAL SIGNS

- Large areas of erythema and necrotizing dermatitis on the ventral surface

DIAGNOSIS

- History and physical examination
- Culture and sensitivity if infected

TREATMENT

- Removal of animal from the heat source
- Silvadene cream application to lesions twice daily
- Systemic antibiotics, depending on culture and sensitivity

INFORMATION FOR CLIENTS

- Hot rocks are not recommended as a cage heat source. A safer method of heating the enclosure would be a floor warmer or a heat lamp placed outside the cage.

Hyperthyroidism

Hyperthyroidism has been associated with frequent ecdysis cycles in snakes, especially corn snakes.

CLINICAL SIGNS

- Excessive number of ecdysis cycles (up to one every 2 weeks)

DIAGNOSIS

- Clinical signs
- Thyroid tests are often ambiguous

TREATMENT

- Tapazole daily may reduce the frequency of shedding.

Neoplasia

Neoplasms of all body systems have been reported in Squamata (snakes). Tumors most often associated with the integumentary system include fibrosarcomas, melanomas, squamous cell carcinomas, sarcomas, and histiocytomas. It is important for the veterinarian to differentiate a tumor from other masses found in the epidermis (most commonly abscesses and granulomas or parasitic swellings).

CLINICAL SIGNS

- Lump or mass palpated or observed on the surface of the animal

DIAGNOSIS

- Physical examination and history
- Fine-needle aspiration or biopsy
- Impression smears

TREATMENT

- Surgical excision *or*
- Cryosurgery *or*
- Photodynamic therapy (has been used in some cases)

INFORMATION FOR CLIENTS

- Report any lump or bump on your snake to your veterinarian.

- A diagnosis can be made only with histopathologic analysis.
- Surgical excision is the common treatment for tumors of the integumentary system.
- The rate of metastasis of these tumors is unknown. Further treatment may be required at a later date.

Iguanas

Lizards have a fairly thick skin covered by scales. They shed their skin periodically just like snakes, except they usually shed the skin in pieces. Rapidly growing lizards may shed as often as every few weeks. Iguanas have femoral pores on the ventral aspect of the thigh—male lizards have large pores, whereas female lizards have smaller ones (Fig. 42-6). Dewlaps and spines are also present in the iguana. These secondary sex characteristics are useful for attracting mates and for appearing ferocious when attacked. Iguanas have large, sharp claws that must be trimmed frequently to prevent injury to humans. Iguanas have tail autotomy (they can shed the tail when needed.) Never grasp an iguana by the tail while restraining it.

Failure to Shed

Dysecdysis, or difficulty shedding, may occur in iguanas (Fig. 42-7). Most shedding problems may be related to environmental humidity levels that are too low (<60% to 70%). Iguanas entering a shedding period will usually become dull in color.

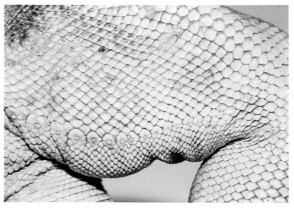

Figure 42-6 Sex differences in femoral pores. (From Mader DR: *Reptile medicine and surgery*, ed 2, St. Louis, MO, 2006, Saunders, by permission.)

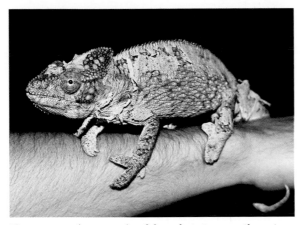

Figure 42-7 An example of dysecdysis in a reptile patient. (From Mader DR: *Reptile medicine and surgery*, ed 2, St. Louis, MO, 2006, Saunders, by permission. Courtesy of D. Mader.)

CLINICAL SIGNS

- Retained pieces of skin on the iguana
- ± Necrosis of the digits or tail where bands of dried tissue remain

DIAGNOSIS

- Physical examination and history of recent shedding
- History of poor environment or dietary conditions

TREATMENT

- Soak the iguana in warm water to facilitate the removal of skin tags.
- Mist the iguana daily to prevent dehydration.
- Lubricants such as K-Y jelly or mineral oil may be used to aid in shedding.

INFORMATION FOR CLIENTS

- Decrease the incidence of dysecdysis by maintaining proper humidity levels in the iguana's environment.
- Daily misting will help maintain skin hydration.
- Provide a bathing pool for soaking in the cage.
- Do not attempt to remove retained skin before soaking and loosening; you may tear the underlying tissue.
- Failure to remove dead skin may result in constriction of digits and limbs, followed by tissue death and dry gangrene.

Abrasions, Abscesses, and Other Sores

Abrasions and sores are frequently seen on the rostral portion of the head and on the plantar area of the feet in lizards kept in wire cages (Fig. 42-8). Abscesses resulting from open wounds may develop as a consequence of a contaminated environment and the normal bacterial flora of the reptile. Reptilian abscesses are caseous in nature as in the bird and must be curetted surgically before treatment. Thermal burns from heat lamps and hot rocks may also be a problem in iguanas. These thermal burns may also become infected, leading to systemic disease.

CLINICAL SIGNS

- Presence of a penetrating or superficial wound
- ± Swollen or painful on palpation
- ± Local joint involvement
- Presence of a bite wound

DIAGNOSIS

- Physical examination and history
- Palpation and exploration of the wound
- Culture and sensitivity if infected

TREATMENT

- Clean the wound: chlorhexidine or dilute povidone-iodine (Betadine) solution
- Surgical curettage and repair, if necessary

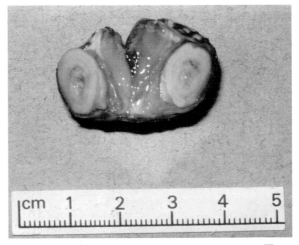

Figure 42-8 Caseous abscess in the green iguana. (From Mader DR: *Reptile medicine and surgery*, ed 2, St. Louis, MO, 2006, Saunders, by permission.)

- Systemic antibiotics based on culture and sensitivity
- Correction of caging problems

INFORMATION FOR CLIENTS

- Animals housed exclusively on rough wire cage floorings are prone to develop sores on their feet, and these sores can easily become infected.
- Bacterial infections are common as a result of reptile wounds. Have all wounds treated promptly to avoid infection.
- Keep heat lamps out of the reptile's reach in the cage. Avoid using hot rocks.

Color Changes

Color changes are seen frequently in iguanas (see Fig. 37-2). Some changes are normal and may be associated with breeding season. Male iguanas become more brightly colored during breeding season, with some taking on a bright orange color. This coloration may last for a few months. Female iguanas may develop an orange color also, but it is not usually as pronounced as that in male iguanas. Stress may also produce a color change. Iguanas may become almost white, bright yellow, green, or very dark in color, depending on the stress level and the individual animal. When exposed to sunlight, their color may darken and dark spots may appear on their backs. When they feel too hot, they lighten their color (less heat absorption). Some color changes, however, are related to diseases.

Infectious black spots on the skin are related to fungal diseases in the iguana. These spots will be of a different texture than that of normal scales and are dry and crusty. Dry gangrene may also produce black areas on skin. A correct diagnosis is necessary before beginning treatment.

CLINICAL SIGNS

- Color of the skin changes
- ± Other signs of systemic disease (animal color usually brownish)

DIAGNOSIS

- Complete history (including breeding history)
- Physical examination
- CBC and serum chemistries
- Fecal examination

- Scraping and fungal culture
- ± Skin biopsy

TREATMENT

- No treatment necessary if color change is normal
- Positive fungal culture: antifungal creams applied to lesions
- Systemic illness: treatment for specific problem
- Dry gangrene may require surgical amputation

INFORMATION FOR CLIENTS

- Know your iguana! Note color changes in your animal under varying conditions.
- Any acute color changes that do not appear to be normal for your pet should be reported to your veterinarian. It may be a sign of illness.

Ascariasis (Ticks and Mites)

External parasites seen in iguanas include ticks and mites. This is usually a problem when animals are kept in unsanitary conditions.

CLINICAL SIGNS

- Excessive scratching
- Shedding problems
- Abnormal-looking scales
- Visible parasites walking on the surface of the animal

DIAGNOSIS

- Visual observation of parasites on skin
- Clinical signs

TREATMENT

- Ivermectin
- Manual removal of ticks
- Topical products to eradicate fleas or ticks, and mites (pyrethroids are best) applied to a towel and wiped onto the iguana; powders may be dusted on the animal and then wiped or washed off
- Olive oil or mineral oil: cover the animal's body lightly to suffocate mites
- Submerge the animal in water—and repeat until mite-free
- Treatment of the environment to prevent reinfestation:
  - Discard any substrate materials and cage accessories that are replaceable. Scrub the habitat and

other accessories with a solution of ½ cup bleach to 1 gallon water. Soak bowls and perches in this solution for 8 hours. Bake wooden toys and platforms at 200°F for 2 to 3 hours to kill any mites or eggs. Treat the enclosure with a pyrethroid pesticide spray; then wait for 15 to 20 minutes before wiping it out. Air out the cage well before placing the animal back into the area.

INFORMATION FOR CLIENTS

- *Never* use pesticides on your iguana without the approval of the veterinarian. Avoid over-the-counter products used for dogs and cats.
- You must treat both the animal and the cage at the same time to avoid reinfestation.
- New additions to your collection should be treated for mites and ticks before placing the new animals with other members of your collection.
- When treating lizards with topical preparations, avoid the eyes because iguanas have no protective eye cap.

Turtles

Beak lesions, shell fractures, and skin problems are common in turtles. Many of these problems may be related to improper housing and diet, and some to trauma caused by predators.

Shell Fractures

Shell fractures are common in turtles, usually as a result of trauma. Predators such as dogs and coyotes cause many of these injuries, as do automobiles (Fig. 42-9), lawn mowers, and other moving vehicles. Shells have a remarkable ability to heal, and scars of old injuries are visible in many wild turtles (Fig. 42-10). Whenever the shell is damaged, additional damage to the underlying soft tissues should be investigated.

CLINICAL SIGNS

- Damage to the shell seen on examination
- ± Signs of systemic trauma, pulmonary contusions, or both

DIAGNOSIS

- History of trauma
- Complete physical examination

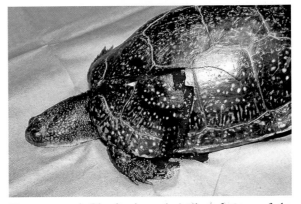

Figure 42-9 A Blanding's turtle with a fracture of the carapace as a result of being struck by an automobile. (From Mader DR: *Reptile medicine and surgery*, ed 2, St. Louis, MO, 2006, Saunders, by permission.)

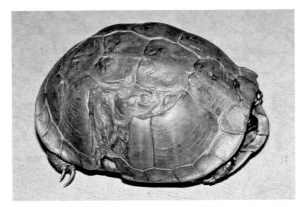

Figure 42-10 A wild-caught three-toed box turtle with a healed fracture of the carapace. (From Mader DR: *Reptile medicine and surgery*, ed 2, St. Louis, MO, 2006, Saunders, by permission.)

- Radiography
- Neurologic examination if area involves spinal area

TREATMENT

- Flush fresh wounds with large amounts of sterile saline for fresh wounds.
- Administer topical and parenteral antibiotics if wounds are more than a few hours old.
- Apply honey or sugar bandages or wet-to-dry bandages daily until a healthy granulation bed forms.
- Primary shell repair may be attempted using acrylics such as Superglue or dental acrylics used for

hoof repair (use carefully because they generate heat when curing).

- Metal bridges may be formed using wire and orthopedic screws or strips of metal adhered using epoxy glue.
- Cable-tie method of shell repair uses nylon cable ties to secure the shell fragments.

● TECH ALERT

Healing of the turtle shell may take up to several years. These wounds will need to be managed properly until complete healing is accomplished.

INFORMATION FOR CLIENTS

- Avoid injury to turtles by keeping them in a protective environment.
- Teach children how to handle turtles. Remind anyone who wishes to handle your turtles that turtles often urinate when handled. If warned, they will be less likely to drop the turtle when surprised!

Myiasis

Turtles are commonly presented for "fly-strike." Sarcophaga flies are commonly implicated in the infestation.

CLINICAL SIGNS

- Crusty black discharge at the shell–skin margins
- Swollen lesion with a visible air hole

DIAGNOSIS

- Complete physical examination
- Presence of cystic lesions containing air holes

TREATMENT

- Maggots should be carefully removed from the cysts under general anesthesia.
- Wounds should be flushed until clean.
- Topical and systemic antibiotics should be administered, as necessary

INFORMATION FOR CLIENTS

- Fly control helps prevent myiasis.
- Maggots must be removed whole to avoid anaphylaxis.

Thermal Burns

Turtles are heliotherms and love to bask in the warm sunlight. However, many owners do not allow their turtles outdoors and, instead, seek to provide warmth with the use of hot rocks or heating lamps. These devices may reach temperatures that can burn the flesh of any animal resting on them.

CLINICAL SIGNS

- Depend on the duration of exposure and the temperature of the heat source
- Burn lesions varying from first degree to third degree
- Edema of the tissue, blistering, oozing from lesions

DIAGNOSIS

- Visual confirmation of a burn lesion
- History of exposure to external heat source

TREATMENT

- Cold-water compresses for first-degree burns
- Topical burn dressing applied after a gentle cleansing (silver sulfadiazine)
- Therapy for shock in severe burn cases
- Intravenous (IV) fluids
- IV antibiotics
- Daily cleansing and debridement of unhealthy tissues

INFORMATION FOR CLIENTS

- Treatment for second-degree and third-degree burns may be prolonged and expensive.
- Avoid thermal burns by not using hot rocks in the cage.
- Reptiles have great ability to heal. The prognosis for less severe burns is good.

REVIEW QUESTION

1. The term *dysecdysis* means:
   a. A type of dystocia
   b. A difficult shed
   c. Inflammation of the hemipenis
   d. A lack of tear duct formation

2. The most effective treatment for dysecdysis in the snake is to:
   a. Use oil to loosen the skin
   b. Increase the humidity by soaking
   c. Rub the snake with a terry towel
   d. Wait until the next shedding
3. Dry, scaly black spots on the skin of the iguana may be caused by:
   a. Bacteria
   b. Viruses
   c. Fungi
   d. Parasites
4. When sexing iguanas, one can see that the males have _____ femoral pores compared with females.
   a. Larger
   b. Smaller
5. The most common cause of shell damage in turtles is:
   a. Fungal disease
   b. Bacterial infection
   c. Predator trauma
   d. Poor husbandry

6. Turtles often _____ when handled.
   a. Defecate
   b. Bite
   c. Urinate
7. Hot rocks are useful for maintaining the environmental temperature in snake cages.
   a. True
   b. False

Answers found on page 556.

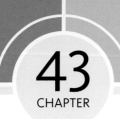

43 CHAPTER

Diseases of the Musculoskeletal System

LEARNING OBJECTIVES

When you have completed this chapter, you will be able to:
1. Recognize metabolic bone disease (MBD) and its causes.

2. Discuss with owners how to correct the diet and environment of reptiles affected by MBD.

Snakes

Metabolic Bone Disease

The most common disease of the musculoskeletal system of snakes is metabolic bone disease (MBD), which is the result of poor diet and husbandry practices. This disease is the result of a dietary deficiency of calcium, vitamin D, or both; a negative calcium to phosphorus (Ca/P) ratio; or lack of exposure to ultraviolet light. MBD is usually a disease of young, rapidly growing reptiles. Lack of circulating calcium stimulates resorption of bone to correct the imbalance and, over time, bones become soft and easily fractured. Diets that lack calcium-containing bone are a common cause of MBD (all-meat diets, dog-food diets); for this reason, the disease is rare in mice-eating snakes.

CLINICAL SIGNS

- Deformities of bony structures (head, spine, ribs, etc.)
- "Rubber jaw": softening of bones of the mandible and maxilla

DIAGNOSIS

- Dietary history and physical examination
- Radiography: lack of bone density, stress fractures
- Ca/P serum levels

TREATMENT

- Improved diet
- Calcium supplementation; calcium glubionate orally or by injection
- Parenteral vitamin D
- Calcitonin when patient is normocalcemic (calcium levels between 8 and 11 mg/dL)
- Cage rest and careful handling to prevent further fractures
- Tube feeding, if necessary

INFORMATION FOR CLIENTS

- Because the carnivorous diet of the snake usually provides the proper level of calcium and phosphorus, snakes rarely acquire MBD.
- The prognosis for MBD depends on the owner's ability to treat the reptile on a long-term basis.

Neoplasia

Osteosarcomas of the mandible and spinal area have been reported in snakes. As with tumors of the integumentary system, the veterinarian must rule out other causes of lumps and bumps before treatment.

CLINICAL SIGNS

- Firm swelling over a bony surface
- ± Loss of condition

DIAGNOSIS

- Other causes of lumps and bumps (abscesses, granulomas) ruled out
- Radiology
- Biopsy

TREATMENT

- Surgical excision
- ± Radiation therapy

INFORMATION FOR CLIENTS

- The prognosis for this type of tumor is poor. Metastasis may occur.

Iguanas

Metabolic Bone Disease

MBD is primarily a disease of long-term deficiency of calcium, vitamin D, or both; a lack of exposure to sunlight, and an improper Ca/P ratio. The disease is commonly seen in young, fast-growing reptiles. Over time, a diet low in calcium or lack of vitamin D and sunlight will cause increased bone resorption and a weakening of all the bones within the body. Affected animals experience development of pathologic fractures, and healing bone is replaced by fibrous tissue. As a result of their herbivorous dietary requirements (low calcium and high phosphorus levels), iguanas are quite susceptible to MBD.

CLINICAL SIGNS

- Lack of ability to lift the trunk off the ground when attempting to walk (Fig. 43-1)
- Swelling around the long bones of the legs ("Popeye" legs)
- Pliable mandible or maxilla
- Lameness or reluctance to move

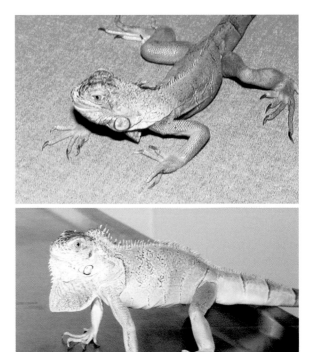

Figure 43-1 Evidence of metabolic bone disease in the iguana in the upper image, compared with the healthy iguana in the bottom image. (From Mader DR: *Reptile medicine and surgery*, ed 2, St. Louis, MO, 2006, Saunders, by permission.)

- Weight loss
- ± Paralysis

DIAGNOSIS

- Complete blood cell count (CBC), serum chemistries
  - Calcium levels less than 8.5 mg/dL
  - Increased phosphorus levels
  - Ca/P ratio reversed from normal
- History
  - Lack of exposure to sunlight
  - Lack of calcium supplementation in all-herbivorous diet
- Insufficient vitamin D_3 supplementation
  - Physical examination
  - Radiography
- Transverse fractures of long bones may be present
- Decreased bone density

TREATMENT

- Correct all dietary and environmental deficiencies.
- Correct all medical problems: fractures, dehydration, among others.
- Tube-feed, if the animal is not eating (Emeraid II, Lafeber Company, Cornell, IL).
- Administer calcium glubionate syrup (Neo-Calglucon).
- Administer vitamin D_3 injection (at least two doses).
- Give calcitonin injections as calcium levels return to normal.

PREVENTION

- Exposure to sunlight is extremely important for green iguanas.
- Supplement low-calcium diets with calcium.
- Make sure vitamin supplements contain vitamin D_3.

⦿ TECH ALERT

Handle iguanas with MBD with care because their bones are easily fractured and spinal injuries may occur.

INFORMATION FOR CLIENTS

- All iguanas need sunlight. Glass filters out necessary wavelengths, so the iguana needs either full-spectrum lighting or exposure to outside sunlight.

- Make sure that the vitamin supplement you are giving contains the proper balance for your reptile. Ask your veterinarian to review the product with you.
- Do not allow affected animals to climb or be handled until the imbalances can be corrected.
- Make sure to provide foods that contain a Ca/P ratio of about 1:1 to 2:1.

Tail Autotomy

Many lizards, including the green iguana, are capable of losing their tails. This provides a means of escape when grabbed by a predator. The iguana's tail has a vertical fracture plane through the body and part of the neural arch of each vertebra in the caudal portion of the tail, allowing the tail to come loose when needed. As the iguana ages, these planes tend to ossify, resulting in a more stable tail. Tails that come loose may be replaced in young iguanas, but the resulting tails are usually smaller and of a different color from that of the original tail.

CLINICAL SIGNS

- Tail breaking off as a result of trauma (Fig. 43-2)

DIAGNOSIS

- Fractured tail separated from the animal

TREATMENT

- Stop the bleeding; use styptic powder.
- Disinfect the stump, and apply antibiotic ointment.

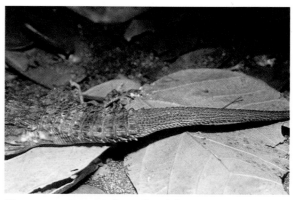

Figure 43-2 Iguanas have the ability to regenerate their tails after traumatic amputation. (From Mader DR: *Reptile medicine and surgery*, ed 2, St. Louis, MO, 2006, Saunders, by permission.)

- Suturing of the stump will usually delay or prevent regeneration.
- If the lesion occurs in the proximal tail or the tissue is severely damaged, amputation may be necessary.

INFORMATION FOR CLIENTS

- Never grab your iguana by the tail for restraint.
- If your iguana's tail is injured, have it examined by your veterinarian. Tail infections may become a serious problem.

⬤ TECH ALERT

Never grab an iguana's tail for restraint.

Fractures of the Extremities

Fractures, other than those related to MBD, do occur in iguanas, usually as a result of trauma. Healing in reptiles is slow, and healing of fractures may require up to 2 years. Internal or external coaptation may be used. External coaptation methods frequently used include splints, slings, Kirschner apparatus, and bandages. Internal coaptation using intramuscular (IM) pins may be required in severe long-bone fractures.

CLINICAL SIGNS

- Lameness or disuse of limb
- Swelling
- Pain on palpation
- Signs of trauma (bruising, torn skin, hemorrhage)

DIAGNOSIS

- History of trauma, physical examination
- Radiography
- CBC and serum chemistries to rule out MBD

TREATMENT

- Stabilization of the fracture site (method will depend on the size of the animal and the location of the fracture):
  - Ball bandage for fracture of the digits
  - Spica splint for fractures of the femur or humerus
  - Tubular splint for distal femoral or humeral fractures

- Body splint (taping the leg to the body as a splint)
- IM pins (Kirschner wires [K-wires] or needles may be used as IM pins)
- K-wires or needles with dental acrylic may be used to construct a Kirschner apparatus
- Bone plates used in large lizards
- Splints and casts may need to be changed frequently in young, growing animals
- Systemic antibiotics if infection is suspected

INFORMATION FOR CLIENTS

- Care must be taken that the external device does not become entangled in cage furniture or basking limbs.
- Splints and casts should be kept dry and clean.
- Splints and casts may need to be replaced frequently during the healing process.
- It may take up to 2 years for proper healing to occur.

Turtles

Diseases of the musculoskeletal system in turtles usually involve trauma or nutritional problems. The most frequently seen disease is MBD, or nutritional secondary hyperparathyroidism.

Metabolic Bone Disease (Nutritional Secondary Hyperparathyroidism)

MBD, or "rubber jaw," is a result of a diet deficient in calcium or vitamin D, a Ca/P imbalanced diet, or inadequate exposure to ultraviolet light (sunlight). The disease is seen in all reptiles and amphibians but is most common in aquatic turtles and lizards.

CLINICAL SIGNS

- Neuromuscular twitching
- Soft bones, soft shells, deformed shells
- Thickening or swelling of long bones, pathologic fractures
- Weakness
- ± Cloacal prolapse

DIAGNOSIS

- Complete physical examination and environmental history

- CBC, serum chemistries: low calcium levels
- Radiography indicates decreased bone density, fractures

TREATMENT

- Correct the underlying dietary and husbandry problems.
- Use calcium glubionate orally and vitamin D to correct deficits.
- Calcitonin can be used if blood calcium levels are corrected first.

Supportive Care

- Treatment for any dehydration
- Calorie supplementation
- Prevention of further fractures

INFORMATION FOR CLIENTS

- Nutritional secondary hyperparathyroidism can be avoided by feeding diets with a proper Ca/P balance and ensuring turtles receive adequate exposure to sunlight.
- The prognosis for this disease depends on the severity of the lesions. Many turtles will heal and do well, but younger, more severely affected animals may never recover completely.
- If malocclusion of the beak occurs, constant trimming may be necessary.
- Female animals with this disease may have trouble passing eggs because of spinal deformities.

REVIEW QUESTIONS

1. Metabolic bone disease (MBD) is a frequent problem in green iguanas. It is related to imbalances of:
   a. Vitamin D and potassium
   b. Calcium and sodium
   c. Phosphorus and potassium
   d. Calcium and phosphorus

2. Another name for metabolic bone disease is:
   a. Hyperthyroidism
   b. Hyperadrenalcortism
   c. Nutritional secondary hyperparathyroidism
   d. Calcemic tetany

3. The _____ should never be used as the sole means for restraint of the iguana.
   a. Caudal body
   b. Dewlap
   c. Tail
   d. Dorsal spines

4. Reptiles with metabolic bone disease may present with:
   a. Multiple limb fractures
   b. Inability to eat
   c. "Popeye-shaped" limbs
   d. All of the above

5. To prevent metabolic bone disease, owners must:
   a. Feed a properly balanced diet
   b. Give antibiotics in the food
   c. Increase exercise
   d. Change the cage substrate

Answers found on page 556.

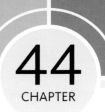

Diseases of the Nervous System

Boid
Enophthalmos

Eustachian
Flaccid

Panniculus

OUTLINE

Snakes
    Nervous System Trauma
    Spinal Osteopathy
    Toxic Neuropathies
    Inclusion Body Disease of Boids
Turtles
    Thiamine Deficiency (Nutritional)

Toxic Chemicals and Drugs
    Chlorhexidine 2%
    Ivermectin
    Heavy Metal Toxicity
Middle Ear Infection

LEARNING OBJECTIVES

When you have completed this chapter, you will be able to:
1. Recognize neurologic disease in reptiles.

2. Relate possible causes to clinical signs.

Snakes

The anatomy of the nervous system in the snake and other reptiles is similar to that in mammals, with some differences. The reptile is the first vertebrate to have developed a cerebral cortex with two hemispheres, the spinal cord extends to the tip of the tail, and there is no cauda equina. The locomotor centers within the spinal cord give it functional autonomy from the brain. It is often difficult to assess the neurologic function of the snake; however, a history of movement difficulties (lack of ability to strike prey, head tilt, tremors) should alert one to the possibility of neurologic disease.

Nervous System Trauma

Head trauma or spinal cord trauma may result in neurologic dysfunction in the snake.

CLINICAL SIGNS
- Related to the site of trauma:
  - Head: seizures
  - Spine: lack of panniculus reaction caudal to lesion, paralysis or paresis

DIAGNOSIS
- Neurologic examination, physical examination
- Radiography

TREATMENT

Supportive Care

- Corticosteroids to decrease inflammation
- Spinal support if the spinal column is fractured

Spinal Osteopathy

The exact cause of spinal osteopathy is unknown; however, it is believed to be related to exposure to a virus that affects mice fed as prey or to a virus of snakes spread by mice. Some think it may be caused by a slowly developing neoplasm or by septicemia. Many suppositions can be found in the literature.

CLINICAL SIGNS

- Multifocal swellings along the dorsum of the spine that are painful on palpation
- Progressive remodeling of the vertebra with ankylosis of the spine
- Finally, inability of the snake to move, constrict, or swallow
- Injury to the spinal cord

DIAGNOSIS

- Physical examination and history
- Radiography
- ± Blood cultures to rule out septicemia

TREATMENT

- If cultures are positive, long-term antibiotic treatment and surgical debridement of lytic bone

INFORMATION FOR CLIENTS

- The prognosis for the patient with spinal osteopathy is guarded, especially if spinal cord damage has occurred.

Toxic Neuropathies

The following substances have been shown to produce neurotoxicity in reptiles:

- Insecticides
- Metronidazole
- Aminoglycosides
- Lead
- Nicotine
- Wood shavings with a high resin content (cedar shavings)

Reptiles, including snakes, are highly sensitive to many insecticides used to treat parasites. Care should be taken when exposing snakes and other species to these chemicals.

CLINICAL SIGNS

- Nonspecific (depends on the toxin):
  - Head tilt
  - Seizures
  - Paralysis
  - Vestibular signs

DIAGNOSIS

- History of exposure
- Lead: blood lead levels

TREATMENT

- Supportive: fluids, force-feeding, if necessary
- Removal of animal from source of toxin

INFORMATION FOR CLIENTS

- Use caution when exposing reptiles to any topical insecticides or oral antiparasitic agents.
- Have your pet examined immediately if any signs of toxicity develop after use of any insecticide.

Inclusion Body Disease of Boids

Inclusion body disease of boids is caused by a retrovirus and affects both boas and pythons. Because boas may be carriers of the disease, it is recommended that they not be housed with pythons.

CLINICAL SIGNS

- Multisystemic disease, including gastrointestinal, respiratory, and neurologic signs
- Acute death preceded by a flaccid paralysis
- Chronic regurgitation
- Inability to strike prey, constrict, or apprehend food
- ± Pneumonia
- Loss of righting reflex and motor coordination
- Disorientation +/− blindness

DIAGNOSIS

- Histology or electron microscopy of tissue (necropsy)

TREATMENT

- No treatment for inclusion body disease is available.

INFORMATION FOR CLIENTS

- Avoid housing pythons and boas together.
- This disease is almost always fatal in pythons, whereas boas may exhibit a mild form of the disease and become carriers.

Turtles

Neurologic disorders are not frequently seen in captive turtles. When these disorders do appear, trauma, toxicity, or nutritional causes should be suspected. Hypothiaminosis has been reported in chelonians fed vegetables high in phytothiaminases. Hypocalcemia and hypoglycemia may also be the cause of neurologic symptoms in turtles.

Thiamine Deficiency (Nutritional)

CLINICAL SIGNS

- Enophthalmos (thiamine deficiency in turtles)
- Muscle twitching
- ± Blindness, incoordination
- Difficulty eating

DIAGNOSIS

- Complete physical examination and dietary history

TREATMENT

- Correction of diet
- Subcutaneous supplementation with thiamine (B_1)

Toxic Chemicals and Drugs

Chlorhexidine

Chelonians are extremely sensitive to chlorhexidine solutions (stock 2% solutions).

CLINICAL SIGNS

- Acute flaccid paralysis
- Diminished withdrawal reflexes
- Possible loss of righting reflex

DIAGNOSIS

- History of exposure

TREATMENT

- No treatment is available.

⦿ TECH ALERT

Do not use undiluted chlorhexidine solutions on turtles.

Ivermectin

Ivermectin is extremely toxic to all chelonians and should never be used in this species.

CLINICAL SIGNS

- Neuromuscular weakness
- ± Death from paralysis of the respiratory muscles

DIAGNOSIS

- History of exposure

TREATMENT

Supportive Care
- Ventilatory support for several days
- Maintenance of hydration and caloric needs

⦿ TECH ALERT

Avoid the use of ivermectin in all chelonians.

Heavy Metal Toxicity

Turtles may ingest lead-based paint chips or lead-containing foreign bodies, which results in lead toxicity.

CLINICAL SIGNS

- Generalized central nervous system dysfunction

DIAGNOSIS

- History of ingestion of lead-containing substances
- Radiology
- Increased lead levels

TREATMENT

- Gastric lavage or enemas to remove lead-containing materials
- Treatment with calcium ethylenediamine tetraacetic acid (EDTA) intramuscularly twice daily

Middle Ear Infections

Aural abscesses or abscessation of the middle ear is a common problem in chelonians, especially box turtles.

The occurrence of abscesses is commonly linked to poor husbandry practices.

CLINICAL SIGNS

- Unilateral or bilateral swelling of the tympanum (Fig. 44-1)
- Discomfort when opening the mouth

DIAGNOSIS

- Complete physical examination and history
- Digital pressure on the tympanum resulting in expression of caseous material within the tympanic cavity
- Culture and sensitivity of material from the abscess

TREATMENT

- Surgically debride the tympanic cavity under general anesthesia using a small ear loop or curette.
- Flush the eustachian tube with sterile saline.
- Pack the wound daily with topical antibiotic ointment, and allow to heal by second intention.
- Correct any underlying hypovitaminosis A problems.

INFORMATION FOR CLIENTS

- Avoid aural abscesses with effective sanitation, proper diet, and good husbandry.

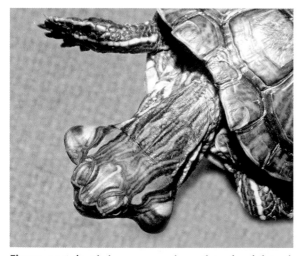

Figure 44-1 Aural abscesses may be unilateral or bilateral, as seen in this young red-eared slider. (From Mader DR: *Reptile medicine and surgery*, ed 2, St. Louis, MO, 2006, Saunders, by permission. Courtesy of D. Mader.)

- Recurrence does occur with failure to correct the underlying causes.

REVIEW QUESTIONS

1. Lack of this reflex is often useful in localizing the site of a spinal cord injury.
   a. The scratch reflex
   b. The panniculus reflex
   c. The withdrawal reflex
   d. The righting reflex
2. Aural abscesses in turtles often present with this sign.
   a. Circling and head pressing
   b. Anorexia and regurgitation
   c. Swelling on the side of the head
   d. Inability to swim or float
3. This species of snake often is a carrier of a retrovirus that may be fatal to other snakes.
   a. Boa
   b. Python
   c. Corn snake
   d. Anaconda
4. Avoid the use of this disinfectant with chelonians.
   a. Betadine
   b. Hydrogen peroxide
   c. Chlorhexidine
   d. Roccal-D
5. Never use this antiparasitic agent in turtles.
   a. Strongyd T
   b. Pyrethrins
   c. Ivermectin
   d. Permethrins
6. Lack of this substance may result in neurologic signs in the turtle.
   a. Thiamine
   b. Alanine
   c. Taurine
7. A swelling on the side of the turtle's head will usually be related to _____.
   a. Bite wounds
   b. Aural abscesses
   c. Parasites

Answers found on page 556.

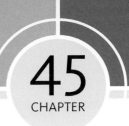

Diseases of the Reproductive System

LEARNING OBJECTIVES

When you have completed this chapter, you will be able to:
1. Recognize problems of the reproductive system that are clinically significant in reptiles.

2. Demonstrate a basic knowledge of husbandry practices that affect reproduction in reptiles.

Snakes

Diseases of the reproductive system in the snake include dystocias, prolapsed of the oviduct and cloaca, and prolapse of the penis. Some species of snakes such as pythons, king snakes, milk snakes, rat snakes, and corn snakes are oviparous (lay eggs), and others, including boas, vipers, and garter snakes, are viviparous (live bearing). The testes of the male snake are found internally in the dorsomedial portion of the coelomic cavity.

Snakes do not have an epididymis. The hemipenes are located in pouches lateral on each side of the cloaca. The location of the ovaries is similar to that of the testes. The oviducts have both an albumin-secreting function and a shell-secreting function, and a true uterus does not exist. The oviducts empty into the cloaca.

The onset of sexual maturity in snakes is affected by size, care, and diet more so than age. Snakes fed well and forced to grow rapidly may reach sexual maturity faster compared with snakes that are fed poor diets and have slower growth rates. When raised under optimal conditions, many snakes will mature between 2 and 3 years of age.

The majority of reptiles have a distinct breeding season, usually triggered by environmental stimuli such as light, temperature, rainfall, and the amount of food present. Many will begin breeding in the spring as temperatures warm; however, tropical snakes (boas and pythons) tend to breed during the cooler periods of the year. The female must be in good health with energy reserves to breed; if not, breeding may not occur. A great deal of maternal energy is used for egg production or live births. Snakes that bear live young usually produce one clutch per year, whereas egg-laying snakes may produce a clutch several times. Female snakes may suspend feeding while giving birth and lose weight. Snakes provide no maternal care for their offspring except in choosing the site in which to deposit them. Neonates usually need no assistance in hatching and are ready to live on their own immediately after birth.

Methods used or sexing a snake include probing the pouches that contain the hemipenes (the deeper pouches are found in the male), by everting the hemipenes, or by observing the spurs found just lateral to the vent (larger in male snakes). Ultrasonography or endoscopy is used to determine the presence of ovaries in the female snake.

Dystocia

Dystocia is the most common reproductive system problem seen in captive snakes. Dystocias may be divided into two groups: (1) obstructive and (2) nonobstructive. Obstructive dystocias result from an inability to pass one or more eggs or fetuses through the oviduct and the cloaca. This may result from extra-large or malpositioned eggs or fetuses, be caused by maternal abnormalities, or be a result of other masses obstructing the path. Nonobstructive causes may result from poor physical condition of the female snake, poor husbandry, improper nesting site, malnutrition, improper temperatures, and other environmental conditions.

CLINICAL SIGNS

- Visual presence of a mass in the cloaca or caudal abdomen
- ± Prolonged straining or prolapsed of the cloaca
- Often no clinical signs are obvious

DIAGNOSIS

- Physical examination and history
- Ultrasonography or radiography

TREATMENT

- Physical manipulation to remove the retained egg or fetus
- Hormonal stimulation; use of oxytocin or arginine vasotocin
- Percutaneous ovocentesis—aspirate the contents of the egg through the ventrum of the snake to decrease the size of the egg
- Surgery to remove retained eggs or fetuses
- Supportive treatment with fluids and warmth

INFORMATION FOR CLIENTS

- Snakes must be kept at optimal conditions to facilitate reproduction.
- Dystocia, although not a true emergency, should be corrected as soon as it is recognized.
- Snakes with retained eggs may repeat the dystocia on future breeding.
- Components of a good breeding program include two snakes of opposite sexes, adult snakes in good health, optimal environmental conditions, and a good diet. Absence of one or more of these may affect the snake's ability to reproduce.

Prolapse of the Oviduct and Cloaca (Colon)

Prolapse occurs with prolonged straining to pass eggs or fetuses, but it may also be caused by excessive straining for any reason (Fig. 45-1). With a shell gland or oviduct prolapse, the shell gland or oviduct will have a lumen, but no feces will be present (as opposed to a prolapse of the colon with feces), and

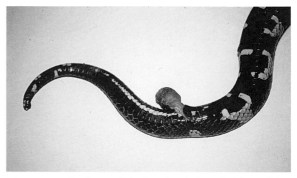

Figure 45-1 Prolapse of the hemipenis in a California king snake. (From Mader DR: *Reptile medicine and surgery*, ed 2, St. Louis, MO, 2006, Saunders, by permission.)

longitudinal striations appear on the surface of the shell duct that are not present on the colon.

CLINICAL SIGNS

- Mass of reddish, moist, or dry tissue protruding from the vent
- Straining
- Lack of fecal or urinary elimination

DIAGNOSIS

- Physical examination and history of egg laying or straining

TREATMENT

- The prolapsed tissue should be cleaned gently.
- Lubrication and manual reduction should be done; purse-string suture of the vent may be required to temporarily maintain the reduction until swelling decreases.
- If manual reduction is not possible, surgical amputation of necrotic material and repair of oviduct should be performed; ovariohysterectomy may be required to prevent further occurrences.

INFORMATION FOR CLIENTS

- Prolapses should be reduced as soon as possible to prevent further damage to the tissues involved.
- If the animal is not used for breeding, ovariohysterectomy should be considered.

Iguanas

Iguanas are oviparous; they lay eggs. Dystocias are common in iguanas and are often the result of inadequate nesting sites. Eggs require anywhere from 90 to 130 days of incubation time before hatching, and the young are hatched totally independent of the parents. Male iguanas typically have large femoral pores, two hemipenes, and a larger dew lap compared with that of female iguanas. Female iguanas tend to be smaller and have small femoral pores (see Fig. 42-6). Both ovaries of the female iguana are active. Large lizards usually mature between 3 and 4 years of age, but reproduction is a costly process for the female iguana; if the female is not in good physical condition before breeding, it can be detrimental to her overall health.

In general, animals in poor physical condition will not breed or reproduce.

Dystocia

Dystocia in the iguana is commonly a result of lack of proper nesting sites (Fig. 45-2). Dystocia lasting for more than several days may be fatal to most lizards. It is possible for lizards to lay eggs without the presence of a male lizard, although these eggs will be infertile.

CLINICAL SIGNS

- Anorexia
- Depression, unresponsive (healthy gravid lizard will be alert and active)
- Distended abdomen

DIAGNOSIS

- Physical examination and history
- Radiography: gravid uterus

TREATMENT

- Manual removal of the eggs if retained in the cloaca
- Hormone therapy: oxytocin, arginine vasotocin
- Surgical removal:
  - Removal of up to 30 eggs has been reported in green iguanas
  - Ovariosalpingectomy recommended if the animal is not to be used for breeding at a later date

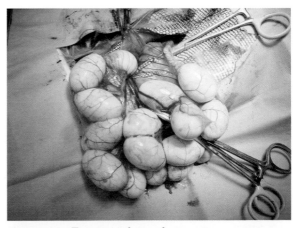

Figure 45-2 Exteriorized gravid uterus in a green iguana. (From Mader DR: *Reptile medicine and surgery*, ed 2, St. Louis, MO, 2006, Saunders, by permission.)

INFORMATION FOR CLIENTS

- Female iguanas lay eggs without the presence of a male iguana.
- You should contact your veterinarian immediately if signs of depression develop in a gravid female iguana.
- Removal of the uterus and ovaries will prevent the recurrence of the dystocia in animals not specifically used for breeding.

Prolapse of the Oviduct, Cloaca, and Hemipenis

Prolapse of the oviduct or the hemipenis is seen in iguanas (Fig. 45-3 and Fig. 45-4). Treatment depends on the severity of the prolapse and the tissue involved.

CLINICAL SIGNS

- Tissue protruding from the vent (tissue may be red and congested or black and necrotic, dry or moist)

DIAGNOSIS

- Physical examination and history

TREATMENT

- Gently clean externalized tissue.
- Invert and replace it back through the cloaca.

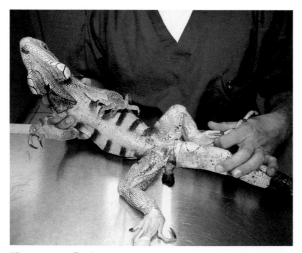

Figure 45-3 Prolapse of the hemipenis in a green iguana. (From Mader DR: *Reptile medicine and surgery*, ed 2, St. Louis, MO, 2006, Saunders, by permission.)

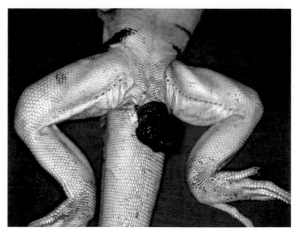

Figure 45-4 Prolapse of the Cloaca in the iguana. (From Mader DR: *Reptile medicine and surgery*, ed 2, St. Louis, MO, 2006, Saunders, by permission.)

- Apply a purse-string suture to hold the tissue until swelling decreases (if needed)
- Surgical replacement should be attempted if the tissue cannot be reduced and invertedinto the proper position.

INFORMATION FOR CLIENTS

- Prompt treatment of any prolapse is required to decrease tissue damage.

Turtles

Egg binding and penile prolapse are the most frequently seen reproductive system problems of turtles.

Egg Binding

Many stresses in chelonians result in failure to lay eggs. Nutritional secondary hyperparathyroidism, dehydration, hypovitaminosis A, hypocalcemia, and failure to find an adequate nesting area are some of the problems that may cause this type of reproductive failure.

CLINICAL SIGNS

- Owners' report that the turtle laid several eggs and then quit or was laying an egg intermittently (normally eggs are laid all at one time)
- ± Signs of systemic disease

DIAGNOSIS

- History of egg passage
- Complete physical examination and environmental history
- Palpation of egg in cloaca
- Radiography

TREATMENT

- Increase hydration (fluids and soaking of animal)
- Manual removal of egg
- Ovocentesis of the egg, with careful shell removal
- Providing proper nesting materials
- Correction of deficiency of vitamin A and calcium, if present
- Oxytocin effective in chelonians
- Correct preferred optimal temperature zone (POTZ)
- Surgery if not corrected by the above therapy

INFORMATION FOR CLIENTS

- Provide proper nesting materials for breeding turtles.
- Make sure that the animals are kept at proper POTZ and that the diet is adequate.
- Seek veterinary assistance if a female turtle stops laying eggs abruptly.

Penile Prolapse

Male chelonians have a single, large, fleshy penis that varies in color from pink to deep purple. The penis may become engorged and evert when the turtle is excited. Penile prolapse is common in chelonians. Trauma, straining, breeding, infection or inflammation, nutritional secondary hyperparathyroidism, and the presence of gastrointestinal foreign bodies may all contribute to this condition.

CLINICAL SIGNS

- Presence of a large, fleshy mass protruding from the cloaca
- ± Straining

DIAGNOSIS

- In any cloacal prolapse, the organ prolapsed should be identified:
  - Intestinal tract—muscular with a lumen; fecal material present
- Bladder—thin walled; fluid filled
- Penis—male animal; muscular solid tissue mass with a central groove
- Oviduct—female animal; lumen with no fecal material
- History and physical examination

TREATMENT

- Sedation often is necessary.
- Clean and lubricate the tissue and gently replace it into the cloaca.
- Purse-string suture vent may prevent recurrence of prolapse.
- Amputation may be necessary if the tissue is necrotic.
- Correct any underling nutrition and husbandry problems.
- Oviduct prolapse may be treated in a similar manner.

INFORMATION FOR CLIENTS

- Prolapse of any organ should be considered an emergency.
- Owners should wrap the cloacal area with a clean, damp towel or cloth and bring the animal to the clinic immediately. The sooner the prolapse is reduced, the better will be the outcome.

REVIEW QUESTIONS

1. A reptile that is viviparous produces:
   a. Eggs
   b. Live young
   c. Both live young and eggs
2. Waiting a few days for the swelling to decrease with an oviduct prolapse will make treatment safer for the patient.
   a. True
   b. False
3. Snakes may be sexed by identifying that:
   a. Males are heavier than female snakes
   b. Females have a deep hemipenis pouch
   c. Females have a shallow hemipenis pouch
   d. Males have a large external penis
4. Obstructive dystocia may result from:
   a. Poor diet
   b. Malposition of an egg
   c. Malnutrition
   d. Systemic disease

5. Most well-maintained snakes will mature around:
   a. 6–12 months
   b. 2–3 years
   c. 6–8 years
   d. 4–6 months
6. Iguana eggs take _____ days to hatch.
   a. 30–40
   b. 80 100
   c. 90–130
   d. 100–160

7. Owners noticing tissues protruding out of the cloaca of their reptile should _____.
   a. Cover the tissue with a clean, wet towel and come to the clinic
   b. Apply lubricant to the tissue and replace it using a finger
   c. Soak the tissue in warm water and wait for swelling to decrease

Answers found on page 556.

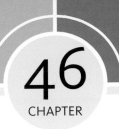

Diseases of the Respiratory System

LEARNING OBJECTIVES

When you have completed this chapter, you will be able to:

1. Recognize the clinical signs of respiratory disease in reptiles.
2. Explain to clients why these conditions need to be treated aggressively and for long periods.

3. Realize that oxygen therapy may not be the best treatment for dyspnea in reptiles.

Snakes

Pneumonia

Pneumonia is a common presenting sign in the sick reptile patient. Although pneumonia is primarily a disease of the respiratory system, its cause may be multifactorial. A number of infectious agents may cause pneumonia, and if linked to poor husbandry, an inadequate diet, and poor sanitation, a serious and often life-threatening disease may result. The respiratory system of the reptile is unlike that of the mammal. The glottis of snakes is situated rostrally in the oral cavity, allowing for respiration while eating large meals. Most snakes have only one functional lung, the left one being absent. Reptiles, unlike mammals, may function by using anaerobic metabolism, which allows them to compensate for progressive respiratory disease until it is well advanced. Respiration is usually controlled, not by blood carbon dioxide levels and pH but by the temperature and the partial pressure of oxygen (PO_2) in tissues. As the temperature increases, so does the oxygen demand, which the patient meets by increasing tidal volume, not respiratory rate. Environments rich in oxygen (oxygen cages) may, therefore, suppress ventilation in the sick animal. Together, the poor ability of the reptile lung to move inflammatory exudates out of the lung, the suppressed tidal volumes resulting from pulmonary infiltrates and exudates, and the ability of the reptile to shift to anaerobic metabolism may make early diagnosis of disease quite difficult.

CLINICAL SIGNS

- Dyspnea (open-mouth breathing)
- Extension of the neck to facilitate breathing
- Increased respiratory rate
- ± Nasal discharge
- Abnormal respiratory sounds
- Cyanotic mucous membranes
- Depression, lethargy
- Reluctance to feed

DIAGNOSIS

- Physical examination and history
- Radiography
- Transtracheal wash (catheter inserted via the glottis)
- Culture and sensitivity; wet mount for parasites
- Complete blood cell count (CBC) and serum chemistries

TREATMENT

- Will depend on the diagnostic laboratory results
- Antibiotic therapy:
  - Usually begins with a combination therapy of aminoglycoside and β-lactam antibiotic while waiting for culture results
  - Nebulization using antibiotics: 10 to 30 minutes three to four times daily
- Increase environmental temperatures to top of the preferred optimal temperature zone (POTZ)
- Maintenance of hydration (1% to 2% body weight subcutaneously daily)
- Force-feeding, if not too stressful
- Often difficult to know when to stop treating the patient; antibiotics should be used for a minimum of 3 weeks or until the hemogram and patient appear to be improving (eating, breathing better, etc.)

Iguanas

The respiratory system of lizards is different from that of mammals. The position of the glottis is variable in lizards, being more rostral in carnivorous lizards and at the base of the tongue in others. The tracheal rings are incomplete, and the trachea bifurcates near the base of the heart. Lizard lungs are equal in size, and gas exchange occurs in the cranial portions. The caudal portions function similar to the air sacs of birds, being poorly vascularized and not used for respiratory functions. Both inspiration and expiration are active processes in the lizard, and no diaphragm exists to facilitate respiration. As in snakes, lizards have the ability to function with anaerobic metabolism and may be able to conceal disease until it is advanced.

Pneumonia

Pneumonia is common in reptiles. It may be the result of bacterial, viral, fungal, or parasitic infections.

CLINICAL SIGNS

- Dyspnea; open-mouthed breathing
- ± Nasal discharge
- Increased respiratory sounds on auscultation
- Anorexia
- ± Cyanotic mucous membranes
- Depression
- Lethargy

DIAGNOSIS

- CBC and serum chemistries
- Radiography (lateral view is most important)
- Transtracheal wash (done by passing a catheter through the glottis and injecting sterile saline into the lung, then retrieving the fluid for culture and sensitivity)
- Culture and sensitivity testing of tracheal wash
- Wet mount and cytology of the fluid

TREATMENT

General Treatment
- Force-feeding (avoid if too stressful for the animal)
- Fluid therapy to correct dehydration
- Vitamin supplementation
- Supplemental oxygen therapy to be avoided because it may decrease the respiratory rate

Bacterial Pneumonia
- Many gram-negative bacteria have been demonstrated to cause pneumonia in reptiles. Disease may be primary or secondary to bacterial disease in the oral cavity or elsewhere in the body.
- Systemic antibiotic use should be based on culture and sensitivity results. Currently recommended

antibiotics include the following (given for up to 28 days):

- Amikacin
- Ceftiofur
- Cefotaxime
- Enrofloxacin
- Piperacillin
- Ticarcillin

Viral Pneumonia

- Viral pneumonia is not seen as commonly in iguanas as in snakes and turtles. If found, treatment is supportive.

Fungal Pneumonia

- Fungal pneumonia may occur when antibiotics are overused or environmental conditions are unsanitary.
- Surgical excision of any fungal granuloma is recommended, when possible.
- Provide nebulization with amphotericin B and oral ketoconazole
- Correct husbandry problems

Parasitic Pneumonias

- Lung worms, pentastomids, trematodes, and some migrating nematodes may cause respiratory infections.
- Antiparasitic medication is given.

INFORMATION FOR CLIENTS

- Proper husbandry aids in the prevention of respiratory disease in the iguana.
- Treatment, when necessary, will be prolonged and expensive.
- Have your animal examined by your veterinarian at any sign of respiratory distress.

Turtles

Respiratory disease is all too common in turtles. The anatomy of the respiratory tract predisposes the turtle to pneumonias and upper respiratory diseases.

Mycoplasmosis in Tortoises

Mycoplasmosis has been documented in both captive chelonians and in wild desert tortoises. The bacterium *Mycoplasma agassizii* has been the proven agent in this disease. The disease may be spread by direct contact.

CLINICAL SIGNS

- Nasal discharge (rhinitis)
- Conjunctivitis
- Ocular discharge
- Palpebral edema
- Chronic symptoms may appear cyclically

DIAGNOSIS

- Complete physical examination and environmental history
- Direct culture of *Mycoplasma*
- Polymerase chain reaction testing for *Mycoplasma*
- Enzyme-linked immunosorbent assay (ELISA) positive for *Mycoplasma* antibodies in plasma

TREATMENT

- Several different protocols reported in the literature
- Antibiotic therapy; enrofloxacin or clarithromycin, which appear to work well
- Topical antibiotic-cortisone products applied directly into the nares or used in nasal flushes every 48 to 72 hours

Supportive Care

- Maintain hydration.
- Keep turtle in the POTZ.
- Provide nutritional support.

INFORMATION FOR CLIENTS

- After resolution of the acute infection, turtles may become chronically infected. These animals may have increased susceptibility to secondary infections and may have recurrent bouts of symptoms.
- Consider any animal that has been infected to be a source of infection for other chelonians; they should be isolated from noninfective turtles.

Pneumonia and Lower Respiratory Disease

Pneumonia is not uncommon in reptiles of all types. The anatomy of the respiratory system, the high bifurcation of the trachea, and the long, narrow bronchi do not allow for easy removal of accumulated debris.

Many of these animals have a history of recent transportation through the retail pet trade, parasitism, malnutrition, being kept at suboptimal temperatures in unsanitary conditions, or all of these conditions. The animal with lower respiratory disease is often in critical condition by the time the owner notices signs of illness. Treatment must be aggressive if it is to be successful.

CLINICAL SIGNS

- Dyspnea, open-mouth breathing, neck extended
- Anorexia
- Lethargy
- Mucous membranes may be cyanotic
- ± Nasal discharge (if an upper respiratory component is present)
- Abnormal lung sounds
- Asymmetric swimming may be seen in aquatic turtles

DIAGNOSIS

- A complete physical examination and history
- Radiography
- Endoscopy (need special techniques in turtles)
- Tracheal wash with culture and sensitivity
- CBC
- Computed tomography (CT) or magnetic resonance imaging (MRI)

TREATMENT

- Therapy depends on the organism causing the disease.
- All patients must be maintained at the upper limit of the POTZ.
- Fluids should be administered to maintain hydration.
- Supplemental feeding should be given.
- Correct all deficiencies in husbandry and nutrition.

Bacterial

- Most will be gram-negative bacteria
- Antibiotics based on culture and sensitivity results:
  - Aminoglycosides and β-lactams
  - Enrofloxacin or clarithromycin if mycoplasma is isolated
- Nebulization two to four times daily

Fungal

- Antifungal drugs used in nebulization or orally at doses extrapolated from other species (use with caution)

Viral

- Supportive care

◉ TECH ALERT

One of the driving forces for respiration in the reptile is PO_2. Increased oxygen levels may inhibit respiration. Avoid giving these animals supplemental oxygen unless it can be delivered at levels of 30% to 40% and can be humidified.

INFORMATION FOR CLIENTS

- These animals are critically ill, and many do not survive.
- Treatment may be prolonged and costly.
- Treatment is doomed to failure if husbandry conditions are not improved.
- These animals must be quarantined from others in the collection.
- Repeated clinical and laboratory examinations will be needed to determine when treatment may be discontinued.

REVIEW QUESTIONS

1. All dyspneic reptiles should be placed in an oxygen-enriched environment immediately upon hospitalization.
   a. True
   b. False
2. Disease of the diaphragm is a common problem in reptiles.
   a. True
   b. False
3. When treating respiratory diseases in reptiles, treatment should be continued for at least:
   a. 7 days
   b. 21 days
   c. 36 days
   d. 10 days

4. Older reptiles should not be allowed to develop: (Choose all that apply.)
   a. Dehydration
   b. Vitamin A or D deficiencies
   c. Calcium deficiencies
   d. Bacterial infections

5. All reptiles have a bladder and a cloaca.
   a. True
   b. False

Answers found on page 556.

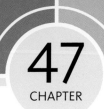

Diseases of the Urinary System

LEARNING OBJECTIVES

When you have completed this chapter, you will be able to:
1. Discuss the differences between mammalian and reptilian renal systems.

2. Describe why visceral gout is frequently seen as a cause of death in reptiles.

Anatomy and Physology of the Reptilian Renal System

The urinary system of reptiles comprises two kidneys and, in some species, a bladder. In general, the reptilian kidneys are elongated and lobulated. The arterial supply for the kidney is via the renal artery and venous drainage via the portal veins. Each reptilian kidney contains fewer nephrons than those of the mammalian kidney, but the glomeruli are well developed and occur at right angles to the long axis of the kidney. The nephron is composed of the glomerulus, a proximal tubule, a short distal tubule, and a collecting duct. The ureters open into the urodeum of the cloaca.

The primary job of the kidney is control of the extracellular fluid volume and composition. The bladder (where one exists), the cloaca, and the nasal salt glands also help regulate fluid volume and composition. Uric acid is excreted from the proximal tubule along with varying amounts of protein.

Reptilian urine is clear to straw colored with a specific gravity between 1.003 and 1.014. The urine pH depends on diet just like in mammals. Usually, only few cells are present, and no bilirubin or protein and, no ketones or glucose exist, but bacteria are common (contamination from the cloaca). Crystals of urates are common.

TECH ALERT

Because of the renal portal system, medications injected into the caudal half of the reptile will pass through the kidney and be eliminated from the body without being distributed to the rest of the body. For this reason, never inject medications or fluids into the rear half of the reptile.

Snakes

Gout

The most frequently seen disorder of the renal system in snakes is gout, a disease routinely associated with dietary imbalances. Snakes require animal protein in their diet, and their system is adapted to handle that form of protein. In some reptiles, the end product of protein breakdown is uric acid, whereas in others, it is allantoin or urea. The uric acid is cleared from the blood through the renal tubules. When uric acid levels increase in blood, uric acid crystals begin to precipitate out in body fluids such as synovial fluid and other body tissues. Deposits in tissues such as cartilage, tendons, and soft tissues are called *tophi*. In reptiles, tophi can be found in the pericardial sac, kidneys, liver, spleen, lungs, subcutaneous tissues, and other soft tissues. Risk factors for the formation of gout include dehydration, renal disease, excessive protein intake, and misuse of nephrotoxic antibiotics (aminoglycosides).

CLINICAL SIGNS

- Firm, white swellings around joints or in soft tissues (often oral membranes)

DIAGNOSIS

- Physical examination and history
- Demonstration of monosodium urate crystals in tophi lesions (Fig. 47-1 and Fig. 47-2)

TREATMENT

- Correct deficiencies in diet and husbandry practices.
- Provide access to clean water at all times.
- Use human medications used to treat gout (doses extrapolated from humans):
  - Allopurinol
  - Probenecid
  - Colchicine

INFORMATION FOR CLIENTS

- The overall prognosis for animals with severe gout is poor.
- Patients with moderate gout can be managed on medications, but the condition may quickly become painful if the medication is stopped.

Iguanas

Cystic Calculi

Iguanas have a bladder and cystic calculi may form from urate salts.

CLINICAL SIGNS

- Lethargy
- Depression
- Anorexia
- Dehydration
- Constipation
- Hind-limb paresis or paralysis

DIAGNOSIS

- Physical examination (palpation); history of stress and water deprivation
- Radiography (calcium urate stones are radiodense, whereas ammonium urate stones are less dense)

TREATMENT

- Correction of dehydration with fluid therapy
- Cystotomy

INFORMATION FOR CLIENTS

- The formation of cystic calculi has been linked to improper nutrition and limited access to water. Make sure that your iguana has free access to clean water at all times.

Turtles

Urinary Calculi

Urinary calculi are seen in chelonians. Causes include hypovitaminosis A and D, excessive calcium and dietary protein, excess feeding of oxalates (spinach), and bacterial infections. Dehydration may predispose the animal to the formation of stones in the bladder.

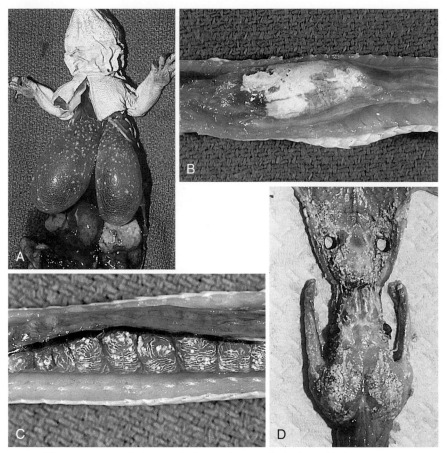

Figure 47-1 Urates in tissue. **A,** Lungs. **B,** Pericardial sac. **C,** Kidneys. **D,** Liver, spleen, and subcutaneous tissues. (From Mader DR: *Reptile medicine and surgery*, ed 2, St. Louis, MO, 2006, Saunders, by permission.)

CLINICAL SIGNS

- Many urinary calculi diagnosed during routine examinations; and present with no signs of urinary distress
- ± Anorexia
- ± Signs of constipation
- ± Egg binding
- ± Dysuria
- ± Hindlimb paresis

DIAGNOSIS

- Palpation of the bladder through the inguinal fossa

- Radiology (Fig. 47-3)
- Complete presurgical workup: complete blood cell count (CBC) serum chemistry, urinalysis

TREATMENT

- Surgical removal of larger stones; smaller stones may be removed by endoscopy

Supportive Care

- Correction of dehydration
- Supplemental feeding if anorexic
- Antibiotics given before surgery because bladders are not sterile in these animals

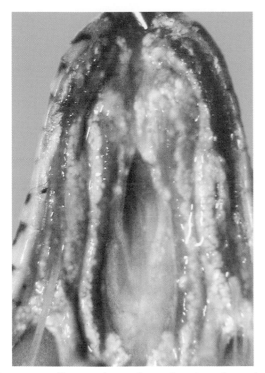

Figure 47-2 Gout tophi in the oral cavity of a python. (From Mader DR: *Reptile medicine and surgery*, ed 2, St. Louis, MO, 2006, Saunders, by permission.)

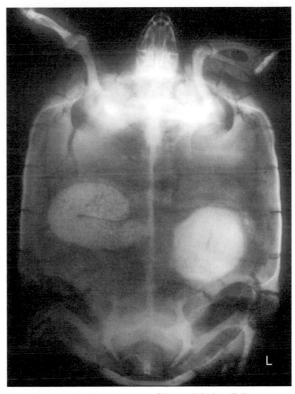

Figure 47-3 Bladder stones. (From Mader DR: *Reptile medicine and surgery*, ed 2, St. Louis, MO, 2006, Saunders, by permission.)

INFORMATION FOR CLIENTS

- Chelonians with bladder stones often show no clinical symptoms.
- Removal of all small stones is necessary because small stones will become large ones. Large stones may be life-threatening to the animal.
- Proper diet and husbandry may be able to prevent the formation of bladder stones. Keep all animals well hydrated. Provide adequate water sources for soaking and drinking.

Gout

All reptiles need protein. Carnivores best utilize animal protein, whereas herbivorous reptiles require plant proteins. Although each can utilize both types of proteins, overingestion of improper types of protein may have adverse health effects on the animal. Proteins are broken down into uric acid in some reptiles and to allantoin (which then is broken down into urea and allantoic acid) in others. Salts of uric acid are removed from blood by excretion via the renal tubules. These salts are relatively insoluble in water, and when dehydration occurs, they readily precipitate into joints and other tissues throughout the body. Two types of gout are recognized: (1) primary (overproduction of uric acid) and (2) secondary (disruption of normal balance between production and excretion from disease).

CLINICAL SIGNS

- Swollen, painful joints
- ± Urate deposits in tendons, soft tissue, around joints
- ± Signs of systemic problems such as renal disease, starvation
- ± History of drug therapy that may affect the kidneys

DIAGNOSIS

- Complete physical examination and history
- Radiography
- Identification of monosodium urate crystals in the joint or tissue

TREATMENT

- Allopurinol treatment to reduce the serum uric acid levels
- Surgical removal of tophi from the joint
- Correction of the diet and environmental temperatures
- Correction of dehydration and maintain good hydration

INFORMATION FOR CLIENTS

- Proper diet and temperatures are mandatory to prevent the formation of crystals in joints and soft tissue.
- All animals must have continuous access to fresh water.
- The overall prognosis for gout is poor, but many animals may be comfortable maintained on long-term allopurinol treatment.

REVIEW QUESTIONS

1. Firm, white swellings around the joints and in the soft tissues of reptiles may be a collection of:
   a. Calcium soap
   b. Fat
   c. Urates
   d. Protein
2. Which of the following have a bladder? (Mark all that apply.)
   a. Green iguana
   b. Red-tailed boa
   c. Turtle
   d. Python
3. To avoid renal gout in reptiles, limit the use of this class of antibiotics.
   a. Penicillins
   b. Cephalosporins
   c. Aminoglycosides
   d. Quinolones

Answers found on page 557.

Diseases of the Cardiovascular System

KEY TERMS

Auscultate
Bradycardia
Endocarditis

Fibrillation
Holter monitor
Tachycardia

Thromboembolus
Thrombophlebitis

OUTLINE

LEARNING OBJECTIVES

When you have completed this chapter, you will be able to:

1. Auscultate the heart in an equine patient and appreciate normal versus abnormal sounds.
2. Explain to owners the value of diagnostic testing in cases of heart disease in their pets.
3. Explain how small lesions may progress to large problems in the equine patient.

The Equine Companion

Is there anything more beautiful than a horse galloping free across a field of green grass? Not in my book! Humans have enjoyed a relationship with horses for thousands of years. The horse of today has moved from a working farm animal to a companion animal, loved and pampered by owners of all ages.

Horses today are living longer, healthier, more useful lives than ever before. As our companions get older, the need for better health care is important, and veterinarians are being called on to provide this advanced care. As a technician, you may be lucky enough to work with these magnificent animals.

⦿ TECH ALERT

If you are not a "horse person" spend time watching horses, learn about their interactions, and listen to suggestions on safety. Respect the fact that they are "fight or flight" animals that are large enough to do serious damage to anyone handling or working around them. Remember to put safety first when handling any horse.

⦿ TECH ALERT

Knowing how to speak "horse language" will aid the technician when dealing with equine clients. Learn these special terms.

Anatomy and Physiology of the Equine Cardiovascular System

Cardiovascular disease is common in the horse and has been estimated to be the third most common cause of poor performance. The equine heart is designed exactly like those of other mammals. There are two atria (left and right) and two ventricles. Valves between the atria and ventricles divide the heart into four chambers. The right atrioventricular (AV) valve is known as the *tricuspid valve*, and the left AV valve is called the *mitral valve*. The valves are attached to the muscular walls of the ventricles with chordae tendinae, literally the "strings of the heart."

The left and right sides of the heart are separated by the AV septum. The auto-rhythmic cells of the sinoatrial (SA) node set the rate for contractions, which can be augmented by input from the central nervous system (CNS). From the SA node, electrical impulses travel across the atria, down the septum to the AV node, where they are slowed. From there the impulses pass through the AV Bundle (Bundle of His) and out over the ventricles on the Purkinge fibers. The resulting depolarization of the cardiac muscle cells causes contraction of the entire heart muscle. The heart rate of the resting horse is slower than that of the dog or the cat, normal rates usually between 25-and 40 beats per minute (beats per minute). Larger chambers found in the equine heart require a longer time to fill, hence the slower heart rate. As in small animals, cardiac output depends on the heart rate and the stroke volume (the volume of blood pumped out of the heart each contraction). Any defect that reduces either can affect the circulating volume of blood to other organ systems.

Heart Sounds

Heart sounds are generated when the valves close, causing turbulence in the blood flow around the valve. The first heart sound (S_1) is the result of closure of the right and left AV valves. S_2, the second heart sound, occurs as a result of closure of the pulmonic and aortic valves. If these valves fail to close in synchronous fashion, the third and fourth heart sounds may be heard.

⦿ TECH ALERT

When auscultating the equine heart, the technician may have to reach behind the shoulder blade along the left side of the chest to better hear the cardiac sounds. In many horses, it may be possible to hear the third and fourth heart sounds.

Electrocardiography

The electrical activity of the heart can be measured at the body wall using any electrocardiography (ECG). Below are several examples of equine ECG. The rhythmicity of the heart may be determined by ECG, and it can be used to indicate cardiac enlargements

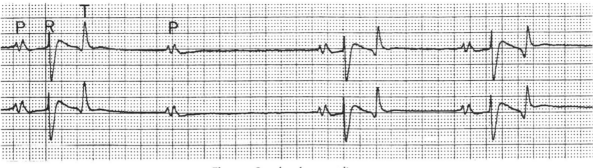

Figure 48-1 An electrocardiogram.

as well. The most common arrhythmia seen in fit horses is a second-degree AV block (Fig. 48-1). Atrial fibrillation is also a common finding in older horses, being related to the large size of the heart's atrial chambers.

Valvular Disease

Valvular disease is common in foals (congenital) and in mature horses (degenerative or infectious). Diseased valves may either impede normal flow (stenosis) or allow backflow (insufficiency), which increases the workload of the heart and decreases cardiac output. Common causes of valvular disease in the horse include endocarditis and ruptured cordae tendinae.

CLINICAL SIGNS

- Murmur on auscultation
- Increasing exercise intolerance
- ± Fever (with endocarditis)
- ± Weight loss
- ± Intermittent lameness
- ± Arrhythmias
- Development of congestive heart failure (CHF)

DIAGNOSIS

- Clinical findings on physical examination
- ECG
- Echocardiography with Doppler study
- Exercise testing
- If endocarditis:
  - Anemia
  - Decreased blood protein
- Leukocytosis
- Positive blood cultures
- Holter monitoring

TREATMENT

- Will depend on severity of symptoms and location of the lesion

Degenerative Valvular Disease

Degenerative valvular disease in the horse usually results in valvular insufficiency, or a leaky valve. With every contraction (systole), blood is pumped forward out of the ventricles but much of the chamber volume is also pumped backward into the atria. This increases the volume in the chambers for the next contraction (preload). As the chambers become over-stretched they must work harder until they begin to fail (Fig. 48-2).

- Manage the development of CHF and cardiac arrhythmias:
  - Furosemide (a diuretic) orally
  - Digoxin: one to two times daily orally
  - Angiotensin-converting enzyme (ACE) inhibitors: two times daily (avoid use in pregnant mares)

Bacterial Endocarditis

Endocarditis is an inflammatory disease of the lining tissue of the heart. The most common location for lesions is on the left AV valve or on the left side endocardium. Jet lesions from mitral insufficiency or ventricular septal defects typically damage the endothelial lining of the heart. Circulating bacteria begin

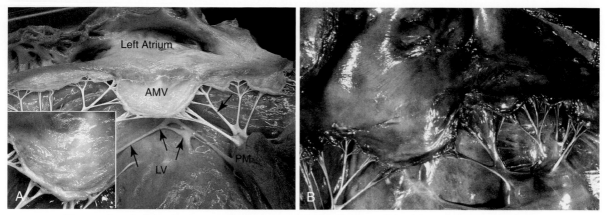

Figure 48-2 A, Mitral valve insufficiency caused by thickening of the valve which prevents proper closure. The body of the valve is very irregular and thick, and changes are most evident in the close-up view (*see inset at lower left*). **B,** Chronic suppurative valvulitis caused by chronic endocarditis has led to scarring, thickening, and distortion of the mitral valve. (From Reed SM: *Equine internal medicine*, ed 3, St. Louis, MO, 2010, Saunders, by permission.)

to colonize the damaged area, attracting inflammatory cells, and cellular debris begins to build up at the site. As the inflammatory process continues cardiac output decreases, creating a shock-like syndrome. Emboli often break loose and migrate to other organs producing organ failure or compromise.

- Intravenous (IV) antibiotic therapy based on culture and sensitivity results for 4 to 8 weeks
- Potassium penicillin every 6 hours
- Gentamicin q24h
- Extremely guarded prognosis in most cases

INFORMATION FOR CLIENTS

- Repeat cardiac examinations will be required to monitor the progress of disease and the efficacy of treatment.
- Owners of horses diagnosed with valvular disease should inquire as to the safety of riding or driving these animals. Sudden death is certainly a possibility in many of these animals.
- The prognosis for these disorders is related to the severity of the lesion and the area affected:
  - Mitral valve regurgitation: generally good in mature horses
  - Aortic valve regurgitation: generally good
  - Tricuspid regurgitation: generally good
  - Endocarditis: generally poor

Ruptured Chordae Tendinae

Clinical symptoms of ruptured chordates depend on the number ruptured. Tearing of the chordate will result in a flapping of the valve leaflet and produce a valvular insufficiency. The greater the number of chordates torn, the worse is the leakage of the valve. Eventually, the horse may develop CHF. (Fig 48-3).

CLINICAL SIGNS

- Increasing exercise intolerance
- Lethargy
- Auscultation of a murmur

DIAGNOSIS

- Complete physical examination
- Serum chemistries
- ECG
- Echocardiography

TREATMENT

- Supportive
- As the valvular insufficiency worsens, treatment for CHF may be needed

INFORMATION FOR CLIENTS

- These horses should not be ridden, as their heart function may worsen suddenly.

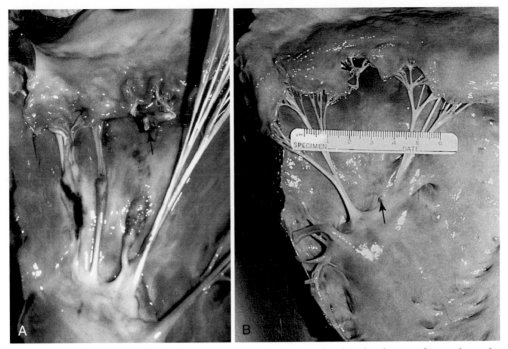

Figure 48-3 A, Acute, and **B,** Chronic, rupture of the mitral valve chordate tendineae (arrow). (From Reed SM: *Equine internal medicine*, ed 3, St. Louis, MO, 2010, Saunders, by permission.)

Vascular Disease

Vascular disorders seen in the horse include thrombophlebitis from catheter placement or IV injections, parasitic thromboemboli in the mesentery arteries, and vascular rupture (Fig. 48-4).

CLINICAL SIGNS

- Thrombophlebitis: heat, pain, swelling at site over vein, fever
- Parasitic thromboemboli: recurrent signs of colic
- Vascular rupture: sudden death

DIAGNOSIS

- Complete physical examination
- Complete blood cell count (CBC): neutrophilic leukocytosis
- Echocardiography: abnormal
- Culture and sensitivity of infected site
- History of poor deworming practices (colics)
- Necropsy (vascular rupture)

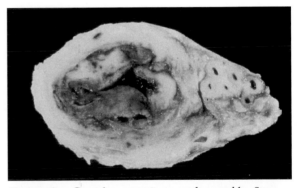

Figure 48-4 Cranial mesenteric artery damaged by *Strongylus vulgaris* migration. (From Reed SM: *Equine internal medicine*, ed 3, St. Louis, MO, 2010, Saunders, by permission.)

TREATMENT

- Broad-spectrum antibiotics
- Non-steroidal antiinflammatories
- Surgically remove the obstruction; may include vascular grafting
- There is no general treatment for parasitic thrombi

Thrombophlebitis

Thrombophlebitis is an inflammation of the lining of a vein with the formation of clots. This condition is often seen in the jugular vein from improper catheter maintenance or from other vascular trauma. It is estimated that 6%-to 22% of all IV catheters placed in the jugular vein will cause some degree of thrombophlebitis. The problem can be minimized by proper selection of catheter materials, aseptic placement of all catheters, proper maintenance, and early removal of unnecessary catheters. Early recognition of the problem and catheter removal will improve the prognosis.

- High doses of broad-spectrum antibiotics or antibiotics based on culture and sensitivity results
- Hot compresses over site of inflammation
- Surgical resection of the vein if medical treatment is unsuccessful

Parasites

Migration of immature strongyles through the anterior mesenteric artery may cause inflammation in the lining of the vessel. Chronic irritation will eventually result in a decrease in blood flow through the vessel and therefore a decrease in blood flow to a portion of the gastrointestinal tract. The result may be frequent bouts of colic.

- Institute an effective deworming plan that includes the use of ivermectin or other wormers. However, damage to the vessels cannot be reversed. It is important that horse owners understand the importance of frequent treatment with equine antiparasitics. Whether a rotational-product program or a one-product-worming program is chosen, horses should be wormed multiple times during the year (at least every 8–12 weeks).

Vascular Rupture

In 2012, spectators at a prestigious equine competition watched in horror as one of the top horses finished a jumping round, collapsed, and died from an aortic rupture. Altough this problem is not common, it does occur, and it is always unexpected. Usually, no predictive signs or symptoms exist, although aneurisms may often be detected on ultrosonography.

- No treatment currently is available. Sudden death is the only common sign.

INFORMATION FOR CLIENTS

- All horses should be dewormed frequently (every 2-3 months) using a rotation schedule of wormers. This treatment should begin early in the horse's life and be maintained in the adult animal. Pasture maintenance is important also for control of intestinal parasites.
- Care should be taken to maintain asepsis when administering IV injections to the horse. Avoid repeated injections in the same area of the vein.
- Horses diagnosed with cardiac disease should be considered unfit and unsafe to ride or drive because of the possibility of sudden death.

⦿ TECH ALERT

Technicians should pay close attention to the health of the vessel, length of time the catheter is to remain in place, and the environment in which the patient will be kept. All catheters should be placed aseptically.

Cardiac Arrhythmias

Abnormal cardiac rhythms are commonly found in healthy horses. Tachycardia maybe the result of fear, anxiety, pain, or exercise, although bradycardia may occur at rest. A second-degree AV block can be commonly demonstrated in fit horses at rest. Although many arrhythmias will produce no clinical symptoms, three may result in clinical signs of cardiac disease.

Atrial Arrhythmias

The size of the equine heart predisposed the horse to atrial arrhythmias, which are fairly common in the horse. Atrial tachycardia, atrial flutter, and atrial fibrillation are the most likely causes of clinical disease. All three causes may be treated similar to atrial fibrillation.

CLINICAL SIGNS

- Auscultation of a rapid, abnormal heart rhythm
- History of poor or declining performance
- Exercise intolerance

- ± Pulmonary hemorrhage
- ± Respiratory distress
- CHF
- Ataxia, collapse, or both

DIAGNOSIS

- Complete physical examination
- CBC and serum chemistry: usually normal but can indicate a hypokalemia in cases where the arrhythmia is electrolyte induced
- Radiography: usually normal
- ECG
- Echocardiography: usually normal unless underlying cardiac disease is present

TREATMENT

- Provide drug therapy for conversion to normal rhythm using drug therapy. (Fig. 48-5):
  - Quinidine sulfate: orally every 2 hours until conversion or until toxicity develops
  - Digoxin: given concurrently if resting heart rate is more than 90 to 100 beats/min or conversion cannot be achieved with quinidine alone
- Consider resting the horse for 1 to 2 weeks after conversion, although racing horses may return to training within 48 hours of conversion.
- Rule out other concurrent cardiac disease as the cause of arrhythmia.

INFORMATION FOR CLIENTS

- Approximately 25% of all horses will have a recurrence of abnormal rhythm within the first year after conversion and will need to be re-treated. Eventually these animals may become resistant to conversion.
- ECG monitoring will be required during treatment to monitor for signs of drug toxicity.
- With conversion, most horses will return to their original level of performance.

REVIEW QUESTIONS

1. The first step in diagnosing cardiac disease in the horse is to:
   a. Perform a complete physical examination and auscultate the heart
   b. Perform thoracic radiography and ECG
   c. Obtain CBC and serum chemistries with electrolytes
   d. Perform an echocardiographic study
2. What arrhythmia is demonstrated by ECG in a healthy, resting performance horse?
   a. Second-degree atrioventricular block
   b. Atrial tachycardia
   c. Ventricular tachycardia
   d. Atrial fibrillation

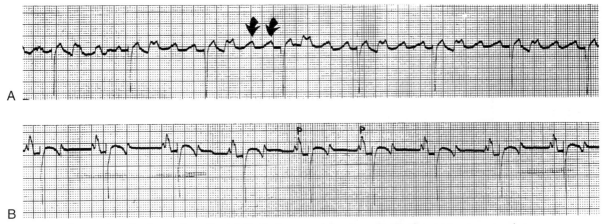

Figure 48-5 A, Conversion of atrial fibrillation to atrial tachycardia. **B,** Conversion to normal sinus rhythm. (From Reed SM: *Equine internal medicine,* ed 3, St. Louis, MO, 2010, Saunders, by permission.)

3. When placing indwelling catheters in the equine patient, the technician must pay close attention to:
   a. Aseptic preparation of the insertion site
   b. The health of the vessel chosen
   c. The time the catheter will be in place
   d. The environment of the patient
   e. All of the above

4. Owners of horses diagnosed with moderate to severe cardiac disease should:
   a. Check with the veterinarian prior to riding or driving these horses
   b. Ride these animals for a limited time daily
   c. Use these animals for driving only
   d. Have these animals euthanized

5. Which of the following would most accurately diagnose a cardiac defect?
   a. Radiography
   b. Electrocardiography
   c. Echocardiography
   d. Computed tomography

6. Some degree of thrombophlebitis occurs when any indwelling catheter is placed into a vessel.
   a. True
   b. False

7. An enlarged atrium may predispose the horse to this arrhythmia.
   a. Atrial tachycardia
   b. Ventricular fibrillation
   c. Ventricular tachycardia
   d. Atrial fibrillation

8. Heart disease accounts for 50% of all horses with poor performance.
   a. True
   b. False

9. The migration of *Strongylus* spp. parasites causes thromboemboli in:
   a. The caudal vena cava
   b. The aorta
   c. The mesenteric artery
   d. The jugular vein

10. Which of the following heart rates would be correct for a healthy horse at rest?
    a. 25–40 beats per minute (bpm)
    b. 30–60 beats per minute (bpm)

Answers found on page 557.

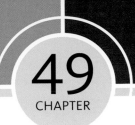

Diseases of the Digestive System

LEARNING OBJECTIVES

When you have completed this chapter, you will be able to:
1. Recognize the signs of colic in the equine patient.
2. Advise clients of management practices that may predispose horses to gastrointestinal (GI) problems.
3. Recognize the zoonotic potential of many equine diarrheas.

Anatomy of the Normal Digestive System

The digestive tract of the horse is that of an animal that was designed for grazing—that is, constant walking and eating. The lips of the horse, designed for prehension of grass, are amazingly sensitive and can sift out powdered medication when it is mixed in with their feed.

The horse's teeth are those of an animal adapted for grazing. Equine teeth have enamel ridges that traverse the chewing surfaces and are constantly erupting throughout the horse's life. As some of the enamel ridges get worn away, they are replaced by the ever-growing tooth. This constant tooth eruption, as well as the fact that the horse's upper jaw is wider than its lower jaw, may lead to dental problems as the horse goes through life.

The horse's esophagus is a long, muscular tube that courses from the animal's mouth to the stomach. The esophagus is mainly made up of two layers of smooth muscle: (1) an inner circular layer and (2) a longitudinal outer layer. These two layers of smooth muscle, and the way they work in concert, enable the horse to swallow its food.

The stomach of the horse is relatively small in comparison with its body size. The stomach of the average 1100-pound horse has the same capacity of a 250-pound hog—roughly 2 to 4 gallons. The stomach has two regions: (1) a nonglandular portion, which takes up roughly the proximal half and (2) the distal half, which is glandular. The small size of the stomach and its constant secretion of hydrochloric acid (HCl) have an impact on the horse's feeding schedule, which the owners need to be aware of. The main function of the stomach is mixing of the feed with digestive juices and the start of protein digestion. The stomach also absorbs small amounts of water, alcohols, and water-soluble medications.

The small intestine is where most of the digestion and absorption of the concentrate portion of the feed occurs. Foodstuffs are broken down by chemical digestion mainly in the duodenum, which is the portion closest to the stomach. The resultant materials are absorbed as they pass through the jejunum and the ileum.

The fibrous portion of the diet empties from the ileum into the cecum. The cecum is a large, comma-shaped organ that occupies much of the right side of the horse's abdominal cavity. The main function of the cecum is fiber digestion. Here, microorganisms break down the fiber portion of the diet into glucose and volatile fatty acids (VFAs). The glucose is used by the gut microorganisms, and the VFAs are used by the horse for energy.

After digestion by the cecum, the remaining material goes into the large colon (Fig. 49-1). The large colon has four portions: the right and left ventral and dorsal colons. The contents then travel into the transverse and then the descending colons. The main function of the colon is to absorb water from the feedstuff.

Many of the digestive system diseases that are seen in horses may be attributed to their somewhat peculiar digestive anatomy.

Dental Considerations: Uneven Tooth Wear

Because of the modification of diet and feeding patterns by domestication, demands on young performance horses, and the lack of selection for dental soundness, most horses need regular dental evaluation and work. Regular dental work improves the horse's comfort, increases the efficiency of feed utilization, and possibly increases the animal's performance.

As stated earlier, the horse's teeth are constantly erupting throughout its life, and its upper jaw is wider than the lower jaw. This may lead to an uneven wear pattern of the occlusal surfaces of teeth (Fig. 49-2).

Common dental abnormalities that need attention include the following:

- Sharp enamel points on the lingual and buccal surfaces
- Sharp hooks that protrude downward from the first or last tooth of the upper arcade
- Sharp ramps that protrude upward from the first or last tooth of the lower arcade
- Wave mouth
- Step mouth that results from a lack of wear of one tooth, allowing it to grow excessively long
- Retained wolf teeth that may cause pain to the tongue when it is displaced because of bit pressure

CLINICAL SIGNS

- Bit avoidance
- Quidding (dropping small, chewed bits of hay)
- Poor performance
- Undigested feed in feces
- Weight loss
- Prolonged eating time

TREATMENT

- If the veterinarian identifies any of the problems described above on a dental examination, he or she should take steps to correct them.
- Hooks, ramps, sharp points, and wave mouths can be corrected by floating the horse's teeth. Basically, a rasp is passed over the tooth to remove unwanted

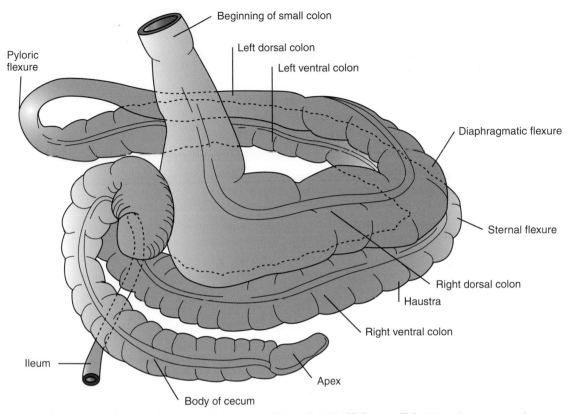

Figure 49-1 Colon and cecum of the horse. (From Colville T, Bassert JM: *Clinical anatomy and physiology for veterinary technicians*, St. Louis, MO, 2008, Mosby, by permission.)

sharp portions. Floats may be either hand floats or power floats. Power floats are becoming more commonly used because they are easier on the user.

INFORMATION FOR CLIENTS

- Yearly dental examinations should be performed on every horse. Older horses may need twice yearly floating to maintain dental health.
- Weight loss and loss of condition may be a sign of dental problems.

🔘 TECH ALERT

Use of a proper mouth gag is important to get a complete examination of the dental arcade. Avoid placing fingers between the horse's teeth when a mouth gag is not being used. Use of the horse's tongue as a mouth gag may damage the tongue and therefore should be avoided.

Choke

Choke refers to a condition in which a partial or total obstruction of the esophagus occurs, usually caused by feed impaction (Fig. 49-3). Horses that choke often have a history of bolting their feed. Choke may also occur if a horse is fed too quickly after sedation. The esophagus may become obstructed because of a number of causes, including the following:

- Feed (often pelleted feeds) expansion when it hits esophagus
- Drugs that cause decrease in smooth muscle motility:
  - Xylazine (Rompun)
  - Detomidine (Dormosedan)
- Trauma, inflammation
- Scar tissue
- Neoplasia

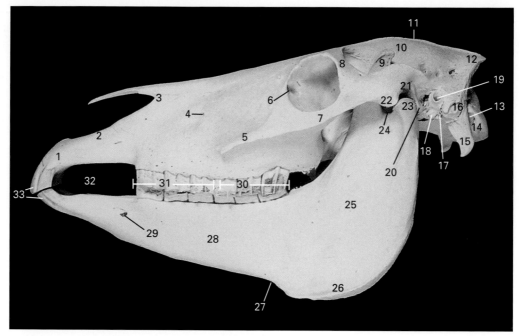

Figure 49-2 Mandible and maxilla of a mare. Note that the upper maxilla is wider than the lower mandible. (From Clayton HM, Flood PF, Rosenstein DS: *Clinical anatomy of the horse*, ed 1, St. Louis, MO, 2005, Mosby, by permission.)

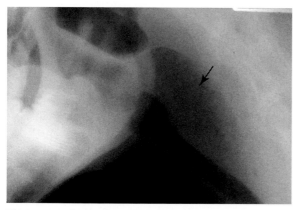

Figure 49-3 Arrow shows impaction of ingesta in the cervical esophagus in a horse with "choke." (From Auer JA, Stick JA: *Equine surgery,* ed 4, St Louis, 2012, Saunders.)

CLINICAL SIGNS

- Difficulty swallowing
- Excessive salivation
- Swelling of throat
- Discharge of food from nostrils
- Neck extension

DIFFERENTIAL DIAGNOSES

- The following conditions should also be considered if a horse is showing clinical signs of choke:
  - Dysphagia due to nerve deficits (rabies should always be included in the differential diagnosis)
  - Cleft palate
  - Dental problems
  - Oral foreign body

DIAGNOSIS

- Definitive diagnosis may be obtained by palpation of the esophagus and passage (or lack thereof) of the nasogastric (NG) tube.
- The veterinarian may also elect to use radiography for visual identification of the obstruction.

TREATMENT

- Ensure that the horse is relaxed, especially its smooth muscles (IV Rompun, IV Dormosedan, lidocaine through tube).
- Lavage with gallons of warm water through the NG tube.
- Perform esophageal massage.

- Provide intravenous (IV) fluid therapy.
- Severe cases may need general anesthesia.
- Antibiotics should be given to combat secondary aspiration pneumonia.
- Nonsteroidal antiinflammatory drugs (NSAIDs) should be used to reduce esophageal inflammation.

INFORMATION FOR CLIENTS

- Do not allow access to feed or hay for 4 hours after sedation.
- If feeding dry feeds that will expand, make sure that the animal consumes the feed slowly, or soak them first.
- When feeding apples, carrots, or other bulky items, cut them into smaller pieces to avoid the horse swallowing them whole.

⬤ TECH ALERT

The signs of choke may range from mild to severe. Get a thorough history, and palpate the entire length of the esophagus.

Gastric Ulcers

Gastric ulcers have become a much more frequently recognized disease in recent years. It is estimated that greater than 80% of show and race horses have some degree of mucosal ulceration.

The prevalence of gastric ulcers in horses is mainly attributed to management techniques. Most heavily worked horses are kept in stalls for 22 or more hours each day. They are fed high-concentrate meals rather than being allowed to graze freely all day.

Horses that have an empty stomach for longer than 6 hours at a time are more prone to develop ulcers compared with those with constant access to grass or hay.

Feeding concentrate meals predisposes a horse to ulcers by two major pathways:
1. Lack of saliva production
2. Constant secretion of HCl acid in the stomach

Saliva contains bicarbonate and acts as a natural buffer to the stomach acids. A horse can salivate only when it has something in its mouth. A grazing horse is salivating nearly constantly, whereas one fed meals salivates only at mealtime. A grazing horse also has a constant physical buffer which protects the stomach from the acid environment. Concentrate feeds also contribute to the problem because concentrates produce one-fourth the amount of saliva compared with an equal amount of forages.

NSAIDs such as flunixin meglumine and phenylbutazone have been shown to cause ulcers in the stomach and other portions of the digestive tract, especially in the right dorsal colon. If possible, the use of NSAIDs should be limited to 5 to 7 days. Oral NSAIDs should also be administered with a meal.

CLINICAL SIGNS

- Chronic, low-grade colic (see later)
- Anemia, if gastric ulcers are severe and chronic
- Loss of condition and decreased endurance

DIAGNOSIS

- Gastric ulcers are diagnosed by an endoscopic examination of the stomach.

TREATMENT

- Treatment of gastric ulcers includes medication and management changes.
- Omeprazole has been found to be the most effective pharmaceutical agent for the treatment of gastric ulcers.
- Management changes that may help the problem are letting the horse out to graze for as many hours as possible during the day; feeding small, frequent meals; and increasing the amount of forage and decreasing the amount of concentrate consumed.

INFORMATION FOR CLIENTS

- Performance horses, young horses in training, and stalled horses are most at risk for development of ulcers. Make sure your training program gives the animal plenty of relaxation time, more forage in the diet, and lots of grazing. If you suspect a problem, have an endoscopic examination performed. Ulcers may have healed before they cause problems.

Colic

Colic is a term that is used to describe a variety of conditions, not a single disease entity. Colic may be defined loosely as a type of abdominal pain, and in many cases, it may be a man-made problem. As in gastric ulcers, management situations are often the cause of this syndrome. The management situation of many modern horses includes being fed two meals per day, feeding more concentrate than is needed, and confinement to a stall, all of which can have adverse effects on the horse's digestive system and lead to colic. In addition, bad management practices such as feeding moldy feed, providing inadequate water, and feeding directly on the ground, among other practices, may lead to colic. Since the cause of colic and the location of the gut affected may not be known, it is important that diagnosis and treatment be performed quickly to prevent further injury to the horse.

Gut sounds in horses with colic may be absent or hyperactive. The absence of gut sounds in both flank areas should signal to the technician that colic is likely a problem. Gas colic often causes hyperactive gut sounds.

Impaction Colic

The anatomy of a horse's gut predisposes it to impactions, especially in or at the following areas:

- Ileocecal junction
- Pelvic flexure
- Diaphragmatic flexure
- Impaction colic can be caused by a variety of factors, including:
  - Sand, which will often accumulate in the cecum
  - Enteroliths (stones)
  - Feed, especially in horses that do not have adequate access to water
  - Dietary indiscretion, when a horse ingests objects such as baling twine, rubber, wood, and so forth

Gas or Spasmodic Colic

Colic is often caused by grain overload when bacteria ferment the concentrate and produce gas. These conditions are typically extremely painful but often resolve spontaneously as the gas works its way out of the digestive tract. In addition, the pain appears to be intermittent in nature—the horse may appear normal and suddenly may throw itself on the ground and roll in pain.

Displacement or Entrapment Colic

Colic occurs when a portion of (GI) tract moves out of normal positioning and may become trapped by another structure. Inguinal hernias and nephrosplenic entrapments are two examples of this type of colic.

Infectious or Inflammatory Colic

Colic occurs as a result of the pain of inflammation of structures in the abdominal cavity. Peritonitis and anterior enteritis are two examples.

Necrotic Colic

Colic occurs because of lack of blood supply to an area of the intestine. That portion of the intestine then dies, and feed does not pass through. Pain may result both from damage to the tissue and the buildup of ingesta proximal to the necrotic area. In the past, the major cause of colic was migration of strongyle larvae (see later), which cause damage to the lining of the intestinal vessels resulting in blood clots that may break off and occlude the blood supply to the intestine. In recent decades, this type of colic has become more uncommon because of the development of more effective deworming practices.

Gastric Ulcers

See earlier text for a detailed description of gastric ulcers.

CLINICAL SIGNS

Clinical signs of colic are *any* signs of abdominal pain, including (but not limited to) the following:

- Pawing
- Rolling
- Lying down more than normal
- Sweating
- Kicking at abdomen
- Looking at sides
- Tachycardia

DIAGNOSIS

- Clinical signs, in addition to the following:
  - Gray to brick-red mucous membranes, poor capillary refill time (CRT)
  - Increased body temperature (often up to 106°F)
- Increased packed cell volume

⬤ **TECH ALERT**

Heart rate over 60 beats per minute strongly suggests that the horse is experiencing severe pain and may be a candidate for surgery.

TREATMENT

- Prevent the horse from rolling, which may cause displacement and torsion. Some say that walking a horse will stimulate GI tract motility and help relieve impactions or gas; others claim that it tires the animal.
- Pain relief:
  - Buscopan (Hyoscine Butylbromide) 0.3 mg/kg intravenously (IV) once
  - Flunixin meglumine (higher doses may mask the worsening of pain over 24 hours. Use lower doses, when needed)
  - Xylazine (although this will impair gut motility)
- Administering the following via an NG tube:
  - Water
  - Electrolytes
  - Mineral oil—helps to relieve impaction (*Note:* If a horse may be headed to surgery, mineral oil should not be given through the NG tube.)
  - Psyllium—especially in sand colic
- Dipyrone—injectable for fever and pain
- IV fluids to maintain hydration and relieve impaction
- Horses that do not respond to NG treatment and pain medication should have further work up including the following:
  - Rectal palpation
  - Abdominal tap with culture and sensitivity of the fluid
  - Complete blood cell count and differential of abdominal fluid, when present
- Surgery in severe cases

INFORMATION FOR CLIENTS

- Fortunately, many cases of colic can be prevented by following these management practices:
  - Increase the forage portion of the diet, and decrease the concentrate portion.
  - Let the horse graze as much as possible.
  - Feed many small meals throughout the day.
  - Allow access to fresh, clean water at all times.
- Encourage water intake by horses that do not drink much, especially during cool weather:
  - Soaking the hay
  - Providing electrolytes
  - Making warm mashes out of feed
  - Following a proper deworming schedule
- With today's surgical techniques, surgery for colic is more likely to be successful than in the past.

⬤ **TECH ALERT**

Flunixin meglumine (Banamine) has a long half-life in the horse and may mask serious symptoms of intestinal disease. Avoid using it as the first line of treatment in horses with colic.

Gastrointestinal Parasitism

Horses live in contaminated environments; pastures, stalls, and turnouts may all become contaminated with parasite eggs over time. It would not be unusual for any horse to harbor some intestinal parasites. Many different parasites may infest the equine GI tract. These parasites live in different locations of the tract and have different physiologic or pathologic effects. However, some generalities do occur.

Large Strongyles

- Three species of large strongyles affect horses:
  - *Strongylus vulgaris*
  - *Strongylus edentatus*
  - *Strongylus equinus*
- Regarded by many experts to be the most pathogenic of all internal equine parasites
- Life cycle:
  - Adults attach themselves to cecum and colon and lay eggs
  - Eggs hatch, and larvae crawl in grass
  - The horse ingests and swallows larvae
  - Larvae migrate through vessels and gut wall
  - Prepatent period (from ingestion to egg laying) is 6 to 12 months, depending on species
- Pathophysiology:
  - Disease is caused by the migration of worms, causing inflammation in blood vessels and leading to formation of clots; clots may occlude the

vessels, resulting in lack of blood supply to the area and causing local tissue death
  - Liver disease and peritonitis also possible
- Effective dewormers: pyrantel, ivermectin, moxidectin, and fenbendazole.

Small Strongyles

- Also known as *cyathostomes*
- More than 50 species of small strongyles affect horses
- Life cycle:
  - Adults in colon lay eggs
  - Eggs hatch; infective larvae are consumed by horse
  - Larvae invade the wall of the cecum and large colon
  - Larvae form cysts in the walls of the gut for 1 to 2 months
  - Larvae emerge and mature into adults
- Pathophysiology:
  - Direct damage to the gut wall, impairing digestion and absorption
- Effective dewormers: pyrantel, ivermectin, moxidectin, and fenbendazole

Threadworms

- *Strongyloides westeri*
- Life cycle:
  - Adults lay eggs in the small intestine
  - Larvae are ingested by the horse
  - Larvae migrate
- Problems mainly in foals:
  - Ingestion of larvae in mare's milk
  - Implicated in foal heat diarrhea
- Some immunity by 12 to 16 weeks of age; infections minimal
- Effective dewormers: pyrantel, ivermectin, moxidectin, and fenbendazole

Roundworms

- *Parascaris equorum* (Fig. 49-4).
- Most common in foals, clinically irrelevant in horses older than 2 years
- Life cycle:
  - Adults live in small intestine and lay eggs
  - Foals ingest embryonated eggs
  - Liver and lung migration

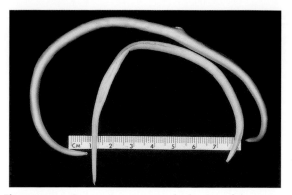

Figure 49-4 *Parascaris equorum*—the largest of the equine nematodes. (From Hendrix CM, Robinson E: *Diagnostic parasitology for veterinary technicians*, ed 4, St. Louis, MO, 2012, Mosby, by permission.)

- Pathophysiology:
  - Intestinal blockage
  - Worms actually use the nutrients instead of the horse
  - May cause intussusception
- Effective dewormers: pyrantel, ivermectin, moxidectin, and fenbendazole

Pinworms

- *Oxyuris equi*
- Life cycle:
  - Adults live in large and small colon
  - Female parasites migrate to the anus, rupture, and spew eggs into the environment
  - Infective eggs are ingested; larvae hatch and migrate
- Pathophysiology is mostly from irritation of the perineum; the horse itches and rubs its tail head
- Effective dewormers: pyrantel, ivermectin, moxidectin, and fenbendazole

Tapeworms

- *Anoplocephala perfoliata, Anoplocephala magna*
- Life cycle involves a mite in which the larvae must develop:
  - The horse ingests the mite
  - Larvae are released from the mite and attach themselves to the cecum and small intestine

- Adults release proglottids into the environment; proglottid releases the eggs, which are consumed by mites
- Previously, little clinical disease attributed to tapeworms; with newer, more effective dewormers, competing parasite populations are removed and tapeworms are able to flourish
- Effective dewormer: praziquantel

Bots

- *Gastrophilus* spp.
- Life cycle:
  - Adult fly lays eggs on the horse
  - The horse licks the eggs and ingests larvae
  - Larvae migrate through the oral cavity and tongue
  - Bots are located in the stomach
- Pathophysiology:
  - Usually does not cause too many problems
  - May cause ulceration, perforation, peritonitis
- Effective dewormer: ivermectin, after the first hard frost

CLINICAL SIGNS

- Diarrhea
- Rough hair coat
- Weight loss
- Anemia
- Colic

DIAGNOSIS

- Fecal flotation and egg counts

TREATMENT AND PREVENTION

- Regular deworming (every 8–12 weeks)
- Rotation of classes of dewormers:
  - Most common dewormers: pyrantel pamoate or tartrate, ivermectin, moxidectin, fenbendazole, and praziquantel
- Pasture and manure management:
  - Not forcing horses to eat near fecal piles
  - Composting manure
  - Breaking up and spreading manure, which exposes eggs to ultraviolet radiation and drying
  - Disposing of manure

⦿ TECH ALERT

All horses will be found to have some eggs on fecal flotation. The goal of routine deworming is to decrease the worm load of the individual horse and to decrease pasture contamination.

Diarrhea

In general, *diarrhea* is defined as an increase in the frequency of defecation and the volume of feces, and it is often accompanied by soft feces. The presence of soft feces does not necessarily mean that the animal has diarrhea. Soft feces may be normal for that animal. What you should look for is a change in the normal consistency of feces, together with an increase in frequency and volume. Diarrhea can be a serious problem in a horse, especially in young foals. Severe, prolonged diarrhea may lead to dehydration and electrolyte imbalances.

Disease entities which are all common causes of diarrhea are discussed below.

Salmonellosis

Salmonellosis may affect horses of all ages, but it mostly affects the young. It is usually seen in horses that are crowded, stressed, or both. The causative agent is *Salmonella* spp. The organism is present in most horses, but it usually causes disease only when the animal is immunocompromised such as in times of stress. Illness is caused by a toxin that the bacteria release.

CLINICAL SIGNS

- Profuse, foul-smelling, often bloody diarrhea
- May become septic, with the following symptoms:
  - Inappetence, depression
  - Fever
  - Abdominal pain
  - Increased heart and respiratory rates
  - Injected sclera
  - Dehydration

DIAGNOSIS

- A diagnosis is made on the basis of the results of a fecal culture.

TREATMENT

- Correction of fluid loss—IV fluids with electrolytes, then oral fluids through NG tube
- Antiserum
- NSAIDs
- Diarrhea control—bismuth salicylate (Pepto)
- ± Antibiotics
- Probiotics

⊙ TECH ALERT

Salmonella is contagious to everyone who interacts with the horse infected by the organism. Wear protective clothing, mask, and gloves when handling these animals, and make sure that all bedding is disposed of as a biohazard. These horses must be quarantined in the hospital to prevent transmission to other patients.

INFORMATION FOR CLIENTS

- Because the causative organism is present in the gut of most horses, little can be done to prevent the disease other than taking steps to minimize stress.
- This is a zoonotic disease and may be transmitted to humans through contact with feces and other bodily fluids. Use protective clothing when handling and cleaning these animals.

Clostridial Infections

Clostridial infection is similar to salmonellosis but much more severe. Animals often die before the onset of diarrhea. This disease is most often seen in foals. The disease is caused by *Clostridium perfringens* type A. These bacteria release a toxin that erodes the gut wall.

CLINICAL SIGNS

- Profound depression and inappetence
- Severe pain
- Injected sclera
- Shock, with the following symptoms:
  - Pale mucous membranes
  - Rapid heart rate
  - Weak, thready pulse
- Fever

- Profuse, bloody diarrhea, although horses die before diarrhea is seen

DIAGNOSIS

- Fecal culture

TREATMENT

- IV fluid therapy
- Pain control
  - Banamine
  - Ketoprofen
  - Xylazine
- Penicillin

Ehrlichiosis (Potomac Horse Fever)

Ehrlichiosis is more commonly found in horses living near large waterways and is also more commonly seen in the summer months. The disease is caused by *Neorickettsia (Ehrlichia) risticii*. The exact method of transmission remains unknown. What is known is that it involves a fluke (larval stage of snail), and it also appears to involve insects that feed on the secretions of snails and flukes. This disease causes inflammation of the colon, impaired water absorption, and diarrhea.

CLINICAL SIGNS

- Fever, depression
- Mild abdominal pain
- Slowed gut movements
- Diarrhea
- Some horses experience toxic signs
- Laminitis is a common sequel

DIAGNOSIS

- Based on clinical signs and serum antibody levels

TREATMENT

- Oxytetracycline
- Maintenance of hydration, possibly by IV fluid therapy
- Banamine may help to prevent laminitis

INFORMATION FOR CLIENTS

- Prevention is by vaccination. However, the vaccine has only one strain of the causative organism, so it may be of limited utility. Also, protection is short lived (3–6 months).

◉ TECH ALERT

Overuse of antibiotics has many negative side effects. Diarrhea is often the result of inappropriate or prolonged antibiotic use and may affect any horse that has been receiving antibiotic therapy. Antibiotics severely decrease the number of favorable gut microflora, thus allowing unfavorable organisms to flourish. The unfavorable organisms then cause diarrhea. It is for this reason that injectable antibiotics are preferred, whenever possible, in the horse. In addition, maintaining the normal gut microflora is necessary for proper digestion of feedstuffs. Diarrhea may result if the feedstuffs are not properly digested.

TREATMENT

- Treatment is accomplished by stopping antibiotic therapy and administering probiotics.

INFORMATION FOR CLIENTS

- Ehrlichiosis may be prevented by removing horses from areas where flukes and snails live.

REVIEW QUESTIONS

1. Which of the following parasites has historically been considered the most pathogenic of all equine intestinal parasites?
   a. *Strongylus* spp.
   b. *Strongyloides* spp.
   c. *Parascaris* spp.
   d. *Oxyuris* spp.
2. One of the most common causes of explosive diarrhea in stressed, hospitalized horses is:
   a. *Escherichia coli*
   b. *Salmonella*
   c. *Pseudomonas*
   d. *Ehrlichia*
3. One possible consequence of feeding horses soon after sedation or anesthesia is:
   a. Choke
   b. Diarrhea
   c. Constipation
   d. Aspiration
4. Which of the following might predispose a horse to gastric ulcers?
   a. Chronic administration of NSAIDs
   b. Intense training
   c. High-concentrate diets
   d. All of the above
5. It is recommended that all horses have their teeth examined and floated:
   a. Every 6 months
   b. At least yearly
   c. Every 2 years
   d. When clinical signs develop
6. Long-term use of NSAIDs may result in:
   a. Esophageal smooth muscle dysfunction
   b. Gastric ulceration
   c. Chronic diarrhea
   d. Malabsorption of nutrients
7. In which of the following are you most likely to find round worms?
   a. a nursing foal
   b. a yearling colt
   c. a three-year-old horse
   d. an adult horse
8. Which of the following parasites may result in damage to the tail of the horse?
   a. *Strongylus vulgaris*
   b. *Oxyuris* spp.
   c. *Parascaris* spp.
   d. *Gastrophilus* spp.

Answers found on page 557.

50
CHAPTER

Diseases of the Endocrine System

LEARNING OBJECTIVES

When you have completed this chapter, you will be able to:
1. Recognize common endocrine disorders in the equine patient.
2. Discuss signs and symptoms with owners.

3. Explain treatment and husbandry practices for equine patients with endocrine disorders.

The endocrine system is a complex system of glands producing hormones that affect all of the body's functions. A discussion of the entire system is beyond the scope of this book, but the three organs involved most commonly in the horse will be discussed here.

The endocrine system comprises the hypothalamus, the pituitary gland, the thyroid, the adrenal glands, and the pancreas, as well as the ovaries and the testes. The kidneys and the heart also play a part in the endocrine system of humans and other animals. Hormone levels circulating within the body are under the control of the hypothalamus, which produces releasing hormones, and the pituitary, which produces stimulating hormones in response to the hormones released by the hypothalamus. Equine endocrine disease involves, most commonly, the pituitary, the thyroid, and the

pancreas. The pituitary gland is responsible for producing stimulating hormones that are released into the bloodstream and are transported to their target organs elsewhere in the body. The target organ then produces its specific hormone, which affects specific functions of the body. Thyroid-stimulating hormone (TSH) is produced in the anterior portion of the pituitary, and it signals the thyroid gland to increase the production of the two thyroid hormones, triiodothyronine (T_3) and thyroxin (T_4). These two hormones affect almost all of the body's normal functions. The middle region of the pituitary gland, the pars intermedia, is more active in the horse than in the dog or the cat and is typically involved in endocrine dysfunction seen in horses. Adenomas in this region result in production of excess amounts of endogenous adrenocorticotropic hormone (ACTH), which accounts for the clinical signs seen in the affected horses. The pancreas is both an endocrine organ and an exocrine organ. The islets of Langerhans (the endocrine portion) are composed of α-cells that secrete glucagon, β-cells that secret insulin, and δ-cells that produce somatostatin. Blood glucose and amino acid levels determine the amount of insulin and glucagon secreted by the islet cells. Insulin is necessary for absorption of glucose into body cells, which also depends on the function of insulin receptors at the cell membrane. Abnormalities in any of these hormonal pathways may result in the clinical signs seen with endocrine disease in the horse. Fortunately, few problems are routinely seen in this system.

Equine Cushing Syndrome (Pars Intermedia Dysfunction)

Equine Cushing syndrome is one of the more common endocrine diseases that affect horses. This disease is more commonly found in older horses, that is, those in their late teens to early twenties. The disease is a result of hypertrophy and hyperplasia of the *pars intermedia* of the pituitary gland (it gets bigger). The body experiences a decrease in dopamine production and an increase in ACTH secretion. ACTH causes increased cortisol concentrations. Cortisol causes a number of changes in the body, including decreased immune response, loss of the muscle mass due to catabolism, and increase in blood glucose concentrations. The first signs of this disease in the older horse may be the presence of a long, shaggy coat that is not shed normally in the spring (Fig. 50-1).

CLINICAL SIGNS

- Weight loss and muscle wasting
- Thick, long-hair coat that does not shed normally
- Lethargy
- Sweating
- Excessive urination and water consumption
- Recurrent laminitis
- Recurrent infections

DIAGNOSIS

- Clinical signs are suggestive of the disease
- Response to a dexamethasone suppression test

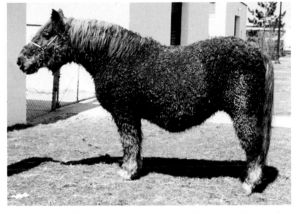

Figure 50-1 Hypertrichosis and potbelly caused by endocrine imbalance of pituitary and *pars intermedia* dysfunction (PPID) (From Scott DW, Miller WH: *Equine dermatology,* ed 2, St. Louis, MO, 2011, Saunders, by permission.)

TREATMENT

- Good management (optimal nutrition, hoof care, body clipping)
- Pergolide, bromocriptine (dopamine receptor agonists)
- Pracend Tablets®; Boeringer—pergolide licensed for use in horses
- Cyproheptadine—less expensive, but does not work as well

INFORMATION FOR CLIENTS

- Because of the heavy hair growth, or lack of shedding, the horse requires special care during the warm months. Body clipping the horse is best. If the horse cannot be clipped, it should be kept under a fan during the warm months.
- The horse's diet needs careful monitoring so that it is less likely to develop laminitis.

Hypothyroidism

Hypothyroidism is one of the most diagnosed conditions in horses and, some would argue, one of the most overdiagnosed. Hypothyroidism may affect horses of any age, breed, or sex and is one of two types:
- *Primary hypothyroidism* refers to inadequate activity of the thyroid gland.

- *Secondary hypothyroidism* refers to a disorder of the anterior pituitary, which does not produce enough TSH.

CLINICAL SIGNS

Foals
- Weakness, incoordination
- Signs of dysmaturity:
  - Poor suckling response
  - Fine-hair coat
  - Joint and tendon laxity
  - Poor righting reflexes
  - Low body temperature
  - Poor muscle development, umbilical hernias
  - Incomplete ossification of bones

Adults
- Exercise intolerance
- Lethargy
- Low heart rate
- Obesity and laminitis

DIAGNOSIS

- A diagnosis made by two methods
- Blood work:
  - Measuring circulating thyroid hormone levels: not reliable
  - Alternative (thyrotropin-releasing hormone response test): expensive and rarely used
- Response to thyroid hormone supplementation

TREATMENT

- Thyroid hormone supplementation
- Weaning horses off supplements rather than stopping them abruptly

Insulin Resistance

Insulin resistance may be defined as a decreased response to endogenous insulin levels associated with increased blood glucose concentrations. Insulin resistance results from changes in the sensitivity of the insulin receptors at the cellular level. Since a number of these receptors must be activated to achieve the desired effect, with an increase in the number of nonfunctional receptors, higher insulin levels will be required to activate the remaining functional

receptors. Insulin resistance is seen in horses with pars intermedia dysfunction, granulose cell tumors, and hyperlipidemia. The development of the clinical signs of insulin resistance is poorly understood. Laminitis is a frequent sign of insulin resistance, and many horses improve when placed on low carbohydrate rations. Some experts believe that laminitis may be the result of elevated levels of glucocorticoids seen with pars intermedia dysfunction.

CLINICAL SIGNS

- Signs of pars intermedia dysfunction
- Laminitis made worse by increased carbohydrate in the diet (spring and fall grasses)

DIAGNOSIS

- Positive response to low-carbohydrate diets
- Positive diagnosis of pars intermedia dysfunction

TREATMENT

- Pergolide for equine Cushing syndrome
- High-fiber, low-carbohydrate diet
- Muzzle to limit grass intake in pastured horses

INFORMATION FOR CLIENTS

- Pituitary tumors in horses are not surgically accessible, so a cure is not possible.
- Every horse will respond differently to pergolide, and doses may require adjustment as the disease progresses.
- Laminitis, when it occurs, may necessitate special shoeing and may be the limiting factor to the survival time of the patient.

REVIEW QUESTIONS

1. Which gland in the endocrine system is involved in equine Cushing disease?
   a. The thyroid gland
   b. The pancreas
   c. The pituitary gland
   d. The hypothalamus
2. Cushing syndrome is most commonly seen in horses that are:
   a. Less than 1 year of age
   b. Between 5 and10 years of age
   c. Over 10 years of age

3. Signs of dysmaturity in foals may be linked to dysfunction of:
   a. The pancreas
   b. The ovary
   c. The thyroid
   d. The pituitary
4. Horses with recurring laminitis may have:
   a. Cushing syndrome
   b. Pancreatitis
   c. Insulin resistance
   d. Thyroid dysfunction

5. Diets low in _____ are recommended for insulin-resistant horses.
   a. Lipids
   b. Proteins
   c. Carbohydrates
   d. Fiber

Answers found on page 557.

51
CHAPTER

Diseases of the Eye

LEARNING OBJECTIVES

When you have completed this chapter, you will be able to:
1. Diagram the structure of the eye.
2. Assist the veterinarian with a complete eye examination.
3. Discuss treatment difficulties and alternatives with clients.

Anatomy of the Equine Eye

The equine eye is large and beautiful and, for many horse-loving people, is the window to the soul of the horse. The structure of the eye is the same as for other mammals. The three distinct layers to the globe are: (1) the fibrous layer, the cornea and sclera; (2) the vascular layer, the choroid or uvea; and (3) nervous layer, the retina. Less of the globe is protected by the bony orbit, so damage to the cornea is common in horses. The *cornea* is clear and is composed of the epithelial surface cells, stroma, and Descemet's membrane. The cornea is avascular but is well supplied with sensory nerve fibers. The cornea is the anterior boundary of the *anterior chamber* of the globe. Fluid that circulates through the anterior chamber provides nutrition for the cornea. The

caudal border of the chamber is the uvea, which is responsible for the production of the aqueous humor, gives the *iris* its color, and is the location of the *pupil*. The lining tissue of the uvea is highly pigmented and vascular. It serves to decrease scatter as light passes into the back of the eye through the pupil and lens. The *tapetum* is located in the choroid layer. This highly colored, reflective area reflects light back onto the retina, which results in maximizing the use of available light.

The *pupil* in the eye of the horse is elliptical, not round. The dorsal and ventral margins contain pigmented prominences known as the *corpra nigra*. Pupillary light response in the horse is both consensual and direct. The *fundus* of the retina is partially vascularized with 30 to 60 retinal vessels radiating

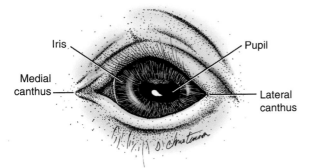

Figure 51-1 Equine eye structures. (From Christenson DE: *Veterinary medical terminology*, ed 2, St. Louis, MO, 2009, Saunders, by permission.)

from the *optic disk*. The optic disk is located in the non-tapetal area of the fundus and is oval and salmon-pink in color. The *lens*, that separates the anterior chamber from the posterior vitreous, acts to focus light on the retina (Fig. 51-1).

In general, any ocular disease is considered an emergency. Some of these conditions may progress from a seemingly minor problem in the morning to a sight-threatening emergency that afternoon. As a rule, if a horse has an eye problem, a veterinarian should be contacted as soon as possible. Signs of ocular disease include cloudy eyes, blepharospasm, photophobia, and discharge. If these signs are observed, the first action that should be taken is to bring the horse inside, out of the sunlight. A veterinarian should then be called.

Entropion

Entropion is a condition that involves the rolling inward of the horse's eyelids and subsequent corneal irritation. Entropion is either unilateral or bilateral. Entropion may be congenital or secondary to other conditions.

CLINICAL SIGNS

- Excessive tear production
- Blepharospasm
- Photophobia
- Inversion of the eyelid
- Corneal ulcers

DIAGNOSIS

- Visual examination of the eye
- A corneal stain to rule out corneal ulcers

TREATMENT

- Eye ointments
- Manual eversion with tissue glue
- Surgery

> ## ● TECH ALERT
>
> Advise clients to discard old eye medications after the treatment has been completed. Old medications may become contaminated, and their use may result in damage to the eye.

Sarcoid

See Chapter 53 for detailed information about equine sarcoid.

Squamous Cell Carcinoma

See Chapter 53 for detailed information about squamous cell carcinoma in horses.

Conjunctivitis

Conjunctivitis, or inflammation of the conjunctiva, is associated with a wide variety of disease processes. It is more commonly seen in the summer, during dry, dusty conditions, and when flies are present.

CLINICAL SIGNS

- Ocular discharge
- Pruritus
- Red, swollen conjunctiva
- May be associated with upper respiratory infections
- Parasites; May be more prevalent in young horses; *Thelasia, Habronema, Onchocerca* spp.

TREATMENT

- Stain the eye to rule out corneal ulcers.
- Treat the underlying cause.

- Clean the discharge, and keep flies away from the eyes.
- Apply eye ointment or drops

Corneal Ulcers

Corneal ulcers are one of the most common causes of ocular disease in horses. Major causes of corneal ulcers include trauma and scratching of the cornea, bacteria, and fungi.

CLINICAL SIGNS

- Photophobia
- Blepharospasm
- Cloudy cornea or blue eye (Fig. 51-2).
- New blood vessels in cornea

DIAGNOSIS

- Stain the cornea with fluorescein stain.
- It is also advisable to look for a foreign body.

TREATMENT

- Atropine—relaxes ciliary muscles, controls pain

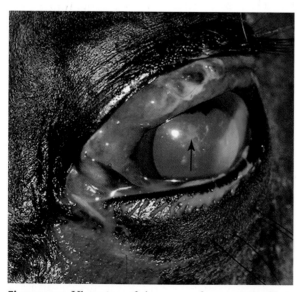

Figure 51-2 Ulceration of the cornea from trauma. Note the swollen conjunctiva and corneal stain (*arrow*). (From Gilger BC: *Equine Ophthalmology*, ed 2, St. Louis, MO, 2011, Saunders, by permission.)

- Antibacterial ointment, antifungal ointment, or both *without steroids*

> **◉ TECH ALERT**
>
> Topical treatment of the equine eye is difficult. It is often necessary to place a catheter sub-conjunctivally to facilitate multiple daily treatments.

INFORMATION FOR CLIENTS

- *Never* put anything that contains steroids into an animal's eye without first consulting a veterinarian because steroids may cause a corneal ulcer to worsen.

Moon Blindness (Periodic Ophthalmia, Recurrent Uveitis)

Moon blindness got its name because it tends to come and go. The exact cause of the disease remains undetermined. Many animals with recurrent uveitis also have a high antibody titer to leptospirosis. Some authors also believe that the disease may be immune mediated.

CLINICAL SIGNS

- Cloudy eye (cornea appears blue or white and opaque) (Fig. 51-3)
- Blepharospasm
- Excessive tears

DIAGNOSIS

- Visualization of protein flare in fluid of anterior chamber
- Affected eye appearing smaller than the unaffected globe
- Can measure antibody titers against leptospirosis
- Corneal stain to rule out ulcers

TREATMENT

- Topical corticosteroids
- Long-acting steroids, which can be injected under the conjunctiva
- Atropine
- Flunixin meglumine (Banamine)

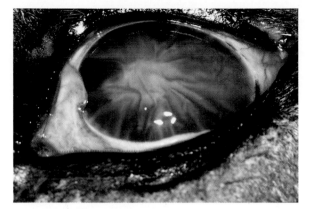

Figure 51-3 Horse with signs of active equine recurrent uveitis. (From Holtgrew-Bohling K: *Large animal clinical procedures for veterinary technicians*, ed 2, St. Louis, MO, 2012, Mosby, by permission.)

 TECH ALERT

Quick treatment of this disease helps prevent permanent damage in many cases. Consider this a "must see vet today" type of condition.

Cataracts

A *cataract* is an opacity that causes the lens to lose its ability to allow the passage of light. Cataracts may be congenital or acquired, and some evidence suggests that a hereditary component may exist.

CLINICAL SIGNS

- Visual deficits
- Cloudy appearance to lens

DIAGNOSIS

- Visual examination

TREATMENT

- Surgery (prognosis is good for foals)
- Atropine (dilates pupil, lets more light in, may focus light on clear part of lens)

TECH ALERT

Many blind horses can be ridden safely if the owners do not overstep the ability and comfort level of the animal.

REVIEW QUESTIONS

1. What step should be taken when a horse with an eye problem is seen in the pasture?
   a. Put antibiotic ointment in the eye
   b. Bring the horse out of the light; then call the vet
   c. Put steroid ointment in the eye
   d. Call the vet and leave the horse in the pasture
2. The most common cause of eye problems in horses is:
   a. Corneal ulcers
   b. Retinal degeneration
   c. Entropion
   d. Periodic ophthalmia
3. Used eye medications should be:
   a. Refrigerated for future use
   b. Disposed of when treatment has ended
   c. Kept in case the problem recurs
   d. Given to friends for their horses
4. _____ stain should be used to rule out a corneal ulcer prior to treatment.
   a. Dif-quik
   b. Fluorescein
   c. Rose Bengal
5. Long-term use of ophthalmic atropine might result in some horses developing _____.
   a. Colic
   b. Dry eye
   c. Corneal damage

Answers found on page 557.

Hematologic Diseases

OUTLINE

Equine Infectious Anemia   **Red Maple Toxicosis**

LEARNING OBJECTIVES

When you have completed this chapter, you will be able to:
1. Explain to clients the need for the Coggins test for all horses on a yearly basis.

Blood disorders are a serious, although rare, problem in horses. As an animal's blood cells become weakened or destroyed, they start losing their ability to carry oxygen and nutrients to tissues. Such an instance, if allowed to progress unchecked, is incompatible with life.

Equine Infectious Anemia

Equine infectious anemia (EIA) is a disease that affects horses throughout the world. No age, breed, or sex predilection is associated with this disease. The causative organism is lentivirus that is spread via blood transmission.

Biting flies are the most common method of transmission, although sharing needles and surgical instruments between horses may also spread the disease.

CLINICAL SIGNS

- Fever
- Depression
- Anemia
- Clotting disorders

- Chronic carriers show little sign of the disease; these horses typically will have recurrent bouts of clinical disease

DIAGNOSIS

- Draw a blood sample and perform the Coggins test.

TREATMENT

- No treatment exists for EIA.

⬤ TECH ALERT

All horses should be tested yearly for EIA. Horses housed in clinics should have a negative Coggins test before hospital admission, whenever possible.

INFORMATION FOR CLIENTS

- Prevention of EIA consists of typical biosecurity measures—not sharing needles or instruments between horses, fly control, and so forth.
- If a horse tests positive, it must be reported to the State Veterinarian. The horse will then be retested.
- A horse that tests positive must be euthanized or branded and quarantined *for the rest of its life*.

- As a responsible horse owner, you should have your horses tested yearly.

Red Maple Toxicosis

Red maple toxicosis is caused by a toxin that accumulates in wilted or dried red maple (*Acer rubrum*) leaves. When ingested, the toxin causes oxidation damage to the red blood cells (RBCs). At first, the toxin causes methemoglobinemia, and the erythrocytes are not able to carry oxygen efficiently. This is followed by Heinz body formation, that is damage to the RBC membrane, and eventual rupture of the erythrocyte.

CLINICAL SIGNS

- Jaundice
- Brown urine
- Weakness, depression
- Petechiae

DIAGNOSIS

- Clinical signs, together with examination of a blood smear

TREATMENT

- The condition is treated with supportive care and blood transfusions. The animal should be kept in a calm, quiet environment, and supplemental oxygen should be given, if necessary.

INFORMATION FOR CLIENTS

- Every effort should be made to prevent the ingestion of wilted red maple leaves by cleaning up the leaves while they are still fresh on the ground or by not pasturing horse near red maple trees.

REVIEW QUESTIONS

1. How is a case of equine infectious anemia (EIA) diagnosed?
   a. With Coombs test
   b. With Coggins test
   c. With card agglutination test
   d. EIA cannot be diagnosed accurately
2. If an animal tests positive for EIA, what is the next step for the animal?
   a. Quarantine
   b. Retesting by State Veterinarian
   c. Euthanasia
   d. Antibiotic therapy

Answers found on page 557.

Diseases of the Integumentary System

LEARNING OBJECTIVES

When you have completed this chapter, you will be able to:
1. Recognize differences among the common skin problems in the equine patient.

2. Advise clients on preventive measures required to limit the spread of skin diseases.

Reporting of skin diseases in horses is quite common. It is not unusual for the owner to notice various lesions as the horse is being groomed and prepared for work. Following are important questions in the history of a horse presented for skin problems:
- How old is the horse?
- What season of the year is it?
- Is the horse in a stable or on pasture?
- Is the horse maintained in a herd, or singly?
- Are other horses showing signs of skin disease?
- Where is the horse located?

Answers to these questions can help narrow down the list of potential diseases that may be affecting the animal.

Insect Hypersensitivity

Insect hypersensitivity is a systemic, allergic reaction to the bite of an insect. The condition is usually seen during the summer months and is first noticed in animals 4 years of age or younger. The most common insects to cause the condition are those of the genus *Culicoides*, also known as biting gnats (Fig. 53-1).

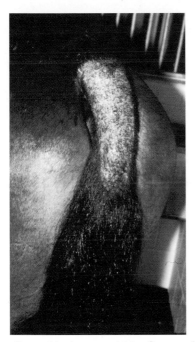

Figure 53-1 Insect-bite hypersensitivity. Severe self-induced hypotrichosis of the tail. (From Scott DW, Miller WH: *Equine dermatology*, ed 2, St. Louis, MO, 2011, Saunders, by permission.)

CLINICAL SIGNS

- Intense pruritus
- Alopecia, excoriation, erythema, scaling
- Urticaria (hives)
- Lesions most common along mane, ventral body

DIAGNOSIS

- Clinical signs
- Presence of the insects in the environment

TREATMENT

- Insect control, fly sprays
- Steroid therapy
- Antihistamines do not appear to be effective
- If lesions are severe animal will need antibiotic therapy as well

INFORMATION FOR CLIENTS

- The occurrence and severity of insect hypersensitivity may be prevented with good management.

Insect control, fly sprays, and fans may keep the gnats off the horses.
- If the animals are kept in a small paddock, manure removal may reduce the number of gnats present.

Fly Bite Dermatitis

Lesions are seen as a result of the bite of the fly. Fly bite dermatitis is usually seen during the warmer months of the year.

CLINICAL SIGNS

- Wheals
- Pustules
- Nodules

TREATMENT

- Feed-through fly control
- Fly sprays
- Appropriate care of any wounds that may appear

Lice (Pediculosis)

Lice are one of the most common ectoparasites that affect horses. Lice are host specific, and two species affect horses. Sucking lice (*Haematopinus asini*) are more damaging to the animal and live off its blood. Biting or chewing lice (*Damalinia equi*) live off the dead cells and other debris in the horse's skin. Lice infestation is usually seen in the winter months. The reasons may be that the horse's hair is longer and grooming may not be as thorough, and horses may congregate for warmth. Transmission of lice is through direct horse-to-horse contact, or they may be carried on inanimate objects.

CLINICAL SIGNS

- Intense pruritus, especially around mane and tail (Fig. 53-2).
- Presence of adults or eggs (nits) in the hair

DIAGNOSIS

- Visualization of adults and eggs in the hair coat

TREATMENT

- Topical shampoos (pyrethrins and organophosphates, although organophosphates should be avoided, if possible, for safety reasons)

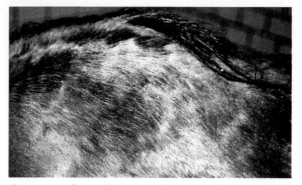

Figure 53-2 Lice infestation: alopecia and scaling of the mane. (From Scott DW, Miller WH: *Equine dermatology*, ed 2, St. Louis, MO, 2011, Saunders, by permission.)

- Treatment of the environment
- Clipping
- Treatment of all horses on the premises
- Ivermectin: more effect against sucking lice than against biting lice

Mites

Many different species of mites are normal inhabitants of the horse's skin, and some are free-living in the environment. Disease caused by mites is most often seen when an animal becomes immunocompromised.

CLINICAL SIGNS

- Intense itching
- Distribution of lesions depends on species of mite

DIAGNOSIS

- Microscopic examination of skin scrapings

TREATMENT

- Lime sulfur dips
- Pyrethrin dips
- Ivermectin

Ticks

Four predominant types of blood-sucking ticks affect horses, mainly in the warmer months of the year: *Otobius megnini*, the spinous ear tick; *Dermacentor* spp.; *Ixodes* spp. (deer tick); and *Amblyomma* spp.

CLINICAL SIGNS

- Bite sensitivity, found most often in the following areas:
  - Ears
  - Face
  - Neck
  - Groin
  - Tail
  - Distal limbs
- Some severe systemic hypersensitivity
- Tick paralysis

DIAGNOSIS

- Presence of ticks on the horse

TREATMENT

- Removal of ticks
- Pyrethrin dips

Onchocerciasis

Onchocerciasis is caused by a nematode parasite, the adults of which live in the ligamentum nuchae. The larvae migrate through skin and cause dermatitis. Small insects are implicated in the spread of the disease, which is usually nonseasonal in occurrence.

CLINICAL SIGNS

- Pruritic lesions, especially in area of ventral abdomen
- "Bull's-eye" lesions, especially on face (Fig. 53-3)
- Uveitis is often seen concurrently

DIAGNOSIS

- Histopathology can be performed, but a more common method of diagnosis is by observing response to treatment.

TREATMENT

- Administer oral ivermectin, repeated in 3 weeks.
- Death of microfilariae can cause intense itching, and steroids may be prescribed.

Rain Scald, Rain Rot

Rain rot is one of the more common skin diseases of horses. When the disease occurs on the palmar and

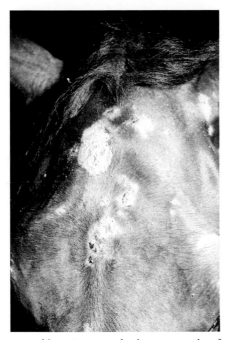

Figure 53-3 Alopecic crusted plaques on the forehead with onchocerciasis. (From Scott DW, Miller WH: *Equine dermatology*, ed 2, St. Louis, MO, 2011, Saunders, by permission.)

plantar aspects of the pasterns, it may be referred to as "dew poisoning," "mud scratches" or "scurf." This disease has both fungal and bacterial components. The causative bacterium is *Dermatophilus congolensis*, and this condition may also be referred to as *dermatophilosis*. This condition is usually seen during moist conditions, and in a large portion of the United States, it is most common in the winter months.

The causative organisms become trapped in the hair and reproduce in a moist environment. The condition may be transferred by direct contact or through inanimate objects.

CLINICAL SIGNS

- Matting of hair, followed by alopecia and crusting
- "Paintbrush" lesions—hair epilates in clumps that resemble a paintbrush
- Lesions most often found along back of the leg, the rump and back of the horse
- Mud scratches most often on white legs
- Often nonpruritic, but may be painful

DIAGNOSIS

- The clinical signs and history are highly suggestive, and definitive diagnosis of the condition is made by observing an impression smear of the lesions.

TREATMENT

- Treatment usually consists of bathing with one of the following:
  - Iodine-based shampoos
  - Chlorhexiderm washes
  - Dilute bleach solution
  - Antifungal powder
  - Ketoconazole or chlorhexidine pads

INFORMATION FOR CLIENTS

- Rain rot can be prevented by daily grooming.
- If a horse does experience development of rain rot, its brushes, blankets, and so on need to be washed in an iodine-based solution before being used on another horse.

● TECH ALERT

In many areas of the United States, rain rot is a common problem among long-haired horses (winter hair) outside in the wet spring weather. Clipping the coat or using a good shedding blade allows the coat to dry faster.

Ringworm

The fungal infection ringworm is one of the most common dermatoses in stabled horses (Fig. 53-4). Two genera of fungi cause ringworm, *Trichophyton* and *Microsporum*. Usually, affected animals have some sort of compromise to the skin or the immune system. The fungi may be transmitted via direct contact or inanimate objects.

CLINICAL SIGNS

- Multifocal lesions of alopecia scaling, crusting
- Lesion may start as classic round areas of hair loss, but is just as often seen over a larger area (Fig. 53-5).
- May or may not be pruritic

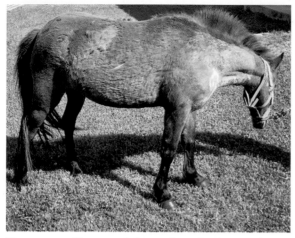

Figure 53-4 Dermatophilosis often develops in horses in wet environments. (From Sellon DC, Long MT: *Equine infectious diseases*, St. Louis, MO, 2007, Saunders, by permission.)

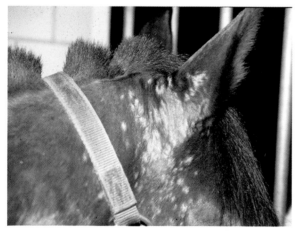

Figure 53-5 Dermatophytosis caused by *Trypanosoma equinum*. Annular areas of alopecia on the face and at the base of the ears. (From Scott DW, Miller WH: *Equine dermatology*, ed 2, St. Louis, MO, 2011, Saunders, by permission.)

DIAGNOSIS

- History and clinical signs are suggestive
- Definitive diagnosis is made by a fungal culture

TREATMENT

- Disease is often self-limiting, so benign neglect often works

- Disinfection of blankets, brushes, and so on
- Topical antifungals
- Miconazole
- Iodine
- Chlorhexiderm
- Griseofulvin for those animals that do not respond to topical treatments

⦿ TECH ALERT

Ringworm is contagious to humans that come in contact with the animal or contaminated tack or blankets.

INFORMATION FOR CLIENTS

- Make sure that blankets and brushes are thoroughly disinfected before using them on unaffected horses.

Scratches (Pastern Dermatitis)

Scratches, also called "mud fever" or "greasy heel," is seen in horses kept in wet, unhygienic conditions. It is more common in breeds with heavy feathering on the legs. The condition is more frequent in the spring when the pastures are wet and muddy.

CLINICAL SIGNS

- Swelling of the pastern skin on the rear of the leg
- Hair loss
- Scab formation
- Painful skin, in severe condition the skin may ulcerate

DIAGNOSIS

- Location of the lesions

TREATMENT

- Clip the feathering on legs to open the area to air.
- Wash the area with an antiseptic shampoo or dry well.
- Remove the scabs.
- Apply antifungal or antiseptic pads to raw area.
- Keep the horse in a clean, dry stall until the lesions heal.

⦿ TECH ALERT

The horse's skin may be very painful to the touch, so be prepared for the horse to react.

INFORMATION FOR CLIENTS

- Keep feathering short during wet conditions.
- Stall horses on clean, dry bedding.
- Dry the pastern area well after bathing.

Sweet Itch

Sweet itch is a warm weather skin disease caused by hypersensitivity to the bites of midges (small "no-see-um" flies). Lesions are seen along the topline of the horse, around the mane and tail, and on the face and ears. These flies are usually are more active around dawn and sunset.

CLINICAL SIGNS

- Pruritus
- Scaly lesions along the topline or at the base of the tail

DIAGNOSIS

- Position of the scaly, itchy lesions
- History of exposure to the outside during the evening and morning hours

TREATMENT

- Corticosteroids *or*
- Oral antihistamines
- Stalling horse during times when flies are most active; use of a fan to keep flies away

INFORMATION FOR CLIENTS

- Fly sheets and masks to prevent flies from biting the horse
- Frequent applications of fly spray or wipes
- Use of fans in stalls to keep flies away
- Stalling horse during times when flies are most active

Sarcoids

Sarcoids are the most common skin tumor of horses (Fig. 53-6). They are slow growing and locally invasive, but nonmetastatic. The onset of the tumors is mainly seen in younger horses (<10 years old). It is currently believed that a papovavirus may be responsible for these tumors. Deoxyribonucleic acid (DNA) testing suggests that these tumors are caused by bovine papillomaviruses type 1 and 2. The tumors tend to occur

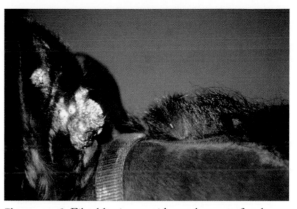

Figure 53-6 Fibroblastic sarcoid on the ear of a horse. (From Sellon DC, Long MT: *Equine infectious diseases*, St. Louis, MO, 2007, Saunders, by permission.)

at sites of previous trauma but may spread to other areas of the body or to other horses. Sarcoids occur as single tumors or multiple nodules (Fig. 53-7). The best treatment for sarcoids is benign neglect. The tumors have been found to get worse after biopsies have been performed. If they must be removed, cryosurgery with

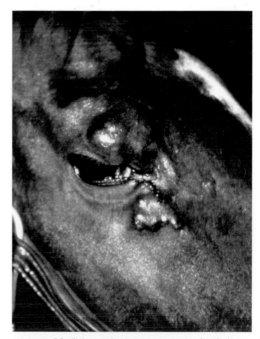

Figure 53-7 Nodular, subcutaneous sarcoid of the eyelid. (Courtesy Dr. Melissa Hines. IN Sellon DC, Long MT: *Equine infectious diseases*, St Louis, 2007, Saunders)

surgical debulking of the tumor has been shown to reduce recurrence rates.

DIAGNOSIS

- Biopsy

TREATMENT

- Sarcoids are most often treated by surgical excision, injection of chemotherapeutic agents into the tumor, or cryotherapy.
- XTerra (Larson Laboratories): -a caustic substance with extract of the bloodroot plant

Proud Flesh

Proud flesh is the red, protruding flesh that is found on the distal limbs after an injury. Essentially, proud flesh is granulation tissue growing out of control, or "exuberant granulation tissue." Proud flesh is red, cauliflower-like growth over a wound that bleeds easily.

TREATMENT

- Apply powdered meat tenderizer to lesion
- Enzyme sprays
- Surgical removal
- Avoid the use of caustic substances that delay healing

INFORMATION FOR CLIENTS

- Measures to prevent proud flesh formation:
  - Wrapping
  - Chlorhexidine diacetate (Nolvasan) or steroid ointment
  - Enzyme sprays
  - Avoiding the use of caustic substances that will delay healing
  - Furacin ointment may cause an increase in the development of proud flesh
- When the proud flesh is cut off, it will bleed profusely. However, the horse will show few signs of being aware of the procedure. Although rich in blood vessels, scar tissue is devoid of sensory nerve endings, so the animal does not feel any pain.

Warts (Papillomatosis)

Warts are common in a variety of animal species (Fig. 53-8). They most often affect horses younger than 3 years. Warts are caused by a papillomavirus and are transmitted by direct contact.

CLINICAL SIGNS

- Papillomatosis lesions are typical wartlike growths, usually multifocal, and found most commonly around the muzzle and lips of horses.

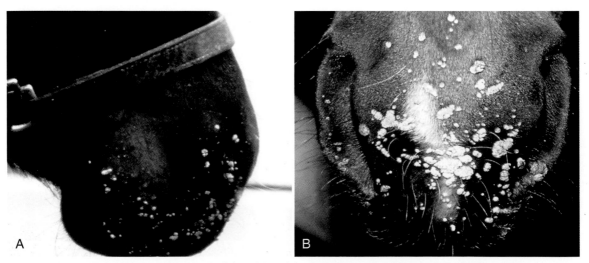

Figure 53-8 Warts on the muzzle (*A*) and lips (*B*) of a young horse. (Courtesy Dr. Melissa Hines. IN Sellon DC, Long MT: *Equine infectious diseases,* St Louis, 2007, Saunders)

TREATMENT

- Warts are usually self-limiting, so benign neglect is a common course of action.
- In severe cases, autogenous vaccines may be used.
- In addition, immunostimulants may be used, especially when warts appear in older horses.
- Separation of affected animals may prevent spread to the rest of the herd.

INFORMATION FOR CLIENTS

- Avoid using the same tack, feed buckets, and water buckets for other horses.

⊙ TECH ALERT

Avoid spreading warts by not using the same bridles and bits, feed buckets, and water buckets for multiple horses. Wear gloves when treating the lesions.

Wounds

Wounds to the skin may be from any external source of trauma, and the specific treatment for the wound may depend on the source. General steps taken in the treatment of wounds include stopping blood loss, clipping the hair from the area, and thorough cleansing. The wound may then be evaluated to determine whether sutures or staples are necessary. Puncture wounds should be flushed thoroughly and allowed to heal from the inside outward. Any puncture wound close to a joint needs careful evaluation by a veterinarian to determine whether the joint capsule has been compromised. Most wounds will benefit from antibiotic therapy. Whenever a horse has a wound, tetanus prophylaxis needs to be considered.

⊙ TECH ALERT

If an injured horse is current on tetanus vaccination, give a tetanus toxoid booster. Avoid using tetanus antitoxin in vaccinated horses because severe anaphylactic reactions have been reported.

Snake Bite

Rattlesnakes, copperheads, and water moccasins are the most common snakes causing bites in horses.

The venom from snakes is hemotoxic and proteolytic and bites result in profound local swelling with tissue and blood cell destruction. Most bites occur in the summer months and are usually on the nose, head, or neck. Swelling on the head may compromise respiration. As with other species, treatment of the horse is symptomatic; hydrotherapy is used to decrease swelling, with or without non-steroidal antiinflammatories. Antivenom, while available, is of limited use.

Fire Ant Bites

Fire ants, found mostly in the southern United States, produce painful bites that develop into papules on the legs, nose, or ventrum. Horses may roll into anthills and be bitten by hundreds of ants. If many ant bites have occurred antibiotics and nonsteroidal antiinflammatories may be necessary to decrease pain and combat infection of the bites.

CLINICAL SIGNS

- Localized swelling on the nose or face; maybe extreme
- Necrosis of the tissue associated with the swelling
- Usually will not be able to find puncture marks due to swelling
- Many painful papules on the legs and body; horse may be manic because of the pain

DIAGNOSIS

- Complete blood cell count (CBC), serum chemistries
- Seeing the animal bitten

TREATMENT

- Hydrotherapy to reduce swelling
- Non-steroidal antiinflammatories
- ± antibiotics
- Surgical debridement if tissue is necrotic

REVIEW QUESTIONS

1. Which of the following conditions has both a bacterial and a fungal component?
   a. Ringworm
   b. Rain rot
   c. *Rhodococcus* pneumonia
   d. Recurrent uveitis

2. The most common tumor of the skin is _____.
   a. Squamous cell carcinoma
   b. Sarcoid
   c. Cutaneous adenoma
3. Which of the following could be used for treatment of rain rot?
   a. Iodine shampoo
   b. Ketoconazole shampoo
   c. Dilute chlorox solution
   d. All of the above
4. Why do most snake bites occur on the head of the horse?

5. How might a technician prepare and autogenous wart vaccine? (Check all that apply.)
   a. _____ Grind up a few warts in a sterile liquid medium, and inject subcutaneously into the horse
   b. _____ Scrape the warts with a scalpel blade until they bleed
   c. _____ Surgically remove the wart with wide excision
   d. _____ All of the above

Answers found on page 557.

Diseases of the Musculoskeletal System

LEARNING OBJECTIVES

When you have completed this chapter, you will be able to:
1. Assist the veterinarian in the diagnosis of musculoskeletal diseases.
2. Explain the value of proper nutrition and maintenance of the horse to clients.

3. Appreciate how conformation affects musculoskeletal diseases seen in horses.

Anatomy and Physiology of the Musculoskeletal System

The skeleton of the horse is somewhat similar to that of dogs and cats but with some major differences. The vertebral column is longer than that of the dog even though the horse still has only 7 cervical vertebrae. There are 16 thoracic vertebra and 16 ribs.

The lumbar, sacral, and pelvic bones are just like those of the canine only larger. The femur and humerus are shaped as in other mammals but from the elbow and stifle the bones are different. Horsemen through the ages have had special names for the bones of the lower legs. The technician should learn both the anatomic and the common names for these bones. The carpus, in the front legs, is called the *knee*. It comprises a series of bones stacked on top of one another, as in other animals, plus the ulna and the radius. The "knee" in the rear leg is known as the *stifle*. That joint is made up of the femur, patella, fibula, and tibia. Distal to the carpus, the horse stands on the third metacarpal bone in the front leg and the third metatarsal bone in the rear leg. These bones are commonly known as the *cannon bones*. Medial and lateral to the cannon bone are the *splint bones*, remnants of the second and fourth metacarpal and metatarsals. In the rear leg the *hock* is like the heel of the human foot. That joint is made up of the tibia, the fibula, and the tarsal bones. Below the hock is the rear cannon bone. Distal to the cannon bones are the pastern bones: the fetlock joint comprises the third metacarpal or metatarsal bone plus the

long *pastern* bone or the third proximal phalanx. The long pastern bone articulates with the *short pastern* bone, the third middle phalanx, which articulates with the *coffin* bone, the third distal phalanx, within the hoof (Fig. 54-1).

Anatomy of the Equine Limb

Most veterinary technicians are familiar with the bones of dogs and cats but have not been exposed to "horse" terminology. When listening to clients or when discussinsg disease problems with owners, the technician needs to be fluent in the terminology of "equine" anatomy.

Since most of the differences in terminology occur in the limb and since most musculoskeletal problems also occur there, the limb anatomy of the horse is important to the technician. The horse front leg consists of the scapula, humerus, radius and

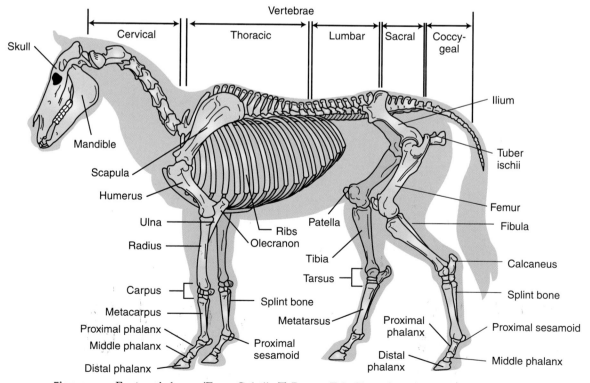

Figure 54-1 Equine skeleton. (From Colville T, Bassert JM: Clinical anatomy and physiology for veterinary technicians, St Louis, 2002, Mosby, by permission).

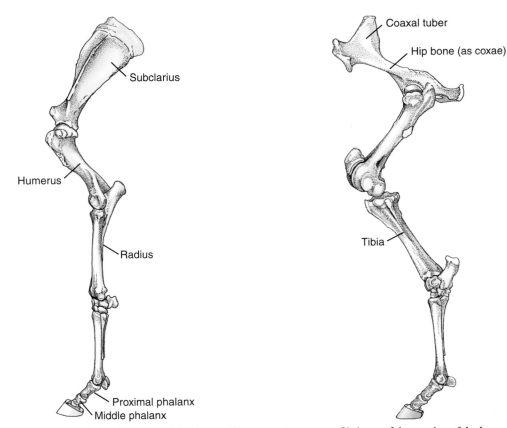

Figure 54-2 Skeleton of the front leg of the horse (From Dyce KM, Sack WO, Wensing CJG: *Textbook of veterinary anatomy*, ed 4, St. Louis, MO, 2010, Saunders, by permission.)

Figure 54-3 Skeleton of the rear leg of the horse (From Dyce KM, Sack WO, Wensing CJG: *Textbook of veterinary anatomy*, ed 4, St. Louis, MO, 2010, Saunders, by permission.)

ulna, knee (the carpus), cannon bone (the third metacarpal bone), long pastern (the proximal phalanx), short pastern (the middle phalanx), and coffin bone (the distal phalanx). The rear leg consists of the femur, stifle, tarsus (the hock), tibia and fibula, cannon bone (the 3rd metatarsal bone), long pastern (the proximal phalanx), short pastern (the middle phalanx), and coffin bone (the distal phalanx) (Fig. 54-2 and Fig. 54-3).

Disorders of the musculoskeletal system are of great importance to the equine industry. The main purpose of a horse is to work, and if it has problems related to the skeletal system it will not be able to do much work. One of the first things that must be understood is the difference between a *blemish* and *unsoundness*. A blemish is an alteration in the appearance that does not affect the horse's serviceability. Unsoundness, in contrast, does affect the horse's ability to do its job. In most cases unsoundness occurs in the horse's front limbs, distal to the knee.

Subsolar Bruising ("Corns")

The hoof is the shock absorber of the equine limb. Its construction allows a 1200-pound animal to move over a variety of surfaces without damage to the internal bony structures (Fig. 54-4). Problems with the hoof account for much of the lameness problems seen in pleasure horses.

Sole bruises are usually caused by trauma to the sole with subsequent hemorrhage between the

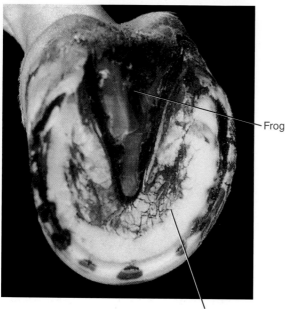

Frog

Sole

Figure 54-4 The sole of the hoof (From Clayton HM, Flood PF, Rosenstein DS: *Clinical anatomy of the horse*, ed 1, St. Louis, MO, 2005, Mosby, by permission.)

sensitive and insensitive soles. Some factors that make an animal more likely to have bruising include the following:

- Exercise on hard ground
- Thin, flat soles
- Coffin bone rotation

CLINICAL SIGNS

- Horses may or may not show acute onset of lameness
- The lameness is usually chronic and low grade
- Bruises are often bilateral
- Sole pain is evident with hoof testers

DIAGNOSIS

- Visualization of bruise

TREATMENT

- Make sure of proper shoeing or trimming to support foot and protect sole
- Nonsteroidal antiinflammatory drugs (NSAIDs) to control pain

INFORMATION FOR CLIENTS

- The condition may be prevented by maintaining proper foot conformation so that the sole is concave and non–weight-bearing.

Hoof Abscesses

Hoof abscesses are the most common cause of acute, severe lameness in horses. Horses with a history of foreign body penetration into the hoof capsule and those with chronic laminitis are more likely to experience development of hoof abscesses. The condition occurs when bacteria gain access to hoof structures and form abscesses. Pain occurs because abscesses cannot expand due to the hoof's rigid structure. Pain is relieved when abscesses rupture.

CLINICAL SIGNS

- Acute, severe lameness (3–5 out of 5)
- ± Heat in foot and over coronary band
- ± Palmar digital pulses
- ± Fetlock and pastern swelling
- Localized pain with hoof testers

DIAGNOSIS

- Visualization of draining tract
- Radiography of the hoof to visualize how deep the tract extends

TREATMENT

- Localize pain and pare out abscess
- Epsom salt soaks
- ± Drawing agent (Ichthammol)
- Antibiotics usually not indicated, unless the horse has been kept in dirty, unsanitary conditions
- *Be aware of tetanus prophylaxis! A tetanus booster should be given any time a puncture wound occurs.*

Navicular Syndrome

Navicular syndrome is most common in large-bodied horses, especially of Quarter horse, Thoroughbred, and Warmblood breeds. Onset is most often seen in 6- to 8-year-old horses. The condition may occur when excessive stress and strain on flexor tendons puts pressure on navicular bursa *or* excessive concussion on coffin joint leads to inflammation of the navicular bursa. This leads to inflammation and erosion of navicular bone. Heavily muscled horses with small feet, horses with short, upright pasterns, and horses with improperly trimmed hooves (long toe, low heel) are more likely to acquire the condition.

CLINICAL SIGNS

- Chronic, low-grade lameness, often bilateral
- Lameness may be intermittent
- Pointing
- Pain over frog with hoof testers

DIAGNOSIS

- Palmar digital nerve blocks
- Radiography (Fig. 54-5).

TREATMENT

- NSAIDs (use caution!); some will cause gastric ulceration)
- Correct hoof imbalance
- Support heels
- Isoxsuprine
- Suspensory ligament desmotomy
- Palmer digital neurectomy

INFORMATION FOR CLIENTS

- Although no reliable way to prevent occurrence of the condition exists, the likelihood of its occurrence may be reduced by maintaining proper hoof balance.

Thrush

Thrush is a bacterial infection of the sulci of frogs and is usually found in horses that are kept in wet conditions. The most common bacterium isolated from horses with thrush is *Fusarium necrophorum*. A horse is more likely to contract thrush if it is kept in wet, dirty conditions, especially if the feet are not properly maintained (Fig. 54-6).

CLINICAL SIGNS

- Foul-smelling black discharge from frog sulci
- Horse is usually not lame, unless the infection is severe
- Deep erosion of frog sulci

DIAGNOSIS

- Visual signs and smell
- Treatment
- Cleaning of feet, removal of necrotic tissue
- Application of topical astringents such as Koppertox, iodine, and others.

INFORMATION FOR CLIENTS

- Thrush is easily prevented by keeping the horse's living conditions clean and sanitary. Daily cleaning of the feet will also reduce the occurrence.

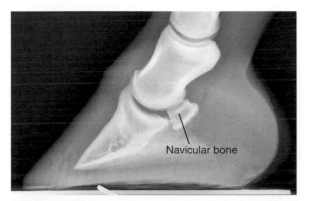

Figure 54-5 The arrow points to the avicular bone (distal sesamoid). (From Floyd AE, Mansmann RA: *Equine podiatry*, ed 1, St. Louis, MO, 2007, Saunders, by permission.)

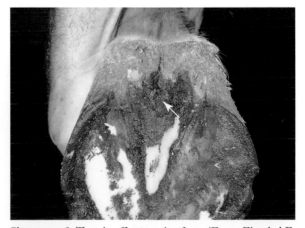

Figure 54-6 Thrush affecting the frog. (From Floyd AE, Mansmann RA: *Equine podiatry*, ed 1, St. Louis, MO, 2007, Saunders, by permission.)

Side Bone (Calcification of Lateral Cartilages)

Sidebone is usually found in the front feet of older horses. Draft breeds are overrepresented in the population of affected horses. Sidebones usually start as unsoundness and then regress to a blemish. The inciting cause for a horse to experience development of sidebones is direct trauma to the foot.

CLINICAL SIGNS

- Lameness in the initial stages
- Evidence of trauma
- Occasionally, a bulge just distal to the coronary band may be seen

DIAGNOSIS

- Radiography of the affected foot (Fig. 54-7).

TREATMENT

- NSAIDs
- Rest (sometimes for as long as 6 months)
- Immobilize foot with bar shoe

Pastern Chip Fractures

Chip fractures of the pastern generally involve the long pastern bone. Repetitive stress and overflexing of the hock may cause these fractures. Horses that have long, weak pasterns are more likely to experience these fractures.

CLINICAL SIGNS

- Slight lameness, if any
- Swelling around dorsal aspect of fetlock joint
- Slight pain on fetlock flexion

DIAGNOSIS

- Radiographic evaluation

TREATMENT

- Most often accomplished by arthroscopic chip removal

Proximal Sesamoid Fracture

Sesamoid bones are part of the suspensory apparatus. Wear and tear occurs at the abaxial surfaces where suspensory ligaments pass over the bone. Sesamoid bone fractures are most commonly seen in athletic horses. Stress and strain on the fetlock joint, often from repeated overextension of the joint, puts force on the suspensory ligaments, which, in turn, pull on the sesamoid bones, causing them to fracture. Performance horses with long, weak pasterns are more likely to experience fracture of their proximal sesamoids compared with other horses.

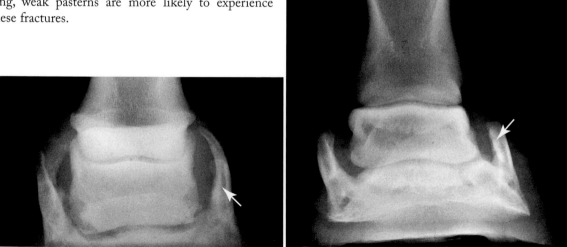

Figure 54-7 Side bone: ossification of the collateral cartilages. (From Floyd AE, Mansmann RA: *Equine podiatry*, ed 1, St. Louis, MO, 2007, Saunders, by permission.)

CLINICAL SIGNS

- The condition is more common in the fore-limbs.
- A variable degree of lameness exists.
- Pain is evident on flexion of the fetlock and palpation of the sesamoid bones.

DIAGNOSIS

- Radiographic examination
- Ultrasonography of the suspensory apparatus

TREATMENT

- Surgery
  - Removal of fragment
  - Casting with rest for up to 1 year
  - Internal fixation
- Prognosis more favorable if the fracture is diagnosed early

Sesmoiditis

Sesmoiditis is an osteitis of the proximal sesamoid bones, and it is most often encountered in racehorses. These horses often present with a history of gait restriction during training. Extreme stress and strain and repetitive loading lead to tearing of suspensory ligament attachments. This, in turn, leads to inflammation of the proximal sesamoid bones. Horses with long, weak pasterns are more likely to be affected by sesamoiditis.

CLINICAL SIGNS

- The condition is more common in the forelimbs.
- A variable degree of lameness exists.
- Pain is evident on flexion of the fetlock and palpation of the sesamoid bones.

DIAGNOSIS

- Radiographic examination
- Ultrasonography of the suspensory apparatus

TREATMENT

- Prognosis guarded at best
- NSAIDs
- Isoxsuprine
- Rest

Bucked Shins

The term *bucked shins* refers to the condition where new bone has been produced on the dorsomedial aspect of cannon bones. Bucked shins are one of the most common types of lameness of 2-year-old Thoroughbreds. The condition is often found in animals with a history of a sudden onset of hard training or of trauma. It occurs when the periosteum tears and subsequent new bone deposited. Stress fractures of the dorsal cortex are also likely. Training a young horse without adequate conditioning increases the likelihood of this condition.

CLINICAL SIGNS

- Usually bilateral
- Most common in forelimbs
- Variable degree of lameness
- Hard, warm, painful swelling on dorsal aspect of cannon

DIAGNOSIS

- Clinical signs
- Radiographic evidence

TREATMENT

- Rest (30 days)
- NSAIDs
- For milder cases, decrease high-speed training

INFORMATION FOR CLIENTS

- Bucked shins can be prevented by modifying the training regimen (when increasing speed, decrease distance). This will allow bones to adapt to the increased stress. Also, changing the training surface may help. Incidence of the condition is less on turf.

Splints

Splints occur when osteitis and periostitis of splint bones exist. This condition is most commonly seen on the medial surfaces of the front limbs in younger horses at the start of their performance careers. Splints are caused by excessive concussion and stress or by direct trauma to the metacarpus or the metatarsus. Periosteal tearing and subsequent inflammation and calcification occur. Horses are predisposed to development of this condition in the presence of mineral and vitamin imbalances (calcium, phosphorus, vitamins A and D) in the diet, or if the horses have faulty conformation such as bench knees, offset knees, or buck knees.

CLINICAL SIGNS

- Swelling usually on medial aspect of cannon
- Variable degree of lameness

DIAGNOSIS

- Clinical signs
- Radiographic evaluation

TREATMENT

- Rest
- Correction of diet
- Application of pressure bandages

Fracture of Splint Bones

Splint bone fractures often occur in young horses when they are boisterous and sustain injury. Splint bone fractures are most often a result of direct trauma to bone, and fractures of the lateral splint bone are more common than those of the medial bone.

CLINICAL SIGNS

- Mild (2–3 out of 5) lameness
- Swelling over splint bones
- Pain on palpation of fracture site

DIAGNOSIS

- Radiographic evaluation

TREATMENT

- Benign neglect and rest (most fractures heal in 3–6 months)
- Amputation of bone (no more than distal two thirds)
- Internal fixation (screw)
- Pressure bandages

Suspensory Ligament Desmitis

Suspensory ligament desmitis refers to inflammation of any branch of the suspensory (interosseus) ligament. The condition is caused by stress and strain throughout the ligament. Long, low pasterns place additional strain on the ligaments and predispose a horse to the condition.

CLINICAL SIGNS

- Mild (1–2 out of 5) lameness
- Lameness is more pronounced on soft surfaces
- Pain on palpation of affected area

DIAGNOSIS

- Radiography to rule out any pathology of the bony column
- Ultrasonography of the affected tendon

TREATMENT

- Rest, then slowly return to work (6–10 months)
- If concurrent with splint fracture, remove fractured bone
- NSAIDs
- Cold hosing, pressure bandage

Bowed Tendon

A bowed tendon is a result of an injury to the deep flexor tendons, superficial flexor tendons, or both, and of their sheaths. Bowed tendons are more commonly found in the forelimbs and are classified as high, middle, or low. Bowed tendons are most often seen in horses used for high-intensity work. Bows are caused by severe strain to the tendons, and the tendons may actually rupture. Bowed appearance is caused by fibrinous attachments. The following factors predispose a horse to development of the condition:
- Long, weak pasterns
- Forced training procedures on unconditioned legs
- Improper trimming or shoeing (long toe, low heel)
- Heavy muscles and small legs

CLINICAL SIGNS

- Bowed appearance to palmar or plantar aspect of the leg
- Heat and pain on palpation
- Mild-to-moderate (2–4 out of 5) lameness

DIAGNOSIS

- Clinical appearance
- Ultrasonographic evaluation

TREATMENT

- Rest (at least 6 weeks)
- Poultices
- ± Steroid injections
- Surgery
  - Tendon splitting
  - Superior check ligament desmotomy
- Prognosis unfavorable for return to previous level of performance

INFORMATION FOR CLIENTS

- A bowed tendon may be prevented if the horse is conditioned properly before being put into hard work.
- Proper trimming of the foot to ensure that the hoof–pastern axis is correct may also help prevent occurrence.

Infectious Tenosynovitis

Infectious tenosynovitis caused by a cut or penetrating injury to the palmar or plantar aspect of cannon area. This injury then introduces bacteria into the tendon and tendon sheath.

CLINICAL SIGNS

- Lameness (3–5 out of 5)
- Pain, heat, swelling of affected area
- Distention of tendon sheath

DIAGNOSIS

- Ultrasonographic examination of the affected area
- Examination of the synovial fluid from the tendon sheath
- Complete blood cell counts (CBC)

TREATMENT

- Broad-spectrum antibiotics
- Irrigation of the tendon sheath
- NSAIDs

Laminitis

Laminitis may be described as avascular necrosis of the sensitive laminae. Laminitis is usually secondary to other conditions, such as (but not limited to the following:
- Grazing lush pastures

- Grain overload
- Metritis or retained placenta
- Excessive weight bearing by contralateral limb

Laminitis occurs when an insult causes blood to bypass dermal laminae via shunts. One theory is that this may be caused by endotoxins. Extreme vasoconstriction follows, and the lack of blood supply causes sensitive laminae to die. Sensitive laminae separate from insensitive laminae, and the coffin bone rotates away from hoof wall because of pull of the deep digital flexor tendon.

CLINICAL SIGNS

- Bounding pulses in the palmar digital arteries
- Feet may feel warm
- "Saw-horse" stance (Fig. 54-8)
- Pain over toe with hoof testers

DIAGNOSIS

- Lateral foot radiography, which may show rotation of the coffin bone

TREATMENT

- Correction of underlying or predisposing factors
- Phenyibutazone or pain control
- Flunixin meglumine (Banamine) initially to bind endotoxins

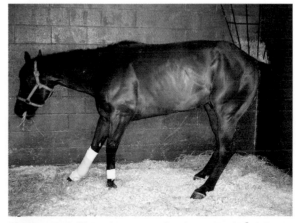

Figure 54-8 Typical stance of a horse with laminitis. (From Reed SM, Bayly WM, Sellon DC: *Equine internal medicine*, ed 3, St. Louis, MO, 2010, Saunders, by permission.)

- Cold water hosing initially
- Shoeing with proper padding
- Elevation of heels
- Deep bedding
- Isoxsuprine
- Acepromazine for vasodilation
- Nitroglycerin around coronary bands

INFORMATION FOR CLIENTS

- To prevent their horses from getting laminitis, may use some management techniques, including the following:
  - Securing grain in locked bin
  - Limiting springtime grazing
  - Ensuring that the mare expels all fetal membranes

Sweeney

Technically, sweeney is not a musculoskeletal condition; rather, it is a neurologic problem. The problem arises from damage to the suprascapular nerve. Horses that exhibit signs of sweeney usually have a history of trauma to the shoulder region, such as might be caused by an ill-fitting draft collar. This trauma causes inflammation of and damage to the suprascapular nerve.

CLINICAL SIGNS

- Atrophy of the muscles in the shoulder region
- Gait abnormalities; in chronic cases, the gait abnormalities are caused by mechanical restriction, rather than pain

DIAGNOSIS

- Clinical signs

TREATMENT

- Steroid injections
- NSAIDs
- Surgery
  - *Note:* Improvement, if it happens, will be gradual.

Bog Spavin

Bog spavin is soft swelling of the hock that is generally considered a blemish, rather than unsoundness.

This condition is often seen in young horses. It is defined as a distension of the sheath of the tarsocrural (tibiotarsal, or hock) joint. The underlying causes are trauma, strain to the joint, or both.

CLINICAL SIGNS

- Swelling of the dorsolateral and dorsomedial aspects of the hock

DIAGNOSIS

- Clinical signs
- Radiography to rule out other causes

TREATMENT

- Rest
- Steroid injections
- Withdraw fluid
- Correction of diet imbalances

Bone (Jack) Spavin

Bone spavin is defined as osteoarthritis of the medial hock. Bone spavins are among the most common cause of hindlimb lameness in performance horses. This is a progressive disease that may result in fusion of the joint. This condition is more common in older (>10 years of age) horses.

The condition is caused by stress on the hock as a result of trauma and concussion. This leads to arthritic changes in the hock. Animals with faulty conformation such as sickle hocks and cow hocks are more likely to be affected.

CLINICAL SIGNS

- Chronic, mild-to-moderate lameness (1–3 out of 5)
- Positive flexion test

DIAGNOSIS

- Injecting the hock with local anesthesia
- Radiographic examination

TREATMENT

- Intraarticular injections
- NSAIDs
- If the condition progresses to the point of joint fusion, the horse may become serviceably sound and pain-free

Upward Fixation of Patella

Upward fixation of patella is a condition where the patella "locks," keeping the stifle in extension; it is more common in unconditioned horses. As the leg flexes, the patella normally moves over the femoral trochlea. At extension, the medial patellar ligament "hooks over" the medial ridge of the femoral trochlea. Normally, the patella disengages when the leg is flexed. When upward fixation of the patella occurs, the medial patellar ligament does not disengage from the trochlea, and the leg stays in extension. Animals that are postlegged or exhibit poor muscle tone appear to be more likely to experience this condition compared with animals.

CLINICAL SIGNS

- This condition is easy to recognize when a horse takes a step but cannot flex the stifle.

DIAGNOSIS

- Based on the typical gait of a horse affected by this condition
- When palpated, the patella is easily moved medially and proximally

TREATMENT

- Exercise—for strengthening of quadriceps muscles; performing work up and down hills is often effective
- Surgery—medial patellar ligament desmotomy if the exercise regimen yields no results

Rhabdomyolysis

Rhabdomyolysis, also known as "azoturia," "tying up," and "Monday morning sickness," is a muscular problem seen in working horses. Animals affected by the disease often have a history of being hardworking animals that had not worked for a few days but still received a full grain ration. The disease becomes apparent when the animal returns to work. The exact cause and physiology of the condition is unknown. Indeed, several causes of rhabdomyolysis may exist. Some theories include sodium deficiency potassium deficiency, or both; muscle glycogen storage problems; vitamin E deficiency or selenium deficiency; and thiamine deficiency. An animal is more likely to exhibit signs of the disease if the training or conditioning schedule has been inconsistent.

CLINICAL SIGNS

- Reluctance to move
- Stiffness, sore muscles on palpation
- Tremors
- Colic symptoms
- Red urine (from muscle breakdown)

DIAGNOSIS

- Clinical signs
- Blood work (creatine phosphokinase and aspartate aminotransferase, electrolytes)
- Urinalysis (myoglobinuria and electrolyte excretion)

TREATMENT

- Tranquilization
- NSAIDs
- Muscle relaxers
- Vitamin B
- It is unwise to force the horse to move if it is severely "tied up"

> ### 🔘 TECH ALERT
>
> Certain breeds of horses (Draft horses, Quarterhorses) may have signs of "tying up" caused by muscular diseases related to genetic defects in metabolism. These diseases must be ruled out by performing a muscle biopsy.

Nutritional Secondary Hyperparathyroidism

Nutritional secondary hyperparathyroidism is a problem with the calcium to phosphorus ratio in the feed. Horses that exhibit signs of this condition have a history of grazing certain types of plants that are high in calcium-binding substances such as oxalates. The condition may also occur from an owner feeding a diet that is high in phosphorous and low in calcium. The lack of available calcium causes parathyroid gland to release greater than normal amounts of parathyroid hormone. This may be either an actual lack of calcium or a perceived lack of calcium because of a high phosphorus level.

Parathyroid hormone causes calcium to be absorbed from the bones. As stated earlier, a horse that has a dietary calcium and phosphorous imbalance is more likely to exhibit signs of the disease. The proper calcium to phosphorus ratio in the diet should be at least 1.5:1, preferably 2:1.

CLINICAL SIGNS

- Intermittent shifting leg lameness, inability to rise if severe
- Facial bones may enlarge
- Spontaneous bone fractures

DIAGNOSIS

- Fractional excretion of calcium in the urine

TREATMENT

- Correct the mineral imbalance in the diet, and supplement calcium. Often, a calcium-to- phosphorous ratio as high as 5:1 is used in the initial treatment of the condition.

REVIEW QUESTIONS

1. Where do most lameness conditions in horses originate?
   a. In the hind limb, above the hock
   b. In the front limb, above the knee
   c. In the front limb, below the knee
   d. In the hind limb, below the hock
2. Splints and bucked shins are common conditions in young racehorses. Which of the following is a cause or predisposing factor for these conditions?
   a. Faulty conformation
   b. Inadequate mineral balance in diet
   c. Concussion
   d. All of the above

3. What is the most likely cause of acute, non–weight-bearing lameness in a horse?
   a. Hoof abscess
   b. Fractured sesamoid bone
   c. Fractured coffin bone
   d. Canker
4. Which of the following is most important in preventing musculoskeletal problems in performance horses?
   a. Weight restriction
   b. Proper breeding
   c. Limiting grain feeding
   d. Proper conditioning
5. A horse found standing in his stall will not move. He exhibits pain when touched. Which of the following might be the cause of his problem?
   a. Rhabdomyolysis
   b. Fractured splint bone
   c. Bowed tendon
   d. Navicular disease
6. Which of the following should be restricted in a horse experiencing laminitis?
   a. Water
   b. Grain
   c. Hay
   d. Pasture
7. The best way to prevent thrush is to _____. (Check all that apply.)
   a. Keep the horse in a dry area
   b. Clean the feet daily
   c. Have the horse shod
   d. Soak the feet

Answers found on page 557.

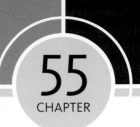

Diseases of the Nervous System

LEARNING OBJECTIVES

When you have completed this chapter, you will be able to:
1. Recognize common causes for neurologic diseases in the horse.
2. Discuss the importance of vaccines in the prevention of neurologic diseases in the equine patient.

Diseases of the nervous system have a large impact on the equine industry. Neurologic diseases may progress from fairly minor (alteration in gait and performance) to very serious (inability to rise and death). The effects of these diseases may be brought about by trauma to nerves, inflammation around nerves, or alterations in neurotransmitters. In most instances, no specific treatment for a disease of the nervous system exists, and effective nursing care is all that is possible. Fortunately, many neurologic diseases can be prevented by vaccination.

Rabies

Rabies is a zoonotic disease with the greatest public health implications. Most states have laws mandating the vaccination of dogs and cats, and some states have mandated the vaccination of horses; the vaccine is available only through licensed veterinarians. Even if not dictated by state laws, it is advisable to have yearly rabies vaccination given to horses. Any animal that is showing neurologic signs, especially one with a known history of having been bitten by another animal, should be suspected of having rabies.

The infectious agent is a Lyssavirus. An infected animal, usually a raccoon, skunk, fox, or bat, bites the victim and passes the virus in the saliva. The virus migrates through the body and the nervous system and localizes in the central nervous system (CNS). The virus may affect the cerebrum, brainstem, or spinal cord.

CLINICAL SIGNS

• If the virus settles in the brain, extreme behavioral changes, often aggressive, are seen.

- If the brainstem is affected, behavioral changes that involve the animal becoming more subdued and quiet are seen.
- If the spinal cord is affected, the animal exhibits ataxia, which progresses to paralysis.
- Signs are rapidly progressive, and the animal usually dies within 5 to 10 days of the onset of signs.

DIAGNOSIS

- Brain tissue examination

TREATMENT

- No treatment exists for rabies.

TECH ALERT

Wear gloves when examining *any* horse exhibiting neurologic signs.

INFORMATION FOR CLIENTS

- If a vaccinated animal has been bitten by a rabid animal, the animal should be revaccinated and observed for 45 days.
- An unvaccinated animal that has been bitten by a suspected rabid animal should be euthanized. If the owner is unwilling to perform euthanasia, the animal needs to be watched closely for 6 months and *handled with extreme caution*.
- Euthanize any horse that has been exposed to rabies and shows signs of neurologic disease.
- A yearly rabies vaccine will prevent the disease.

Sleeping Sickness

The tern *sleeping sickness* refers to three different diseases that occur in the United States: (1) eastern equine encephalomyelitis, (2) western equine encephalomyelitis, and (3) Venezuelan equine encephalomyelitis. Venezuelan equine encephalomyelitis has only rarely been seen, and then only in the southernmost states along the Mexican border. Of the three disease entities, western equine encephalomyelitis is the least fatal. This disease is seen more commonly in the hot, humid parts of the country. It is seen primarily in horses that have a history of not being vaccinated properly. The causative agent is a togavirus, which

occurs in wild bird populations. The disease is transmitted by a mosquito that bites a bird and ingests the virus in the bird's blood. The mosquito then passes the virus to a horse (or a human). Horses are dead-end hosts (i.e. the disease is not passed between horses or from a horse to a human).

CLINICAL SIGNS

- Weakness
- Ataxia
- Inability to rise

DIAGNOSIS

- History
- Clinical signs
- Antibody titers suggestive of exposure
- Definitive diagnosis made by virus isolation from brain tissue and cerebrospinal fluid

TREATMENT

- No specific treatment exists for sleeping sickness; only effective supportive care is given. The disease is fatal in most cases.

INFORMATION FOR CLIENTS

- Sleeping sickness can be prevented by maintaining a regular vaccination schedule.
- In the southern parts of the country, where mosquitoes survive throughout the year, biannual vaccination is recommended.
- Controlling mosquito populations may also aid in the prevention of the disease.

West Nile Encephalitis

West Nile virus infection with encephalitis is similar to the sleeping sicknesses in that the virus is found in the wild bird population and is spread by mosquitoes. The major difference is that more than 90% of animals affected by western and eastern and equine encephalomyelitis die, whereas the mortality rate for animals infected with West Nile virus is approximately 30% to 40%. No specific treatment exists for West Nile virus, but effective vaccines are available. Again, in the warmer, moister parts of the country, horses should be vaccinated twice yearly.

Narcolepsy

Narcolepsy is a disease characterized by inappropriate sleep activity, often taking the appearance of "fainting." The condition is usually seen in horses younger than 1 year of age. Owners report a history of the horse collapsing. The collapse may be initiated by stimulation of herd mates. Suffolk and Shetland ponies appear more likely to suffer from narcolepsy compared with other breeds. The disease is caused by a biochemical imbalance in the sleep–wake centers of the brain. Serotonin, dopamine, and norepinephrine all are involved in this condition.

CLINICAL SIGNS

- Signs can range from mild muscle weakness to full-blown sleep.
- Horse's knees may buckle, and the horse may become ataxic.
- The frequency of episodes is variable, and the horse appears clinically normal between episodes.

DIAGNOSIS

- A presumptive diagnosis is based on clinical signs and history.
- Physostigmine may be used to elicit an attack.
- Atropine may reverse the signs in an attack.

TREATMENT

- Treatment is usually unrewarding. Serotonin uptake inhibitors and antidepressants have been tried with limited success.

INFORMATION FOR CLIENTS

- These horses should be ridden carefully because they may suddenly fall, producing serious injury to the rider.

Wobbler Syndrome

In Wobbler syndrome, the spinal cord is compressed by a narrowing of the vertebral canal, resulting in neurologic deficits. The condition is usually seen in young, fast-growing horses. On average, owners notice onset of clinical signs in horses as early as 18 months of age. The condition is more common in Thoroughbreds and Quarterhorses than in other breeds. Male horses appear to be more affected than female horses. The most common presenting complaints are a history of poor performance, weakness, and stumbling. Abnormal growth, articulation of the cervical vertebrae, or a combination of both results in narrowing of the vertebral canal. The narrow vertebral canal causes pressure on the spinal cord. The condition may be congenital, a result of rapid growth or mineral imbalances, or both.

CLINICAL SIGNS

- Ataxia and weakness
- Stumbling, toe dragging
- Hind-limbs usually more affected
- Signs: usually bilateral
- Progression: variable

DIAGNOSIS

- Clinical signs
- History
- Radiography

TREATMENT

- Decrease pain and inflammation (nonsteroidal antiinflammatory drugs (NSAIDs)
- Dietary management:
  - Feed adjusted for a slow growth rate
  - Correction of mineral imbalances
  - Vitamin E and selenium supplementation
- Surgery
- Euthanasia if the horse is a danger to itself or handlers
- Surgical stabilization, if possible

TECH ALERT

Use caution when handling these horses. Bending the horse's neck, backing, or turning may result in the horse falling on the handler. These horses should *not* be ridden.

INFORMATION FOR CLIENTS

- Feeding young animals for moderate growth rates while ensuring proper mineral balance may help to prevent the disease when the condition is not congenital.

Equine Protozoal Myeloencephalitis

Equine protozoal myeloencephalitis (EPM) has become a fairly common disease, with some estimates claiming exposure of up to 50% of all horses. However, EPM is also one of the most misdiagnosed diseases of horses! In some locations, any horse that appears lame is thought to have EPM. Since treatment is fairly expensive and some horses go without a correct diagnosis, it is important that diagnostic work be done to ensure a correct diagnosis. Horses are dead-end hosts to the parasite; thus, the disease is not passed from one individual to another. The onset of the disease is often seen in 1- to 5-year-old horses. Often, a stressful event is present in the animal's history. Ponies appear to be resistant to the disease. Thoroughbreds and Standardbreds are over-represented in the population of EPM victims. The causative agent is a protozoal parasite, *Sarcocystis neurona*. In North America, the definitive host of this parasite is the opossum. The horse ingests cysts in the water or feed that has been contaminated, most often with opossum feces. Organisms divide in nerve tissue, causing damage. Migration of organisms may cause inflammation, necrosis of tissue, or both. Clinical signs of the disease depend on the number of migrating parasites and the amount of neurologic tissue affected. Signs may be acute or insidious and often include asymmetry of gait, sore back, excessive bucking, and failure to maintain gaits.

CLINICAL SIGNS

- Ataxia
- Gait abnormalities
- Muscular atrophy
- Head tilt
- Progression of signs over time, culminating in the animal's inability to rise

DIAGNOSIS

- Analysis of cerebrospinal fluid for antigens from the organism
- Serum immunofluorescent antibody tests: proven to be more accurate in diagnosis
- All other possibilities ruled out with CBC, serum chemistries
- Complete physical and lameness examination

TREATMENT

- Nitazoxanide (Naviator)
- Ponazuril (Marquis)
- Sulfadiazine and pyrimethamine (Daraprim)
- Long-term medication (1 month or longer) is required

INFORMATION FOR CLIENTS

- Pastured horses should be fed off the ground in areas rich in opossum populations, although any grazing horse could become infected.
- Vaccine is no longer available.
- Management techniques such as keeping feed and water sources protected to prevent the disease being passed to other animals.

Tetanus

Of all domestic animals, horses are the most susceptible to tetanus, which is a result of the release of a bacterial toxin. Horses that are affected often have a history of a lack of routine vaccination. They usually have a history of puncture wounds, stiffness, or both. The disease occurs when *Clostridium tetani*, an anaerobic type of bacteria that is present in the environment, releases a toxin. This toxin prevents release of γ-aminobutyric acid (GABA). GABA normally inhibits nerve impulse propagation. In the absence of any inhibition on nerve impulse conduction, nerves continuously are firing, causing constant muscle contraction (Fig. 55-1).

CLINICAL SIGNS

- Muscle stiffness and spasms
- Increased sensitivity to noise and touch
- Overall stiffness of body
- Eventually this progresses to rigid paralysis and death caused by asphyxiation
- Death usually occurs within 10 days

DIAGNOSIS

- Wound history
- Clinical signs

TREATMENT

- Effective supportive care; prevention of the disease is easier than treatment.

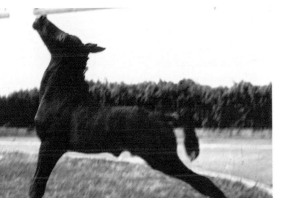

Figure 55-1 Extensor rigidity in a foal with tetanus. (Courtesy Dr. John Barnes. IN Sellon DC, Long MT: *Equine infectious diseases,* St Louis, 2007, Saunders)

INFORMATION FOR CLIENTS

- Regular yearly vaccination schedule with tetanus toxoid is recommended.
- With a history of regular vaccination, a wound that occurs within 6 months of vaccination should cause minimal concern for the horse's health. A booster vaccine may be given as a precaution.
- If the wound occurs within 6 months to a year following vaccination, then a booster vaccine should be given.
- If the last vaccine is overdue, then a booster vaccine and tetanus antitoxin should be administered. These two injections should be given at opposite ends of the horse—that is, one injection in the neck and the other in the semitendinosus muscle. This protocol can also be followed if the horse's vaccine status is unknown.
- Two injections are given so that tetanus toxoid stimulates antibody production, and tetanus antitoxin consists of antibodies that will bind the toxin. (Toxoid provides active immunity, and antitoxin provides passive immunity.)

Hyperkalemic Periodic Paralysis

Hyperkalemic periodic paralysis is a genetic disease, found only in the descendants of one Quarterhorse sire named Impressive. The condition is usually seen in young, well-muscled horses. This is an inherited condition that causes an abnormality of sodium channels, resulting in constant depolarization of muscle cells.

CLINICAL SIGNS

- An episode is often brought on by stressful situations such as a halter class in the show ring.
- Muscle tremors, sweating, rapid breathing, and weakness are observed during an episode.
- Animals remain conscious during episodes.

DIAGNOSIS

- Clinical signs and history
- Blood tests: may show hyperkalemia
- Deoxyribonucleic acid (DNA) testing to support diagnosis

TREATMENT

- Hand walking
- Intravenous fluids (*no potassium*)
- Decreased potassium in diet

INFORMATION FOR CLIENTS

- All descendants of Impressive should undergo DNA testing to prevent the disease; positive animals should not be used for breeding.
- Check with your breeding association to determine whether offspring with one positive parent can be registered. Regulations are currently changing.

Headshaking

This frequently seen disorder is characterized by persistent or intermittent spontaneous movements of the head unrelated to external stimulation. Often, the horse will also sneeze, snort, or rub the nose against a stationary object during the episode. Some animals are so badly affected that they become unsafe to ride or handle. Thoroughbreds and geldings appear to be overrepresented. Affected horses are typically between 7 and 9 years of age, and the disorder appears to be seasonal, with more cases seen in early spring and summer. The exact cause of the disorder is unknown, but trigeminal neuralgia and photophobia have been found to be the two most common causes. However, over 60 other possible diagnoses are found in the literature!

CLINICAL SIGNS

- Head shaking with no apparent external stimuli
- Rubbing nose against the ground or other stationary objects
- Facial twitching
- Bizarre behavioral patterns

DIAGNOSIS

- Complete physical examination including ophthalmologic, dental, and otoscopic examinations
- Blindfolding the horse or placing the animal in darkness may improve symptoms
- Seasonality of the shaking

TREATMENT

- Cyproheptadine orally
- NSAID's or corticosteroids
- Acupuncture
- Nerve blocks: infraorbital nerve or the posterior ethmoidal nerve
- Face masks to block sunlight

INFORMATION FOR CLIENTS

- The exact cause of this disorder may not be found.
- Severe head shaking makes the horse unsafe to ride or to handle.
- Fly masks with a drawstring closure over the nostrils may help by placing pressure on the upper lip and restricting air passage into the nostrils.

REVIEW QUESTION

1. Which of the following conditions that affect horses can also affect humans? (List all that apply.)
   a. Rabies
   b. Equine infectious anemia
   c. Moon blindness
   d. Eastern, western, and Venezuelan equine encephalomyelitis
   e. West Nile encephalitis
   f. Equine protozoal myeloencephalitis (EPM)

Answers found on page 557.

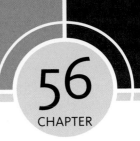

Diseases of the Reproductive System

Caslick operation
Dysmature
Endophyte

Endotoxin
Metritis

Placentitis
Toxicoxis

OUTLINE

Bacterial Abortions
Viral Abortions
Contagious Equine Metritis
Dystocias
Endometritis
Retained Placenta
Ovarian Cell Tumors
Rupture of the Uterine Artery

Uterine Prolapse
Rectal Tears
Rupture of the Prepubic Tendon
Cryptorchidism
Penile Tumors
Penile Paralysis
Fescue Toxicosis

LEARNING OBJECTIVES

When you have completed this chapter, you will be able to:
1. Recognize reproductive disorders as they occur in clients' mares.
2. Discuss the needed changes in management of breeding mares.

3. Explain prescribed therapies to owners.

Of all our domestic animals, it appears that successful reproduction is most difficult in the mare. Even with all the advances in reproductive technologies (artificial insemination, embryo transfer, hormonal manipulation), the mare's reproductive efficiency remains about 60% to 75%. This is partially attributable to the mare's estrous cycle. The mare has a 21-day estrous cycle and is in estrus for 5 to 7 days. Unlike most animals, the mare ovulates 24 to 48 hours *before* the end of estrus, making timing of insemination more difficult in the mare. Because of the low reproductive efficiency, reproductive disorders may have a significant impact on a breeder's operation.

Bacterial Abortions

A wide variety of bacteria cause abortions, most often as a result of placentitis. Bacterial abortions are more commonly seen in older mares. The most common bacteria isolated are *Escherichia coli*, *Salmonella* spp., *Klebsiella* spp., and *Actinobacillus* spp.

CLINICAL SIGNS

- Abortion
- Discharge
- Mare returns to estrus
- Premature milk letdown

DIAGNOSIS

- Bacterial culture and sensitivity

TREATMENT

- After a bacterial abortion, the mare's uterus should be flushed, with antibiotics placed in the final liter of flush.
- Systemic antibiotics may also be administered.

Viral Abortions

The most common cause of equine viral abortion is equine herpes virus type 1 (EHV-1). Abortions usually occur in the last trimester, and more than one mare on the farm is affected. This condition closely resembles abortions caused by bacterial and fungal organisms.

DIAGNOSIS

- Virus isolation from aborted fetus and placenta

⬤ TECH ALERT

Wear gloves when handling any aborted fetal material and the placenta.

INFORMATION FOR CLIENTS

- Pregnant mares should be vaccinated with a killed vaccine at 5, 7, and 9 months of gestation to prevent viral abortions.

Contagious Equine Metritis

Equine metritis is a highly contagious disease that was first described in England and Ireland. The disease has since been eradicated from the United States. Presenting history is often limited to the animal being infertile. The causative organism is a gram-negative bacterium, *Taylorella equigenitalis*. The organism is usually passed from the stallion to the mare during breeding.

CLINICAL SIGNS

- A copious mucopurulent discharge from the vulva is seen 10 to 14 days after breeding.
- Discharge usually stops within 2 weeks and mares become inapparent carriers (Fig. 56-1).

DIAGNOSIS

- Bacterial culture and sensitivity: the urethral fossa and diverticulum in the stallion and the clitoral fossa in the mare often the most rewarding sites from which to collect a sample

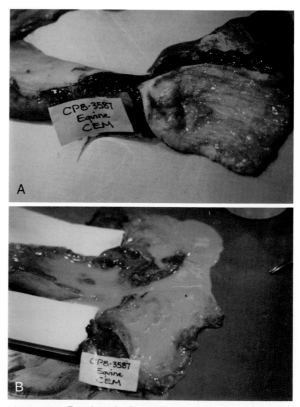

Figure 56-1 Purulent discharge from a mare with contagious equine metritis (**A**), caudal vagina, and uterus postmortem (**B**) (Courtesy Maryland Department of Agriculture. IN Sellon DC, Long MT: *Equine infectious diseases*, St Louis, 2007, Saunders)

TREATMENT

- Antibiotics may not be effective.
- The main goal in treatment is to clear the organism from the uterus and clitoral fossa in the mare and from the sheath, urethral fossa, and urethral diverticulum in the stallion; treatment involves washing the affected areas at least once daily for 1 week with chlorhexidine scrub.

Dystocias

Dystocia is defined as difficulty during parturition. In mares, the second stage of labor (defined as the time from when the amniotic sac ruptures to the time the foal is delivered) should last *no more than 20 minutes!* Dystocias appear to occur more in maiden mares.

Of the many possible reasons for difficult parturition in mares, the three most common are as follows:
- Mare–foal size mismatch
- Malpresentation of foal
- Twins

A dystocia is said to occur if the amniotic fluid rushes out and 20 minutes later the foal is still not delivered. It becomes serious if the mare is straining, with no progress in foal delivery.

TREATMENT

- Correct the position of the foal in the birth canal.
- If the fetus cannot be re-positioned because of the straining of the mare, the mare may be anesthetized to increase muscle relaxation.
- If it is determined on vaginal examination that the foal is dead, a fetotomy may be performed.
- A cesarean section may be performed as a last resort, preferably at a surgical referral center.
- The procedure may be performed on the farm if referral is not an option; at this point, the main goal is to save the foal because most mares will not survive an on-farm cesarean section.

TECH ALERT

The placenta separates from the maternal blood supply early in the foaling process. Most equine foaling occurs within 30 minutes of the start of contractions. Any mare taking longer to deliver a foal may need immediate assistance to avoid the loss of the mare, the foal, or both.

Endometritis

Endometritis is one of the most common diseases of the reproductive system in mares. Endometritis is categorized into four classes. A higher class number indicates a smaller likelihood of the mare becoming pregnant. The condition is more often seen in older mares, both those that have had many offspring and maiden mares. Underlying causes of endometritis include the following:
- Repeated breeding:
  - At each breeding, semen elicits a mild inflammatory response. A result of this inflammation is a small amount of fibrosis.
  - After repeated mating, these small pathologic changes start to combine into a larger problem.
- Chronic infections:
  - Infections of the uterus may occur when the mare's physical barriers to infection are compromised.
  - *Streptococcus zooepidemicus*, *Escherichia coli*, *Pseudomonas* spp., *Klebsiella* spp., *Staphylococcus* spp., yeast, and fungi are common disease-causing organisms.
  - Mares with poor vulvar conformation are more likely to contract uterine infections.
- Sexually transmitted diseases: the inflammatory response to venereal diseases may cause fibrosis of the uterine mucosa.
- Degeneration is caused by aging.

CLINICAL SIGNS

- Failure to conceive
- ± Vulvar discharge
- Fluid accumulation in uterus

DIAGNOSIS

- Culture and sensitivity
- Ultrasonography
- Uterine biopsy

TREATMENT

- Uterine lavage with antibiotics
- Oxytocin

INFORMATION FOR CLIENTS

- Breed mares as few times as possible during a cycle. This necessitates skill in determining as accurately as possible the timing of ovulation.

- Surgically correct the problems in the conformation of the vulva (Caslick operation).

Retained Placentas

All of the placenta should be passed within 3 to 6 hours (Fig. 56-2). Owners are often instructed to call the veterinarian if the placenta has not passed within 3 hours. After assessing the situation, the veterinarian may give instructions to wait a while longer. Mares with a retained placenta often have a history of dystocia. After a prolonged or difficult labor, the placenta may rip, and parts may stay in the uterus.

CLINICAL SIGNS

- Placental membranes seen protruding from the vulva after 3 hours
- Vaginal discharge if a small remnant of placenta remains in the uterus for days
- ± Signs of laminitis after 48 hours
- Mare shows systemic signs of illness

DIAGNOSIS

- Palpation of the uterus and placenta through the vulva
- Visualization of placental remnants

TREATMENT

- Oxytocin to assist uterine contraction and expulsion of contents

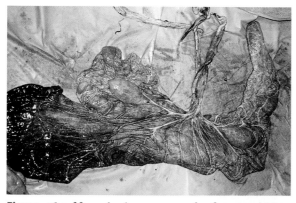

Figure 56-2 Normal placenta passed after parturition. (From Samper JC: *Equine breeding management and artificial insemination*, ed 2, St. Louis, MO, 2009, Saunders, by permission.)

- Uterine lavage
- *Gentle* traction such as by hanging a half-full milk jug (containing water) from the protruding tissue
- If the placenta is hanging after a few hours, a knot tied so that the mare does not step on the placenta, to prevent it acting as a wick for environmental bacteria
- Flunixin meglumine (Banamine) to bind endotoxins
- Systemic antibiotics, if needed

Ovarian Cell Tumors

Ovarian tumors are generally benign, steroid-producing growths. These tumors may be primarily of the granulosa cells, mixed, or predominantly thecal cells. Causes of clinical syndrome include the following:
- Tumor arises on ovary.
- If a greater number of granulosa cells are involved, excess estrogen with little progesterone is produced.
- If a greater number of thecal cells are involved, excess testosterone is produced. This is because thecal cells convert progesterone to testosterone, which is converted to estrogen in granulosa cells.

CLINICAL SIGNS

- Persistent estrus (granulosa cell involvement)
- Anestrus
- Aggressive behavior (thecal cell involvement)
- Mares exhibiting pain when ridden or handled

DIAGNOSIS

- Ultrosonography
- Rectal palpation: the affected ovary noticeably larger than the unaffected one

TREATMENT

- Removal of the affected ovary

◉ TECH ALERT

Use caution when handling these mares, especially when they are in season. They can be extremely volatile, and some have even fallen on handlers when pressure is put over the affected ovary.

Rupture of the Uterine Artery

It is not uncommon for a mare to experience tearing of the uterine artery. Such an occurrence, although rare, may be fatal. This condition is usually seen in older mares. Straining during parturition, pressure from the foal, or both may cause an arterial tear. If blood slowly diffuses through the broad ligament, a hematoma may form, which causes clot formation and stops the bleeding; otherwise, the mare may bleed out.

CLINICAL SIGNS

- The mare found dead in her stall
- Pale mucous membranes
- Colic signs
- Weakness

DIAGNOSIS

- Palpation of the broad ligament, feeling for a tear or hematoma formation

TREATMENT

- The mare *must* be kept in a quiet state; otherwise, treatment will be unrewarding. It may be best to move her into a dark stall, and chemical sedation may also be used.

Uterine Prolapse

Uterine prolapse is a condition that is rarely seen in mares that have had difficult deliveries. Often, the owner will report that the mare is still straining after the foal is born, and tissue can be seen protruding from the vulva. Prolapses of other organs such as the bladder, vagina, or rectum have a similar appearance. The identity of the protruding tissue needs to be ascertained to correct the problem.

DIAGNOSIS

- Visual confirmation and palpation

TREATMENT

- Keep the uterus moist. Hypertonic saline will keep the uterine mucosa moist and will also pull fluid out from tissues and perhaps shrink the prolapsed organ so that it is easier to push it back in. In the past, sugar was spread on the organ to get it to shrink.
- Administer sedation, anesthesia, or both to reduce straining.
- Replace the uterus (this is easier said than done).
- Oxytocin will promote contraction and uterine involution; do not give oxytocin until the uterus is securely back in place.
- Administer systemic antibiotics.

Rectal Tears

Rectal tears are a potentially serious condition that may lead to the death of the mare. Rectal tears are graded from I to IV, with grade IV being the most serious. A rectal tear is most likely to be seen in a mare that has just foaled or one that has just been rectally palpated. At foaling, the foal's foot may go through the uterus or the vagina. Most often, tears are caused by rectal palpation.

Any time a mare is palpated, a risk for a rectal tear exists, and the owner should be aware of this. With a severe tear, peritonitis may develop quickly and the mare may die if the condition is not treated properly.

CLINICAL SIGNS

- Blood on the sleeve after palpation
- Signs of colic
- Septicemia

TREATMENT

- Immediate referral to a hospital facility, if available
- Antibiotic therapy
- Flunixin meglumine
- ± Intravenous fluids
- Surgical correction
- Wet, soft feeds

INFORMATION FOR CLIENTS

- Rectal palpation requires adequate restraint to prevent damage. It should never be attempted by untrained personnel.

Rupture of the Prepubic Tendon

Rupture of the prepubic tendon usually occurs in late pregnancy probably because of the increase in weight of the fetus placing stress on weak abdominal muscles. It occurs more frequently in older mares or in mares that are in poor shape. These mares may require assistance during delivery because they may be unable to contract the abdominal muscles firmly enough to move the fetus through the birth canal.

CLINICAL SIGNS

- Physical examination of the pregnant mare shows tipped pelvis and a sawhorse stance (Fig. 56-3).
- The udder is swollen and congested.
- The mare is reluctant to move.
- A drop in the abdominal margin is apparent

DIAGNOSIS

- Mare in late pregnancy
- Rectal palpation revealing the abdominal floor falling away from the brim of the pelvis

TREATMENT

- Support wraps for the abdomen may be used to enable the mare to carry the fetus to delivery.

INFORMATION FOR CLIENTS

- Keep breeding mares in good condition; make sure that they get plenty of exercise and good nutrition.
- Avoid breeding older mares that are multiparous.
- Have palpation and ultrasonography performed on bred mares to make sure they are not carrying twins.

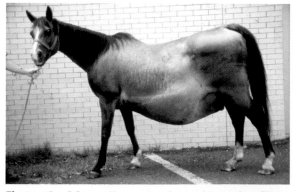

Figure 56-3 Mare with a ruptured prepubic tendon. (From Brinsko SP, Blanchard TL, Varner DD, et al: *Manual of equine reproduction*, ed 3, St. Louis, MO, 2011, Mosby, by permission.)

- Avoid re-breeding mares with a ruptured prepubic tendon.

Cryptorchidism

Cryptorchidism is a condition in which one or both testes have not descended into the scrotum. Usually, testes descend by age 6 months, but sometimes it is as long as 2 years before they drop. Often, the first time an owner is aware of the condition is when the animal is presented for evaluation before castration. A strong genetic link exists in the occurrence of the condition, so *animals with cryptorchidism should not be used for breeding.*

The condition is treated by performing an abdominal surgery to remove the retained testicle. *It is unethical to remove the descended testicle while leaving the retained testicle in place.* Although such an animal would not likely be able to produce viable sperm, it would still exhibit undesirable stallion-like behaviors.

Penile Tumors

Penile tumors are usually squamous cell carcinoma or sarcoid tumors (see Chapter 53 for a more detailed discussion).

Penile Paralysis

Penile paralysis is a condition in which the penis drops and does not retract. Affected animals often have a history of sedation with acepromazine. The condition may be caused by administration of acepromazine, damage to third and fourth sacral nerves, and certain neurologic diseases such as rabies, EHV-1, and trauma.

CLINICAL SIGNS

- The penis drops and does not retract.
- The stallion does not achieve erection.
- A portion of penis distal to sheath becomes edematous and swollen.

TREATMENT

- Treatment of underlying causes
- Hydrotherapy
- Furosemide
- Amputation of the penis

INFORMATION FOR CLIENTS

- Although penile paralysis is a rare condition, owners should avoid giving acepromazine to stallions and geldings.

Fescue Toxicosis

Fescue toxicosis is a problem that occurs in mares grazing endophyte-infested tall fescue pastures. Tall fescue is a cold and insect-tolerant, tough, nutritious grass. Endophyte-free varieties do exist, but they lack some of the vigor of the entophyte-infested varieties. If infested and endophyte-free varieties are planted in adjacent pastures, the endophyte-infested grass will grow more than the endophyte-free grass and take over the pasture.

The endophyte produces ergovaline, which has undesirable effects. Some of the effects may be traced back to vasoconstriction and prolactin inhibition caused by the ergovaline.

CLINICAL SIGNS

- Prolonged gestation (sometimes as long as 13 months)
- Dysmature foals
- Thickened placentas
- Agalactia:
  - Weak foals due to lack of energy from milk
  - Immunocompromised foals due to lack of colostrum

DIAGNOSIS

- Clinical signs
- Presence of the endophyte in the pasture; a forage sample is brought to the county extension office and then send the sample to the proper laboratory

TREATMENT

- Removal of mares from pasture 60 to 90 days before foaling
- Assistance at foaling
- Keeping colostrum on hand
- Tube-feeding of foal
- Domperidone

REVIEW QUESTION

1. To prevent the effects of fescue toxicosis, which of the following are possible options for the management of broodmares grazing endophyte-infested tall fescue pastures? (List all that apply.)
   a. Muzzle the mares.
   b. Remove the mares from the pasture 30 to 90 days before foaling.
   c. Administer domperidone.
   d. Supplement selenium.
   e. Increase protein in the concentrate portion of the diet.
2. Within what period of time (from the beginning of parturition) should foals be delivered?
   a. 60 minutes
   b. 45 minutes
   c. 90 minutes
   d. 20 minutes
3. Which of the following may cause penile prolapse?
   a. Xylazine
   b. Dormosodan
   c. Acepromazine
   d. Diazepam
4. Mares ovulate 24 to 48 hours _____ of estrus.
   a. before the end
   b. before the beginning
   c. after the end
5. Granulosa cells in the ovary of the mare produce:
   a. Testosterone
   b. Progesterone
   c. Estrogen
6. All mares used for breeding should be vaccinated against this disease.
   a. Equine encephalitis
   b. Herpes virus infection
   c. West Nile virus infection
   d. Equine flu
7. Multiparous mares may be more prone to problems of the reproductive system.
   a. True
   b. False

Answers found on page 558.

Diseases That Affect the Neonate

Colostrum   Lysis   Multiparous
Isoerythrolysis

Perinatal Asphyxia Syndrome   **Neonatal Isoerythrolysis**
Failure of Passive Transfer   **Combined Immunodeficiency Syndrome**

When you have completed this chapter, you will be able to:
1. Explain neonatal problems to clients.
2. Use basic knowledge of these disorders to aid in
   the development of treatment regimes.

Perinatal Asphyxia Syndrome

Perinatal asphyxia syndrome (PAS), more commonly known as "dummy foal syndrome," is seen in
foals deprived of oxygen during dystocias or when
premature separation of the placenta occurs during
normal births. The syndrome is also seen in foals
that have no prenatal problems, and these foals are
believed to undergo some sort of hypoxia in utero.
These "dummy foals" appear normal at birth but
show signs of central nervous system abnormalities
within a few hours after birth (Fig. 57-1). The syndrome affects the cardiovascular system, the renal
system, the gastrointestinal (GI) system, and the
central nervous system (CNS).

Treatment involves support for all the systems
involved; control of seizures, correction of electrolyte
imbalances, maintenance of tissue perfusion, caloric
intake and maintenance of the GI tract, and maintenance of renal perfusion. These foals require
24-hour intensive care. If PAS is recognized early,
the prognosis for foals is good to excellent. The
prognosis worsens with late recognition or inadequate treatment.

CLINICAL SIGNS

- Development of CNS signs in a newborn foal;
  seizures
- Absence of the suckling reflex
- Depression

DIAGNOSIS

- CNS signs that develop soon after birth

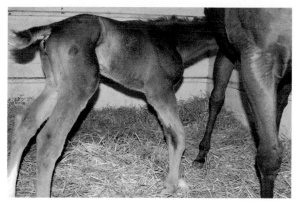

Figure 57-1 Foal exhibiting typical "dummy" behavior and having difficulty searching for the mare's udder. (Courtesy Dr. Tom Seahorn, Lexington, KY. IN From Brinsko SP, Blanchard TL, Varner DD, Schumacher J, Love CC, Hinrichs K, Hartman DL: *Manual of equine reproduction*, ed 3, St Louis, 2011, Mosby)

- Clinical symptoms related to other organ systems in the foal
  - Complete blood count (CBC), serum chemistry abnormalities
  - Cardiovascular abnormalities or decreased perfusion

TREATMENT

- Supportive care of all systems involved
- Anti-seizure medication (diazepam, Phenobarbital, Gabapenntin)
- Enteral feeding if GI function is abnormal
- Heat lamps, padding to prevent decubital ulcers, frequent turning
- Intravenous (IV) fluids to maintain organ perfusion, correction of electrolyte abnormalities

○ TECH ALERT

Foals with PAS require intense treatment 24 hours of the day. They do best when placed in intensive care units of larger equine clinics.

Failure of Passive Transfer

Failure of passive transfer is a condition in which a foal does not receive adequate amounts of immunoglobulins from the mare's colostrum. This condition may occur any time the foal does not receive enough colostrum, for example, when a mare rejects the foal, a mare has not produced milk, or a foal cannot stand on its own. Colostrum (first milk) contains antibodies against any antigens to which the mare has been exposed. The foal's intestine will not absorb the antibodies more than 18 hours after parturition, so it is important that the foal receive colostrum as soon as possible.

CLINICAL SIGNS

- The mare may have a distended udder.
- The foal appears septicemic (usually seen a few days after birth).
- The foal appears maladjusted (may be seen hours after birth).

DIAGNOSIS

- If a foal is suspected of having failure of passive transfer, the diagnosis can be confirmed by performing a simple immunoglobulin G (IgG) test.

TREATMENT

- If the results of the foal's IgG test are low, the animal may be given colostrum from a nurse mare, as long as it receives the colostrum within 18 (preferably 12) hours after birth. After 18 hours or if no colostrum is available, plasma transfusions can be given (Fig. 57-2).

INFORMATION FOR CLIENTS

- Colostrum can be frozen for future use in breeding operations where failure of passive transfer causes a problem.

Neonatal Isoerythrolysis

Neonatal isoerythrolysis is a condition in which the mare's antibodies attack the foal's red blood cells (RBCs). The condition is usually seen only in foals from multiparous mares, and it is most often seen in Thoroughbreds. The disease occurs after a mare is mated to a stallion with a different blood type. If the resultant foal carries the sire's blood type, and if the mare's and foal's blood mix (as can happen at parturition), the mare will produce antibodies against the foal's erythrocytes. If the breeding is repeated the

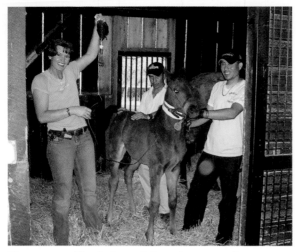

Figure 57-2 Tranfusion of hyperimmune plasma to a 28-day-old foal. (From Brinsko SP, Blanchard TL, Varner DD, et.al: *Manual of equine reproduction*, ed 3, St. Louis, MO, 2011, Mosby, by permission.)

next year, antibodies in the colostrum will attack the foal's erythrocytes, causing lysis.

CLINICAL SIGNS

- A foal that is affected with this condition becomes listless and weak because of the diminished oxygen-carrying capacity of its blood.
- Mucous membranes and sclera take on a yellowish tint as the foal becomes icteric because of the lysis of its erythrocytes.

TREATMENT

- Affected foals are treated with blood transfusions from a cross-matched mare or gelding. One should also be sure to check for failure of passive transfer in these foals.

INFORMATION FOR CLIENTS

- If neonatal isoerythrolysis is suspected, the foal should be muzzled for 48 hours to prevent ingestion of nursing colostrum from the mare (can use stored or frozen colostrums, if necessary).
- It is advised that breeding not be repeated.

Combined Immunodeficiency Syndrome

Combined immunodeficiency syndrome (CID) occurs only in Arabian and Arabian cross foals. This is a hereditary condition (it is estimated that 25% of the Arabian population carries the gene for this disease) that causes a foal not to produce T- or B-lymphocytes. This lack of lymphocytes leads to a lack of immunoglobulin production and illness.

CLINICAL SIGNS

- Clinical signs usually present at about 3 to 5 months of age because this is when the protective effect of antibodies from colostrum is declining.
- Signs may be any signs of illness.
- CID should always be suspected in a sick Arabian or Arabian cross foal.

TREATMENT

- No treatment for this condition is available. Bone marrow transplants have been attempted with little success.

INFORMATION FOR CLIENTS

- CID can be prevented by performing DNA testing of the mare and the stallion. If both (or even one) of the parents carries the gene, then the animals should not be used for breeding.

REVIEW QUESTIONS

1. Which white blood cell line is affected in the foal with CID?
   a. Neutrophils
   b. Lymphocytes
   c. Basophils
   d. Monocytes
2. The foal's intestine cannot absorb antibodies after_____ hours postpartum.
   a. 12
   b. 8
   c. 18
   d. 10
3. Neonatal isoerythrolysis occurs in foals having _____.
   a. A blood type the same as the mare
   b. A blood type the same as the stud
   c. With any blood type

4. Lack of oxygen during foal development may result in _____.
   a. Prenatal isoerythrolysis
   b. Hypoimmunization
   c. Dummy foal syndrome

5. Foals cannot be given stored colostrum at birth.
   a. True
   b. False

Answers found on page 558.

58
CHAPTER

Diseases of the Respiratory System

LEARNING OBJECTIVES

When you have completed this chapter, you will be able to:
1. Recognize symptoms and causes related to equine respiratory diseases.
2. Discuss environmental conditions that promote the spread of respiratory disease.
3. Understand that other systems in the body may also be affected by some of the organisms that cause respiratory disease in the equine patient.

Respiratory diseases of horses are a problem for owners because of the effect of these diseases on animal performance. A slight respiratory problem may cause a small impairment in the performance of the animal, but that small degree of impairment may make the difference between finishing a race in the money or going home with empty pockets. For diseases that cause coughing and nasal discharge as noticed by the owner, resting the animal has been promoted as one part of the treatment. However, while the animal is being rested, training time and performance time are being lost.

Epiglottic Entrapment

Epiglottic entrapment is a relatively common condition that occurs more often in Standardbreds and Thoroughbreds than in other breeds. The exact cause of the condition is unknown. It is possible that a congenital formation defect exists in the tissue of the pharynx. The condition is apparent when the epiglottis is trapped by soft tissue in the pharynx. This leads to a less efficient breathing system, with subsequent effects on performance.

CLINICAL SIGNS

- Coughing
- Respiratory noise
- Poor performance

DIAGNOSIS

- Endoscopy

TREATMENT

- Epiglottic entrapment may be treated surgically if the horse's performance is adversely affected.
- If the disease has no effect on performance, then benign neglect (ignoring the disease) is the treatment of choice for many cases.

Epistaxis

Epistaxis is defined as bleeding from one or both nostrils. Epistaxis is usually secondary to some other condition. Nosebleeds affect all horses equally, and they are often seen in racehorses. Among the many different causes of epistaxis are the following:
- Trauma such as from nasogastric intubation or blunt trauma
- Infections or abscesses
- Exercise-induced pulmonary hemorrhage
- Tumors

DIAGNOSIS

- Clinical signs
- Thorough physical examination
- Endoscopy to visualize the underlying cause
- Complete blood cell count (CBC) to rule out infectious causes

TREATMENT

- Treat the underlying cause.

Left Laryngeal Hemiplegia

Left laryngeal hemiplegia affects the left side of the larynx, making it unable to retract properly during increased respiratory effort. The condition is more commonly seen in Thoroughbreds and draft horses. The most common (or owner-noticed) onset of clinical signs is at 2 to 3 years of age. The heritable basis to the condition is the result of demyelination of the left recurrent laryngeal nerve, leading to a loss of nervous control of laryngeal muscles and partial airway obstruction.

CLINICAL SIGNS

- Inspiratory noise during exercise
- Poor performance
- Noise becoming progressively worse

DIAGNOSIS

- Endoscopic examination (sometimes with the horse on a treadmill)

TREATMENT

- Surgical correction

Soft Palate Dislocation

Soft palate dislocation is an intermittent condition seen mostly during peak exercise. The condition is most common in racehorses. Problems may occur when the soft palate gets displaced dorsally. This narrows the airway and leads to partial obstruction. The exact cause of soft palate dislocation is unknown, although a problem with the vagus nerve is suspected.

CLINICAL SIGNS

- Gurgling noise
- Poor performance
- Dyspnea during exercise

DIAGNOSIS

- Endoscopy with the horse exercising on a treadmill
- Ruling out other diseases, plus clinical signs and history

TREATMENT

- Alter the horse's tack. Tongue ties and "figure-of-eight" nose bands are often used with varying degrees of success.
- If the tack changes do not alleviate the condition, then surgery is performed.

Primary Sinusitis

Sinusitis is defined as infection and inflammation of the sinuses. The ones most affected are the maxillary and frontal sinuses. Primary sinusitis is most often seen in younger horses. Other upper respiratory infections are often present when a horse is affected by primary sinusitis.

The infection may be caused by any number of bacteria or fungi. Inhalation of these pathogens is a common mode of infection of the sinuses.

CLINICAL SIGNS

- Chronic, persistent mucopurulent nasal discharge
- Often unilateral
- If the condition is severe enough, the animal may be dyspneic
- Occasionally, systemic illness

DIAGNOSIS

- For the disease to be treated properly, the condition must be differentiated from secondary sinusitis, such as that caused by an infected tooth root
- Percussion of sinuses, listening for fluid line
- Radiography of the skull
- Bacterial and fungal culture and sensitivity obtained from sinuses

TREATMENT

- Lavage and drainage of sinuses; antibiotics or antifungals should be mixed in the lavage fluid (depending on culture and sensitivity results)
- Systemic antibiotic therapy usually unrewarding

Secondary Sinusitis

The most common underlying cause of secondary sinusitis is infection of the roots of upper teeth. Secondary sinusitis is most common in mature, rather than young, horses. Anything that affects and causes infection of tooth roots, such as fractures, abscesses, tumors, and so forth, may lead to a secondary sinusitis.

CLINICAL SIGNS

- Unilateral, mucopurulent nasal discharge
- Malodorous breath
- If severe enough, distortion of facial contours

DIAGNOSIS

- Radiography
- Endoscopy

TREATMENT

- Removal of the tooth and lavage of the socket or abscess pocket
- Drainage of the sinus

Strangles

Strangles is a highly contagious disease caused by the bacterium *Streptococcus equi* (Fig. 58-1 and Fig. 58-2). The disease is transmitted by aerosol inhalation. Horses may carry the organism in the respiratory tract, especially in the guttural pouches, and act as a nidus for infection of other horses. All horses with a purulent nasal discharge and high fever should be isolated and have the nasal cavity cultured for *S. equi*. Horses that have had strangles tend to develop a strong immunity against the organism. Some infected horses will develop complications. "Bastard strangles" is the term used for abscesses that develop in internal organs throughout the body. "Bastard strangles" carries a poor prognosis and may be fatal.

CLINICAL SIGNS

- Fever >103°F
- Thick, creamy, yellow nasal discharge

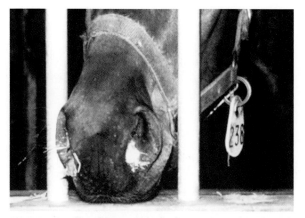

Figure 58-1 Purulent nasal discharge in a horse with strangles. (From Sellon DC, Long MT: *Equine infectious disease*, St. Louis, MO, 2007, Saunders, by permission.)

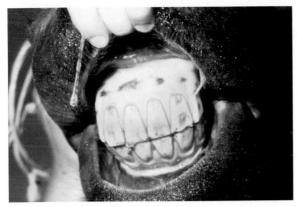

Figure 58-2 Oral mucosa in a horse with purpura hemorrhagica secondary to *S. equi* infection. (From Sellon DC, Long MT: *Equine infectious disease*, St. Louis, MO, 2007, Saunders, by permission.)

- Swollen retropharyngeal lymph nodes
- Inappetence

DIAGNOSIS

- Clinical signs
- Results from a bacterial culture and sensitivity

TREATMENT

- Lance the abscesses, let them drain, and flush them with a chlorhexidine solution.
- Penicillin may be given to horses that have a fever but are not showing signs of abscesses.
- Isolation of affected horses may help prevent a farm-wide outbreak.
- Vaccination of unaffected horses may also prevent a farm-wide outbreak.

⊙ TECH ALERT

The disease may be spread from horse to horse through tack, water or feed buckets, and your clothing. When handling an infected horse, wear protective clothing and gloves, and treat the affected horses last. Isolate them in the clinic, if possible. Stalls must be sanitized and left unused after housing an infected horse.

INFORMATION FOR CLIENTS

- Disease outbreaks can be prevented in two ways:
  - Bio-security: Wash your hands and clothes after working with a horse that has strangles;

work with these horses as the last job of the day; and wash areas with chlorhexidine solution.
  - Vaccination: An intranasal vaccine is available.
- *Even if the horse is vaccinated, it may still contract the disease.* However, the disease will most likely be of lesser severity.
- At-risk horses should be vaccinated four times yearly.
- Young horses taken to horse shows are most at risk for infection.

Guttural Pouch Empyema

Guttural pouch empyema, the accumulation of pus in the guttural pouches, is a disease that is secondary to a previous respiratory infection. Its exact pathogenesis is unknown.

CLINICAL SIGNS

- Poor performance
- Nasal discharge, which is seen in greater amounts when the horse lowers its head

DIAGNOSIS

- Endoscopic examination of the guttural pouches

TREATMENT

- Local and systemic antibiotic therapy
- Surgery to remove chondroids (hardened bits of pus)

Guttural Pouch Mycosis

Guttural pouch mycosis is a condition in which fungal plaques are located in the guttural pouches. These plaques are often associated with underlying vessels and may occasionally compromise the function of the vessels. Guttural pouch mycosis is more common in the northern hemisphere than in the southern hemisphere. Many fungal species have been found in the condition. *Aspergillus* is a common isolate from affected horses.

CLINICAL SIGNS

- Epistaxis
- Dysphagia (difficulty swallowing)
- Nasal discharge

DIAGNOSIS

- Endoscopic examination

TREATMENT

- Systemic antifungal therapy
- Local and systemic antibiotic therapy

Chronic Obstructive Pulmonary Disease ("Heaves")

Chronic obstructive pulmonary disease is an allergic condition most commonly seen in older horses that are kept in dry, dusty environments. The allergic reactions, similar to asthma in humans, may cause loss of elasticity of alveoli and inflammation and constriction of airways.

CLINICAL SIGNS

- Respiratory effort, especially on expiration
- Presence of heave line
- Crackles and wheezing
- Cough
- Clinical signs often resolving or becoming less severe when the animal's environment is changed

DIAGNOSIS

- Clinical signs
- CBC
- Bronchoalveolar lavage

TREATMENT

- Changing the horse's environment
- Soaking the hay, and feeding from ground-level feeders
- Antihistamines (however, they are not always effective in horses)
- Steroid injections
- Bronchodilators such as clenbuterol (Ventipulmin)

⊙ TECH ALERT

Make owners aware that some of the drugs used for treating respiratory problems in horses are not allowed in competition.

INFORMATION FOR CLIENTS

- Chronic obstructive pulmonary disease may be prevented or alleviated by careful management of the horse's environment, ensuring proper ventilation and air flow.
- Feeding pelleted feeds and placing hay in ground feeders will decrease the amount of dust inhaled while feeding.
- Hay may also be moistened to decrease dust.
- Horses should be able to lower their head when trailering to allow for clearing of the respiratory tract.
- Stall bedding should be dust free; avoid any cleaning procedures that produce excessive dust in the barn (leaf blowers for sweeping)

Exercise-Induced Pulmonary Hemorrhage

Exercise-induced pulmonary hemorrhage (EIPH) is a common occurrence in hardworking racehorses. Thoroughbreds are most commonly affected. The exact cause is unknown, but one theory is that high cardiac output and vascular blood pressure lead to rupture of capillaries in the lungs. Blood from the burst capillaries is then expelled through the nostrils.

CLINICAL SIGNS

- Unilateral or bilateral epistaxis
- Decreased performance
- Increased swallowing
- Respiratory distress

DIAGNOSIS

- Endoscopic examination of lungs after a race

TREATMENT

- No reliable treatments or preventive measures are available, although many horses are given furosemide before racing in the hope of preventing EIPH.

Foal Pneumonia

Foal pneumonia affects foals approximately 1 to 3 months of age but is not limited to that age range. The disease is caused by the bacterium *Rhodococcus equi*. The organism is found in the soil of almost every horse farm. It grows readily in soils contaminated with manure. This hardy bacterium, once it is in the environment, can persist for months or even years. Foals are thought to be exposed to the bacteria during the first few days of life. The organism has a specific affinity for macrophages and may become distributed throughout the foal's body. The survival rate for foals with *R. equi* is between 60%-90% with aggressive treatment.

CLINICAL SIGNS

- Dyspnea
- Cough
- Inappetence
- Fever
- Diarrhea

DIAGNOSIS

- Clinical signs
- Thoracic radiography
- Transtracheal wash

TREATMENT

- A combination of erythromycin and rifampin is effective in treating foal pneumonia.
- Azithromycin or clarithromycin may also be used in place of erythromycin, which has many adverse effects when used in foals.

INFORMATION FOR CLIENTS

- Ensuring that the foal has adequate amounts of colostrum and giving plasma transfusions to foals born on a farm where *Rhodococcus* has been present the previous year may help prevent the disease.
- Vaccines may prevent the disease.
- Avoid spreading manure on pastures unless it has been composted.
- Keep manure picked up daily from stalls and pasture turn-outs.
- *Rhodococcus equi* can infect humans, especially immunosuppressed individuals.

Equine Influenza

Equine influenza is one of the most debilitating respiratory viral diseases of horses. It usually affects younger animals, especially those that are subjected to high levels of stress. High animal densities and movement also increase the risk of contracting the disease. The disease is caused by a myxovirus.

CLINICAL SIGNS

- Fever
- Cough
- Lethargy
- Inappetence
- Nasal discharge

DIAGNOSIS

- Clinical signs
- Ruling out other causes

TREATMENT

- *Rest* the horse.
- Administer antibiotics to cover secondary bacterial invaders.

INFORMATION FOR CLIENTS

- Prevention is by regular vaccination.
- An intramuscular or intranasal vaccine is available.
- Vaccine protection is short-lived.
- At-risk horses should be vaccinated four times yearly.

Equine Viral Rhinopneumonitis

Equine viral rhinopneumonitis is the most common viral respiratory disease in horses. Reproductive and neurologic forms of the disease also exist. Viral rhinopneumonitis usually affects horses 2 years of age or younger, although older animals may also be affected. The disease is caused by the equine herpes virus (EHV-1 and EHV-4).

CLINICAL SIGNS

- Nasal discharge
- Clinical signs not as severe as with flu
- Mid- to late-term abortions (EHV-1)

DIAGNOSIS

- Clinical signs

TREATMENT

- Rest
- Supportive care

INFORMATION FOR CLIENTS

- Regular vaccination helps to prevent viral rhinopneumonitis. Protection from the vaccine is short-lived, so twice yearly vaccination is recommended.

- At-risk horses should be vaccinated four times yearly.
- Pregnant mares should be vaccinated with a killed virus to prevent abortions at 5, 7, and 9 months of gestation.

REVIEW QUESTIONS

1. The most common viral respiratory disease seen in horses is _____.
   a. Rotaviral sinusitis
   b. Equine influenza
   c. Equine viral rhinopneumonitis
   d. Equine encephalitis
2. Strangles is caused by:
   a. *Streptococcus equi*
   b. *Staphylococcus aureus*
   c. *Streptococcus pneumoniae*
   d. *Staphylococcus epidermis*
3. Another name for chronic obstructive pulmonary disease is _____.
   a. Bronchitis
   b. Sinusitis
   c. Heaves
   d. Atopy
4. Equine rhinopneumonitis is caused by:
   a. A herpes virus
   b. A rotavirus
   c. An influenza virus
   d. A rhinovirus
5. Pulmonary hypertension can be reduced by use of:
   a. Furosemide
   b. Penicillin
   c. Mannitol
   d. Cortisone
6. Equine strangles may be transferred to uninfected horses by humans.
   a. True
   b. False
7. When hauling a horse in a trailer, make sure the horse can lower its head.
   a. True
   b. False
8. What type of bacteria is *S. equi*?
   a. Gram-positive
   b. Gram-negative

Answers found on page 558.

Diseases of the Urinary System

LEARNING OBJECTIVES

When you have completed this chapter, you will be able to:
1. Recognize the signs of urinary tract disease in the horse.

2. Understand that urinary tract disease in the horse is uncommon.

Primary urinary tract problems are rare in horses because of the pH of the equine urine, the sterility of the system, and the fact that voiding of urine serves to wash out any infectious organisms that may be ascending the tract. Urinary tract problems, therefore, are more often secondary to other problems. If a horse does have a urinary tract problem, the following are pertinent questions to ask the owner:
- What is the color of the urine?
- Is there any history of illness?
- Is the amount of urine produced normal?
- What is the animal's water intake?
- Is urine flow normal?
- Is there a possibility of exposure to toxins?

Cystitis

Cystitis is defined as inflammation of the urinary bladder. Primary cystitis is rare in horses. Cystitis is more common in mares, especially those in late gestation and early after birth.

Cystitis may be caused by anything that can lead to urine stasis in the bladder, such as the following:
- Nerve damage
- Obstructions (although *rare*)
- Neoplasia

CLINICAL SIGNS

- Frequent passage of small amounts of urine
- Urine scald
- ± Pain
- Hyperthermia, tachycardia

DIAGNOSIS

- Urinalysis
- Bacterial culture and sensitivity
- Ultrasonography of the bladder

TREATMENT

- Treatment of underlying causes
- Indwelling catheters
- Antibiotic therapy

Urinary Bladder Prolapse

Urinary bladder prolapse is an unusual condition that is most often seen in postpartum mares. Relaxation of the pelvic muscles, dilation of sphincter muscles, and strain during parturition all work together to prolapse the bladder.

CLINICAL SIGNS

- Bladder, poking out through the vagina
- If the bladder ruptures, intestines may stick through
- Colic signs

TREATMENT

- Cleaning and replacing the bladder
- ± Surgery to keep bladder in place
- Antibiotic therapy
- ± Indwelling catheter

Pyelonephritis

Pyelonephritis is a bacterial infection of the kidney and is seen most often in adults. This is usually an ascending infection from lower in the urinary tract. Pyelonephritis is usually a secondary condition to urine pooling or stasis because urine flow typically washes bacteria down and out of the tract. Bacteria are usually the same as those of the predisposing cystitis.

CLINICAL SIGNS

- Same as those for cystitis, together with possible signs of systemic disease

DIAGNOSIS

- Blood work
- Urinalysis
- Ultrasonography of kidneys

TREATMENT

- Pyelonephritis is treated much in the same way as cystitis, although the course of treatment for pyelonephritis is of much longer duration.

Urinary Bladder Rupture

Urinary bladder rupture is usually a secondary condition, which is more common in foals than in adults. A history of trauma or urethral obstruction may exist. This may also be found in postpartum mares. Rupture may be caused by direct trauma to bladder or intense straining, or the bladder may fill so full of urine that it bursts. Male foals may be predisposed to bladder rupture because of the narrowness of the urethra and the internal pressures that develop during foaling.

CLINICAL SIGNS

- Decreased, or total, lack of urine output
- Depression
- Foals: standing with the back in ventral flexion, back and front feet not close together

DIAGNOSIS

- Abdominocentesis (belly tap); if the bladder is ruptured, urine will be seen in the peritoneal fluid
- The peritoneal fluid will also contain more creatinine than does the serum

TREATMENT

- Small defects may heal on their own
- Surgery to repair the defect
- Intravenous (IV) fluids with no potassium

Incontinence

Incontinence refers to the inability to control urination. Often, more than one horse in the herd is affected, and a history of grazing sorghum, Sudan grass, or both may exist.

Causes for incontinence include the following:
- Neurologic disease, with loss of control of bladder, urethral sphincters, or both
- Equine herpes virus
- Cauda equina neuritis
- Equine protozoal myeloencephalitis
- Trauma
- Neoplasia

CLINICAL SIGNS

- Passage of small amounts of urine, anytime
- Dribbling of urine

- Absence of urine
- May show other signs of neurologic disease

DIAGNOSIS

- Rectal palpation and ultrasonography

TREATMENT

- Underlying cause may be difficult to treat, symptomatic treatment may be the only option
- Manual bladder expression
- Treatment of urine scald
- Phenoxybenzamine
- Bethanechol

Urolithiasis (Stone)

Uroliths may form in the bladder, kidney, ureters, or urethra, and they rarely cause obstruction. If obstruction is caused, it is most likely in a male horse. A urolith forms when a change occurs in the urine pH. A nidus forms, and the stone accumulates around it, similar to the way that an oyster forms a pearl (Fig. 59-1).

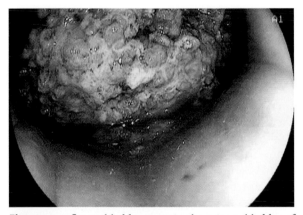

Figure 59-1 Large bladder stone in the urinary bladder of a horse. (From Sellon DC, Long MT: *Equine infectious disease*, St. Louis, MO, 2007, Saunders, by permission.)

CLINICAL SIGNS

- Small amounts or no urine
- Blood in urine
- Straining
- Colic signs

DIAGNOSIS

- Ultrasonography or radiography if the animal is small enough

TREATMENT

- The stone needs to be removed. This can be accomplished by manual evacuation in mares, passage of a urinary catheter, or surgical intervention. Intravenous fluids should also be administered.

REVIEW QUESTIONS

1. Urinary tract infections in the horse are usually the result of:
   a. Hematogenous bacterial spread
   b. Ascending bacterial infections
   c. Viral infections
   d. Trauma
2. A ruptured bladder should be suspected in a male foal that:
   a. Fails to produce urine
   b. Has an altered stance while straining
   c. Has a distended abdomen
   d. All of the above
3. Urinary bladder prolapse is most commonly seen in the:
   a. Stallion
   b. Prepartum mare
   c. Postpartum mare
   d. Gelding

Answers found on page 558.

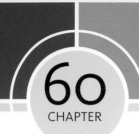

Sheep and Goat Husbandry

KEY TERMS

Herbivore   Ruminant

LEARNING OBJECTIVES

When you have completed this chapter, you will be able to:
1. Appreciate how goats and sheep live and exist.

Although including a section on sheep and goats in a book devoted to companion animals may seem odd, the fact is that more and more people are keeping a small number of these animals as pets. Because they look on them as pets, owners expect the greatest level of care for these animals.

Sheep and goats are flock-dwelling or herd-dwelling ruminant herbivores. Goats and sheep need the proximity of others of their species, although sheep are more connected to the group compared with goats.

Both sheep and goats may be grouped into one of three major types: (1) Those that are bred specifically for meat, (2) those that are bred for fiber (mohair, cashmere, wool), and (3) those that are bred to produce milk. More people in the world drink goat's milk than cow's milk.

Sheep and goats have some similarities with regard to their eating. Both are ruminants; that is, they graze, or browse in the case of goats, and then lie down to chew their cud. The food is regurgitated from the rumen, and the animal re-chews it until the particle size is small enough for digestion. Both goats and sheep will respond quite well to no more than high-quality pasture and a mineral mix. Whereas sheep prefer to graze on grasses and succulent broad-leafed plants, goats have a more varied diet, browsing on twigs, shrubs, brushy weeds, and some grass. When in times of increased production, such as growth, breeding, or lactating, a grain supplement may be given to the animals to meet energy requirements. One must take care, however, not to give too much grain to male sheep and goats because this may predispose them to urinary calculi. Also, sheep are susceptible to copper toxicity and need a lower level of this mineral in their diets. And, goats cannot survive by eating tin cans and paper!— they need high-quality feed just as other domestic animals do.

Although most sheep and goats live quite well out on the range, in some situations it would be advantageous to confine them. Most of these animals are quite hardy, and as long as they have some shelter from wind and rain, their housing needs are modest. Greater attention needs to be paid to the type of fencing that is used. Goats are extremely clever at escaping from confinement, so fences need to be secure and strong. Goats can climb or wriggle through many fences. Electric fences work well for containment, but if the power goes out, goats will walk through the fence. Some goats like to stick their heads through wire fences; then their horns get caught in the wire and they cannot escape. Goats have been severely injured by marauding dogs when they have had their head caught through a fence.

One major concern for sheep and goat producers is protection from predators. Coyotes and free-running domestic dogs may wreak havoc on a group of sheep or goats. Electric fences work well to keep the stock in and also deter predators. Another option is to use guard animals. Several breeds of dogs are specifically designed to be guardians of livestock. In recent years, donkeys and even llamas are gaining popularity as guardians.

Confining the animals close to the house at night also helps prevent predation by coyotes, although not by domestic dogs, which typically attack during the day.

REVIEW QUESTIONS

1. Diets high in grain may predispose male goats to:
   a. Rickets
   b. Urinary calculi
   c. Diarrhea
   d. Gas colic
2. Diets for sheep should contain limited amounts of this element.
   a. Iron
   b. Selenium
   c. Copper
   d. Phosphorus
3. Which of the following would present the greatest danger to goats kept as pets?
   a. Poor-quality diets
   b. Lack of exercise
   c. Viral diseases
   d. Predators

Answers found on page 558.

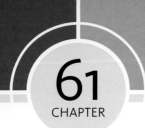

Diseases of the Digestive System

LEARNING OBJECTIVES

When you have completed this chapter, you will be able to:

1. Recognize the causes of digestive system diseases in the small ruminant.

2. Discuss the value of proper diet and feeding practices with owners of small ruminants.

Sheep and goats are ruminants; that is, they have four chambers to their "stomach": (1) the rumen, (2) reticulum, (3) omasum, and (4) the abomasum (Fig. 61-1). The abomasum is the portion of the tract that is most similar in function to the monogastric stomach. As an animal grazes, it swallows the forage material, which goes into the rumen. After the animal is done grazing, it finds a spot and lies down in sternal recumbency. The animal then regurgitates what it has eaten and proceeds to chew it. Sheep and goats typically chew approximately 40 times; then they swallow the bolus again. They repeat the procedure, and when the particle size is small enough, the animal swallows it and the chewed food proceeds into the reticulum.

Although the ruminant digestive system is fairly adaptable and a ruminant can eat a lower quality of forage, they still need a reasonably good-quality diet. Fortunately, digestive system diseases in ruminants are uncommon.

🔘 **TECH ALERT**

Goats and sheep have no upper incisors!

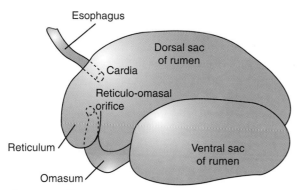

Figure 61-1 Digestive system of the small ruminant as seen from the left side. (From Colville T, Bassert JM: *Clinical anatomy and physiology for veterinary technicians*, ed 2, St. Louis, MO, 2008, Mosby, by permission.)

Bloat

Bloat is the accumulation of free gas or froth in the rumen. Bloat is less common in small ruminants than in cattle, and it occurs less frequently in goats than in sheep. Bloat may be caused by ingestion of diets such as high-legume diets or cereal grains that promote the formation of froth in the rumen. Some other diets such as those high in grain promote the formation of free gas. Sometimes, an animal will have an accumulation of free gas in the rumen because of a failure to eructate.

CLINICAL SIGNS

- Abdominal distension, especially apparent in the left paralumbar fossa
- Signs of abdominal pain
- Anxiety
- Respiratory distress

DIAGNOSIS

- Observation of obvious abdominal distension
- In the case of free gas bloat, a "ping" can be heard in the left paralumbar fossa
- If an orogastric tube is passed, free gas can be heard (and smelled) escaping through the tube. Frothy bloat will result in froth being seen on the tube.

TREATMENT

- Bloat is an emergency situation and requires immediate attention

- Passage of orogastric tube
- Diocctyl sodium succinate (DSS), mineral oil, vegetable oil for frothy bloat
- Trocarization of the rumen
- Rumenotomy

INFORMATION FOR CLIENTS

- Bloat can be prevented by implementing sensible feeding practices:
  - Avoid diets that are high in concentrate and low in forages.
  - Limit availability of bloat-inducing feedstuffs.
  - When introducing animals to a new, lush pasture, do so slowly so that the animals can adjust.

Rumen Acidosis

Rumen acidosis is caused by the rapid fermentation of highly digestible carbohydrates. The problem occurs more often with finely ground grains because the bacteria can more rapidly ferment the carbohydrate. The condition is more commonly seen in animals that have been fed a primarily forage-based diet and then have received a large amount of concentrate feed. As the carbohydrates are digested, the pH declines. The decline in pH causes the normal resident microfauna and microflora of the rumen to die. Water is drawn into the rumen, and the animal becomes dehydrated and may die. The acid buildup causes damage to the rumen epithelium. This allows the leakage of bacteria into the system, and the animal may become septic.

CLINICAL SIGNS

- Vary with the amount and type of feed
- Signs first appear from 12 to 36 hours after ingestion of feed
- Signs include shock, anorexia, weakness, depression
- Severe dehydration
- Signs of sepsis
- Diarrhea

DIAGNOSIS

- Examination of rumen fluid shows the following:
  - pH < 5.5
  - Protozoa reduced in number
  - Large, gram-positive rods

TREATMENT

- Treatment to reverse hypovolemia and shock, remove offending feedstuffs, and correct the acidosis and sepsis
- Intravenous (IV) fluids containing sodium bicarbonate
- Flunixin meglumine
- Rumenotomy to remove feedstuffs
- Transfaunation of rumen microflora
- Thiamine subcutaneously (SQ)

INFORMATION FOR CLIENTS

- Rumen acidosis may be avoided by following sound feeding practices:
  - If increasing the concentrate portion of the diet, do so slowly so that the gut microflora can adjust to it.
  - Buffering agents may also be added to the diet when feeding high-concentrate diets.

Diarrhea

Diarrhea involves loose to runny stools and is defined as the increase in the volume and frequency of defecation. Dehydration and electrolyte imbalances are the concerning sequelae to diarrhea, especially in very young kids and lambs. Animals of certain ages are more prone to specific infectious causes of diarrhea (Fig. 61-2).

Enterotoxigenic *Escherichia coli*

Enterotoxigenic *E. coli* causes diarrhea mainly in neonatal lambs and, to a lesser extent, in kids. This type of bacteria has two main methods by which it causes disease. The first is by attachment and colonization of the intestinal villi. As these villi are destroyed, the intestine loses its absorptive capabilities. The second method is by production of an enterotoxin, which interferes with normal gut function. *E. coli* causes disease in young animals younger than 10 days, with 1 to 4 days of age being the most common age of onset.

CLINICAL SIGNS

- Usually presents as an outbreak, rather than in a single animal
- Diarrhea
- Dehydration
- Recumbency
- Many animals die before development of diarrhea

DIAGNOSIS

- Fecal culture and serotyping for K99 and F41 antigens
- Histopathology from necropsy confirms

TREATMENT

- Fluid therapy: PO (orally), IV, SQ
- Antibiotics (amoxicillin, ampicillin, neomycin, trimethoprim or sulfa [TMS]) may be beneficial but may also kill off beneficial gut flora
- Flunixin meglumine

> ### ⊙ TECH ALERT
>
> Use caution when handling the feces of any animal exhibiting signs of diarrhea.

Rotavirus

Lambs and kids are infected by group B rotaviruses, in contrast to other species that are infected by group A. These viruses infect the cells at the tip of the intestinal villi, causing a malabsorptive diarrhea. The virus usually infects animals 2 to 14 days of age. Older animals are occasionally infected.

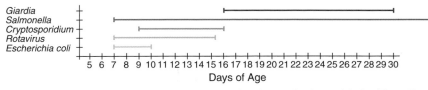

Figure 61-2 Ages at which infectious agents cause diarrhea in lambs and kids. (From Pugh DG: *Sheep and goat medicine*, Philadelphia, PA, 2002, Saunders, by permission.)

CLINICAL SIGNS

- Diarrhea
- Depression
- Dehydration

DIAGNOSIS

- Electron microscopy of fecal and colon samples

TREATMENT

- Supportive care

Cryptosporidiosis

This condition is caused by a protozoal organism, *Cryptosporidium parvum.* These organisms can sporulate in the gut and immediately infect nearby villi. This may result in severe, sustained disease. Oocysts are immediately infectious when shed in the feces, which enables extremely rapid spread. This organism typically affects lambs and kids 5 to 10 days of age.

CLINICAL SIGNS

- Animals often show no systemic signs of illness; they can be bright, alert, and continue to feed
- Liquid, yellow feces
- Diarrhea may be mild and self-limiting or severe; relapses are not uncommon

DIAGNOSIS

- Staining of air-dried fecal samples and microscopic examination shows the parasites in feces. It is possible, but difficult, to find the organisms on fecal flotation.

TREATMENT

- No consistently reliable treatment for cryptosporidiosis is available. Isolation of affected animals and thorough cleaning of the premises may prevent widespread infection of the herd.

INFORMATION FOR CLIENTS

- This is a zoonotic disease, and affected animals need to be handled with great care.

Salmonellosis

Bacteria of the genus *Salmonella* may affect lambs and kids of any age. These bacteria produce an enterotoxin and also cause inflammation and necrosis of the mucosa of both the large and small intestine.

CLINICAL SIGNS

- Sudden death, most often in animals younger than 1 week
- Diarrhea
- Fever, depression
- Shock
- Bloody feces

DIAGNOSIS

- Fecal culture

TREATMENT

- Supportive care
- ± Antibiotic therapy

INFORMATION FOR CLIENTS

- Salmonellosis is a potential zoonotic disease, and proper sanitary precautions should be observed after handling an affected animal.

Clostridium Perfringens

Types A, B, C, and D *Clostridium perfringens* all cause diarrhea, but type D is most often the causative agent. This condition is also known as *enterotoxemia* and *overeating disease.* In type C infection, a β-toxin causes hemorrhagic enteritis mainly in animals younger than 3 weeks. Type D infection results in illness caused by an ε-toxin. The disease is often associated with feeding changes, and it is most commonly seen in the fastest growing animals.

CLINICAL SIGNS

- Three forms—acute, peracute, and chronic (more common in goats)
- Sudden death
- Profuse, bloody diarrhea
- Neurologic signs (more common in sheep)

DIAGNOSIS

- Clinical signs
- Can culture from intestinal tissue at necropsy

TREATMENT

- Aggressive supportive care

- Type D antitoxin
- Treatment is rarely successful

INFORMATION FOR CLIENTS

- A vaccine is available.
- Vaccinate at 4 to 6 weeks of age, then in 4 weeks.
- Yearly vaccinations are recommended, preferably a few weeks before parturition.
- Goats may need vaccinations two or three times a year.
- Reducing energy value of diet and avoiding changes in diet may help prevent infection.

Coccidiosis

Coccidiosis is a problem caused by protozoa of *Eimeria* spp. Clinical disease often manifests itself during times of stress such as weaning, shipping, dietary changes, among others. Oocysts must sporulate outside the host to become infective, and both sporulated and nonsporulated oocysts may survive in the environment for months, if not years. Lambs and kids from 1 to 4 months of age are most susceptible.

CLINICAL SIGNS

- Diarrhea—usually not bloody, but may contain mucus and blood
- Anorexia, weakness, dehydration, rough hair coat may be seen

DIAGNOSIS

- Coccidia may be seen on fecal flotation or direct smear. It is not unusual to see a few coccidia in the feces of a clinically normal animal, so care must be used when interpreting the results.

TREATMENT

- Sulfa drugs are effective in treating an animal with coccidiosis.
- If an animal in the herd is affected, the rest of the animals should be given coccidiostats to prevent disease outbreak.

INFORMATION FOR CLIENTS

- Incidence of the disease can be lessened with thorough sanitary measures and judicious use of coccidiostats. If possible, minimize exposure to stressful situations.

Nematode Infestation

The most common nematode parasites of sheep and goats are those of the *Haemonchus, Ostertagia, Trichostrongylus, Cooperia, Nematodirus, Oesophagostomum,* and *Bunostomum* species. The parasites may affect the abomasums or the intestines of the animals, and clinical disease is often seen during and after times of stress and with overgrazing of the pasture. Larvae can over-winter (survive inhospitable conditions), but hot, dry weather conditions reduce larval survivability.

CLINICAL SIGNS

- Anemia
- Ventral edema
- Poor growth
- Weight loss
- Diarrhea

DIAGNOSIS

- Examination of a slide from fecal flotation will show the presence of eggs but will not determine the load or clinical significance.
- Fecal egg counts, determining eggs per gram of feces, gives a more reliable estimate of the parasite load.

TREATMENT

- Treatment of parasitized animals may be done with one or more of a wide variety of anthelmintics. When deworming a herd or flock, dosage should be based on the weight of the heaviest animal to avoid underdosing and subsequent parasite resistance.

INFORMATION FOR CLIENTS

- Effective sanitation and waste management may decrease the likelihood of parasitism.
- Avoid overgrazing a pasture, and practicing rotational grazing will help prevent parasitism.
- If the pasture is relatively small, manure removal will help reduce the parasite load.

Pregnancy Toxemia or Fatty Liver Syndrome

Fatty liver syndrome may occur when an animal is in a negative energy balance. The body then starts to break down its fat stores, and the products are transported to the liver. The breakdown of fats leads to free fatty acids (FFAs) in the liver. These FFAs are not broken down; instead, they are converted to ketone bodies or lipoproteins. The lipoproteins accumulate in the liver together with ketone bodies. This disease is often seen in the last month of gestation and with multiple births.

CLINICAL SIGNS

- Anorexia
- Depression
- Behavioral alterations
- Recumbency
- Ketone smell to breath
- Dystocia

DIAGNOSIS

- Clinical signs and the presence of multiple fetuses
- Ketoacidosis, hypocalcemia, hypokalemia
- Proteinuria and ketonuria

TREATMENT

- Early cases treated with oral or IV glucose
- Balanced electrolyte solution
- Sodium bicarbonate
- Rumen transfaunation
- Increasing energy level

INFORMATION FOR CLIENTS

- Fatty liver syndrome can be prevented through proper nutrition and ensuring an adequate energy intake, especially during the last month of gestation.

Copper Toxicosis

Copper toxicosis is more common in sheep than in goats, and it often occurs when sheep are fed a diet that is formulated for goats. When the copper-to-molybdenum or copper-to-sulfate ratio is greater than 10:1, copper will accumulate in the sheep's liver.

Disease is seen when the copper is released from the liver, often during times of stress.

CLINICAL SIGNS

- Anorexia
- Depression
- Diarrhea
- Weakness
- Death, with evidence of hemolysis and icterus

DIAGNOSIS

- Increased copper concentrations in serum
- Anemia
- Hyperbilirubinemia
- Increased liver enzymes
- Azotemia
- Isosthenuria

TREATMENT

- Supportive care for renal failure and anemia
- Ammonia tetrathiomolybdate
- D-penicillamine
- The rest of the flock should be treated with ammonium molybdate and sodium thiosulfate

INFORMATION FOR CLIENTS

- Avoid giving high-copper diets.
- Consider other sources of copper in the environment.

● TECH ALERT

Never feed sheep food formulated for use in goats. Make sure owners are advised of this when deciding to raise sheep.

REVIEW QUESTIONS

1. Which of the following treatments may be effective for bloat?
   a. Trocarization
   b. Passage of an orogastric tube
   c. Administration of mineral or vegetable oil
   d. All of the above

2. A late-term pregnant doe exhibiting neurologic signs and having sweet smelling breath might be suffering from:
   a. Pregnancy toxemia
   b. Diabetes mellitus
   c. Pancreatitis
   d. Copper toxicosis

3. "Overeating disease" is caused by which of the following conditions?
   a. *Salmonella* infection
   b. *Clostridium* infection
   c. *E. coli* infection
   d. *Pasturella* infection

4. Diarrhea in lambs or kids 2 to 14 days of age may be related to:
   a. Rotavirus
   b. *Salmonella*
   c. *Clostridium*
   d. *E. coli*

5. The "ping" heard when percussing a bloat is best heard in:
   a. The right paralumbar fossa
   b. The left paralumbar fossa
   c. The right sternal border
   d. The left sternal border

6. Which of the following organisms are zoonotic? (Check all that apply.)
   a. *Salmonella*
   b. *Clostridium*
   c. *Coccidia*
   d. *Cryptosporidium*

Answers found on page 558.

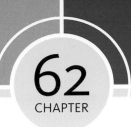
Diseases of the Endocrine System

Lactation   Pseudopregnancy

Goiter
Nutritional Secondary Hyperparathyroidism

Inappropriate Lactation Syndrome

When you have completed this chapter, you will be able to:

1. Recognize the importance of a diet with the proper calcium–phosphorus balance.

2. Recognize three of the most common endocrine dysfunctions seen in small ruminants.

As in other species, the endocrine system of sheep and goats exerts some level of control over many metabolic processes. Fortunately, relatively few endocrine disorders are encountered in sheep and goats.

Goiter

Goiter is the enlargement of the thyroid gland. The most common causes of goiter are iodine deficiency and grazing of certain plants that cause an increase in thyroid size. The physiologic cause appears to be a low concentration of circulating thyroid hormones, which leads to an increased thyroid-stimulating hormone output from the anterior pituitary, resulting in an enlarged thyroid. Goiter may also be a congenital problem.

CLINICAL SIGNS

- Poor wool and hair quality
- Dry skin

- Tendon laxity
- Poor reproductive function

DIAGNOSIS

- Clinical signs
- May also be a low concentration of iodine with increased triglycerides, cholesterol, and phospholipids

TREATMENT

- Supplement iodine in the diet.

Nutritional Secondary Hyperparathyroidism

Nutritional secondary hyperparathyroidism is a problem with the calcium-to-phosphorus (Ca/P) ratio in the feed. Animals that exhibit signs of this condition may have a history of grazing certain types of plants that are high in calcium-binding substances such as oxalates. The condition may also be caused by a diet that is high in phosphorous and low in calcium. The lack of available calcium causes the parathyroid gland to release greater than normal amounts of parathyroid hormone. This may be either an absolute lack of calcium or a perceived lack of calcium caused by a high phosphorus level. Parathyroid hormone causes calcium to be absorbed from the bones.

CLINICAL SIGNS

- Intermittent shifting leg lameness, inability to rise if severe
- Loose teeth
- Spontaneous bone fractures
- Enlarged bones in the skull

DIAGNOSIS

- Fractional excretion of calcium in urine
- Radiographic evaluation
- Dietary analysis

TREATMENT

- Correct the mineral imbalance in the diet.
- Supplement calcium; often Ca/P ratios as great as 5:1 are used in the initial treatment of the condition.

INFORMATION FOR CLIENTS

- The condition can be prevented by maintaining a proper Ca/P ratio in the diet.
- Providing trace mineralized salt and dicalcium phosphate may be beneficial for the animals.

Inappropriate Lactation Syndrome

Occasionally, sheep and goats will appear to have a full udder with no history of being bred. The condition is more common in pet does. The udder is enlarged and nonpainful, although it may be so large that it interferes with locomotion and may lead to secondary musculoskeletal disease. Pseudopregnancy may be a cause of inappropriate lactation. If this is the case, prostaglandin F2-α may be used. If the condition occurs in a pet goat that will not be bred, a mastectomy may be performed. Inappropriate lactation may also be a sign of a more serious reproductive system problem.

REVIEW QUESTIONS

1. Nutritional secondary hyperparathyroidism involves a dietary imbalance in:
   a. Potassium and sodium
   b. Calcium and phosphorus
   c. Potassium and selenium
   d. Sodium and phosphorus
2. Nonbred pet does with enlarged udders may be suffering from:
   a. Mastitis
   b. Mammary neoplasia
   c. Pseudopregnancy
3. Goiter may be seen in animals whose diet is low in:
   a. Calcium
   b. Sodium
   c. Selenium
   d. Iodine
4. Which of the following medications should be avoided if the cornea is ulcerated?
   a. Neomycin
   b. Tetracycline
   c. Atropine
   d. Dexamethasone

Answers found on page 558.

Diseases of the Eye

Blepharospasm　　　　Lacrimation　　　　Photophobia
Epiphora　　　　　　　Neonatal　　　　　Retrobulbar
Incipient

OUTLINE

Entropion　　　　　　　　　　　　**Cataracts**
Infectious Conjunctivitis (Pink Eye)

LEARNING OBJECTIVES

When you have completed this chapter, you will be able to:
1. Discuss common causes of eye problems in small ruminants.

As in other species, eye problems in sheep and goats should be considered an emergency. Eye conditions deteriorate rapidly, and quick attention can make a difference in the animal being able to use its eyes again. If an eye problem is noticed, the first thing that the owner should do is move the animal indoors, out of the sunlight; then veterinary care should be sought immediately.

Entropion

Entropion is a condition where the eyelid rolls inward and cause eyelashes to rub on the cornea, which results in an ulcer. Entropion is reported to be the most common ocular abnormality in neonatal lambs. Entropion may be congenital or secondary to trauma, dehydration, loss of the retrobulbar fat pad, and painful conditions that cause the contraction of the retrobulbar muscles.

CLINICAL SIGNS

- An inward deviation of the lower eyelid, upper eyelid, or both
- Blepharospasm
- Photophobia
- Lacrimation

TREATMENT

- Topical ocular antibiotic ointments and manual eversion of lid
- Placement of sutures or staples to hold the lid in an everted position
- Surgical correction

INFORMATION FOR CLIENTS

- Because a hereditary basis for congenital entropion exists, affected animals should not be used for breeding.

Infectious Conjunctivitis (Pink Eye)

Many different organisms cause conjunctivitis; fortunately, most respond to a commonly avialable medication. These organisms include *Mycoplasma*, *Chlamydia psittaci*, *Listeria monocytogenes*, and *Branhamella ovis*. The condition may occur with or without ulceration of the cornea.

CLINICAL SIGNS

- Reddened conjunctiva
- Blepharospasm
- Photophobia
- Epiphora

TREATMENT

- Tetracycline ophthalmic ointment may be applied.
- Ensure that no ulcer is present if steroids are to be used.
- Third eyelid flaps may be used if severe ulceration of the cornea has occured.

Cataracts

Cataracts are the most common lens abnormality in sheep and goats. Most cataracts are congenital. Cataracts are defined as any opacity in the lens except that which occurs during normal aging.

Cataracts may be categorized by appearance, location, and size:

- Incipient cataracts cover less than 5% of total lens.
- Early immature cataracts cover 6% to 50% of the lens.
- Late immature cataracts cover 51% to 99% of the lens.
- Mature cataracts cover the entire lens.
- Hypermature cataracts are characterized by wrinkling of the lens capsule and formation of dense plaques on the lens capsule.

Congenital, nonprogressive cataracts do not interfere with vision and should be of no concern to owners.

REVIEW QUESTIONS

1. Which of the following is the most common eye disorder in sheep and goats?
   a. Cataracts
   b. Corneal ulcers
   c. Entropion
2. The recommended treatment for pinkeye in sheep and goats is:
   a. Tetracycline ophthalmic ointment
   b. Gentamicin ophthalmic ointment
   c. Triple antibiotic ophthalmic ointment
   d. Any ophthalmic ointment with steroid
3. The first thing the owner should do when discovering an eye problem in an animal is to:
   a. Treat the eye
   b. Call the veterinarian
   c. Move the animal out of the sunlight
   d. Collect laboratory samples

Answers found on page 558.

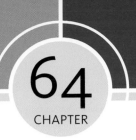

Hematologic and Lymphatic Diseases

LEARNING OBJECTIVES

When you have completed this chapter, you will be able to:
1. Discuss the common bacterial causes of hematologic and lymphatic diseases with owners.

2. Describe the benefits of vaccination to prevent these diseases.

Several conditions may affect the hematologic and lymphatic systems. These conditions include those that lead to anemia, swollen lymph nodes, and multisystemic diseases. These conditions are often difficult to diagnose and treat, especially if they are affecting more than one body system.

Caseous Lymphadenitis

Caseous lymphadenitis is not uncommon in sheep and goat herds. Certain breeds and management practices predispose a herd to this disease. Caseous lymphadenitis is caused by the bacterium *Corynebacterium pseudotuberculosis*. The infection usually spreads through breaks in skin such as when shearing, tail docking, and running through dip tanks. The organism may survive for long periods in damp, dark areas such as soil and manure.

CLINICAL SIGNS
- Swelling of superficial lymph nodes (Fig. 64-1)
- In sheep, these abscesses form layers and have the appearance of an onion; in goats, the abscess material is thick and creamy
- If abscesses form in the viscera, chronic weight loss may occur
- Overall signs of poor production

DIAGNOSIS
- Serologic testing and culture of the organism from the necrotic, abscessed area

TREATMENT
- If caseous lymphadenitis is suspected, abscesses should not be allowed to rupture and drain in proximity to the flock or herd.
- Affected animals should be isolated for treatment.

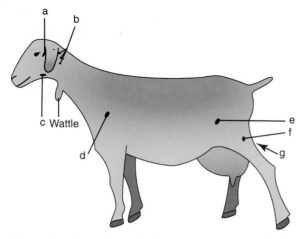

Figure 64-1 Locations of the most common palpable lymph nodes that can become enlarged in caseous lymphadenitis. The parotid (*A*), retropharyngeal (*B*), mandibular (*C*), prescapular (*D*), prefemoral (*E*), and popliteal (*F*) nodes are shown; the arrow points to the superficial inguinal lymph node (*G*). The most common location for wattles is also shown. However, wattles also may be found in other areas of the cervical region. (Adapted from Williams CSF: Routine sheep and goat procedures, Vet Clin North Am Food Anim Pract 6:753, 1990. IN Pugh DG: *Sheep and goat medicine*, Philadelphia, 2002, WB Saunders)

- Antimicrobial therapy is often unrewarding.
- When the abscess is open, it should be drained and flushed with either iodine or chlorhexidine solution.

INFORMATION FOR CLIENTS

- Affected animals should be removed from the flock or herd.
- The environment should be kept free from sharp objects that may compromise the skin barrier.
- Vaccination may reduce the incidence of the disease but may not eradicate it.

⬤ **TECH ALERT**

Pus in abscesses in goats and sheep may be thicker and more caseous and may not drain well via the syringe and needle.

Malignant Edema

Clostridium septicum is the most common cause of malignant edema, although mixed infections do occur. Usually, a history of a wound is present, and the organism then contaminates the wound.

CLINICAL SIGNS

- Local and regional pain
- Edematous swelling in the area of the original wound
- Fever
- Shock
- Death

DIAGNOSIS

- Malignant edema is difficult to diagnose antemortem. A neutrophilic leukocytosis is present, with a left shift, metabolic acidosis, azotemia, and change in liver and muscle enzymes; these changes are not diagnostic of the disease because they occur with other conditions as well.
- Lesions typically involve the head and neck area in young rams. The rams will be febrile and may die within 72 hours.

TREATMENT

- Supportive care such as intravenous fluids, antiinflammatories, and nutritional support are used to treat the disease. No specific treatment exists.

INFORMATION FOR CLIENTS

- Aseptic techniques and hygiene during invasive procedures such as injecting, dehorning, castration, and so forth are important in preventing malignant edema.

Blackleg

Blackleg is most often caused by *C. chauvoei*, although mixed infections can and do occur. As in other clostridial diseases, infection occurs when a wound becomes contaminated. Disease is caused by a toxin that causes local tissue necrosis and systemic toxemia. This organism may also cause gangrenous mastitis in ewes.

CLINICAL SIGNS

- Local and regional pain
- Cutaneous emphysema
- Edematous swelling in the area of the original wound
- Fever
- Shock
- Death

DIAGNOSIS

- Blackleg is difficult to diagnose antemortem. A neutrophilic leukocytosis exists, with a left shift, metabolic acidosis, azotemia, and change in liver and muscle enzymes; these changes are not diagnostic of the disease because they occur with other conditions as well.
- The disease progresses rapidly, and animals may be found dead with few signs.

TREATMENT

- Wound management
- Penicillin
- Supportive care

INFORMATION FOR CLIENTS

- Aseptic techniques and hygiene during invasive procedures such as injecting, dehorning, castration, and so forth, are important in preventing the disease.

Red Water Disease

Red water disease is caused by *C. hemolyticum*. This organism will colonize the livers of affected animals and produce a β-toxin, leading to intravascular hemolysis. The condition is often seen secondary to liver disease caused by migrating liver flukes.

CLINICAL SIGNS

- Red urine and feces
- Weakness
- Depression
- Icterus

DIAGNOSIS

- Laboratory findings suggestive of this condition include anemia, hemoglobinemia, and hemoglobinuria.
- A mature neutrophilia with a left shift may be evident.

TREATMENT

- Penicillin
- Flukicides
- Supportive care
- Antiinflammatories

Vaccination Recommendations

Goats

- *C. perfringens*, type C and D
- *C. tetani*
- *Chlamydia* and *Campylobacter* for breeding does

Sheep

- *C. perfringens* type C,D
- *C. novi*
- *C. sordelli*
- *C. chauvoei*
- *C. septicum*
- *C. tetani*
- *Chlamydia* and *Campylobacter* for breeding ewes
- Leptospirosis and rabies in endemic areas

REVIEW QUESTIONS

1. Which of the following is an effective way to treat or control caseous lymphadenitis in a goat herd?
   a. Daily prophylactic antibiotics
   b. Keeping wounds clean and disinfected
   c. Culling affected animals
   d. Caseous lymphadenitis cannot be controlled
2. The best way to diagnose a wound infection is with _____.
   a. Response to treatment
   b. Serology
   c. Wound culture
   d. Complete blood cell count
3. Since pus in ruminants may be thicker or caseous in nature, the best way to drain the abscess would be _____.
   a. Surgical opening with curettage
   b. Draining with a syringe and needle
   c. Waiting for the abscess to rupture spontaneously

Answers found on page 558.

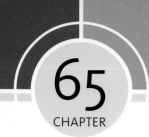

65 CHAPTER

Diseases of the Integumentary System

Dermatophilosis   Papule   Pruritus

LEARNING OBJECTIVES

When you have completed this chapter, you will be able to:
1. Recognize the most common skin diseases in goats and sheep.

2. Advise clients on proper husbandry for goats and sheep.

Skin problems are not uncommon in sheep and goats. These conditions may lead to loss of production through decreased growth, damage to the fiber, and weight loss. History, clinical signs, and a thorough physical examination are critical in determining the cause of the skin problems.

Contagious Ecthyma (Sore Mouth, Orf)

Contagious ecthyma is caused by a parapoxvirus and shows a preference for attacking epithelial tissue. The virus is present throughout the world and remains active in the environment for months, if not years. Transmission is through direct contact or contamination of skin abrasions, and morbidity is greatest in animals that are grazing coarse pasture plants.

CLINICAL SIGNS

* Papules, vesicles, pustules
* Thick crusts, especially around mouth (Fig. 65-1)
* Lesions may spread to oral cavity, eyelids, feet, udder
* Lesions typically resolve in 2 weeks

DIAGNOSIS

* Skin biopsy

TREATMENT

* Treatment of individual animals is generally not needed unless the lesions are severe; if so, supportive care is needed.

● TECH ALERT

This is a zoonotic disease. Wear gloves, and maintain good hygiene when handling infected animals.

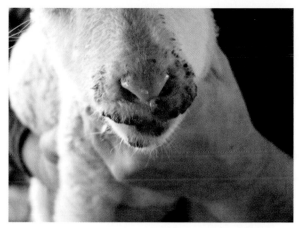

Figure 65-1 Malignant contagious ecthyma. Note the lesions around the mouth and on the face. (From Pugh DG: *Sheep and goat medicine,* ed 2, St. Louis, MO, 2012, Saunders, by permission.)

INFORMATION FOR CLIENTS

- Contagious ecthyma is a highly zoonotic disease, and hygiene is important when handling affected animals.

Dermatophilosis

Dermatophilosis is usually seen during wet or moist conditions; it is caused by the bacterium *Dermatophilus congolensis.* The causative organisms become trapped in hair or wool and reproduce in the moist environment. The condition may be transmitted by direct contact or transfer from inanimate objects.

CLINICAL SIGNS

- Matting of hair, followed by alopecia and crusting
- Lesions most often found along face, muzzle, and ears; in extremely wet or humid environments, lesions on the dorsum are not uncommon

DIAGNOSIS

- Clinical signs and history that are highly suggestive
- Definitive diagnosis by observing an impression smear of the lesions

TREATMENT

- Systemic penicillin or oxytetracycline

- Topical treatment with copper sulfate, zinc sulfate, potassium aluminum sulfate

Ringworm

Ringworm is a common skin condition of all domestic animals. Four species of fungi have been cultured from ringworm lesions in sheep and goats. The condition is transmitted via direct contact or inanimate objects.

CLINICAL SIGNS

- Erythema, alopecia, crusting
- Lesions may be typical circular lesions, especially on face
- Mild-to-moderate pruritus

DIAGNOSIS

- Fungal culture of skin and hair or wool

TREATMENT

- Topical treatment with iodine compounds, chlorhexidine, or antifungals may help limit spread throughout the flock or herd.

⊙ TECH ALERT

Ringworm is a zoonotic disease. Wear protective clothing when handling infected animals.

INFORMATION FOR CLIENTS

- Ringworm is a zoonotic disease, and care must be taken when handling affected animals.

Lice (Pediculosis)

Infestation with lice is most common in the winter months, especially when animals are crowded in their living quarters. The many species of lice that affect sheep and goats are grouped into two main categories: (1) sucking lice and (2) biting lice. Sucking lice live off blood and body fluid, whereas biting lice live on dead skin cells, hair, and debris. Lice are transmitted through direct contact and may be carried on inanimate objects.

CLINICAL SIGNS

- Intense pruritus
- Alopecia

DIAGNOSIS

- Presence of lice and eggs in hair or wool

TREATMENT

- A number of different topical solutions are effective against lice infestations. Ivermectin injections are effective against sucking lice but have limited efficacy against biting lice.

⬤ **TECH ALERT**

Most goats have lice, but they are not contagious to handlers. Lice are species specific.

Mange Mites

Mange is more of a problem for goats than for sheep. A variety of mites affect these animals, but all are treated in the same basic manner. Diagnosis is made by skin scraping or by examination of exudates from nodules caused by demodectic mange. Treatment consists of dipping the animal. Compounds that have been used include coumaphos, lime sulfur, γ-hexachlorocyclohexane (Lindane), and methoxychlor.

REVIEW QUESTIONS

1. Lice found on goats will infect the handler.
   a. True
   b. False
2. Contagious ecthyma is caused by a:
   a. Parapoxvirus
   b. Parvovirus
   c. Paramyxovirus
   d. Papovavirus
3. The diagnosis of mange in goats is made by:
   a. Culture
   b. Skin scrape
   c. Enzyme linked immunosorbent assay (ELISA) test
   d. Gram staining
4. Ringworm in goats can be easily cured by oral medication.
   a. True
   b. False

Answers found on page 558.

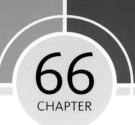

Diseases of the Musculoskeletal System

LEARNING OBJECTIVES

When you have completed this chapter, you will be able to:
1. Recognize the common musculoskeletal problems in goats and sheep.
2. Discuss treatments and correction of husbandry problems with the clients who have lame goats and sheep.

Lameness issues in sheep and goats are noticed mainly when the animals cannot move around to graze and feed efficiently. Some animals, however, are used as pack animals, and their soundness is important to their use. Most of the lameness problems in sheep and goats arise in the feet, with overgrown feet being the most common problem. Like other hooved animals, sheep and goats need regular hoof trimming (Fig. 66-1). Animals that are fed high-quality, high-protein diets and those that are not on hard ground with the opportunity to wear down their hooves are more likely to have hooves that become overgrown (Fig. 66-2).

Infectious Footrot

Infectious footrot is a contagious disease caused by the bacterium *Dichelobacter nodosus*. Animals that have had a previous infection with *Fusobacterium necrophorum*, those kept in small pastures, and those kept in wet conditions with long grass are predisposed to the disease.

CLINICAL SIGNS
- Both claws in multiple feet affected
- Lameness, usually in more than one individual

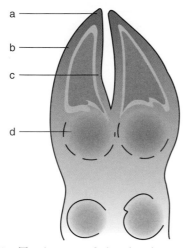

Figure 66-1 The bottom of the sheep's or goat's foot. The toe (*A*) should be cleaned out, and the outer hoof wall (*B*) should be cut to remove all overgrowths, bring the wall down to the sole, and make the outer wall parallel with the coronary band. The inner hoof wall (*C*) is then cut, with more inside wall than outside wall being removed. The heel (*D*) should not be cut unless it is badly overgrown. (From Pugh DG: *Sheep and goat medicine*, Philadelphia, PA, 2002, Saunders, by permission.)

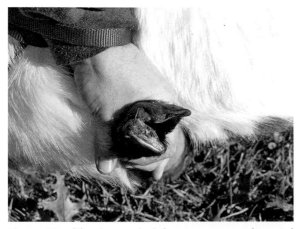

Figure 66-2 The claw on the left is overgrown and in need of trimming. The claw on the right has been trimmed back so that the wall and toe are even with the sole. (From Pugh DG: *Sheep and goat medicine*, Philadelphia, PA, 2012, Saunders, by permission.)

- Horn tissue separates from underlying structures
- Malodorous exudates
- Interdigital dermatitis more common in goats
- Anorexia and weight loss

DIAGNOSIS

- History
- Clinical signs

TREATMENT

- Proper hoof trimming
- Topical antibiotics and antiseptics
- Zinc sulfate, copper sulfate foot baths

⬤ TECH ALERT

Technicians should learn to properly "sit" up a sheep or goat for foot trimming to avoid injury.

INFORMATION FOR OWNERS

- Proper maintenance of feet is important in these animals.

Laminitis

Laminitis is not uncommon in sheep and goats. Animals that have laminitis often have a history of grazing lush pastures or consuming high-concentrate feeds. Systemic illnesses such as pneumonia, mastitis, and metritis predispose an animal to laminitis.

CLINICAL SIGNS

- Lameness
- Warm feet
- Animals prefer to remain recumbent

DIAGNOSIS

- Clinical signs
- Radiography of the feet

TREATMENT

- Nonsteroidal antiinflammatory drugs (NSAIDs)
- Treatment of the primary underlying cause

INFORMATION FOR CLIENTS

- Many instances of laminitis can be prevented by effective management.
- Slowly increasing the feed or turnout time on lush pastures decreases the likelihood of an animal becoming affected.

Septic Arthritis

Septic arthritis occurs most commonly in neonates but may also occur in adults if there is a penetrating wound near a joint. A variety of bacteria has been implicated in this condition.

CLINICAL SIGNS

- Lameness
- Warm swelling of joints
- Anorexia
- Fever

DIAGNOSIS

- Culture and cytology of synovial fluid
- Abnormal appearance to synovial fluid
- Radiography to monitor progression of condition

TREATMENT

- Joint lavage
- Antibiotics

INFORMATION FOR CLIENTS

- Septic arthritis in neonates can be prevented by ensuring adequate quality and quantity of colostrums.
- Dipping of the umbilicus of the neonate is also essential to prevent the condition.

Caprine Arthritis Encephalitis

Caprine arthritis encephalitis is a multisystemic disease caused by a retrovirus. Transmission is most common from doe to kid through nursing. Venereal transmission and transmission by contaminated instruments and equipment are also possible, although insects have not been shown to have a role in the transmission of the disease.

CLINICAL SIGNS

- Chronic progressive arthritis
- Seen in goats older than 6 months
- Carpal swelling
- Lameness and debilitation as disease progresses

DIAGNOSIS

- Serologic testing, the most common being agar gel immunodiffusion test

TREATMENT

- No specific treatment exits. Affected animals may be a source of infection to others, and their condition worsens over time. Supportive care keeps the animals comfortable temporarily, but most affected animals eventually are culled from the herd.

INFORMATION FOR CLIENTS

- Routine serologic testing and culling of positive animals may eradicate the disease from a herd. If a caprine arthritis encephalitis–positive doe has kids, the kid should be removed from the dam immediately and raised as a bottle baby.

Nutritional Muscular Dystrophy (White Muscle Disease)

Nutritional muscular dystrophy is caused by lack of selenium in the diet. Selenium acts as an antioxidant, protecting cell membranes from damage by free radicals. A lack of selenium leads to cell membrane damage. These areas of damage are seen as white areas in the muscle.

CLINICAL SIGNS

Cardiac Form
- Dyspnea
- Recumbency
- Tachycardia

Skeletal Muscle Form
- Stiff gait
- Muscle tremors when standing
- Hunched appearance
- Dysphagia

DIAGNOSIS

- Increased serum levels of creatine kinase and aspartate aminotransferase
- Whole-blood selenium concentrations, from more than one animal

TREATMENT

- Injection of vitamin E or selenium
- Avoidance of exposure to stress and exertion

INFORMATION FOR CLIENTS

- Many areas of the United States are selenium deficient. Supplementation of selenium helps prevent white muscle disease, but care must be taken not to oversupplement to avoid selenium toxicity.

Rickets and Osteomalacia

This disease (rickets in young animals and osteomalacia in adults) is a result of improper mineralization of bone caused by lack of vitamin D, or less frequently, lack of calcium or phosphorus in the diet.

CLINICAL SIGNS

- Affected animals are usually younger than 1 year
- Stiff gait
- Shifting leg lameness
- Recumbency
- Enlargement of costochondral junction

DIAGNOSIS

- Increased alkaline phosphatase
- Hypocalcemia
- Hypophosphatemia
- Radiographic evidence of wide growth plates and thin cortices

TREATMENT

- Vitamin D_3 injections
- Calcium and phosphorus supplementation

INFORMATION FOR CLIENTS

- Rickets and osteomalacia can be prevented by allowing the animals access to sunlight and ensuring the proper mineral content of the diet.

Ergot Toxicosis

Ergot toxicosis results when animals ingest an alkaloid produced by the fungus *Claviceps purpurea*. This fungus commonly affects cereal grains and grasses. The condition may also be caused by grazing endophyte-infested fescue pastures.

CLINICAL SIGNS

- Swelling of distal limbs
- Coolness of distal limbs
- Hair loss
- Discoloration of skin of distal limbs, tail, ears
- Affected skin may slough off
- Lameness, especially of hind-limbs in goats

DIAGNOSIS

- Finding the toxic compounds in the feed

TREATMENT

- Removal of affected animals from the source of the toxin

REVIEW QUESTIONS

1. What is the most common foot abnormality found in sheep and goats?
   a. Hairy heel warts
   b. Laminitis
   c. Hoof abscesses
   d. Overgrowth of hoof wall
2. White muscle disease is caused by lack of:
   a. Calcium
   b. Molybdenum
   c. Selenium
   d. Manganese
3. Which two chemicals must be properly balanced in ruminant diets?
   a. Potassium and sodium
   b. Copper and nickel
   c. Iron and vitamin D
   d. Calcium and phosphorus

4. Footrot can be treated by: (Mark all that apply.)
   a. Copper and zinc sulfate baths
   b. Proper foot trimming
   c. Antibiotics
   d. All of the above

5. This type of pasture should be avoided.
   a. Rye grass
   b. Bermuda grass
   c. Fescue
   d. Blue grass

Answers found on page 558.

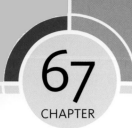

67
CHAPTER

Diseases of the Nervous System

OUTLINE

Scrapie
Rabies
Listeriosis

Menigeal Worm
Tetanus
Polioencephalomalacia

LEARNING OBJECTIVES

When you have completed this chapter, you will be able to:
1. Recognize neurologic diseases in goats and sheep.
2. Be able to explain to owners the need for routine vaccination programs for their herds.

3. Be able to explain the need for owners to purchase good-quality diets for each species.

Neurologic diseases are not common in sheep and goats, but they can be devastating to the animal and its owner. Many neurologic conditions carry a poor to grave prognosis. When determining the cause of a condition, signalment, history, and mental status are all important factors. A thorough neurologic examination is then performed to localize the lesion and have a better idea about what condition is affecting the animal.

Scrapie

Scrapie is a reportable disease in the United States. It is a member of the group of diseases known as *transmissible spongiform encephalopathies*. It is a

progressive, degenerative disorder of the central nervous system (CNS) seen mainly in sheep but occasionally in goats. The exact cause of scrapie is believed to be a prion, a small piece of protein that enters the cells in the brain and alters protein structures, causing the cell to eventually die. The disease is similar to "mad cow disease" and other degenerative encephalopathies.

CLINICAL SIGNS

- Seen most commonly in Suffolk sheep
- Mild apprehension, fixed gaze, aggressiveness
- Exercise intolerance and ataxia
- Intense pruritus
- Recumbency
- Blindness, seizures, death

DIAGNOSIS

- It is difficult to make an antemortem diagnosis because no specific lesions or laboratory test results are specific to the disease.

TREATMENT

- No effective treatment exists.

Rabies

Rabies is a zoonotic disease that has serious public health implications. Most states have laws mandating the vaccination of dogs and cats, and some states mandate the vaccination of horses. No laws exist regarding the vaccination of sheep and goats. Currently, no rabies vaccines have been approved for goats; if goats are vaccinated, they are usually vaccinated with a product approved for sheep. The vaccine is available only through licensed veterinarians. If any animal is showing neurologic signs and has a history of having been bitten by another animal, rabies should be suspected.

The infectious agent is a Lyssavirus. An infected animal, usually a raccoon, skunk, fox, or bat, bites the victim and passes the virus through saliva. The virus migrates through the body and the nervous system and localizes in the CNS. The virus may affect the cerebrum, the brainstem, or the spinal cord.

CLINICAL SIGNS

- If the virus settles in the brain, extreme behavior changes, often aggressive, are seen.
- If the brainstem is affected, behavior changes, with animal becoming more subdued and quiet, are seen.
- If the spinal cord is affected, the animal exhibits ataxia that progresses to paralysis.
- Signs are rapidly progressive, and the animal usually dies within 5 to 10 days of the onset of signs.

DIAGNOSIS

- Examination of brain tissue

TREATMENT

- No treatment currently exists for rabies.

INFORMATION FOR CLIENTS

- If a vaccinated animal is bitten by a rabid animal, the animal should be revaccinated and observed for 45 days.
- If an unvaccinated animal is bitten by a suspected rabid animal, it should be euthanized. If the owner is unwilling to perform euthanasia, the animal needs to be watched closely for 6 months and *handled with extreme caution.*
- Euthanize any animal that has been exposed to rabies and shows neurologic disease.
- A yearly rabies vaccine will prevent the disease.

⬤ TECH ALERT

Treat any animal showing neurologic signs as if has rabies. Wear gloves and protective eye-ware when examining the oral cavity.

Listeriosis

Listeriosis is caused by the bacterium *Listeria monocytogenes.* The bacterium is shed in body fluids in sick and unaffected animals. The bacterium lives for long periods in the environment. Listeriosis has been associated with the feeding of silage and grazing in wet, boggy pastures.

CLINICAL SIGNS

- Loss of ability to eat
- Signs of vestibular disease
- Depression
- Dysphagia
- Recumbency

DIAGNOSIS

- No specific diagnostic test exists for antemortem cases.
- A thorough neurologic examination is necessary to rule out other neurologic diseases.

TREATMENT

- Intensive antibiotic therapy; penicillin, oxytetracycline, and florfenicol are the most commonly used antibiotics.
- Therapy should be for a minimum of 14 days.

- Nonsteroidal antiinflammatory drugs (NSAIDs) are also indicated.

INFORMATION FOR CLIENTS

- *L. monocytogenes* can affect people as well; therefore, caution should be exercised if the disease is suspected in a flock or herd.

Meningeal Worm

The meningeal worm *Parelaphostrongylus tenuis* is a parasite of the white-tailed deer but affects sheep and goats as well. The oocysts are passed in the feces of the deer, and are then ingested by snails and slugs. Small ruminants become affected when they accidentally ingest these intermediate hosts while grazing. The larvae migrate along the peripheral nerves to the spinal canal, where they cause inflammation and destruction, leading to clinical signs of neurologic deficits.

CLINICAL SIGNS

- Animals usually display acute onset of signs.
- They usually remain bright and alert but show progressive hind-limb ataxia which culminates in inability to rise.

DIAGNOSIS

- Clinical signs
- History

TREATMENT

- High doses of ivermectin for 5 days
- Flunixin meglumine

INFORMATION FOR CLIENTS

- In areas where meningeal worms have been known to be a problem, a prophylactic, routine deworming program should be instituted.

Tetanus

All domestic animals are susceptible to tetanus. The causative organism is normally found in the environment and in the gastrointestinal tract. Sheep and goats most often are affected when the bacteria contaminate an open wound. The bacterium *Clostridium*

tetani releases a toxin. The toxin prevents release of γ-aminobutyric acid (GABA). GABA normally inhibits nerve impulse propagation, but without inhibition on nerve impulse conduction, then the nerves are always firing, causing constant muscle contraction.

CLINICAL SIGNS

- Muscle stiffness and spasms
- Increased sensitivity to noise and touch
- Overall stiffness of body
- Eventual progression to rigid paralysis and death due to asphyxiation
- Death usually occurs within 10 days

DIAGNOSIS

- Wound history
- Clinical signs

TREATMENT

- No treatment exists for tetanus. Good supportive care needs to be provided. Tetanus is easier to prevent than to treat.

INFORMATION FOR CLIENTS

- Tetanus can be prevented by yearly vaccination.

Polioencephalomalacia

Polioencephalomalacia is caused by lack of thiamine. Normally, the rumen microbes produce enough thiamine to meet the animal's needs. Sudden diet changes, ingestion of bracken fern, and prolonged anorexia may all lead to lack of thiamine. Thiamine is a necessary cofactor for glucose metabolism. A lack of thiamine leads to lack of glucose. Glucose is needed for energy, which allows the brain to maintain a proper osmotic gradient. Cellular swelling thus results from thiamine deficiency.

CLINICAL SIGNS

- Central blindness
- Strabismus
- Depression
- Incoordination
- Head pressing
- Coma and death

DIAGNOSIS

- Clinical signs
- Response to treatment

TREATMENT

- Thiamine injections: intravenously first, then intramuscular or subcutaneous injections every 6 hours for the first day, and then every 6 to 12 hours for at least 2 days

REVIEW QUESTIONS

1. Which of the following is the treatment for polioencephalomalacia?
   a. Niacin injection
   b. Ascorbic acid injection
   c. Thiamine injection
   d. Vitamin K injection

2. The presence of this bacterium in food may result in food poisoning in humans. In goats and sheep, it is associated with feeding of silage and grazing on wet, boggy pasture.
   a. *Clostridia*
   b. *Listeria*
   c. *Escherichia coli*
   d. *Staphylococcus*

3. No law mandates rabies vaccine for pet goats.
   a. True
   b. False

4. Would you recommend that owners remove the kid or lamb from a female with mastitis and bottle feed them?
   a. Yes
   b. No

Answers found on page 559.

68
CHAPTER

Diseases of the Reproductive System

OUTLINE

Dystocia
Vaginal and Uterine Prolapses
   Campylobacter (Vibriosis)

Chlamydiosis
Brucellosis
Mastitis

LEARNING OBJECTIVES

When you have completed this chapter, you will be able to:

1. Identify obstetric problems in pregnant goats and sheep.

2. Recognize the zoonotic potential of many organisms that cause abortion or dystocias in these animals.

Sheep and goats are seasonally polyestrous. Most are short-day breeders, although some breeds have estrous cycles year-round. Normal gestation length is approximately 153 days. The doe has an estrous cycle length of 21 days, and she stays in estrus for an average of 36 hours. The ewe has an estrous cycle length of 18 days, and she stays in estrus for an average of 30 hours.

Dystocia

Dystocia, or difficult parturition, is a major cause of losses in a small ruminant operation. If a female animal starts contraction and no progress is made within 30 minutes, a veterinarian should be called. If the dam is clinically normal, the vet may elect to wait 30 minutes before any intervention. Female animals should be examined 30 minutes after parturition to determine whether any more fetuses are present in the uterus. Dystocias are most commonly caused by fetal malpresentation, dam-to-fetus size mismatch, and occasionally *ringwomb*, a condition in which the cervix fails to dilate. If the veterinarian's hands are small enough, and copious amounts of lubricants are used, many dystocias may be corrected manually. Otherwise, a cesarean section must be performed.

● TECH ALERT

Be sure to check the dam for a second or third fetus because multiple fetuses are not uncommon in these species.

Vaginal and Uterine Prolapses

Vaginal prolapses are not uncommon in sheep. Uterine prolapsed in goats and sheep, and vaginal prolapse in goats fortunately are quite rare. Nutritional factors have been implicated in vaginal prolapse, whereas many uterine prolapses are caused by hypocalcemia. The tissue that is prolapsed should be scrubbed and replaced. Raising the hindquarters of the doe or ewe facilitates the process as does an epidural. Hyperosmotic solutions may be applied to shrink the mass of tissue. After the tissue is replaced, sutures are applied to retain the tissue. Specific devices are designed to help retain a prolapsed vagina.

Campylobacter (Vibriosis)

Vibriosis, the condition caused by *Campylobacter*, is one of the most significant causes of spontaneous abortion in sheep in the United States. Two species of *Campylobacter* are known to cause abortions. Infection occurs when the pregnant sheep ingests the organism that has been in the digestive tract of another individual.

CLINICAL SIGNS

- Late-term abortions
- Stillbirths
- Weak lambs

DIAGNOSIS

- Isolation of the organism from fetal abomasums, placenta, or dam's vaginal discharge

TREATMENT

- Penicillin, streptomycin, or tetracycline
- During an outbreak, tetracycline or oxytetracycline given in late gestation to prevent abortions

> **TECH ALERT**
>
> Use caution when handling aborted fetuses and placentas.

INFORMATION FOR CLIENTS

- A vaccine that aids in the prevention of abortions is available.

- Zoonotic potential from this disease exists, so care should be taken when handling aborted fetuses.

Chlamydiosis

Chlamydia psittaci infection is a common cause of abortion in sheep and goats. Pigeons and sparrows appear to be reservoirs for the disease. Transmission is through uterine fluids. Once infected, female animals acquire immunity, which may last as long as 3 years.

CLINICAL SIGNS

- Abortions, usually in the last month of gestation
- Anorexia and fever in female animals shortly before abortion

DIAGNOSIS

- History of abortion
- Clinical signs
- Examining an impression smear of the placenta, fetal tissues, or uterine discharge

TREATMENT

- Administration of tetracycline during the last 4 to 6 weeks of gestation helps prevent abortions.

INFORMATION FOR CLIENTS

- A vaccine is available.
- *Chlamydia* is zoonotic, so care must be taken when handling affected animals.

Brucellosis

Brucellosis causes abortions in goats and, occasionally, sheep and epididymitis in rams. The organism is ingested and then becomes localized in tissues. The organism may be passed in semen.

CLINICAL SIGNS

- Abortions, commonly during the last trimester
- Signs of systemic disease—fever, weight loss, depression, and so forth
- Infected ewes are rarely ill

DIAGNOSIS

- Bacterial isolation from aborted fetus
- Serologic tests detect carrier animals

TREATMENT

- No treatment currently is available.
- Affected animals should be culled.

INFORMATION FOR CLIENTS

- New animals should be tested for brucellosis before being added to the breeding flock.
- A vaccine is available but has questionable efficacy.
- The disease has zoonotic potential, so milk products should be pasteurized before consumption.

Mastitis

Mastitis, or inflammation of the udder, may be infectious or noninfectious. Mastitis has a great impact on the herd in terms of both loss of milk for human consumption and loss of milk available to kids or lambs. Microorganisms that are known to be causative agents of mastitis include *Escherichia coli*, *Klebsiella* spp., *Mycoplasma* spp., and *Pseudomonas* spp. Mastitis is a disease entity that may just affect the udder, or it may be toxic and affect the whole system.

CLINICAL SIGNS

- Swollen, red, warm udder
- Gangrenous areas of udder
- Thick, discolored milk
- Signs of septicemia

DIAGNOSIS

- Culture and sensitivity for causative agent

TREATMENT

- Based on results from culture and sensitivity
- Intramammary infusions
- Systemic antibiotics
- Intravenous fluids for severe toxic mastitis
- Udder amputation

REVIEW QUESTIONS

1. How is vaginal prolapse treated?
   a. Amputation of the tissue
   b. Culling of the animal
   c. Estrogen injections
   d. Replacement of tissue and use of a restraining device
2. Which of the following organisms that cause reproductive diseases has zoonotic potential?
   a. *Brucella*
   b. *Campylobacter*
   c. *Chlamydia*
   d. All of the above
3. Would you recommend that owners remove the kid or lamb from a female with mastitis and bottle feed them?
   a. Yes
   b. No

Answers found on page 559.

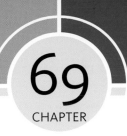

Diseases of the Respiratory System

Emaciation
Malaise

Morbidity

Tachypnea

***Oestrus ovis* Infestation**
Sinusitis
Pasteurellosis

Parainfluenza Type 3
Contagious Caprine Pleuropneumonia
Ovine Progressive Pneumonia

When you have completed this chapter, you will be able to:
1. Recognize the relationship between respiratory disease and decreased herd production.

2. Discuss with owners the importance of isolating animals showing signs of respiratory disease to prevent the spread of disease in the herd.

Respiratory diseases can have a significant impact on a flock or herd through decreased milk production, slower growth, and the economics involved in treating the diseases. Respiratory disease may not be noticed by many owners until it has progressed to a fairly serious condition because many owners do not examine individual animals on a daily basis.

Oestrus Ovis Infestation

Oestrus ovis infestation is a condition caused by a fly that deposits larvae around a sheep's or goat's nostrils. The larvae then migrate into the nasal cavity and sinuses; then they fall out and pupate on the ground.

CLINICAL SIGNS
• Secondary bacterial infections

• Sinusitis
• Shaking of the head
• Rubbing of the nose
• Nasal discharge

DIAGNOSIS
• Endoscopy, visualizing the larvae

TREATMENT
• Ivermectin to kill larvae

Sinusitis

Sinusitis is a rare condition in sheep and goats, usually secondary to some other condition. Frontal sinus infections are usually found in animals that have a history of recent dehorning, whereas tooth problems are the most common cause of maxillary sinus infections.

CLINICAL SIGNS

- Discharge
- Facial asymmetry
- Foul odor
- Occasional signs of systemic disease

DIAGNOSIS

- Clinical signs

TREATMENT

- Lavage of the affected sinus
- Systemic antibiotics, if needed

INFORMATION FOR CLIENTS

- Keeping the head bandaged after dehorning may prevent sinusitis.

Pasteurellosis

Pasteurella haemolytica is one of the most important bacterial diseases of sheep and goats. This bacterium causes severe, life-threatening pneumonia. The bacterium is a normal inhabitant of the upper respiratory tract, but during times of stress and when the animal is immunocompromised, it may cause deleterious effects.

CLINICAL SIGNS

- Nasal discharge
- Fever
- Anorexia
- Weight loss
- Sudden death

DIAGNOSIS

- Clinical signs
- History
- Isolation of the organism from tissues, usually at necropsy

TREATMENT

- Oxytetracycline
- Sulfonamides in drinking water

INFORMATION FOR CLIENTS

- The chances of pneumonia can be reduced by minimizing stress to the herd or flock.
- Vaccination with a cattle respiratory complex vaccine may decrease the likelihood of disease.

Parainfluenza Type 3

Most infections with parainfluenza type 3 are inapparent because most sheep are seropositive. Outbreaks of disease, with high levels of morbidity, have been reported.

CLINICAL SIGNS

- Cough
- Serous nasal discharge
- Ocular discharge
- Most common in lambs younger than 1 year

DIAGNOSIS

- Isolation of the virus from nasal swab

TREATMENT

- Antibiotics to control secondary bacterial infections

Contagious Caprine Pleuropneumonia

Caprine pleuropneumonia is caused by *Mycoplasma capricola* subspecies *capri pneumoniae*. The disease is contagious in housed goats, with the morbidity rate approaching 100% and the mortality rate ranging from 60% to 100%.

CLINICAL SIGNS

- Cough
- Fever
- Listlessness
- Anorexia
- Death in 2 days

DIAGNOSIS

- No effective way to diagnose this condition exists.

TREATMENT

- Tylosin

- Enrofloxacin
- Tetracycline

INFORMATION FOR CLIENTS

- Vaccination may prevent caprine pleuropneumonia.
- Tetracycline may minimize disease spread in an outbreak.

Ovine Progressive Pneumonia

The causative agent of ovine progressive pneumonia (OPP) is a lentivirus. OPP is one of the most important diseases affecting sheep in North America. The virus persists in monocytes and macrophages. Ingestion of milk from affected animals appears to be the most common method of transmission.

CLINICAL SIGNS

- Signs often appear shortly after stressful episodes
- Slowly progressive malaise
- Progressive emaciation
- Dyspnea
- Tachypnea
- Cough

DIAGNOSIS

- Enzyme-linked immunosorbent assay (ELISA) testing for viral nucleic acid particles

TREATMENT

- Supportive care

INFORMATION FOR CLIENTS

- Maintaining a closed flock, testing, and culling may all help maintain a disease-free flock.

Review Questions

1. Which parasite deposits larvae around an animal's nostrils?
   a. *Trichostrongylus*
   b. *Dictyocaulus*
   c. *Oestrus ovis*
   d. *Haemonchus contortus*
2. Frontal sinus infections are usually secondary to:
   a. Tooth root abscess
   b. Recent dehorning
   c. *Oestrus ovis* infection
   d. None of the above
3. A large herd of goats was kept housed in a barn all winter to be protected from heavy snowfall. Approximately 99% of them came down with signs of pleuropneumonia. What bacterium is most likely responsible for this outbreak?
   a. *Mycoplasma*
   b. *Streptococcus*
   c. *Bordetella*
   d. *Haemophilus*

Answers found on page 559.

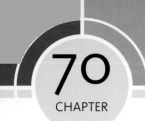

Diseases of the Urinary System

LEARNING OBJECTIVES

When you have completed this chapter, you will be able to:
1. Recognize common urinary problems in sheep and goats.

Fortunately, urinary tract problems are rare in properly maintained sheep and goats. The main concerns are plants that are known to be nephrotoxic and urolithiasis. Ordinarily animals will not graze plants that are toxic, unless they have nothing else to graze. Ensuring plentiful, wholesome forage should ensure that animals do not become exposed to plant toxicities. If plant toxicity does occur, the animal should be removed from the offending plant and supportive care instituted.

Other predisposing conditions include castration at an early age and the normal anatomy of the urethra.

Urolithiasis (Stones)

Urolithiasis is seen mainly in wethers, rams, and bucks that are on high-concentrate diets. It is most common in feedlot and pet animals. The most common site of obstruction is the urethral process and the sigmoid flexure. A thorough dietary history is very important when an animal with urethral calculi is presented in the clinic.

CLINICAL SIGNS

- Hematuria
- Stranguria
- Signs of abdominal pain
- Crystals may be seen on preputial hairs
- Distended bladder

DIAGNOSIS

- Clinical signs
- Urinalysis
- Radiography may show stones

TREATMENT

- Amputation of urethral process
- Penile catheterization and retrograde flushing
- Cystotomy
- Urethrostomy
- Vitamin C or other urinary acidifiers

INFORMATION FOR CLIENTS

- Male sheep and goats should receive most of their energy from forages.
- They should have access to clean, palatable water at all times.
- A proper calcium and phosphorous balance needs to be maintained in the diet.
- Ammonium chloride may be added to the diet to reduce the incidence of some types of stones.

Ruptured Bladder

Ruptured bladder may occur as a sequel to any urinary obstruction. Improper castration of males with elastrator bands may result in urinary obstruction and ruptured bladder. After rupture, animals may appear perfectly normal for longer periods than observed in other species, and they may even eat well.

CLINICAL SIGNS

- Mild colic
- Depression
- Anorexia
- Abdominal distension
- No urine production, dehydration

DIAGNOSIS

- Serum chemistries will show azotemia, hyperphosphatemia, hyperkalemia, and hyponatremia
- Abdominal fluid seen on ultrasonography
- Elevated creatinine levels in abdominal fluid ($> 2\times$ normal levels)

TREATMENT

- Intravenous (IV) normal saline
- Slow evacuation of fluid from the abdominal cavity
- Surgical repair of the damaged bladder

INFORMATION FOR CLIENTS

- Carefully observe any animal that has been treated for urinary obstruction.
- Make sure to observe the animal for normal urination.
- Proper management may decrease the incidence of urinary problems.

Ulcerative Posthitis (Pizzle Rot)

Ulcerative posthitis–balanoposthitis occurs more frequently in males kept on high-protein diets. Reaction of normal preputial bacteria with increased levels of urea in urine results in swelling, necrosis, and ulceration of the prepuce. Signs of the disease may be seen as early as 2 weeks after beginning a high-protein diet. Castration before puberty may result in decreased ability to extend the penis during urination, allowing urine to pool in the prepuce and predisposing the animal to pizzle rot.

CLINICAL SIGNS

- Straining to urinate
- Swelling of the prepuce
- Thick, malodorous urine
- Ulceration of preputial mucosa

DIAGNOSIS

- Examination of the prepuce

TREATMENT

- Reducing protein content of the diet
- Debridement of any necrotic tissue
- Application of topical antibiotics, astringents, or antiseptics to preputial mucosal surfaces
- If scar tissue is obstructing urine flow, surgical remodeling of scar tissue to re-establish flow
- Clip all hair or wool from the area, and burn it or dispose of it as a biohazard material

INFORMATION FOR CLIENTS

- Maintain the proper protein level in the diet (under 12% is recommended).
- Make sure that the animals have clean, fresh water at all times.
- Remove affected animals from the herd to prevent spread of infection.

Review Questions

1. What is the most common predisposing factor for urolithiasis in a buck, ram, or wether?
   a. Too much concentrate in the diet
   b. Too much hay in the diet
   c. Not having access to a mineral salt block
   d. Stress
2. What substance is commonly added to the diet of sheep and goats to prevent urinary stone formation?
   a. Selenium
   b. Aluminum chloride
   c. Propylene glycol
   d. Magnesium

3. Diets for small ruminants should contain no more than _____% protein.
   a. 8%
   b. 16%
   c. 20%
   d. 12%

Answers found on page 559.

Bibliography

Ainsworth D: Rhodococcal infections in foals, *Equine Vet Ed* 32, August 1999.

Arnauld des Lions J, Guillot J, Legrand E et al: Aspergillosis involving the frontal sinus in a horse, *Equine Vet Ed* 326, October 2000.

Baker R, Lumsden JH: *Color atlas of cytology of the dog and cat*, St Louis, 2000, Mosby.

Birchard SJ, Sherding RG: *Saunders manual of small animal practice*, ed 3, St Louis, 2006, Saunders.

Bojrab JM, editor: *Current techniques in small animal surgery*, ed 4, Baltimore, 1998, Williams & Wilkins.

Bonagura J, editor: *Kirk's current veterinary therapy XIII*, St Louis, 2000, Saunders.

Brigham E, Duncanson G: An equine postmortem dental study: 50 cases, *Equine Vet Ed* 79, April 2000.

Brigham E, Duncanson G: Case study of 100 horses presented to an equine dental technician in the UK, *Equine Vet Ed* 84, April 2000.

Brinker WO, Piermattei DL, Flo GL: *Brinker, Piermattei, and Flo's Handbook of small animal orthopedics and fracture treatment*, ed 4, St Louis, 2006, Saunders.

Brown S: *Small animal health series*, VeterinaryPartner.com.

Carlton WW, McGavin MD: *Thompson's special veterinary pathology*, ed 2, St Louis, 1995, Mosby.

Case LP, Carey DP, Hirakawa DA, Daristotle L: *Canine and feline nutrition*, ed 2, St Louis, 2000, Mosby.

Cheek R, Ballard B: *Exotic animal medicine for the veterinary technician*, Ames, IA, 2004, Blackwell.

Colville T, Bassert JM: *Clinical anatomy and physiology for veterinary technicians*, St Louis, 2002, Mosby.

Compendium of veterinary products, Port Huron, MI, 1991, North American Compendiums.

Cowell RL, Tyler RD, Meinkoth JH: *Diagnostic cytology and hematology of the dog and cat*, ed 2, St Louis, 1999, Mosby.

Crow SE, Walshaw SO: *Manual of clinical procedures in the dog, cat, and rabbit*, ed 2, Philadelphia, 1997, Lippincott-Raven Publishers.

de Jaeger E, de Keersmaecker S, Hannes C: Cystic urolithiasis in horses, *Equine Vet Ed* 30, February 2000.

DeLahunta A: *Veterinary neuroanatomy and clinical neurology*, ed 2, St Louis, 1983, WB Saunders.

Dunn J: *Textbook of small animal medicine*, St Louis, 1999, WB Saunders.

Dyce KM, Sack WO, Wensing CJG: *Textbook of veterinary anatomy*, ed 3, St Louis, 2002, Saunders.

Eastman T, Taylor T, Hooper R, Hague B: Treatment of grade 3 rectal tears in horses by direct suturing per rectum, *Equine Vet Ed* 63, February 2000.

Edwards NJ: *Bolton's handbook of canine and feline electrocardiography*, ed 2, St Louis, 1987, WB Saunders.

Edwards NJ: *ECG manual for the veterinary technician*, St Louis, 1993, WB Saunders.

Ettinger SJ, Feldman EC: *Textbook of veterinary internal medicine*, ed 6, St Louis, 2006, Saunders.

Ettinger SJ, Suter PF: *Canine cardiology*, St Louis, 1970, WB Saunders.

Exotic animals, a veterinary handbook, Yardley, PA, 1995, Veterinary Learning Systems.

Fossum TW: *Small animal surgery*, ed 3, St Louis, 2007, Mosby.

Fubini SM, Ducharme N: *Farm animal surgery*, St Louis, 2004, Saunders.

Gillespie JR: *Animal science*, Albany, NY, 1998, Delmar Publishers.

Goehring L, van Oldruitenborgh-Oosterbaan M: The mystery of equine herpes myeloencephalopathy, *Equine Vet Ed* 53, February 2001.

Gorrel C, Derbyshire S: *Veterinary dentistry for the nurse and technician*, Oxford, 2005, Butterworth-Heinemann.

Greene CE: *Infectious diseases of the dog and cat*, ed 3, St Louis, 2006, Saunders.

Hafez ESE, ed: *Reproduction in farm animals*, ed 6, Philadelphia, 1993, Lea and Febiger.

Han CM, Hurd CD: *Practical diagnostic imaging for the veterinary technician*, ed 3, St Louis, 2004, Mosby.

Harcourt-Brown F: *Textbook of rabbit medicine*, Oxford, 2002, Butterworth-Heinemann.

Hendrix CM, Robinson E: *Diagnostic parasitology for veterinary technicians*, ed 3, St Louis, 2006, Mosby.

Hendrix CM, Sirois M: *Laboratory procedures for veterinary technicians*, ed 5, St Louis, 2007, Mosby.

Hoffman A: Bronchoalveolar lavage technique and cytological diagnosis of small airway inflammatory disease, *Equine Vet Ed* 208, December 1999.

Holmstrom SE: *Veterinary dentistry for the technician and office staff*, St Louis, 2000, Saunders.

Holmstrom SE, Frost P, Eisner ER: *Veterinary dental techniques for the small animal practitioner*, ed 2, St Louis, 1998, WB Saunders.

Hudson J, Cohen N, Gibbs P, Thompson J: Feeding practices associated with colic in horses, *J Am Vet Med Assoc* 219:1419, 2001.

Judy C, Chaffin M, Cohen N: Empyema of the guttural pouch (auditory tube diverticulum) in horses: 91 cases (1977-1997), *J Am Vet Med Assoc* 215:1666, 1999.

Katz J, Evans L, Hutto D et al: Clinical, bacterial, serologic, and pathologic features of infections with atypical Taylorella equigenitalis in mares, *J Am Vet Med Assoc* 216:1945, 2000.

Katz L, Ragle C: Repeated manual evacuation for treatment of rectal tears in four horses, *J Am Vet Med Assoc* 215:1473, 1999.

Kesel L: *Veterinary dentistry for the small animal technician*, Ames, 2000, Iowa State University Press.

Kirk RW, editor: *Current veterinary therapy IX: small animal practice*, St Louis, 1995, WB Saunders.

Kittleson MD, Kienle RD: *Small animal cardiovascular medicine*, St Louis, 1999, Mosby.

La Croix NC, van der Woerdt A, Olivero DK: Nonhealing corneal ulcers in cats: 29 cases (1991-1999), *J Am Vet Med Assoc* 218(5):733, 2001.

Lavin LM: *Radiography in veterinary technology*, ed 4, St Louis, 2006, Saunders.

Lester G: Respiratory disease in the neonatal foal, *Equine Vet Ed* 53, August 1999.

Lewington JH: *Ferret husbandry, medicine and surgery*, Oxford, 2000, Butterworth-Heinemann.

Mader DR: *Reptile medicine and surgery*, ed 2, St Louis, 2006, Saunders.

Mair T, Derksen F: Chronic obstructive pulmonary disease: a review, *Equine Vet Ed* 53, February 2000.

McCurnin DM, Bassert JM: *Clinical textbook for veterinary technicians*, ed 6, St Louis, 2006, Saunders.

McGavin MD, Zachary JF: *Pathologic basis of veterinary disease*, ed 4, St Louis, 2007, Mosby.

McKinnon A, Voss J: *Equine reproduction*, Philadelphia, 1993, Lea & Febiger.

Meredith T, Dobrinski I: Thyroid function and pregnancy status in broodmares, *J Am Vet Med Assoc* 224:892, 2004.

Meyer DJ, Harvey JW: *Veterinary laboratory medicine*, ed 3, St Louis, 2004, Saunders.

Morley PH, Townsend H, Bogdan J, Haines D: Risk factors for disease associated with influenza virus infections during three epidemics in horses, *J Am Vet Med Assoc* 216:545, 2000.

Nelson RW, Couto CG: *Small animal internal medicine*, ed 3, St Louis, 2003, Mosby.

Olmstead ML: *Small animal orthopedics*, St Louis, 1995, Mosby.

Orsini J: Gastric ulceration in the mature horse: a review, *Equine Vet Ed* 36, February 2000.

Osborn CA, Low DG, Finco DR: *Canine and feline urology*, St Louis, 1972, WB Saunders.

Pederson NC et al: Feline immunodeficiency virus infection, *Vet Immunol Immunopath* 21:111, 1989.

Plumb D: *Veterinary drug handbook*, ed 5, Ames, 2005, Iowa State University Press.

Porter M, Long M, Getman L et al: West Nile Virus encephalomyelitis in horses: 46 cases (2001), *J Am Vet Med Assoc* 222:1241, 2003.

Proudman C: The role of parasites in equine colic, *Equine Vet Ed* 65, August 1999.

Pugh DG: *Sheep and goat medicine*, St Louis, 2002, Saunders.

Quesenberry K, Carpenter JW: *Ferrets, rabbits, and rodents: clinical medicine and surgery*, ed 2, St Louis, 2004, Saunders.

Ralston S, Stemme K, Guerroro J: *Preventing heartworm disease in cats*, Proceedings of an Innovations Session (Merck), 1997, North American Veterinary Conference.

Reed S, Bayly W, Sellon D: *Equine internal medicine*, ed 2, St Louis, 2004, Saunders.

Rose R, Hodgson D: *Manual of equine practice*, ed 2, St Louis, 2000, WB Saunders.

Rosenthal K, editor: *Practical exotic animal medicine*, Yardley, PA, 1997, Veterinary Learning Systems.

Ryland LM, Bernard SL: *Practical exotic animal medicine, The Compendium Collection*, Yardley, PA, 1997, Veterinary Learning Systems.

Scott DW, Miller WH Jr, Griffin CE: *Muller and Kirk's small animal dermatology*, ed 6, St Louis, 2001, Saunders.

Scrutchfield W, Schumacher J, Martin M: Correction of abnormalities of the cheek teeth, *Proceedings of the American Association of Equine Practitioners* 42:11, 1996.

Sirois M, editor: *Principles and practice of veterinary technology*, ed 2, St Louis, 2004, Mosby.

Slatter D: *Fundamentals of veterinary ophthalmology*, ed 3, St Louis, 2001, Saunders.

Smith B: *Large animal internal medicine*, ed 3, St Louis, 2002, Mosby.

Sodikoff CH: *Laboratory profiles of small animal diseases: a guide to laboratory diagnosis*, ed 3, St Louis, 2001, Mosby.

Stashak T: *Adams' lameness in horses*, ed 5, Philadelphia, 2002, Lippincott Williams & Wilkins.

Thibodeau GA, Patton KT: *Anatomy and physiology*, ed 5, St Louis, 2006, Mosby.

Thrall DE: *Textbook of veterinary diagnostic radiology*, ed 4, St Louis, 2002, Saunders.

Tilley LP Goodwin JK: *Manual of canine and feline cardiology*, ed 3, St. Louis, 2001, Saunders.

Tortora GJ, Grabowski SR: *Principles of anatomy and physiology*, ed 11, New York, 2005, John Wiley & Sons.

Tully TN, Mitchell MA: *A technician's guide to exotic animal care*, Lakewood, CO, 2001, AAHA Press.

Turner AS, McIlwraith CW: *Techniques in large animal surgery*, ed 2, Baltimore, 1989, Williams and Wilkins.

Wollanke B, Rohrbach B, Gerhards H: Serum and vitreous humor antibody titers in and isolation of Leptospira interrrogans from horses with recurrent uveitis, *J Am Vet Med Assoc* 219:795, 2001.

Wyman M: *Manual of small animal ophthalmology*, New York, 1986, Churchill Livingstone.

Zoonosis updates from the Journal of the American Veterinary Medical Association, ed 2, Schaumburg, IL, 1995, American Veterinary Medical Association.

Glossary

Abdominocentesis: Removal of fluid from the abdominal cavity.

Ablation: Removal of a growth or harmful substance.

Adrenocorticotropic: Describes hormones or drugs that stimulate the adrenal cortex to produce corticosteroids.

Aglactia: The inability of the mother to secrete enough milk to support the young.

Allantoin: A diureide of glyoxylic acid.

Alopecia: Partial or complete lack of hair, often due to endocrine disease.

Amelanotic: Pertaining to nonpigmented tissues due to lack of melanin.

Aminoglycoside: An antibiotic belonging to a group in which amino sugars are linked as glycosides, e.g., streptomycin.

Anaphylaxis: An exaggerated, life-threatening reaction of the immune system to a previously seen antigen.

Anasarca: The accumulation of watery fluid in connective tissue and cavities.

Androgen: Male hormone responsible for the development of male sexual characteristics. Testosterone and androsterone are examples.

Anemia: A decrease in hemoglobin levels within the blood to values less than normal.

Antemortem: Preceding death.

Antibody: An immunoglobulin produced by lymphocytes in response to presence of bacteria, virus or any other antigenic substance.

Antigen: A substance, usually a protein, that stimulates the production of an antibody specific to that protein.

Antitussive: Medications used to suppress a cough.

Arboreal: A species that lives in trees.

Arteriosclerosis: Thickening, decrease of elasticity and the presence of calcium deposits within the arterial walls.

Arthrodesis: Fusion of a joint to limit movement.

Arthroplasty: Surgical replacement or reconstruction of a damaged joint to restore mobility.

Ascites: Abnormal accumulation of intraperitoneal fluid high in protein and electrolytes.

Aseptic: Free of pathogenic microorganisms.

Asphyxiation: When the airway is blocked or closed and air cannot enter the lungs.

Ataxia: impaired ability to coordinate movement.

Atony: Lacking normal tone.

Atrophy: A wasting or decrease in size of a body part, tissue, or organ owing to disuse, disease, or injury.

Auscultate: The act of listening to sounds made by internal body organs, usually with a stethoscope.

Auscultation: The act of listening to sounds in the body (especially the heart).

Autogenous: Produced in or with tissue from the body of the animal to whom it will be given; originating from within the organism; e.g., vaccine or toxin.

Avascular: Not associated with or supplied by blood vessels.

Azotemic: A toxic condition caused by failure of the kidneys to remove urea from the blood.

Baroreceptors: A pressure-sensitive receptor nerve ending found in the atria of the heart, the aortic arch and in the carotid sinuses.

Basophilic: Can be stained with basic dyes.

Benign: Noncancerous.

Blepharitis: Chronic inflammation of the eyelid.

Blepharoedema: Swelling of the eyelids.

Blepharospasm: A condition in which there is sustained, forced, involuntary closing of the eyelids.

Boid: Pythons and boas.

Borborygmus: an audible abdominal sound produced by hyperactive intestinal peristaltic activity.

Bradycardia: Slower than normal heart rate.

Buccal: Side of the tooth closest to the cheek.

Cachexia: General ill health and malnutrition, usually associated with chronic disease.

Calculolytic: Able to dissolve urinary calculi.

Cancellous: A lacelike arrangement of bony trabeculae found at the ends of long bones.

Carcinoma: A malignant epithelial tumor that is invasive and will metastasize.

Cardiomegaly: Enlargement of the heart.

Cardiomyopathy: A disease of the heart muscle; any disease that affects the structure or function of the heart; enlargement of the heart muscle.

Caseous: Cheese-like.

Caslick operation: Surgically closes the upper portion of the vulva.

Cataract: An abnormal, progressive disease of the lens of the eye that inhibits sight characterized by loss of transparency.

Cautery: A devise or agent resulting in coagulation of tissue by heat.

Cecotroph: Soft fecal pellets ingested by rabbits directly from the anus during the night and early morning; "night feces"; Fecal material produced in the cecum of the rabbit.

Celiotomy: Incision into the abdominal cavity.

Chelate: Any coordination compound composed of a central metal atom and an organic molecule composed of multiple bonds in a ring structure.

Chemosis: Swelling of the tissue that lines the eyelids and the surface of the eye.

Choanal: A funnel-shaped channel connecting the sinuses of the bird to the oral cavity.

Cholinergic: Pertaining to nerve fibers that liberate acetylcholine at the myoneural junction.

Chondrodystrophic: An abnormal condition in which cartilage is converted to bone, especially in the epiphyses of long bones. Affected dogs have short misshapen legs with long backs.

Chromodacryorrhea: Red tears.

Ciliostasis: Failure of the cilia that line the upper respiratory tract to move normally leaving the deeper structure unprotected.

Cloaca: End of the primitive hindgut before separation of the bladder, reproductive tract and gastrointestinal system; passage for feces, urine, and reproductive tract in avian and reptilian species.

Coaptation: To join and bring together in proper alignment, e.g., broken bones.

Coccidiostat: An antiprotozoal agent that acts on *Coccidia* parasites.

Colostrum: A form of milk produced by the mammary glands during late pregnancy; contains immunoglobulins.

Concretions: A solid mass formed from particles that come together.

Congenital: Present at birth.

Conjunctivitis: Inflammation of the outermost layer of the eye and the inner surface of the eyelids.

Consensual: Of or relating to a reflexive response of one body structure following stimulation of another.

Contralateral: The side opposite the affected side.

Contusion: A bruise.

Coprophagia: Consumption of fecal matter.

Costochondral: The hyaline joints between the ribs and the costal cartilage.

Creatinine: A substance formed from the metabolism of creatine found in muscle tissue, blood, and urine.

Crepitus: Sound resembling a crackling noise.

Cruciate ligaments: Intraarticular ligaments found within the knee joint.

Cryptorchid: A male animal where one or both testicles are not descended into the scrotum.

Cull: To select from a group based on specific criteria.

Curettage: scraping to remove material from the wall of a space, usually an abscess or cyst.

Cyanotic: A condition in which the mucous membranes take on a bluish color because of inadequate oxygen in blood.

Cyclophotocoagulation: Photocoagulation by directing a laser through the pupil to destroy individual ciliary processes.

Cystitis: Inflammation of the bladder.

Cystocentesis: The process of removing urine directly from the bladder with a syringe and needle.

Cystotomy: Incision of the urinary bladder often to remove a bladder stone.

Debride: To remove dirt, foreign objects, or damaged tissue from a wound to promote healing; the first stage of wound treatment.

Debridement: The process of removing dirt, foreign objects, damaged tissue from a wound.

Decussate: To cross in the form of an "X."

Dermatophilosis: A bacterial skin disease of poorly cared for farm animals mainly seen in mild, wet winters; sometimes called "mud fever."

Dermatophyte: Fungal organism that causes skin disease.

Desmotomy: Incision or division of a ligament; the cutting or division of the ligament.

Diaphysis: The shaft of long bones.

Diastolic: Blood pressure at the exact moment of maximum cardiac relaxation.

Dimorphic: Organism that exists in two different forms.

Discospondylitis: Infection of the spinal vertebrae and intervertebral disks.

Diuresis: Increased production and excretion of urine.

Dyschezia: Abnormal passage of feces through the rectum.

Dyscrasia: Pertaining to an abnormal condition of blood or bone marrow.

Dysecdysis: Abnormal shedding of skin in reptiles.

Dysmature: Relating to or characteristic of faulty embryonic development.

Dysphagia: Difficulty swallowing.

Dystocia: Difficult birthing due to obstruction of the birthing canal.

Dysuria: Painful urination.

Ecdysis: Shedding of skin in reptiles.

Echogenicity: The property of a tissue that allows it to reflect ultrasound waves.

Ectoparasites: Parasites that live on the surface of the host's skin.

Ectotherm: An animal that maintains its body temperature by absorbing heat from its environment.

Ectropion: Eversion, most commonly of the eyelid exposing the lining of the eyelid and the surface of the eye.

Edema: A condition of abnormally large fluid volume in the tissues.

Effusion: Escape of fluid into a body cavity.

Electromyogram: A record of the intrinsic electrical activity within a skeletal muscle.

Electroretinogram: Electrodes placed on the cornea measure electrical responses to light to detect abnormal retinal function.

Emaciation: Excessive leanness associated with malnutrition or chronic disease; low body condition score.

Embolism: A blood clot that is formed within the vessel and breaks loose to travel to other tissues where it becomes lodged.

Embryonated: Egg containing an embryo (immature form).

Emphysema: An abnormal condition of the pulmonary system resulting in overinflation of the alveolar tissues.

Empyema: Accumulation of puss in a body cavity, usually the pleural cavity.

Encephalopathy: Disorder or disease of the brain.

Endemic: Indigenous to a specific area.

Endocarditis: Inflammation of the lining of the heart—the endocardium

Endochondral: Pertaining to something within cartilage.

Endocrine: Pertaining to a process by which cells secrete hormone into blood or lymph that affects another tissue in the body.

Endometritis: Inflammation in the lining tissue of the uterus.

Endophyte: A bacterium or fungus that lives within a plant for at least part of its life without causing apparent disease.

Endotoxin: Toxic substance bound to a bacterial wall that is released when the bacteria ruptures or disintegrates.

Enophthalmos: A posterior displacement of the eye within the socket.

Enterotoxigenic: Bacteria producing an enterotoxin.

Entropion: Inversion, most commonly of the eyelid.

Enucleation: Removal of the eyeball.

Epiphora: An overflow of tears onto the face.

Epiphysis: The enlarged proximal and distal ends of long bones.

Epistaxis: To bleed from the nose.

Eructate: The release of gas from the digestive tract through the mouth.

Erythema: An abnormal increase in the number of red blood cells; usually used to denote redness of skin; tissue redness due to congestion of the capillaries.

Eustachian: The tube that links the nasopharynx to the middle ear.

Eversion: Turning inside out.

Excoriation: A lesion to the surface of the body usually the result of scratching or abrasion.

Exudate: Material (fluid or other) discharged from blood vessel or damaged cellular membranes.

Fasciculation: A localized, uncontrollable twitching of a single muscle group enervated by a single motor neuron.

Fibrillation: Rapid chaotic beating of the heart muscle in which the affected heart may stop pumping blood.

Fistula: An abnormal passage from an internal body organ to the outside of the body.

Fistulated: Having an abnormal passage between an internal organ and the surface of the body or between two internal organs.

Flaccid: Weakness or paralysis and reduced muscle tone without obvious cause.

Flaccid paralysis: An abnormal condition of weakening or loss of muscle tone.

Flatulence: Expulsion through the rectum of a mixture of gases that are the byproducts of the digestive process of animals.

Fomite: Nonliving materials that may transmit microorganisms.

Galactostasis: Stopping of milk production in the mother.

Gangrenous: Necrosis or death of soft tissue due to obstructive circulation usually followed by decomposition and putrefaction.

Gastroenteritis: Inflammation of the stomach and the intestines.

Gingivitis: Inflammation of the free gum margins close to teeth.

Glaucoma: An eye disease where increased intraocular pressure results in damage to the optic nerve.

Gluconeogenesis: The formation of glycogen from fatty acids and proteins.

Glycosuria: Sugar in urine.

Gonadotropin: A hormonal substance that stimulates the function of the testes or the ovaries.

Gout: A disease associated with the deposition of uric acid or metabolites within tissue or joints.

Granuloma: A chronic inflammatory lesion characterized by an abnormal accumulation of macrophages.

Gynecomastia: Enlargement of breasts caused by hormonal imbalance or hormone therapy.

Halitosis: Offensive breath usually from poor hygiene or dental disease.

Hematochezia: Passage of red blood through the rectum usually from the colon or the rectum.

Hematuria: The abnormal presence of blood in urine.

Hemilaminectomy: Removal of a vertebral lamina on one side only.

Hemiplegia: Total paralysis of the limbs and trunk on the same side of the body.

Hemopoietic: Related to the process of formation and development of various types of blood cells.

Hemoptysis: Coughing up blood from the respiratory tract.

Hepatomegaly: Enlargement of the liver.

Herbivore: Animal that feeds only on grass or plants.

Herbivorous: Feeding on plants.

Herniations: A protrusion of a body organ or part through an abnormal opening in a muscle, membrane, or other tissue.

Herpetologist: Individuals that specialize in the study of reptiles, amphibians, crocodilians, and turtles.

Holosystolic: Occurring throughout the entire period of systole; usually used to describe heart murmurs.

Holter monitor: A cardiac monitor that records a continuous heart rhythm during a specific time period such as during exercise or normal activity.

Homeostasis: A relative constancy in the internal environment of the body.

Humoral: Aspect of immunity that is mediated by secreted antibodies.

Husbandry: The science, skill, or art of animal keeping.

Hyaline: Pertaining to substances that are clear or glass-like.

Hypercalciuria: The presence of unusually large amounts of calcium in urine.

Hyperechoic: Increased reflection of ultrasound waves.

Hyperemia: Excessive amount of blood in tissues; skin usually is red and warm.

Hyperkeratosis: Overgrowth of the cornified epithelial layer of the skin.

Hyperplasia: Proliferation of cells that results in the gross enlargement of an organ.

Hypertrichosis: Abnormal amount of hair.

Hypertrophic: Pertains to an increase in size, function, or structure.

Hypertrophy: Increase in the size of an organ due to the enlargement of its component cells.

Hypervolemia: An increase in the amount of intravascular fluid, specifically the volume of blood within the vasculature.

Hyphema: Hemorrhage into the anterior chamber of the eye usually from trauma.

Hypovolemia: A decrease in the amount of intravascular fluids.

Icterus: Pertaining to jaundice (a yellow color related to increased levels of bilirubin in the blood or tissue).

Idiopathic: Without a known cause.

Ileus: An obstruction of the intestine; lack of motility in the bowel.

Immunocompetence: The ability of an immune system to mobilize and deploy its antibodies and other responses to stimulation by antigens.

Incipient: Beginning to exist or appear.

Incontinence: Inability to control the bladder or urination.

Infraorbital: Pertaining to the area of tissue beneath the socket of the eye.

Infundibulum: A funnel-shaped structure.

Insidious: Gradual and harmful.

Inspissated: Being thickened, dried, or made less fluid by evaporation.

Interdigital: The area between two digits.

Intraarticular: Within a joint.

Intromittant organ: General term for an external male organ that delivers sperm during copulation.

Intussusception: A medical condition in which part of the intestine telescopes into another part.

Involute: To roll inward on itself.

Isoerythrolysis: A condition in which red blood cells are destroyed by isoantibodies (antibodies produced against the animals own red blood cells).

Keratitis: Inflammation of the cornea of the eye.

Keratoconjunctivitis: Inflammation of the cornea and conjunctiva.

Kindling: Giving birth.

Lacrimal: Paired glands of the eye that secrete the aqueous layer of tear film.

Lacrimation: Secretion and discharge of tears.

Lactation: The production of milk by the mammary glands.

Laminitis: Inflammation of the lamina within the hoof.

Laparotomy: Any surgical incision into the peritoneal cavity.

Lavage: Irrigation or washing out of an organ.

Leukocytosis: Abnormal increase in the number of circulating white blood cells.

Lipolysis: The breakdown of fats.

Luxation: Dislocation (usually of a joint).

Lysis: The breaking down of a cell.

Macules: A small, flat blemish that is level with the surface of the skin.

Malaise: The general feeling of illness often resulting in lethargy.

Malignancy: Describing a cancer.

Malocclusion: An undesirable relative positioning of the upper and lower teeth when the jaw is closed.

Malodorus: Having a bad odor.

Malpresentation: Abnormal presentation of the fetus during the birthing process.

Melena: Abnormal tarry, black stool usually caused by the presence of digested blood.

Mesenchymal: Tissue derived from the mesoderm.

Mesothelioma: A rare malignant tumor of the mesothelium of the pleura or the peritoneum, usually the result of asbestos exposure.

Metabolic: Relating to or typical of metabolism.

Metastasis: The spread of cancer from the original tumor to other parts of the body.

Metastatic: Tumor cells which spread throughout the body.

Methemoglobinemia: A blood disorder in which an abnormal amount of methemoglobin, a form of hemoglobin, is produced.

Metritis: Inflammation of the wall of the uterus.

Mitacide: Chemical that will kill mites.

Morbidity: The presence of illness; the rate that illness occurs within a population.

Mucopurulent: A combination of mucus and pus.

Multiparous: Having given birth two or more times.

Myeloencephalitis: Inflammation of the spinal cord and the brain.

Myelogram: A radiograph taken after the injection of a radiopaque substance into the subarachnoid space to demonstrate any distortion of the spinal cord, spinal nerves, or the subarachnoid space.

Myelosuppression: Bone marrow suppression; suppression of cells that carry oxygen and provide immunity.

Myiasis: Infestation by larvae of flies usually through a wound or ulcer.

Myocarditis: Inflammation of the heart muscle.

Myopathy: An abnormal condition of skeletal muscle characterized by weakness, wasting, and histologic changes.

Myositis: Inflammation of muscle tissue.

Nasopharynx: Cavity of the nose and part of the pharynx.

Nebulization: A method of delivery of a drug by spraying it into the respiratory passages of the patient; to reduce a liquid to a fine spray for medical use.

Necropsy: Term used for autopsy of a species other than human.

Necrosis: Localized tissue death in response to injury or disease.

Neonatal: Pertaining to the first four weeks after birth.

Nephrosis: Inflammation of the kidney.

Neuromuscular junction: Area of contact between the myelinated nerve and skeletal muscle cell.

Neuronophagia: Destruction of nerve cells by phagocytes.

Nidus: The point of origin of a morbid process.

Nodulectomy: Removal of a small, node-like structure.

Nystagmus: Involuntary, rhythmic movement of the eyes.

Obstipation: A condition of extreme constipation caused by obstruction of the intestinal tract.

Obtundation: The use of an agent that soothes or reduces irritation by blocking the sensibility at some level of the central nervous system.

Occlusal: Refers to the masticating (chewing) surface of the tooth.

Olefactory: Pertaining to the sense of smell.

Oliguria: Decreased ability for urine production and excretion.

Omnivorous: Feeding on plants and animal matter.

Oncology: A branch of medicine concerned with the study of cancers.

Oocysts: A stage in the development of a sporozoan in which after fertilization a zygote develops enclosed within a cyst wall.

Opacity: The degree to which light is not allowed to travel through a structure.

Oropharynx: Cavity of the mouth and part of the pharynx.

Ossicle: A small bone.

Osteopathy: Related to disease of bone.

Osteoporosis: A condition involving an abnormal loss of bone density.

Osteotomy: Sawing or cutting of bone.

Otoscope: Instrument used to examine the ear canal.

Ovariohysterectomy: Surgical removal of the ovaries and the uterus.

Ovariosalpingectomy: Surgical removal of an ovary and the corresponding oviduct.

Oviposition: The act of laying or depositing eggs.

Palpebral: Pertaining to the eyelids.

Panleukopenia: Decrease in all white blood cells.

Panniculus: A sheet or layer of tissue; refers to the reflex movement of this layer when stimulated.

Panosteitis: Inflammation of the entire bone.

Pansystemic: Involvement of all body systems.

Papule: A circumscribed, solid elevation of skin with no visible fluid.

Parenteral: Pertaining to treatment other than through the digestive system.

Paresis: Motor weakness or partial paralysis.

Paroxysmal: A marked, usually episodic increase in symptoms.

Passerine: Perching song birds such as jays, finches, canaries, blackbirds; make up more than half of all bird species.

PCR: Polymerase chain reaction; used to identify specific parts of deoxyribonucleic acid (DNA) or ribonucleic acid (RNA).

Pedunculated: Pertaining to a structure with a stalk.

Pericarditis: Inflammation of the pericardial tissue surrounding the heart.

Perineal: Area adjacent to the distal portion of the gastrointestinal and urogenital systems.

Perineum: Portion of the body in the pelvis occupied by the urogenital passages and the rectum.

Periodontal: Pertaining to the area around the tooth (gums).

Periorbital: Surrounding the socket of the eye.

Peritonitis: Inflammation of the lining tissue of the abdomen.

Perivasculitis: Inflammation of the tissue surrounding large blood vessels.

Petechia/Petechiae: A small red or purple spot on the skin caused by the release into the skin of a very small quantity of blood from a capillary.

Phallus: Penis.

Phlebotomy: Incision of a vein for letting of blood (usually by use of a needle).

Photoperiod: Light cycle.

Photophobia: Abnormal intolerance to visual light; discomfort in bright light.

Photopigments: A light-absorbing chemical that converts light into biochemical energy; the rods and cones in the retina of the eye.

Pica: Craving to eat nonfood substances such as clay or dirt.

Placentitis: Inflammation of the placenta.

Plantar: Pertaining to the sole of the foot.

Pleurodont: Describes teeth that are not rooted in the jawbone but are fused to its inner side.

Pliable: Flexible and easily bent or molded.

Pneumatic: Pertaining to air or gas.

Pneumonitis: Inflammation of the lung.

Pododermatitis: Inflammation of feet.

Poikilocytosis: Abnormal variation in the shape of erythrocytes in blood.

Polypeptide: A chain of amino acids linked by peptide bonds.

Polyphagia: Excessive uncontrolled eating.

Postictal: After a seizure.

Postpartum: After giving birth.

Postprandial: After a meal.

Precordial thrill: A vibration of the chest wall located over the heart.

Prolapse: Sliding of an organ from its normal position.

Pruritus: The symptom of itching that causes the desire or reflex to scratch.

Pseudopregnancy: False pregnancy.

Psittacine: Hookbill birds with characteristics of parrots; roughly 372 species in 86 genera make up this order.

Purulent: Producing or containing pus.

Pyoderma: A purulent skin infection.

Pyogranulomatous: An inflammatory process in which polymorphonuclear cells infiltrate into a more chronic area of inflammation characterized by mononuclear cells, macrophages, lymphocytes, and possibly plasma cells.

Regurgitation: Bring up partially digested food from the stomach to the mouth.

Remission: A partial or complete disappearance of clinical and subjective characteristics of a chronic or malignant disease.

Retrobulbar: Behind the eyeball.

Retroperitoneal: Pertaining to organs closely attached to the abdominal wall and partially covered by the peritoneum.

Rostral: A beak or beak-shaped part of an organism situated toward the nasal area.

Ruminant: Any cud-chewing hoofed mammal with an even number of toes and a stomach with multiple chambers.

Sacculated: Divided into a series of sac-like dilations or pouches.

Saprophyte: An organism that lives on dead organic matter.

Sarcoma: A malignant neoplasm of the soft tissues arising from fibrous, fatty, muscular, vascular or neural tissue.

Sarcomere: Contractile unit of skeletal muscle.

Sclerosis: The hardening and thickening of body tissue as a result of unwarranted growth or deposition of minerals, especially calcium.

Scutes: A bony external plate or scale, as on the shell of a turtle or skin of a crocodilian.

Sebaceous: Pertaining to sebum-secreted from glands in the dermis.

Sebum: Oily substance that prevents hair and skin from drying out.

Septic: Related to causing sepsis.

Serosanguinous: Thin and red; composed of blood and serum.

Signalment: The part of the medical history dealing with the animal's age, sex, and breed.

Spavin: A swelling; bone spavin—bony growth; bog spavin—soft tissue swelling.

Spectacles: The clear scale that covers the eye globe of the reptile.

Spherocytes: Abnormally round red blood cell containing more than normal amounts of hemoglobin.

Splenomegaly: Enlargement of the lung.

Spondylosis: A condition of the spine characterized by fixation or stiffening of a vertebral joint.

Spongiform: Resembling a sponge in appearance.

Squamous epithelium: A sheet of flattened, scale-like cells.

Stertorous: Pertaining to a respiratory effort that is strenuous; a snoring sound.

Stomatitis: An inflammatory condition of the mouth.

Strabismus: A disorder in which the two eyes do not line up in the same direction.

Stranguria: Frequent, difficult, and painful passage of urine.

Stratum: A uniform sheet or layer.

Stroma: Connective, supportive framework of a biologic tissue.

Subclinical: Pertaining to disease so mild that it produces no symptoms.

Syncope: A brief lapse in consciousness; fainting.

Syndrome: The association of several clinically recognizable features or signs observed by someone other than the patient.

Syrinx: The vocal organ of the bird.

Systemic: Pertaining to the entire body.

Systolic: Pertaining to or the result of the contraction of the heart.

Tachycardia: A heart rate faster than normal.

Tachypnea: Rapid breathing.

Tachyzoites: A fast multiplication stage of zoites in the life cycle of *Toxoplasma gondii* or *Neospora caninum*; found in tissues.

Tapetum: The reflective part of the choroid layer that reflects visible light in the eye of many mammals.

Taurine: A derivative of the amino acid cysteine used in the synthesis of bile salts.

Tenesmus: Persistent, ineffectual spasms of the bowel or bladder; straining to defecate.

Tenosynovitis: Inflammation of the fluid-filled sheath that surrounds the tendon.

Thoracocentesis: Removal of fluid from the chest cavity.

Thoracostomy: An incision made into the chest wall for the purpose of draining of fluid.

Thrombocytopenia: A decrease in the number of thrombocytes.

Thromboembolus: A blood clot within the blood vessel that may obstruct blood flow in the vessel.

Thrombophlebitis: Vein inflammation caused by a blood clot.

Thrombosis: An abnormal vascular condition in which a thrombus (clot) develops within a blood vessel.

Thrombus: A clot that develops because of an abnormal condition of the blood vessel.

Tophi: A deposit of monosodium urate crystals in tissues.

Torticollis: An abnormal condition in which the head is inclined or pulled to one side because of contraction of muscles in the neck.

Toxicosis: Pathologic condition caused by the action of a poison or toxin.

Transudate: A fluid passed through a membrane or out of a tissue.

Transfaunation: Replacing rumen microorganisms with contents taken from another animal.

Trephination: Surgical excision of a circular piece of bone or other tissue using a cylindrical saw.

Urate: Any salt of uric acid.

Urethrostomy: A surgical procedure creating a permanent opening into the urethra usually to remove obstructions.

Urodeum: Portion of the cloaca that urine flows into.

Urolithiasis: Formation of stony masses in the urinary tract; stones in the urinary tract.

Urticaria: Skin rash usually a result of allergic reaction, marked by itching and swellings (hives).

Uveitis: Inflammation of the uveal tissues of the eye.

Vestibular: Pertaining to the internal structures of the ear that control balance and the sense of spatial orientation.

Visceral: Pertaining to internal organs in the abdominal cavity.

Voracious: Insatiable appetite.

Wether: A castrated male sheep.

Wheals: Itchy swelling on skin that is raised and red; caused by insect sting or exposure to an allergen.

Zoonotic: Diseases that are transferable from animals to humans.

Answers to Review Questions

Chapter 1

1. b. Patent ductus arteriosus
2. c. Atrial fibrillation
3. d. Persistent right aortic arch
4. a. 60-180 beats/min
5. b. Taurine

Chapter 2

1. a. True
2. b. Less than 1 mm
3. c. Papilloma
4. a. Vomiting; b. Seizures; c. Dehydration; d. Anorexia; e. Fever; f. Diarrhea
5. c. Gastric ulceration
6. a. Ventricular arrhythmia
7. c. Lidocaine
8. d. A fecal examination
9. b. Lymphosarcomas
10. b. Large-bowel disease
11. b. 62%
12. a. Stress
13. b. Diabetes mellitus
14. d. Pancreas
15. c. Portosystemic shunt

Chapter 3

1. a. Negative
2. b. Hypothyroidism; hyperthyroidism
3. a. Radioactive iodine therapy
4. c. Serum fructose concentration
5. b. β
6. b. Addison disease

7. Hypothyroidism; hyperthyroidism
8. c. Both types
9. c. Poor
10. d. Postpartum
11. b. Parathyroid gland

Chapter 4

1. a. Collies; b. Golden Retrievers; d. Beagles
2. b. Roll inward toward the cornea
3. b. Chalazion
4. a. True
5. b. Between 12 and 22 mm Hg
6. d. Several hours
7. c. Plasma cells and lymphocytes
8. b. Cataract
9. b. Cyclosporine ophthalmic
10. c. Feline viral rhinotracheitis

Chapter 5

1. b. Absolute reticulocyte count
2. c. *Rhipicephalus sanguineus*
3. b. von Willebrand disease
4. b. False
5. Prednisone, Cytoxan, L-asparaginase, Vincristine, Doxorubicin
6. b. False
7. Vaccinated cats will test positive for the disease in the future.
8. a. Body surface area
9. b. *Mycoplasma hemofelis*
10. c. Red

Chapter 6

1. c. Low on the left rear leg
2. b. Histiocytoma
3. b. False
4. c. *Rhipicephalus sanguineus*
5. b. diphenhydramine
6. a. True
7. c. Sebaceous cysts
8. d. 50%
9. b. Yellow; red
10. a. True

Chapter 7

1. a. Robert Jones bandage
2. c. Anterior cruciate ligament
3. c. 2 years
4. b. False
5. b. Scapulohumeral joint
6. c. Osteosarcoma
7. a. Most patellar luxations seen early in life are medial luxations.
8. c. No relationship exists between excessive growth and the development of hip dysplasia.
9. a. True
10. d. Hip dysplasia cannot develop in puppies born to female dogs without hip dysplasia.
11. No. Fast growth in this breed may predispose the dog to hip dysplasia.
12. To avoid musculo-skeletal injuries, limit pet's weight and make sure the pet has daily exercise.

Chapter 8

1. c. The severity of the spinal cord injury is related to the weight of the animal.
2. d. 75%
3. a. Poor
4. c. Dobermans
5. c. Rabies
6. c. Embolic ischemic myelopathy
7. d. Antibiotics
8. d. Atlantoaxial subluxation
9. b. 7-10
10. e. Radiography

Chapter 9

1. b. A limited number of cats will have antibodies against feline coronavirus.
2. c. Fighting and bite wounds
3. b. False
4. c. Cat
5. d. Several years
6. b. Poor
7. b. Enrofloxacin (Baytril)
8. b. White blood cells
9. a. Longer than 48 hours
10. a. Vomiting
11. b. Fall
12. c. Schiff-Sherrington syndrome
13. a. Faster
14. d. 6 months
15. a. Wet
16. Because many areas of the country do not have Lyme disease and many house dogs will never be exposed to ticks.
17. Retest the cat every 4-6 months. The cat may become negative. Isolate the cat from other cats in the household.
18. Retest the cat every 4-6 months. The cat may become negative. Isolate the cat from other cats in the household.

Chapter 10

1. a. True
2. b. False
3. b. Castration
4. a. 62 and 65 days
5. a. True
6. d. 4
7. b. Castrate the animal at an early age
8. a. True
9. a. True
10. c. Culture and sensitivity of prostatic fluid

Chapter 11

1. b. Radiograph; d. Computed tomography or magnetic resonance imaging
2. b. *Bordetella*
3. c. 2 years

4. b. Vomiting
5. b. False
6. a. True
7. b. Low nucleated cell count; c. Low total protein
8. c. Seventh intercostal
9. b. *Cryptococcus*
10. a. Fungal
11. a. Toxins released by *Bordetella bronchiseptica* bacteria

Chapter 12

1. c. No
2. e. All of the above
3. a. Small concretions of minerals and large amounts of matrix
4. b. Calcium oxalate; and c. Magnesium ammonium phosphate
5. a. Cystine
6. a. Amikacin
7. b. Potassium
8. d. All of the above
9. a. Blood urea nitrogen (BUN)
10. c. The smooth muscle surrounding the entire urethra
11. d. Struvite
12. b. Oxalate
13. c. Normal saline

Chapter 13

1.   Carbohydrates and fiber
2.   Canine distemper and rabies
3. a. Rubber products
4. a. Strict carnivores
5. a. Weight
6. a. Proper nutrition; c. Clean, fresh water; d. Adequate ventilation in housing; e. Yearly dental checkups; g. Exercise
7. d. Onset of seizure
8. b. Porphyrin
9. b. Small
10. c. 8%
11. b. Volatile fatty acids
12. d. 6-8
13. d. The microflora in the rabbit gastrointestinal tract is sensitive to oral antibiotics.

14. a. Induced
15. b. Trimmed

Chapter 14

1. b. False
2. c. Thickening of the walls of the heart
3. a. Heart
4. b. Improve cardiac performance
5. a. Left apex
6. b. False
7. a. True
8. c. 2
9. a. Lack of adequate collateral circulation

Chapter 15

1. a. *Helicobacter* spp.
2. a. True
3. b. Wet tail
4. c. Incisors
5. a. Prolonged anorexia
6. b. Volatile fatty acids
7. a. Grass hay; d. Clean water; e. Fresh vegetables and fruits
8. c. Intestinal motility
9. a. Pain
10. b. False

Chapter 16

1. c. Adrenal disease
2. b. Hyperadrenocorticism
3. b. Sucrose
4. a. Blocked lacrimal ducts; b. Epiphora

Chapter 17

1. c. Progressive loss of vision
2. b. Porphyrin
3. c. *Treponema* spp.
4. b. Skin tumors

Chapter 18

1. b. Lymphoma
2. c. Lymphoma
3. c. Direct contact with infected mice
4. a. Fibroadenoma of the mammary gland
5. b. Western U.S.
6. a. Barbering

Chapter 19

1. e. None of the above
2. c. *Radfordia* spp.
3. a. Gently remove impacted materials
4. a. Constant trauma to the area
5. a. True
6. a. Rubber mat on the exam table

Chapter 20

1. c. 8%

Chapter 21

1. d. Onset of seizures
2. c. *Encephalitozoon cuniculi*
3. b. Head-tilt; c. Paralysis

Chapter 22

1. a. Induced
2. d. Swollen lymph nodes
3. b. False
4. c. Adenocarcinoma
5. a. Open inguinal rings
6. c. Amoxicillin
7. a. True

Chapter 23

1. b. False
2. b. False
3. c. *Pasteurella multocida*
4. a. True
5. b. False

Chapter 24

1. b. 30%
2. c. Struvite stone
3. a. Male
4. c. Calcium carbonate
5. b. Decrease
6. c. porphyrin

Chapter 25

[no review questions]

Chapter 26

1. a. Epinephrine
2. b. Vitamin E and selenium
3. a. The aortic arch in avian anatomy is derived from the right arch and not from the left as in mammals.
   b. Two portal systems affect blood flow through the liver and the kidney.
   c. The avian heart is larger with respect to body weight.
   d. The heart rates for most birds exceed those of mammals.
4. c. Put the bird back into the cage
5. b. Higher

Chapter 27

1. c. Flush the crop using warm saline, and then refill the crop with a balanced electrolyte solution.
2. d. This disease is treatable, but the animal should not be used for breeding.
3. Describe how to determine the difference between "courtship regurgitation" and vomiting from a disease process.
4. a. Watermelon
5. a. ALT
6. a. Gram-positive
7. b. False
8. b. Proventriculus

Chapter 28

1. b. 600 mg/dL
2. a. A seed diet low in iodine
3. c. C-cells
4. b. An iodine-deficient diet
5. c. Hypoglycemia

Chaper 29

1. b. Feathers
2. c. Red
3. b. Pecten
4. b. Gram-positive
5. a. Pinna
6. b. Vitamin A
7. b. False
8. a. True

Chapter 30

1. b. 3.8 mL
2. b. Jugular vein
3. b. Toenail clip
4. b. Nonregenerative

Chapter 31

1. b. The uropygial gland
2. a. Otomax ointment
3. c. Feathers are missing from tracts on the body only.
4. c. Anxiolytics
5. b. Canary
6. c. *Knemidokoptes pilae*
7. a. Improper perch materials; c. Improper perch size

Chapter 32

1. a. Finches and canaries
2. b. Necrosis of the area distal to the band
3. b. Pneumatic bone
4. c. The keel
5. a. Depletion of calcium

Chapter 33

1. a. True
2. a. True
3. b. Vestibular apparatus
4. b. Hypocalcemia
5. a. True
6. a. *Aspergillus* granulomas
   b. *Mycobacterium* granulomas
   c. *Candida* lesions
7. b. *Chamydia*

Chapter 34

1. c. High levels of antibiotics
2. a. Gram-positive
3. d. Psittacosis
4. c. 60 days
5. c. Exotic Newcastle disease

Chapter 35

1. b. Pink
2. c. Reproductive
3. c. Infraorbital sinus
4. c. Vitamin A
5. d. Teflon-coated
6. a. Place the bird in an oxygenated environment before evaluation
7. b. Lower airway

Chapter 36

1. c. Renal portal system
2. b. Solid urates
3. a. Renal, digestive, reproductive
4. c. Uric acid
5. a. Dystocia
6. b. False
7. d. Calcium
8. a. Gonadal tumor
9. b. Visceral gout

Chapter 37

1.   Preferred optimal temperature zone
2. b. Carnivorous
3. d. *Salmonella*
4. a. 75-100°F
5. a. October to April
6. a. Chopped whole animals such as mice, worms, or guppies and vegetables
7. c. Carapace
8. c. 3-4
9. c. Sodium

Chapter 38

1. b. Decreased from normal
2. c. Two; one
3. a. Their red cells are not able to carry as much oxygen

Chapter 39

1. c. Turtle
2. b. Suppression of the immune system
3. c. Poor husbandry
4. b. *Salmonella*
5. d. Vitamin A
6. b. Anorexic
7. b. Fat bodies
8. c. 2 weeks
9. a. More
10. a. True

Chapter 40

1.   carapace (upper); Panstron (lower)
2. b. False
3. b. Broccoli
4. a. Thyroid hormone
5. a. Poor husbandry

Chapter 41

1. b. Low environmental humidity
2. a. True
3. b. Conus papillaris
4. a. Soaking until softened
5. b. Periorbital swelling

Chapter 42

1. b. A difficult shed
2. b. Increase the humidity by soaking
3. c. Fungi
4. a. Larger
5. c. Predator trauma
6. c. Urinate
7. b. Larger
8. b. False

Chapter 43

1. d. Calcium and phosphorus
2. c. Nutritional secondary hyperparathyroidism
3. c. Tail
4. d. All of the above
5. a. Feed a properly balanced diet

Chapter 44

1. b. The panniculus reflex
2. c. Swelling on the side of the head
3. a. Boa
4. c. Chlorhexidine
5. c. Ivermectin
6. a. Thiamine
7. b. Aural abscesses

Chapter 45

1. b. Live young
2. b. False
3. c. Females have a shallow hemipenis pouch
4. b. Malposition of an egg
5. b. 2-3 years
6. c. 90-130
7. a. Cover the tissue with a clean, wet towel and come to the clinic

Chapter 46

1. b. False
2. b. False
3. b. 21 days
4. a. Dehydration
   b. Vitamin A or D deficiencies
   d. Bacterial infections
5. b. False

Chapter 47

1. c. Urates
2. Which of the following have a bladder? (Mark all that apply.)
    a. Green iguana; c. Turtle
3. c. Aminoglycosides

Chapter 48

1. a. Perform a complete physical examination and auscultate the heart
2. a. Second-degree atrioventricular block
3. e. All of the above
4. a. Check with the veterinarian prior to riding or driving these horses
5. c. Echocardiography
6. a. True
7. d. Atrial fibrillation
8. b. False
9. c. The mesenteric artery
10. a. 25-40 beats per minute (bests/min)

Chapter 49

1. a. *Strongylus* spp.
2. b. *Salmonella*
3. a. Choke
4. d. All of the above
5. b. At least yearly
6. b. Gastric ulceration
7. a. Nursing foal
8. b. *Oxyuris* spp.

Chapter 50

1. c. The pituitary gland
2. c. Over 10 years of age
3. c. The thyroid
4. a. Cushing syndrome ; c. Insulin resistance
5. c. Carbohydrates

Chapter 51

1. b. Bring the horse out of the light; then call the vet
2. a. Corneal ulcers
3. b. Disposed of when treatment has ended
4. b. Fluorescein
5. a. Colic

Chapter 52

1. b. With Coggins test
2. b. Retesting by State Veterinarian

Chapter 53

1. b. Rain rot
2. b. Sarcoid
3. d. All of the above
4. Horses use their sensitive nose to investiate any strange object, even a snack.
5. a. Grind up a few warts in a sterile liquid medium, and inject subcutaneously into the horse; b. Scrape the warts with a scalpel blade until they bleed

Chapter 54

1. c. In the front limb, below the knee
2. d. All of the above
3. a. Hoof abscess
4. d. Proper conditioning
5. a. Rhabdomyolysis
6. b. Grain
7. a. Keep the horse in a dry area; b. Clean the feet daily

Chapter 55

1. a. Rabies; d. Eastern, western, and Venezuelan equine encephalomyelitis; e. West Nile encephalitis

Chapter 56

1. b. Remove the mares from the pasture 30 to 90 days before foaling.
2. d. 20 minutes
3. c. Acepromazine
4. a. before the end
5. c. Estrogen
6. b. Herpes virus infection
7. a. True

Chapter 57

1. b. Lymphocytes
2. c. 18
3. b. A blood type the same as the stud
4. c. Dummy foal syndrome
5. b. False
6. c. Dummy foal syndrome
7. b. False

Chapter 58

1. c. Equine viral rhinopneumonitis
2. a. *Streptococcus equi*
3. c. Heaves
4. a. A herpes virus
5. a. Furosemide
6. a. True
7. a. True
8. a. Gram-positive

Chapter 59

1. b. Ascending bacterial infections
2. d. All of the above
3. c. Postpartum mare

Chapter 60

1. b. Urinary calculi
2. c. Copper
3. d. Predators

Chapter 61

1. d. All of the above
2. a. Pregnancy toxemia
3. b. *Clostridium* infection
4. a. Rotavirus
5. b. The left paralumbar fossa
6. a. *Salmonella*; d. *Cryptosporidium*

Chapter 62

1. b. Calcium and phosphorus
2. c. Pseudopregnancy
3. d. Iodine
4. d. Dexamethasone

Chapter 63

1. a. Cataracts
2. a. Tetracycline ophthalmic ointment
3. c. Move the animal out of the sunlight

Chapter 64

1. c. Culling affected animals
2. c. Wound culture
3. a. Surgical opening with curettage

Chapter 65

1. b. False
2. a. Parapoxvirus
3. b. Skin scrape
4. b. False

Chapter 66

1. d. Overgrowth of hoof wall
2. c. Selenium
3. d. Calcium and phosphorus
4. d. all of the above
5. c. Fescue

Chapter 67

1. c. Thiamine injection
2. b. *Listeria*
3. a. True
4. a. Yes

Chapter 68

1. d. Replacement of tissue and use of a restraining device
2. d. All of the above
3. a. Yes

Chapter 69

1. c. *Oestrus ovis*
2. b. Recent dehorning
3. a. *Mycoplasma*

Chapter 70

1. a. Too much concentrate in the diet
2. b. Aluminum chloride
3. d. 12%

Answers to Clinical Cases

Chapter 1

1) Boxer dogs can carry the gene for Familial Ventricular Arrythmia and show no outward signs of disease until they die suddenly. This gene predisposes them to fatal arrythmias which can result at any time during the life of the dog. This is a conduction disease and not a disease of the heart muscle.
2) Since the disease is genetic, if you were to obtain a dog from the same breeding line, you may get a dog with the problem. It pays to research gene lines and ask questions when buying a Boxer dog.
3) Holter heart monitoring over a 24 hour period may show signs of the disease. There is nothing that can prevent this from occurring. Investigate any seizure-like occurrence, any surgical arrythmias, or fainting that occurs in Boxer dogs.

Chapter 2

Three causes of icterus in the cat are a) Hepatic lipidosis b) Red cell distruction c) Bile duct obstruction
Laboratory tests include ALT, AST, ALP, direct/indirect bilirubin, PVC, RBC, and a hand differential. Further testing might include ultrasonography and liver biopsy.

Index